Administering Medications

Pharmacology for Healthcare Professionals

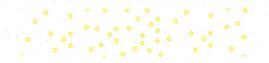

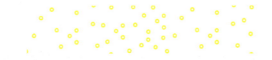

Administering Medications

Pharmacology for Healthcare Professionals

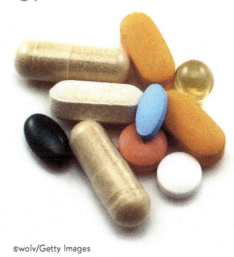

©wolv/Getty Images

ninth edition

Donna F. Gauwitz, RN, MS

Nursing Consultant
Senior Teaching Specialist
School of Nursing
University of Minnesota
Minneapolis, Minnesota

and

Nursing Education Specialist
Mayo Clinic
Rochester, Minnesota

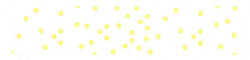

ADMINISTERING MEDICATIONS: PHARMACOLOGY FOR HEALTHCARE PROFESSIONALS, NINTH EDITION

7 8 9 LKV 21

ISBN 978-1-259-92817-8 (bound edition)
MHID 1-259-92817-9 (bound edition)
ISBN 978-1-260-48922-4 (loose-leaf edition)
MHID 1-260-48922-1 (loose-leaf edition)

Executive Portfolio Manager: *William Lawrensen*
Product Developer: *Krystal Faust*
Executive Marketing Manager: *Roxan Kinsey*
Senior Content Project Manager: *Vicki Krug*
Content Project Manager: *Emily Windelborn*
Senior Buyer: *Laura Fuller*
Designer: *Matt Diamond*
Content Licensing Specialist: *Traci Vaske*
Cover Image: *©Glow Images*
Compositor: *MPS Limited*

All credits appearing on page or at the end of the book are considered to be an extension of the copyright page.

Library of Congress Cataloging-in-Publication Data

Gauwitz, Donna F., author.
    Administering medications: pharmacology for healthcare professionals/
    Donna F. Gauwitz, RN, MS, Nursing Consultant, Senior Teaching
    Specialist, School of Nursing, University of Minnesota, Minneapolis,
    Minnesota, and Nursing Education Specialist, Mayo Clinic, Rochester,
    Minnesota.
    Ninth edition. | New York, NY : McGraw-Hill Education, 2020. |
    Audience: 18+ | Includes index.
    LCCN 2018057287 | ISBN 9781259928178 (student edition)
    LCSH: Drugs—Administration. | Pharmacology.
    LCC RM147 .B39 2020 | DDC 615.1068—dc23
    LC record available at https://lccn.loc.gov/2018057287

WARNING NOTICE: The clinical procedures, medicines, dosages, and other matters described in this publication are based upon research of current literature and consultation with knowledgeable persons in the field. The procedures and matters described in this text reflect currently accepted clinical practice. However, this information cannot and should not be relied upon as necessarily applicable to a given individual's case. Accordingly, each person must be separately diagnosed to discern the patient's unique circumstances. Likewise, the manufacturer's package insert for current drug product information should be consulted before administering any drug. Publisher disclaims all liability for any inaccuracies, omissions, misuse, or misunderstanding of the information contained in this publication. Publisher cautions that this publication is not intended as a substitute for the professional judgment of trained medical personnel.

The Internet addresses listed in the text were accurate at the time of publication. The inclusion of a website does not indicate an endorsement by the authors or McGraw-Hill Education, and McGraw-Hill Education does not guarantee the accuracy of the information presented at these sites.

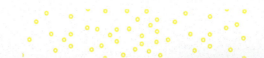

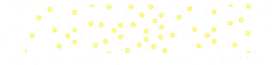

Dedication

I want to thank my husband, William, who is my best friend, for his love and support through all of the phases of this edition. He is my rock and driving force.

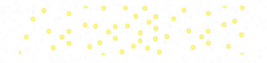

About the Author

Donna Faye Gauwitz, MS, RN, received her diploma in nursing from St. Francis School of Nursing in Peoria, Illinois. After graduation, she worked on medical-surgical nursing units, specifically neurology, and on the psychiatric unit at St. Francis Hospital, a major acute care facility and trauma center in central Illinois. She obtained a bachelor of science degree from Bradley University in Peoria, Illinois. After graduating with a BSN, Donna began her career in nursing education as a staff development coordinator at St. Francis Medical Center, orienting new graduate nurses to the largest medical-surgical unit. She was also an adjunct faculty member at Illinois Central College in East Peoria, Illinois, and at Illinois Wesleyan University in Bloomington, Illinois, teaching medical-surgical and pediatric nursing. While at Illinois Central College, she developed a brand-new college course, Introduction to Eating Disorders, that she taught at the college.

Donna further developed her research and publication interest as a research assistant at the University of Illinois Department of Psychiatry and Behavioral Medicine in Peoria, Illinois, and at Northwestern University College of Nursing in Chicago, Illinois. She did the research and wrote the proposal for an Eating Disorders Clinic and became the director of the clinic at St. Francis Medical Center in Peoria. Her pursuit of advanced education took her to Northwestern University College of Nursing in Evanston, Illinois, to obtain her master's degree. After graduation from Northwestern University, Donna began her full-time teaching career at Methodist Medical Center in Peoria, followed by positions at Barry University in Miami Shores, Florida, and Broward Community College in Pembroke Pines, Florida, teaching medical-surgical, orthopedic, rehabilitation, women's health, and neurology nursing.

During her tenure in education, she had the opportunity to serve as an item writer eight times for the National Council of Licensure in the development of the NCLEX-RN. She published an article in *Insight,* a National Council of Licensure publication. She further pursued her interest in writing by publishing three articles in the *Nursing* journal and one article in the *American Journal of Nursing.* She is also currently the author of *Complete Review NCLEX-RN, and Practice Questions for NCLEX-RN.*

After relocating to Minnesota, she became a nursing education specialist for an acute care surgical unit at the Mayo Clinic in Rochester, Minnesota. Her love of nursing education then took her to the University of Minnesota as a senior teaching specialist and coordinator of the Nursing Skills Laboratory in Minneapolis, Minnesota.

Donna is a member of Sigma Theta Tau and has been listed in *Who's Who in American Nursing.*

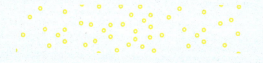

Brief Contents

Contents

Preface xv

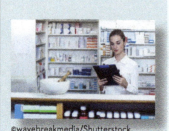
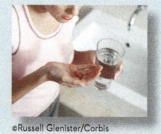
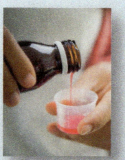

Contents

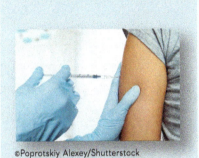
©Poprotskiy Alexey/Shutterstock

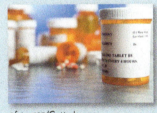
©fstop123/Getty Images

Contents

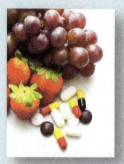
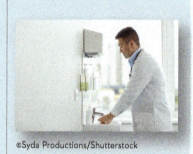
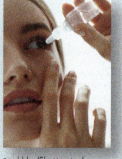
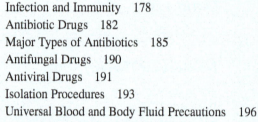

Contents

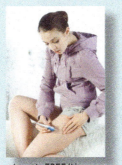
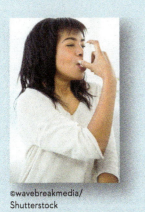

Contents

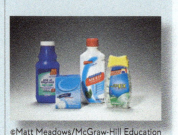
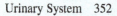
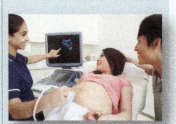

Contents

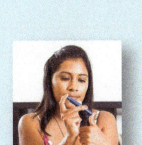
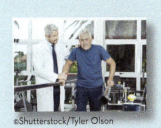
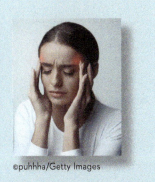

Contents

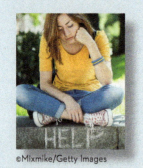
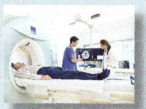
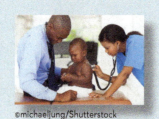

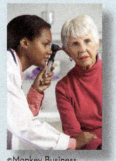

Preface

Administering Medications: Pharmacology for Healthcare Professionals teaches safe medication administration to healthcare students entering nursing, medical assisting, and other allied healthcare professions. Because this textbook speaks directly to students, they can easily identify and apply the concepts they've learned.

The organization of the chapters allows students and instructors to build a knowledge base that starts with the fundamentals of medication administration and progresses through the drugs frequently used to treat most common diseases. Most chapters are organized around a body system to help students fully understand drug actions. For easy identification, the 50 most frequently prescribed drugs are boldfaced in the Representative Drug tables.

The Patient Education, Healthcare for Today and Tomorrow, and Legal and Ethical Issues boxes continue to be highlighted features in this edition. The Patient Education boxes contain important information for the healthcare professional to communicate to the patient. This feature also includes cultural diversity and pediatric and geriatric implications where appropriate. The Healthcare for Today and Tomorrow boxes alert the healthcare professional to issues or problems that may be encountered today or in the future. The Legal and Ethical Issues boxes illustrate the role of the healthcare professional in actual legal and ethical situations pertinent to the content of each chapter.

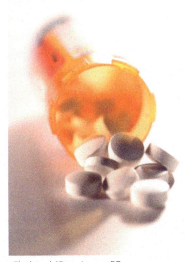
©Thinkstock/Getty Images RF

New to This Edition

The ninth edition of *Administering Medications* has been updated to reflect the most up-to-date information on the safety and education of medications. Revisions are based on updates needed for currency and accuracy, as well as feedback from instructors and students.

General revisions throughout the text include the following:

- **Drugs**—updated and added new drugs throughout tables, feature boxes, and end-of-chapter Representative Drug tables
- **Chapter openers**—visually enhanced layout and updated photos
- **Feature boxes**—updated to stay current along with a new visually enhanced layout
- **End-of-chapter summary points and review assignments**—updated to be consistent with changes to learning outcomes
- **PowerPoints**—now available in an accessible template with updated key points illustrated in each chapter

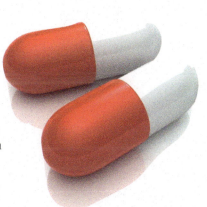
©Burazin/Getty Images

Preface

Chapter Revision Highlights:

- Updated fractions and equations to reflect current practice and systems of measurement
- Figure 3.13 illustration updated to be consistent with Roman numerals and Apothecary System
- Figure 3.15 illustration updated for accuracy to calculate BSA with nomogram
- Added new Table 4.1 Safe Practices for Medical Injections from CDC (Centers for Disease Control and Prevention)
- Table 4.2 updated name to "Standard Precautions for Medical Injection Safety"
- Added new Figures:
  - Figure 4.3 Diagram of the most common needles used
  - Figure 4.5 Jet Injector
  - Figure 4.6 Luer Lock/Luer Slip Systems
  - Figure 4.10 Filter Needle
  - Figure 11.3 Photo of Peak Flow Meter
  - Figure 14.2 Female Uterus and Fallopian Tubes
- New paragraph on immunization and the reemergence of vaccine preventable diseases
- New paragraph on fibromyalgia

Table 4.1 Safe Practices for Medical Injections from CDC (Centers for Disease Control and Prevention)

1. Never administer medications from the same syringe to more than one patient, even if the needle is changed or you are injecting through an intervening length of IV tubing.
2. Do not enter a medication vial, bag, or bottle with a used syringe or needle.
3. Never use medications packaged as single dose or single use for more than one patient. This includes ampules, bags, and bottles of intravenous solutions.
4. Always use aseptic technique when preparing and administering medications.

Figure 4.3

Diagram of the most common needles used.

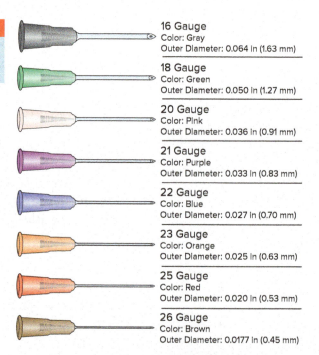

16 Gauge
Color: Gray
Outer Diameter: 0.064 in (1.63 mm)

18 Gauge
Color: Green
Outer Diameter: 0.050 in (1.27 mm)

20 Gauge
Color: Pink
Outer Diameter: 0.036 in (0.91 mm)

21 Gauge
Color: Purple
Outer Diameter: 0.033 in (0.83 mm)

22 Gauge
Color: Blue
Outer Diameter: 0.027 in (0.70 mm)

23 Gauge
Color: Orange
Outer Diameter: 0.025 in (0.63 mm)

25 Gauge
Color: Red
Outer Diameter: 0.020 in (0.53 mm)

26 Gauge
Color: Brown
Outer Diameter: 0.0177 in (0.45 mm)

Acknowledgments

Author Acknowledgment

I wish to express a sincere thanks to the following individuals for their continual support and assistance in this ninth edition:

Thomas Timp, Managing Director
William Lawrensen, Portfolio Manager
Roxan Kinsey, Marketing Manager
Krystal Faust, Product Developer
Vicki Krug, Content Project Manager
Matt Diamond, Designer
Traci Vaske, Content Licensing Specialist
Laura Fuller, Senior Buyer
Jeanne Patterson, Proofreader

Last, I want to express a sincere thank-you to Colleen Marzilli, *The University of Texas at Tyler*, Jane Fritz, *Trinity Valley Community College*, and Jim Mizner, BS, MPA, RPh, *Lori Tyler and Associates*, who served as contributors in reviewing and updating this edition.

Board of Reviewers

Robert Aanonsen, CPhT
Platt College

Cindy A. Abel, BS, CMA, PBT (ASCP)
Ivy Tech State College

Cynthia Allee, MA
Amis Community College

Glenn D. Appelt, PhD, RPh
Columbia Southern University

Laurie S. Barrett, RN
Portland, OR

Alecia Blake, MD
Morehouse School of Medicine

Cynthia Boles, MBA, MT, CMA
Bradford School
Pittsburgh, PA

Paula Manuel Bostwick, RN, MSN
Ivy Tech Community College-Northeast

Dixie Bradbury, MS, CCA
National College of Business and Technology

Lorri Christiansen, AA in Allied Health, RN
Centura College

Sally Christiansen, RN, BSN, MS
Waukesha County Technical College

Molly Cochran Clay, MS, CRNP
Montgomery College

Carmen Cruz, MBA/HCM
Anamarc College

James Dickerson, AAs Computer Networking, NRCMA, AHA instructor/Trainer
Remington College-Dallas Campus

Marian Dixon, RN
Houston Community College

James M. Downey, BA
Abacus Educational Consulting

Terry D. Edwards
Remington College-Houston

Rhonda Epps, RMA, CMA (AAMA), AS
National College of Business and Technology

Theresa Errante-Parrino, CMA (AAMA), CPhT, EMTP, Med
Indian River State College

Kathleen Ewing, NRCMA
Concord Career College

Hobie Etta Feagai, EdD, MSN, FNP-BC, APRN-Rx
Hawaii Pacific University

Rebecca Foyles, RN, MSN
Lenoir Community College

Deborah S. Gilbert, RHIM, MBA, EdS
Dalton State College

Katherine L. Gill, BSN, RN, CNOR
Hutchinson Community College

Margaret Gingrich, RN, MSN
Harrisburg Area Community College

Nancy Glassgow, RN, BSN
Western Dakota Tech

Robyn Gohsman, AAS, RMA, CMAS
Medical Careers Institute

W. Howard Gunning, MSEd, CMA
Southwestern Illinois College

Elaine Lawrence Gwinnett
College of Business

Jena G. Hamra, PhD
Texas A&M University-Commerce

Joanne Holly, MS, RN, CMA (AAMA)
Midstate College

M. Hollis Hutchinson, JD, MSN, RN
Dallas County Community College District

Carol Lee Jarrell, MLT, AHI
Department Chair—Medical
Brown Mackie College

Sherri Kananen, MAEd
Education Affiliates/MedVance Institute

Pat King, MA, RHIA
Baker College

Todd Kudronowicz
Walmart Pharmacy, Platteville, Wisconsin

Naomi Kupfer, CMA
Las Vegas, Nevada

Barbara Lacher
North Dakota State College of Science

Richelle S. Laipply, PhD, MT (ASCP), CMA
University of Akron

Rhonda Lazette, BS, CMA (AAMA)
Stautzenberger College

Kimberly Lowry, RN, BSN
Antonelli College

Maryagnes Luczak
Career Training Academy

Tabitha Lyons, AS, NCMA
Anthem Education Group

Sandy Maas, RN, MSN
Estrella Mountain Community College

Deb McClain
Hagerstown Community College

Michelle C. McCranie
Ogeechee Technical College

Carol E. McMahon
Capitol Community College

Elizabeth McStay, RN
The Salter School

Patty Hawley Mecosta
Osceola Career Center and Ferris State University

Jeanne Miles, RN
Hutchinson Community College

Cynthia H. Myles, BAN, RN, MA
Montana State University-Great Falls, College of Technology

Features List

Older Adult Considerations

Healthcare for Today and Tomorrow

Legal and Ethical Issues

Representative Drug Tables

Practice Procedures

![McGraw Hill Education] **connect**® | Students—study more efficiently, retain more and achieve better outcomes. Instructors—focus on what you love—teaching.

SUCCESSFUL SEMESTERS INCLUDE CONNECT

FOR INSTRUCTORS

You're in the driver's seat.

Want to build your own course? No problem. Prefer to use our turnkey, prebuilt course? Easy. Want to make changes throughout the semester? Sure. And you'll save time with Connect's auto-grading too.

65%
Less Time Grading

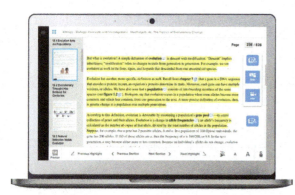

They'll thank you for it.

Adaptive study resources like SmartBook® help your students be better prepared in less time. You can transform your class time from dull definitions to dynamic debates. Hear from your peers about the benefits of Connect at **www.mheducation.com/highered/connect**

Make it simple, make it affordable.

Connect makes it easy with seamless integration using any of the major Learning Management Systems—Blackboard®, Canvas, and D2L, among others—to let you organize your course in one convenient location. Give your students access to digital materials at a discount with our inclusive access program. Ask your McGraw-Hill representative for more information.

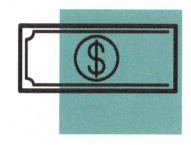

©Hill Street Studios/Tobin Rogers/Blend Images LLC

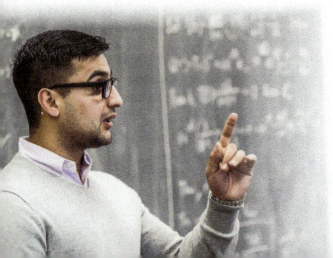

Solutions for your challenges.

A product isn't a solution. Real solutions are affordable, reliable, and come with training and ongoing support when you need it and how you want it. Our Customer Experience Group can also help you troubleshoot tech problems—although Connect's 99% uptime means you might not need to call them. See for yourself at **status.mheducation.com**

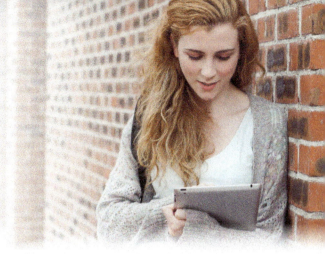

Effective, efficient studying.

Connect helps you be more productive with your study time and get better grades using tools like SmartBook, which highlights key concepts and creates a personalized study plan. Connect sets you up for success, so you walk into class with confidence and walk out with better grades.

©Shutterstock/wavebreakmedia

"I really liked this app—it made it easy to study when you don't have your textbook in front of you."

- Jordan Cunningham, Eastern Washington University

Study anytime, anywhere.

Download the free ReadAnywhere app and access your online eBook when it's convenient, even if you're offline. And since the app automatically syncs with your eBook in Connect, all of your notes are available every time you open it. Find out more at **www.mheducation.com/readanywhere**

No surprises.

The Connect Calendar and Reports tools keep you on track with the work you need to get done and your assignment scores. Life gets busy; Connect tools help you keep learning through it all.

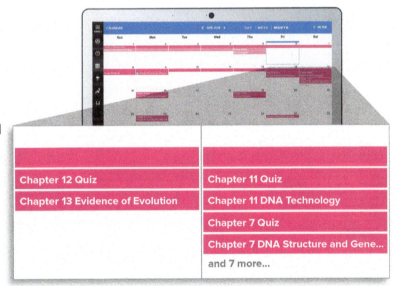

Chapter 12 Quiz

Chapter 13 Evidence of Evolution

Chapter 11 Quiz

Chapter 11 DNA Technology

Chapter 7 Quiz

Chapter 7 DNA Structure and Gene...

and 7 more...

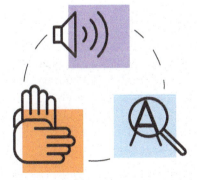

Learning for everyone.

McGraw-Hill works directly with Accessibility Services Departments and faculty to meet the learning needs of all students. Please contact your Accessibility Services office and ask them to email accessibility@mheducation.com, or visit **www.mheducation.com/about/accessibility.html** for more information.

ORIENTATION TO MEDICATIONS

LEARNING OUTCOMES

1-1 Define terms to understanding the administration of medications.

1-2 List the sources and uses of drugs.

1-3 Define *drug standards*, indicating how they are determined and why they are necessary.

1-4 List the names by which drugs are known.

1-5 List drug references and the purpose of each, and purchase drug cards.

1-6 List the major drug laws and their main features.

1-7 List the federal agencies that enforce drug laws and the importance of enforcing them.

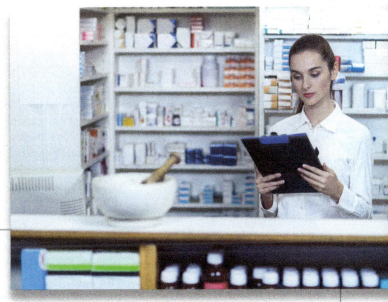

©wavebreakmedia/Shutterstock

In this chapter you will learn where drugs come from, how they are standardized, and how their use is governed by law. You will also learn how to use drug references and drug cards to gather information about medications.

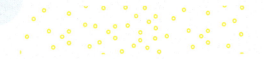

action

adverse reaction

anatomy

brand name

chemical name

contraceptives

contraindications

controlled substances

diagnostic drugs

drug

generic name

indications

over-the-counter (OTC) drugs

palliative drugs

pathology

pharmacodynamics

pharmacokinetics

pharmacology

physiology

precautions

prescription drugs

psychology

side effects

standards

synthetic drugs

therapeutic effect

DEFINITION OF TERMS [LO 1-1]

Not long ago, only doctors and nurses were allowed to administer medications. But times are changing; many other members of the health occupations are now asked to give or know about medications. They are also expected to observe how patients react after taking medications. These are important new responsibilities. They demand that you, a member of the healthcare team working with medications, also have knowledge of many health-related topics. You must know the basic principles of **pharmacology**, which is the study of drugs and their uses. You must understand how the body responds to drugs, or **pharmacodynamics**. You must also understand **pharmacokinetics**, the absorption, distribution, metabolism, and excretion of drugs. These areas require some knowledge of human **anatomy**, the study of body parts, and of **physiology**, the science that deals with the functions of cells, tissues, and organs of living organisms. You must understand the study of disease processes, including changes in the structure and function of the body, or **pathology**, and how drugs change the course of disease. You must also give attention to **psychology**, the study of the normal and abnormal processes of the mind, because a patient's mental state influences how the body reacts to drugs.

This textbook will teach you, step by step, the basics of pharmacology, pharmacodynamics, pharmacokinetics, anatomy, physiology, and pathology. You will also find suggestions for responding to patients' psychological needs, along with information you should tell patients about medications they may be taking. The uses of specific drugs for treatment of disease are discussed in connection with the body systems on which they act. As you learn general principles, most of you will also carry out practice tasks that give you experience in giving medications. Laws, ethics, standards, and guidelines are included in chapters throughout the textbook as they relate to protecting the consumer and the healthcare worker.

PHARMACOLOGY [LO 1-1]

A **drug** is a chemical substance used in the diagnosis, treatment, cure, or prevention of a disease. Pharmacology is the study of drugs: their uses, preparation, routes, and laws. Pharmacology includes the study of how drugs affect the human body. Healthcare professionals are particularly interested in the desired or predicted physiological response that a drug causes, or the drug's **therapeutic effect**.

Pharmacology considers the purpose for taking the drug in contrast with effects of the drug, whether desirable or undesirable. These desirable and undesirable effects are called **side effects**. Pharmacology also focuses on the proper amounts of drugs to give and how to give them. Knowledge of the laws and responsibilities surrounding drug use, along with practical experience in giving medications, will prepare you to play a vital role on the healthcare team.

DRUG SOURCES [LO 1-2]

Drugs come from four sources: plants, animals, and minerals, as well as chemicals **(synthetic drugs)** by means of biotechnology or genetic engineering.

Our ancestors long ago discovered that the roots, leaves, and seeds of certain plants had the power to cure illnesses, ease pain, and affect the mind. Today many drugs are still extracted from parts of plants. An example is digitalis, a cardiac glycoside used to treat congestive heart failure. Digitalis is made from a wildflower, purple foxglove. Drugs from the poppy plant are morphine and codeine, which are potent analgesics. Other drugs of plant origin are gums and oils. An example of a gum is psyllium seed, which is a bulk-forming laxative. Castor oil from the castor bean acts as a stimulant laxative.

Drugs of animal origin are prepared by extracting substances, such as hormones, from animal tissues and organs. Nonsynthetic insulin, for example, is extracted from the pancreases of cattle and pigs. Insulin is a valuable drug used to treat diabetes mellitus by lowering the blood glucose level. Heparin, used to reduce the formation of blood clots, is taken from the intestinal linings of pigs. Careful consideration should be given when considering administering animal-derived medications to people of certain cultural groups. For example, porcine-derived heparin may cause concern and be refused by some Muslim and Jewish patients. In cases such as this, the patient should be encouraged to consult a religious advisor as life-saving medications are typically permitted.

Iron, iodine, calcium, sodium chloride (salt), magnesium hydroxide (milk of magnesia), and magnesium sulfate (Epsom salts) are examples of minerals used in drug therapy. They are derived from rocks and crystals.

Many drugs are made, or synthesized, in the laboratory through chemical processes. Sulfonamide drugs such as *Bactrim* and *Septra* are frequently used in the treatment of urinary tract infections. An advantage of synthetic drugs is that they are generally less expensive than nonsynthetic drugs because they are produced in mass volume. Biotechnology and genetic engineering combine DNA material from different organisms, making new drugs and drug products available. Insulin and vaccines can be produced this way. *Humulin*® insulin is a genetically engineered drug used in the treatment of diabetes mellitus.

DRUG USES [LO 1-2]

The study of drug uses will give you an understanding of one phase of healthcare, drug therapy. The most familiar uses of drugs relate to disease: prevention, treatment, diagnosis, health maintenance, palliative care, and cure. Drugs are also used as **contraceptives**, or drugs to prevent pregnancy.

Disease prevention involves the administration of drugs, such as vaccines, that inoculate the body against disease microorganisms. Health maintenance helps patients maintain or enhance their current levels of health. Drugs such as vitamins and minerals are given for many reasons, including to help keep the body healthy and strong and to keep the body systems functioning normally. Vitamins and minerals are also useful treating certain conditions and improving healing. Vitamin C is used to treat scurvy, burns, delayed fracture healing, wound healing after surgery, and chronic diseases.

Treating disease means relieving the symptoms while the body's natural disease-fighting mechanisms do their work. Aspirin and antihistamines are examples of drugs used to treat disease symptoms. An antihistamine such as *Benadryl Allergy* is an example of a drug used to treat allergy symptoms or motion sickness. Aspirin is used to treat fever and pain. Curing disease often means eliminating disease-causing microorganisms. Antibiotics such as erythromycin and penicillin are drugs given to cure a disease such as pneumonia.

Diagnostic drugs are considered drugs because they are chemical substances used to diagnose or monitor a patient's condition. A diagnostic drug may have side effects and adverse reactions just like any other drug. For example, radiopaque dye (a contrast medium that shows up on fluoroscopes or x-rays) is administered to evaluate various functions of the body, such as to detect gallbladder malfunctions. A radiopaque dye such as iodine may cause anaphylaxis, an immediate, severe, and frequently fatal reaction. It is therefore important to ask patients if they have a shellfish allergy, which indicates a predisposition to an iodine allergy.

Antibiotics are an example of drugs that cure. With drugs that cure, a pathogen is rendered ineffective by the medication. For example, penicillin destroys the cause of a disease such as streptococcal pneumonia.

The prevention of pregnancy is possible with the use of contraceptives, drugs that control fertility. Contraceptive drugs can be administered in a variety of ways, including orally, transdermally, and vaginally.

Drugs often have more than one use. The drug promethazine hydrochloride (*Phenergan*), for example, is used in a variety of ways. It can control allergic reactions, treat motion sickness, induce sleep, and prevent vomiting after surgery. Some drugs have the ability to prevent as well as cure or treat disease. An example of a health maintenance drug is vitamins.

Palliative drugs are used to improve the quality of life but not cure or treat the disease. They are often used in terminal illness such as cancer. Most frequently analgesics are used for pain management in these illnesses. Hospice has been instrumental in helping healthcare professionals realize that opioid dosing frequently exceeds the dose used in other conditions or surgery. In these cases, opioid dependency is not of concern.

DRUG STANDARDS [LO 1-3]

Drugs differ widely in strength, quality, and purity, depending on how they are manufactured. To control these differences, certain rules or **standards** have been set up that products must meet. Drug standards are required by law. The law states that all preparations called by the same drug name must be of a uniform strength, quality, and purity. A drug prepared in Indiana must meet the same standards for strength, quality, and purity as the same drug prepared in California or New Jersey. Because of drug standards, providers who order penicillin, for example, can be sure that patients anywhere in the country will get the same basic substance from the pharmacist. Drug standards also help providers prescribe accurate dosages and predict the results.

Drugs for which standards have been developed are listed in a special reference book called the *United States Pharmacopeia/National Formulary (USP/NF)*. The *USP/NF* is recognized by the U.S. government as the official list of drug standards, which are enforceable by the U.S. Food and Drug Administration (FDA).

Since 1975, the *USP/NF* has engaged in a program to include all drug substances and, to the extent possible, all drug products in the United States. The book is updated regularly, and a new edition is published every five years to keep the information up to date.

DRUG NAMES [LO 1-4]

All drugs have more than one name. In fact, most have four: a chemical name, a generic name, an official name, and one or more brand or trade names.

The **chemical name** describes the chemical composition and molecular structure of the drug. Acetylsalicylic acid is an example of a chemical name.

The **generic name** is the official nonproprietary name assigned by the manufacturer with the approval of the United States Adopted Names (USAN) Council. The generic name is simpler than the chemical name. For example, aspirin is the generic name for acetylsalicylic acid. The official name is usually the same as the generic name.

Also known as the trade or proprietary name, the **brand name** is the name under which the drug is sold by a specific manufacturer. *Flomax* is an example of a brand-name drug. The name is owned by the drug company, and no other company may use it. The symbol ® to the right of the name shows that its use is restricted. A drug that is manufactured by several companies may be known by several different brand names. For example, the drug with the generic name nitroglycerin is sold by several manufacturers under such brand names as *Nitro-Bid,* and *Nitrostat. Bufferin* is an example of a brand, proprietary, or trade name for aspirin.

Brand-Name Drugs versus Generic-Name Drugs

Most drugs are known to the general public by their brand names. For example, *Children's Dimetapp Cold and Cough,* is more familiar-sounding to someone who is not in the profession than is the name brompheniramine. But you and your fellow health workers must be familiar with both the brand and generic names of many drugs. For example, a provider may prescribe a drug by a generic name or a brand name. Because several brand names may exist for the same ingredient, such as acetaminophen, providers are encouraged to order drugs by their generic names. In fact, state and federal governments now permit, encourage, and in some cases mandate that the consumer be given the generic form when buying prescription drugs. Another reason for using generic names is that doing so avoids confusion among similar brand names. A prescription written for a generic product allows the pharmacist to choose among nonbranded drugs available from several companies. Generic drugs are therapeutically equivalent to and much cheaper than brand-name drugs.

Another reason for knowing the generic name is that drugs often have several brand names but only one generic name. If you learn the generic names, you can organize information about several brand-name drugs in your mind. Of course, it is not possible to memorize all the generic and brand names for medications, but you should try to become familiar with both names of the drugs you handle daily in your work.

Where this book mentions specific drugs, generic names are given first and are not capitalized. Brand names are capitalized, italicized, and shown in parentheses following the generic names. Only one or two common brand names are given in each case. Keep in mind that many other brand-name products may be available. Refer to Table 1.1 for five commonly prescribed generic- and brand-name drugs with pronunciation and classification.

Table 1.1 Five Generic- versus Brand-Name Drugs (with Pronunciation and Classification)

Generic Name	Brand Name	Classification
paroxetine hydrochloride (pah-rox-eh-teen high-droh-klor-eyed)	Paxil	Antidepressant (selective serotonin reuptake inhibitor)
escitalopram oxalate (eh-sye-tal-oh-pram ahk-se-layt)	Lexapro	Antidepressant (selective serotonin reuptake inhibitor)
hydrocodone bitartrate with acetaminophen (high-droh-koh-dohn bye-tar-trayt with ah-set-ah-min-oh-fen)	Vicodin	Narcotic analgesic
alprazolam (al-prayz-oh-lam)	Xanax	Antianxiety
tramadol hydrochloride (tram-ah-dol high-droh-klor-eyed)	Ultram	Analgesic

DRUG REFERENCES [LO 1-5]

Several reference books and computer websites provide useful information about drugs on the market. Providers and others in the health occupations often refer to them when planning and administering drug therapy. Drug references can help you understand why and how a particular drug is administered. For each drug, see Table 1.2 for the information included in each drug reference.

Computer websites are rapidly becoming the most popular way to check information on drugs. Websites include:

- www.rxlist.com
- www.fda.gov
- www.safemedication.com
- www.express-scripts.com
- www.drugs.com

Learning how to use the drug references will help provide you with the knowledge healthcare workers need when administering medications.

Table 1.2 Information in a Drug Reference

- *Description*—what the drug is made of.
- *Action*—how the drug works.
- *Indications*—what conditions the drug is used for.
- *Interactions*—undesirable effects produced when drugs are taken with certain foods or with other drugs.
- *Contraindications*—conditions under which the drug should not be used.
- *Precautions*—specific warnings to consider when administering drugs to patients with specific conditions or diseases.
- *Side effects/adverse reactions*—unintended and undesirable effects.
- *Dosage and administration*—correct dose for each possible route of administration.
- *How supplied*—how the drug is packaged and stored.
- *Nursing implications*—medication education to be given and care provided during administration and following. For example, before giving digoxin, the apical pulse should be assessed for one full minute and held if the heart rate is less than 60 bpm.

A common reference book is the *Physicians' Desk Reference (PDR®)*, which is available in many health facilities. The *PDR®* gives information about the drug products of major pharmaceutical companies. It is useful for checking the description, clinical pharmacology, mechanism of **action**, **indications**, **contraindications**, warnings, **precautions**, **adverse reactions**, overdosage, dosage and administration, and how the product is supplied.

The *United States Pharmacopeia Dispensing Information (USPDI)* is another drug reference, first published in 1980 in three volumes. It provides pharmacists and other healthcare workers with easy-to-follow information about official drugs and products. You will find Volume II useful, as this volume is written in nontechnical language that is easy for patients to understand. It is called *Advice for the Patient*. Volume III is the "Orange Book," *Approved Drug Products and Legal Requirements*. This volume includes state and federal requirements for prescribing and dispensing drugs. These volumes are updated each month in the *USPDI Update*.

Another valuable reference is the *Handbook of Nonprescription Drugs*, published by the American Pharmaceutical Association. It deals with over-the-counter information in general categories. Pharmacology textbooks and articles in nursing and other professional journals are also helpful sources of information. Some healthcare facilities keep their own reference lists of the drugs they use most often.

Another reference is the *American Hospital Formulary Service (AHFS) Information Book*. It contains an objective overview, in outline form, of almost every drug available in the United States. This book is updated yearly, and information is easily located with just one index at the back of the book.

In addition, there are many nursing drug reference books on the market, many available as handbooks and more frequently as online references and convenient applications ("apps") for smartphones and tablets. These nursing drug books similarly cover the action, uses, dose and route, adverse effects, contraindications, and precautions of the drug but also focus on nursing considerations, interventions, and patient teaching. Many individuals who are administering medications find it extremely helpful to have the nursing interventions listed, such as monitoring a temperature, measuring intake and output, or encouraging the patient to drink fluids.

No one text is a complete source for all the drug information necessary for the administering of medications. Therefore, it is important that you gather information from the various sources and select the drug reference source that you feel best meets your needs when you administer medications and provide patient and family teaching about those medications.

Understanding and Using the *PDR®*

The current edition of the *Physicians' Desk Reference (PDR®)* contains five sections that are color-coded and contain specific information. The first section is the Manufacturers' Index and is printed on gray pages. This section lists all the pharmaceutical manufacturers that participate in the *PDR®*. Participating manufacturers provide their addresses and phone numbers and show their products along with their corresponding page numbers. The second section is the Brand and Generic Name Index, which is printed on white pages and lists drugs by both their brand and generic names and the page numbers they are listed on. Section three is the Product Category Index, which is printed on gray pages and lists the products by prescribing category. The Product Identification Guide comprises section four. This section provides color photos of the actual size of drugs arranged alphabetically by the manufacturer. These color photos will help you easily identify drugs.

Section five contains Product Information and is also printed on white pages. In this section, you will find detailed information on each drug such as the brand and generic name, description, clinical pharmacology, indications, contraindications, warnings, precautions, adverse reactions, dosage and administration, and lastly how the drug is supplied. The "description" of the drug lists its origin and chemical composition. The "clinical pharmacology" states the effect a drug has on the body and the process by which the drug produces this effect. The diseases or conditions for which a drug is given are listed in the "indications and usage" section. The reasons a specific drug should not be given are included in the "contraindications" section. The potential dangers of a drug are listed under the drug "warnings." The "precautions" state possible undesirable effects a drug may have. Side effects of a drug are listed under "adverse reactions." Under "dosage and administration," you will learn the usual amount of a drug to be given to adults and children and the recommended times for administration. The possible drug forms and their dosages are included in the "how supplied" section.

After understanding the various sections of the *PDR®*, you will be able to look up information on any drug. For example, if the drug you want to give is *Tylenol,* look it up in the white pages or section two (Brand and Generic Name Index). The phonetic spelling is given for the brand name along with the generic name (acetaminophen). The route of administration, such as "for oral use," is also listed. Generally, the manufacturer's name appears in parentheses after the drug name, followed by one or two page numbers. The first page number refers to the Product Identification page number, which provides an actual-size color photo of the drug. The second page number refers to the Product Information page number, which provides all prescribing information.

You may also look for a specific drug by knowing its classification. The blue pages, or Product Category Index, provide the prescribing category. For example, look up antibiotics and you will find a variety of antibiotics such as penicillin.

Other features in the *PDR®* include a list of poison control centers, U.S. Food and Drug Administration agencies, drug information centers, and herb–drug interactions.

Now that you have learned the various sections of the *PDR®* and how to look up drug information, you have all of the information needed to safely administer a drug to your patient.

Electronic resources are available in many healthcare settings and may take the place of paper copies of drug guides and the *PDR®*. The search function in electronic resources can help quickly locate the desired information.

Coping with Technical Language

A problem with many drug references is that they are written in complex language. They use medical terms that may be unfamiliar, especially to new students. The descriptions of drugs assume that the reader has a background in anatomy, physiology, diseases, and pharmacology.

An important aim of this book is to help you learn enough about anatomy, physiology, diseases, and pharmacology to understand what you find in different drug references. You will learn important technical terms, basic principles to help you understand how drugs work, and basic information about various diseases to understand why a particular drug is prescribed.

Coping with Changing Information

Information about drugs is constantly changing. New drugs appear all the time, and old drugs are taken off the market. Drug research turns up better ways of using drugs and administering them. Belimumab (*Benlysta*), approved by the FDA in 2011, is the first drug approved to treat systemic lupus erythematosus since 1955. Propoxyphene HCL *(Darvon)* was recently taken off the market as an analgesic. This means that drug references quickly can become outdated. Some reference publishers such as the *PDR®* send out regular supplements with information updates. These updates should be checked along with the drug reference. Another place to look for current information on drug administration is package inserts. These are printed sheets of information inside the boxes in which drugs are packaged. Package inserts contain the same information that is provided in the *PDR®*.

This text will help you cope with changing information on drugs. After studying the various chapters, you will know general principles about groups or classifications of drugs. Any new information that becomes available should then fit easily into your general understanding of drugs.

PURCHASING YOUR OWN DRUG CARDS [LO 1-5]

Because there are so many drugs and so much information exists about them, no one can expect to keep all of the important facts constantly in mind. Drug cards can be purchased from college or local bookstores. Some students may also prefer to develop a drug file or cards on the computer. Drug cards save time because healthcare workers can find the information more quickly in their card files than in a huge drug reference. The information on drug cards is updated regularly to remain current. Cards should include this information:

Drug name, both generic and brand.

Drug classification, or the group a drug belongs to, such as analgesics (pain relievers), antipyretics (fever reducers), antacids, laxatives, and so on (you will learn the basic drug classifications in later chapters).

Forms in which the drug is available (tablets, capsules, etc.).

Action, or how the drug interacts with the organs or systems that it is supposed to affect.

Uses of the drug.

Side effects and adverse reactions.

Drug interactions.

Signs of drug poisoning (toxicity).

Route of administration.

Dosage range and usual adult dose.

Special instructions for giving the medication, including the interventions required (what to tell the patient about expected side effects, precautions, etc.).

A note on where you got your information (specific drug reference, package insert, etc.).

A sample drug card is shown in Figure 1.1. Beginning with Chapter 6, you will find tables at the ends of chapters listing representative drugs in the major drug categories. These tables can serve as a guide for what to include on your drug cards or drug file. As you study the drugs in Chapters 6 through

Figure 1.1

Sample drug card.

Drug
Acetaminophen (*Tylenol*).

Action
Blockade of prostaglandin stimulation of the central nervous system. Increases peripheral blood flow and sweating.

Uses
Fever reduction, temporary relief of mild or moderate pain.

Doses
Adults and teenagers 325–500 mg oral every 3–4 hours, 650 mg oral every 4–6 hours, 1000 mg oral every 6 hours as needed.

Side Effects
Yellow eyes or skin (rare); bloody or black stools; pain in side and lower back; skin rash, hives, or itching; sores, ulcers, or white spots on the lips or mouth; sore throat; sudden decrease in the amount of urine; unusual bleeding or bruising; unusual tiredness or weakness.

Drug Interactions
Barbiturates, carbamazepine (*Tegretol*), hydantoins, rifampin (*Rifadin*), and sulfinpyrazone may reduce the therapeutic effects and increase the hepatotoxic effects of acetaminophen. Caffeine may increase the analgesic effect of acetaminophen.

Nursing Implications
Instruct patient not to exceed 4 g daily; monitor for acute signs of liver toxicity such as yellow discoloration of skin and eyes, dark urine, itching, and clay-colored stools.

19, make a habit of preparing drug cards or a drug file for the medications you expect to be giving in your health facility.

DRUG LEGISLATION [LO 1-6]

The U.S. government regulates the composition, uses, names, labeling, and testing of drugs. Since the early 1900s, many laws have been passed to enforce the official drug standards and to protect the public from unreliable and unsafe drugs. Federal agencies have been set up to see that these laws are followed. Table 1.3 lists the major drug laws and their enforcing agencies.

The first law, the Pure Food and Drug Act, was passed in 1906. This law states that only drugs listed in the *USP/NF* may be prescribed and sold, because these drugs meet the required standards. Various amendments to this act regulate prescriptions, require testing of new drugs, and call for complete information about drug effects and dangers. The Food, Drug, and Cosmetic Act (FDCA) of 1938, which replaced the 1906 act, spells out additional regulations concerning purity, strength, effectiveness, safety, labeling, and packaging of drugs. It also states that the federal government must review safety studies on new drugs before they can be put on the market. This provision was added after more than 100 deaths resulted from a poorly tested and mislabeled sulfanilamide product. This solution had been marketed as an "elixir" without investigating its toxicity. The FDCA is enforced by the Food and Drug Administration. Since 1962, the FDA has required proof that new drugs are effective as well as safe.

Table 1.3 Major Drug Laws

Legislative Act	Enforcement Agency
Pure Food and Drug Act of 1906 Approves *USP/NF* and requires that drugs meet official standards Requires labeling of medicines containing morphine and other narcotics Amendment of 1912 prohibits making false claims about health benefits of a drug	None
Food, Drug, and Cosmetic Act (FDCA) of 1938 (replaced the 1906 act) Regulates content and sale of drugs and cosmetics Requires accurate labeling and warnings against unsafe use Requires government review of safety studies before selling new drugs Amendment of 1952 allows certain drugs to be dispensed by prescription only and refilled only on a doctor's order; also recognizes OTC drugs as drugs that do not require a prescription Amendment of 1962 requires proof of effectiveness and safety before marketing new drugs and full information on advantages, side effects, contraindications Certain drugs must carry a warning label indicating possible side effects or if drug may be habit-forming Certain drugs must carry the label "Caution: Federal law prohibits dispensing without a prescription."	**Food and Drug Administration (FDA)** Under Department of Health and Human Services Can investigate manufacturers, withdraw approval of drugs, control shipment and testing Enforces FDCA by prosecuting offending firms and seizing goods Drug manufacturers must register with FDA and report to FDA all adverse reactions resulting from use of their products Reviews studies of safety and effectiveness of new drugs
Drug Regulation and Reform Act of 1978 Permits briefer investigation of new drugs, allowing consumers earlier access	FDA
Orphan Drug Act of 1983 Speeds up drugs' availability for patients with rare diseases	FDA
Drug Price Competition and Patent Term Restoration Act of 1984 Permits generic drug companies to prove bioequivalence without duplicating costly clinical trials done by original drug manufacturer Gives longer patent protection for new drugs	FDA
Childhood Vaccine Act of 1986 Requires patient information on vaccines Gives the FDA permission to make necessary recalls	FDA
Controlled Substances Act (CSA) of 1970 Identifies and regulates manufacture and sale of narcotics and dangerous drugs Provides research into drug abuse, prevention, and dependence Provides funding for education on drug abuse, rehabilitation, and law enforcement Classifies drugs into Schedules I–V according to medical usefulness and possible abuse (Table 1.4)	**Drug Enforcement Administration (DEA)** Under Department of Justice May punish violators by fines, imprisonment, or both
Uniform Controlled Substances Act of 1990 A new provision to the original act of 1970 that provides both civil and criminal forfeiture actions Establishes uniformity between federal law and state law in the uniformity among states in the control of narcotics	

(continued)

Table 1.3 *(continued)*

Legislative Act	Enforcement Agency
Nutrition Facts of 1992 Requires basic-serving nutritional information on the nutrition label of most prepackaged food	**United States Department of Agriculture (USDA)**
Nutrition Facts of 2003 Includes trans-fat content in food on the nutrition label	**USDA**
Food Allergen Labeling and Consumer Protection Act of 2004 Requires labeling food if it contains a protein from common allergy-causing foods, such as peanuts, soybeans, cow's milk, eggs, fish, crustacean shellfish, nuts, and wheat	**FDA**
USA Patriot Improvement and Reauthorization Act of 2005 (Combat Methamphetamine Epidemic Act of 2005 [CMEA]) Restricts the sale of over-the-counter products containing pseudoephedrine and ephedrine Makes these products available only by purchase through a pharmacy	**Drug Enforcement Administration (DEA)**

Another important law is the Controlled Substances Act of 1970, also known as the Comprehensive Drug Abuse Prevention and Control Act. It identifies the drugs that are dangerous or subject to abuse, such as narcotics, depressants, and stimulants. This law strictly regulates the manufacture and distribution of controlled substances. It clearly stipulates that possession of a controlled substance is unlawful without a prescription. This law provides research into preventing drug abuse and drug dependence. It also provides for treatment and rehabilitation of drug abusers. It further improves the administration and regulation of the manufacture, distribution, and dispensing of controlled substances.

Controlled substances are grouped into five categories, or schedules, each with its particular restrictions, as shown in Table 1.4. There is a Schedule VI in some states. Drugs with the highest abuse potential are placed in Schedule I. They have no accepted medical use in the United States. Drugs with the lowest abuse potential are placed in Schedule V. You need to be aware that these classifications are flexible. Occasionally, drugs may be added to a schedule or changed from one schedule to another without new legislation. A record is kept of each time a controlled substance is sold and of the amount. There are restrictions on how prescriptions can be refilled. All prescriptions must be signed in ink or sent electronically. Oral emergency orders for Schedule II substances may be filled, but the provider must supply a written prescription within 72 hours.

Pharmacists must carefully follow the rules outlined in the Controlled Substances Act. Violation of the law is punishable by fine or imprisonment or both. The agency that enforces this act is the Drug Enforcement Administration (DEA).

Prescribers must also follow the law in prescribing controlled substances. They need a DEA number from the DEA for each prescriber from which they practice and must inform the DEA of any changes in employment. They are given one tax stamp and number for each license. This number, called the DEA number, must be shown on any prescription for controlled substances.

To keep a supply of controlled substances in an office or a health facility, the staff must fill out special order forms and records. These forms show how many controlled substances are being kept at the facility, as well as who received doses of the drugs and how unused doses were disposed of. A physical inventory of all controlled substances in the office must be made every two years. (You will learn about these forms in Chapter 5.) See Table 1.5 for categories of drugs.

Table 1.4 Drug Classifications under the Controlled Substances Act of 1970

Drugs	Characteristics	Examples
Schedule I drugs	High potential for abuse, severe physical and psychological dependence No accepted medical use To be used for research only Not to be prescribed; unsafe in treatment	Alfentanil, fenethylline, hashish, heroin, lysergic acid diethylamide (LSD), marijuana, peyote, psilocybin, mescaline, benzylpiperazine
Schedule II drugs	High potential for abuse, severe physical and psychological dependence Acceptable medical uses, with restrictions Dispensed by prescription only No refills without new written prescription from a provider	Amphetamines, cocaine, meperidine HCl (*Demerol*), methadone, methylphenidate hydrochloride (*Ritalin*), morphine, opium, pentobarbital (*Nembutal*), hydromorphone hydrochloride (*Dilaudid*), dextroamphetamine, acetaminophen with hydrocodone (*Vicodin*), secobarbital (Seconal)
Schedule III drugs	Moderate potential for abuse, high psychological dependence, low physical dependence Acceptable medical uses By prescription only; may be refilled five times in 6 months if authorized by a provider	Barbiturates, butabarbital (*Butisol*), anabolic steroids, *acetaminophen with codeine* (*Tylenol* with codeine)
Schedule IV drugs	Lower potential for abuse than Schedule III drugs; limited psychological and physical dependence Acceptable medical uses By prescription only; may be refilled five times in 6 months if authorized by a provider	Chloral hydrate, chlordiazepoxide (*Librium*), diazepam (*Valium*), flurazepam HCl, oxazepam, phenobarbital, lorazepam (*Ativan*), meprobamate, pentazocine HCl (*Talwin*), alprazolam (*Xanax*)
Schedule V drugs	Low potential for abuse Acceptable medical uses OTC narcotic drugs, but sold only by registered pharmacists; buyer must be 18 years and show ID	Diphenoxylate HIC with atropine sulfate (*Lomotil*), cough syrups with codeine, e.g., guaifenesin with codeine
Schedule VI drugs	Lower potential for abuse than Schedule IV and limitations on quantities	Cough preparations less than 200 milligrams of codeine (*Robitussin AC*), *Motofen, Lyrica*

ª Requires a prescription.

Source: DEA, U.S. Department of Justice. Check with your local DEA office for current regulations.

Table 1.5 Drug Categories

- **Controlled substances.** These are drugs that have special restrictions as to who can prescribe and sell them and how often they can be prescribed.

  Example: Narcotic
- **Over-the-counter (OTC) drugs.** These can be bought and sold without a prescription.

  Example: Aspirin
- **Prescription drugs.** These drugs are also called legend drugs. They require a provider's prescription (either oral or written) to be bought and sold.

  Example: Lipitor

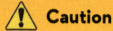
YOU AND THE LAW [LO 1-7]

As a member of the healthcare team, you are responsible for knowing the laws controlling drug use and the names of the regulatory agencies, such as the Federal Trade Commission (FTC) and the Consumer Product Safety Commission. The latter commission enforces the Poison Prevention Packaging Act (PPPA), which mandates "childproof" drug packaging. Claiming ignorance of the law will not stand up in court if you are ever accused of irresponsible handling and administration of drugs.

How can you be sure you understand the law? As a first step, study carefully Tables 1.3 and 1.4. These tables summarize a great deal of information about federal drug laws. Be aware that the specific drugs under each schedule in the Controlled Substances Act may change. Your health facility will have an up-to-date list of controlled substances from the DEA. Get copies of federal drug laws from the library or from the FDA.

As a next step, study the laws of your state. State laws regulate such things as who may give medications, what kinds of training and supervision are required, who may keep the records, and who may take prescriptions over the phone.

Your own health agency will also have regulations for you to follow. There will be special rules, for example, if your agency receives Medicaid or Medicare funds. You should also be aware of the lines of authority in your agency—in other words, who is in charge of what and who supervises whom. You will then be able to go to the right person when you have a legal question about giving a certain drug.

Knowing the law helps protect you from errors and possible lawsuits. But there is a more important benefit—the safety of your patient. By showing your awareness of drug laws, you help educate your patients. You also gain their cooperation in following the law. Drug laws are designed to protect the public. Members of the public depend on your example and your support.

Legal and Ethical Issues | Substituting Drugs

Although the provider or prescriber retains the prerogative to require the dispensing of a particular brand-name drug, every state has a drug substitution law that either mandates or may permit a drug substitution by the pharmacist. The prescriber may give permission to substitute the drug ordered by either checking the "may substitute" box or writing "may substitute" on the prescription. If the prescriber has an objection to a drug substitution, the prescriber will write "do not substitute" or "dispense as written." Some states have a mandatory substitution law to dispense a less expensive drug, and the prescriber must write "medically necessary" to ensure that the more costly brand-name drug is dispensed. Because you care for patients and hand them prescriptions, you need to be informed on the laws for drug substitution.

Summary

Learning Outcome	Summary Points
1-1 Define terms to understanding the administration of medications.	• *Pharmacology* is the study of drugs and their uses. • *Pharmacodynamics* is the study of how the body responds to drugs. • *Pharmacokinetics* is the absorption, distribution, metabolism, and excretion of drugs. • *Anatomy* is the study of body parts. • *Physiology* is the science that deals with the function of cells, tissues, and organs of living organisms. • *Pathology* is the study of how drugs change the course of disease. • A *drug* is a chemical substance used in the diagnosis, treatment, cure, or prevention of a disease. • A *therapeutic effect* is the desired or predicted physiological response the drug causes. • *Side effects* are a drug's desirable or undesirable effects apart from the primary reason for giving the drug.
1-2 List the six sources and uses of drugs.	• The major drug sources are plants, animals, minerals, and chemicals, or synthesized drugs. An example of a plant source is the wildflower purple foxglove, from which digitalis is made. Insulin is extracted from an animal source, cattle and pigs. Sodium chloride is derived from a mineral drug source, rocks. *Bactrim* and *Septra* are synthetic drugs made from chemical sources. • Prevention, treatment, diagnosis, health maintenance, palliative care, and cure are the six uses of drugs.
1-3 Define *drug standards,* indicating how they are determined and why they are necessary.	• Drug standards are certain rules that products must meet. Drug standards are required by law. • The law states that all preparations called by the same drug name must be of uniform strength, quality, and purity. • Drug standards are necessary because drugs differ in strength, quality, and purity. All preparations called by the same drug name must be of uniform strength, quality, and purity.

Learning Outcome	Summary Points
1-4 List the names by which drugs are known.	• The *chemical name* describes the chemical composition and molecular structure of the drug. • The *generic name* is the official, nonproprietary name assigned by the drug manufacturer with the approval of the United States Adopted Names (USAN) Council. • The *official name* is usually the same as the generic name. • The *brand* or *trade name*, also known as the *proprietary name*, is the name under which the drug is sold by a specific manufacturer.
1-5 List drug references and the purpose of each, and purchase drug cards.	• *Physicians' Desk Reference (PDR®)* • *United States Pharmacopeia Dispensing Information (USPDI)* • *Handbook of Nonprescription Drugs* • Many of these drug references contain the drug description along with the action, indication, interactions, contraindications, precautions, side effects/adverse reactions, dosage, and administration, as well as how they are supplied. Look at the designated area for the specific information needed (e.g., Dosage). • The drug name, classification, action, use, dose, interactions, and side effects should be included on the drug card.
1-6 List the major drug laws and their main features.	• Since 1906 with the passage of the Pure Foods and Drug Act, Congress has regulated the manufacture of prescription drugs. • There are many different laws that affect medication creation, distribution, and administration. • It is important to understand the policies and protocols in place that affect your role in medication administration.
1-7 List the federal agencies that enforce drug laws and the importance of enforcing them.	• Food and Drug Administration (FDA) • Drug Enforcement Administration (DEA) • Knowing the laws helps health workers protect themselves from errors and possible lawsuits, provide patient education, and enhance patient safety.

Chapter 1 Review

Define each of the terms listed.

1. (LO 1-1) Drug _____

   _____

2. (LO 1-1) Pharmacology _____

   _____

3. (LO 1-1) Anatomy _____

   _____

4. (LO 1-1) Physiology _____

   _____

5. (LO 1-3) Drug standards _____

_____

6. (LO 1-5) *PDR*® _____

_____

7. (LO 1-3) *USP/NF* _____

_____

8. (LO 1-7) Congress _____

_____

9. (LO 1-1) Pharmacokinetics _____

_____

Answer the questions in the space provided.

10. (LO 1-2) Name four sources of drugs, and give an example of a drug that comes from each source.

   Source   **Example**

   _____   _____

   _____   _____

   _____   _____

   _____   _____

11. (LO 1-2) Name the six therapeutic uses of drugs. Give an example of each.

   Use   **Example**

   _____   _____

   _____   _____

   _____   _____

   _____   _____

   _____   _____

   _____   _____

12. (LO 1-6) Name the three major drug laws and the agencies that enforce them.

   Law and Date   **Enforcing Agency**

   _____   _____

   _____   _____

   _____   _____

13. (LO 1-7) Differentiate between these legal classifications for drugs.

OTC drugs _____

_____

_____

_____

Prescription drugs _____

_____

_____

_____

Controlled substances _____

_____

_____

_____

From Column 2, select the term or phrase that best matches each item in Column 1.

	Column 1	Column 2
_____	14. (LO 1-2) Chemical name	a. *Bufferin*
_____	15. (LO 1-4) Generic name	b. aspirin
_____	16. (LO 1-4) Brand name	c. acetylsalicylic acid
_____	17. (LO 1-5) *PDR*®	d. contains information about drug products provided by pharmaceutical companies
_____	18. (LO 1-4) USAN	e. same as generic name
_____	19. (LO 1-4) Official name	f. system that adopts generic names

Match the drugs to their schedules or classes as spelled out in the Controlled Substances Act of 1990 (original 1970) (LO 1-7).

	Schedule	Drugs
_____	20. I	a. barbiturates, *Butisol, Tylenol* with codeine
_____	21. II	b. opium, morphine, *Demerol,* amphetamines, *Dilaudid*
_____	22. III	c. cough syrup with codeine, *Lomotil*
_____	23. IV	d. *Valium,* phenobarbital, *chlordiazepoxide, flurazepam*
_____	24. V	e. heroin, hashish, LSD, peyote, alfentanil

Multiple Choice—Circle the correct letter.

25. (LO 1-6) Which major drug law speeds up drugs' availability for patients with rare diseases?
    a. Drug Regulation and Reform Act of 1978
    b. Orphan Drug Act of 1983
    c. Pure Food and Drug Act of 1906
    d. Food, Drug, and Cosmetic Act (FDCA) of 1938

26. (LO 1-5) What information is covered in a drug reference book?
    a. Type of providers who can prescribe the drug
    b. Interactions with the drug the drug
    c. Which healthcare workers can administer the drug
    d. Color of the drug

27. (LO 1-2) What are two uses of drugs?
    a. Produce side effects and adverse reactions
    b. Change the genetic and chemical makeup of the body
    c. Prevent and treat disease
    d. Test the knowledge and skill of the healthcare worker

28. (LO 1-3) Who requires the use of drug standards?
    a. Hospitals
    b. Patients
    c. Providers
    d. The law

29. (LO 1-4) Which drug is listed by a generic name?
    a. Acetylsalicylic acid
    b. *Bufferin*
    c. *Nitro-Bid*
    d. *Nitrostat*

Chapter 1 Case Studies

30. You want to understand the sources of drugs before you administer them. What are the four sources of drugs? Your patient has been prescribed *Metamucil,* digitalis, insulin, *Bactrim,* and iron. What are these drugs, and what are their sources? _____

_____

_____

_____

_____

31. Nitroglycerin is prescribed by the healthcare provider, and *Nitrostat* was dispensed by the pharmacy. The patient tells you he is confused and wants to know what the difference means. What should you tell him? _____

_____

_____

_____

_____

Critical Thinking

Respond to the questions in the space provided.

32. (LO 1-7) Janie has just been hired for a new job in a nursing home. She wants to make sure that she knows what she is and is not allowed to do with regard to giving medications. What advice would you give her?

_____

_____

_____

33. (LO 1-7) Why do we have drug standards and drug laws?

_____

_____

_____

Applications

Obtain an electronic drug guide, a current copy of the *PDR*®, and a medical dictionary from your school, health facility, or clinic. Use them to answer the questions that follow.

34. You are giving Mr. Jones regular-strength *Tylenol* every few hours after surgery. You would like to know something more about the drug, so you consult the drug guide or *PDR*®. *Tylenol* is a brand or trade name. Find the section in the *PDR*® that lists drugs alphabetically by brand names. What is the generic name of this drug and how do you know?

_____

35. Look up *Tylenol* in the section you turned to in question 34. How many different forms of *Tylenol* are listed there? _____ Is there a small diamond to the left of any *Tylenol* form? If so, the diamond means there is a photograph of the drug in the Product Identification section in the *PDR*®. If you are using a different drug guide, how do you know that you are administering *Tylenol* if you do not know what it looks like? Find the photograph.

36. How is *Tylenol* supplied? What type of drug are you administering? _____

You may want to do the next activity as a collaborative learning activity. Each student should gather all drug information from a different drug reference; then students meet collaboratively and compare and contrast information.

37. You have an order to give Mrs. Lopez her daily *Cardizem CD* and to provide her with the education necessary for her to begin taking this medication at home. Consulting the various drug reference sources available to you, compare and contrast the advantages and disadvantages of these resources; discuss clinical situations for which each source might be the best one to consult.

PRINCIPLES OF DRUG ACTION

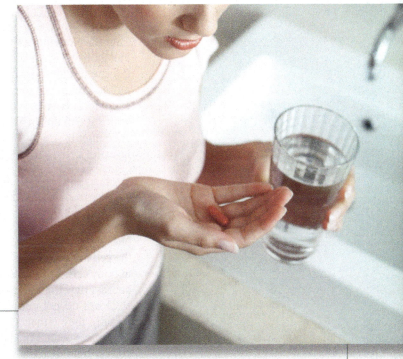

©Russell Glenister/Corbis

In this chapter you will learn what happens to drugs when they enter the human body and how they produce their effects. You will study how drugs are affected by normal body processes, by characteristics of individual patients, and by the method and time of administration. You will also become familiar with the adverse reactions that can occur with drug administration.

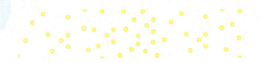

absorption

allergy

anaphylaxis

antagonism

antibody

antigen

cumulative effect

dependence

detoxify

distribution

drug abuse

excretion

histamine

idiosyncrasy

local

metabolism

placebo

potentiation

synergism

systemic

tolerance

withdrawal symptoms

PHARMACOKINETICS [LO 2-1]

Pharmacokinetics is the study of a drug during absorption, distribution, metabolism, and excretion. It refers to how the body handles a drug from the site of administration to the elimination of the drug. The extent to which a drug completes the processes of absorption, distribution, metabolism, and excretion depends on its ability to cross the cell membrane and the rate at which it can do so. Some drugs are free to cross the membrane, while others encounter barriers. Barriers can include either a single layer of cells or several layers of cells, such as the skin.

DRUG ACTION [LO 2-1]

Drugs are chemicals that are known to have specific effects on the body. When one of these chemicals comes in contact with body cells, it causes changes in the cell molecules. That is, the chemical combines with or alters the molecules in body cells to change the way the cells work. The four main drug actions are depressing, stimulating, destroying cells, and replacing substances.

Drugs do not cause cells to function in entirely new and different ways. Usually they either slow down or speed up the ordinary processes that the cells carry out. For example, depressants such as antihistamines slow the body's natural reaction to irritation, and stimulants speed up the energy-producing functions of cells.

Some drugs destroy certain cells or parts of cells. For example, some antibiotics kill disease microorganisms, and fluorouracil (5-FU) and doxorubicin are given to kill cancer cells. Other drugs, such as potassium chloride and calcium carbonate, act to replace or supplement natural substances that the body lacks because of an organ malfunction or poor nutrition. Insulin is a drug taken, in insulin-dependent diabetes mellitus, because the pancreas is unable to produce sufficient insulin to maintain normal blood glucose levels.

Once a drug is taken, it enters into certain processes that go on in the body at all times. These processes are the body's normal means of using food and oxygen to produce energy. Energy is needed for cell growth and repair, for warmth, and for movement. Drugs are treated just like any other substance that enters the body, such as food, drink, and air. The only difference is that each drug interacts in a different way with the normal processes carried on by body cells.

These interactions are determined by many things: the size and shape of the drug molecules, their ability to dissolve in water or fat, the pH balance of drugs and cells, and the electrical charges of molecules. You should have an understanding of four basic body processes that affect drug action: absorption, distribution, metabolism/biotransformation, and excretion (**Figure 2.1**).

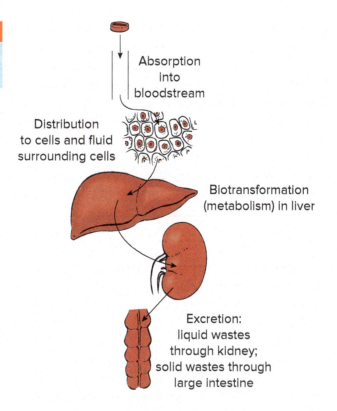

Figure 2.1

How the human body handles drugs.

Absorption into bloodstream

Distribution to cells and fluid surrounding cells

Biotransformation (metabolism) in liver

Excretion: liquid wastes through kidney; solid wastes through large intestine

Absorption

The passage of a drug from the site of administration into the bloodstream is known as **absorption**. How quickly a drug is absorbed is important because it determines how soon a drug becomes available to exert its action. The rate of absorption is influenced by the route of administration, the ability of the drug to dissolve, and the conditions at the site of absorption. The various routes of absorption include, but are not limited to, sublingual, oral, subcutaneous, intramuscular, intravenous, and topical. Most drugs, except topical drugs (those that are applied to the skin), must enter the bloodstream to have a therapeutic effect.

If the drug is not properly absorbed, it may not reach the organs or tissues that it is supposed to affect. The speed of absorption and the amount of absorption are important in pharmacodynamics. Drug action depends on how quickly and completely the drug is absorbed. When an exact serum level is important, blood tests can be ordered to find out how much drug is present in the bloodstream after absorption.

Sublingual drugs are placed under the tongue to dissolve and are absorbed into the bloodstream directly through the lining of the mouth. Buccal drugs are placed and dissolved in the cheek. Oral drugs are swallowed and enter the bloodstream through the walls of the stomach or intestine. Subcutaneous drugs that are injected just below the skin are absorbed more slowly than intramuscular (IM) drugs, which are injected into the muscle. Intravenous (IV) drugs are administered directly into the bloodstream and have the fastest and most dependable absorption (Table 2.1).

Distribution

After a drug is absorbed, the transportation of that drug from the bloodstream to the body tissues and intended site of action is known as **distribution**. Some of the drug passes out of the bloodstream through the thin walls of tiny vessels called capillaries.

Some drugs tend to collect in certain organs or tissues called drug reservoirs. If drugs do collect in reservoirs, they are released into the body

Principles of Drug Action **23**

Table 2.1 Drug Absorption

Route of Administration	Absorption Begins	Examples
Sublingual	Under the tongue	Nitroglycerin, *Levsin*
Buccal	In the cheek	Methyltestosterone
Oral	In the stomach/intestine	Ibuprofen
Intramuscular (IM)	In the muscle	Prochlorperazine
Subcutaneous	Under the skin	Epinephrine, insulin
Intravenous (IV)	In the bloodstream	Antibiotics, antineoplastics
Topical	Through the skin	Hydrocortisone ointment
Rectal	In the rectum	Bisacodyl rectal

more slowly than drugs that are evenly distributed at the start. For example, common sulfonamide drugs, such as *Bactrim* and *Septra,* often prescribed for urinary tract infections, are released slowly from tissues and are therefore considered long-lasting antibiotics.

The same dose of a drug will have a higher drug concentration in an older person than in a younger person. As a result, the drug dosage should be reduced in an older person. Decreased body water, lean body mass, and plasma proteins, along with increased fat content, increase plasma drug concentrations and pharmacological effects. The percentage of adipose tissue (body fat) increases with age, making lipid-soluble drugs more widely distributed in body organs that have a high fat content such as muscle and away from the liver and kidneys, slowing elimination of the drug from the body. Water-soluble drugs have less fluid in the body in which to dissolve and are distributed less to organs with a high fat content. As a result of this, higher plasma drug levels and greater pharmacological effects occur. The concentration of plasma proteins, namely albumin, decreases with age, which increases the overall intensity of the drug.

Metabolism/Biotransformation

Metabolism, or biotransformation, is a series of chemical reactions that inactivate a drug by converting it into a water-soluble compound so that it can be excreted by the body. This is a natural process much like the digestion of food. It is necessary so that the body can rid itself of the waste products left over after the cells make use of nutrients or drugs.

The process of metabolism occurs under the influence of enzymes, which are proteins. They cause chemical changes in a drug. These enzymes not only break down the drug but also **detoxify**, or eliminate substances that are toxic to the body. Most of the metabolism and detoxification of drugs takes place in the liver. Some metabolism also takes place to some extent in the lungs, the intestines, the kidneys, and the blood.

If a person is an older adult, is pediatric, or has a decrease in liver function, there may be insufficient metabolism of the drug, and the risk for drug toxicity increases. As a member of the healthcare team, it is important for you to be aware of the common signs of drug toxicity.

Excretion

Excretion is the body's way of removing the waste products of ordinary cell processes. Drugs are excreted in the same way as other waste products.

Most drugs leave the body through the kidneys and the large intestine. In the kidneys, blood is filtered and liquid waste products collect in the form of urine. In the large intestine, undigested solid wastes collect in the form of feces.

Excretion also takes place in the lungs, where gaseous wastes, such as carbon dioxide and some types of drugs, are collected from the bloodstream. These are excreted when the person exhales. Some drugs are excreted in the sweat and some even in hair. Milk glands also excrete some types of drugs. This is an important fact to know when giving medications to nursing mothers. Drugs that leave the body in breast milk may cause harm to the baby.

If a drug is excreted quickly, its effects are short-lived. If it is excreted slowly, its effects last longer. The rate of excretion depends on the chemical composition of the drug, the rate of metabolism, and how often the drug is administered. The condition of the excreting organs also determines how quickly and completely excretion takes place.

When a person is an older adult, is pediatric, or has kidney disease, there is an increased risk of toxicity from exposures to high doses of a drug. The dose may have to be reduced. As a member of the healthcare team, it is important for you to be prepared to teach patients about the excretion of drugs.

 Patient Education Excretion of Drugs

- Increase fluid intake to aid in excretion of drugs.

- Avoid taking laxatives, because they speed up drug excretion.

- Improper diet and lack of activity slow excretion of drugs.

- After general anesthesia, coughing and deep breathing help eliminate the anesthetic more quickly.

- Keep the skin clean to avoid irritation from drugs eliminated through the sweat glands.

- Chew gum or suck hard candy, such as lemon drops, to decrease the unpleasant effects of drugs eliminated through the saliva.

- Pregnant women should discuss all drugs, including over-the-counter drugs, with their providers to avoid possible risk to the fetus.

FACTORS AFFECTING DRUG ACTION [LO 2-2]

No two people are exactly alike, and no drug affects every human body in exactly the same way. Likewise, an individual may not react the same way to two doses of the same drug. Responses to drug action differ according to age, size, sex, genetics, physiological and pathological conditions, and psychological factors. These personal characteristics may cause slightly different drug actions in different people who receive the same drug.

Factors surrounding the administration of medications may also cause differences in people's responses to a drug. The route of administration, the time of day, the number and size of doses, diet, and environmental conditions all play a role in drug action. Providers take these factors into account before deciding which drug to prescribe and how much to prescribe.

Age

All drugs have standard doses that are considered safe for infants, children, and adults. Drug doses are carefully calculated based on the physiological development, measured in age, for infants and children. Drug doses may be prescribed by the chronological age of the patient.

Infants' body systems are not fully developed. They lack the necessary enzymes to metabolize drugs. Growing children must not take drugs that might affect their development. The body systems of the older adult may not function as efficiently as they did in middle age. Older adults have decreases in kidney and liver function, which result in failure to completely metabolize or excrete drugs. For these reasons, smaller doses and different drugs are required in treating the young or the older adult.

Size

A person's physical stature and body mass index (BMI) factor into drug action and metabolism. The goal of drug therapy is to maintain a certain concentration of a drug to achieve a desired result in the body. The proper adult dose is calculated according to a specific formula based on age and body weight.

As a result of this standard formula, drug dosages for children, adults, and older adults, and patients under- and overweight, may require adjusted drug doses. An obese individual requires a higher dose of a drug to achieve the desired result because of the high percentage of body fat. A drug works more quickly and effectively in a thin individual with a lower amount of body fat. An older adult usually requires a smaller dose of a drug because of decreased size.

Diet

Combining certain drugs with certain foods can alter the drug's effects. For example, the effects of tetracycline (an antibiotic) are decreased when it is taken with milk and milk products. Foods rich in vitamin K, such as green leafy vegetables, decrease the effects of *Coumadin* on blood clotting. The absorption of the fat-soluble vitamins (A, D, E, and K) is decreased when the patient is taking mineral oil for constipation.

Sex

The sex of an individual can influence drug action. Women may react more strongly to certain drugs than men. This is partly because of their generally smaller size and their higher proportion of body fat. Pregnant women must be extremely careful about taking any medication and must avoid taking medications without first consulting with their provider because some drugs may harm the fetus.

Genetic Factors

Each person's individual genetic makeup causes slight differences in basic processes like metabolism and excretion, which affect drug action. Some people are more sensitive to a drug because they lack the naturally occurring enzymes to break down drugs for excretion.

Pathological Conditions

Diseases can strongly affect how patients respond to drugs. Disease may impair the organs necessary for metabolism and excretion. Diseases of the liver and kidneys, especially, affect the processing and elimination of drugs. Heart disease, kidney failure, diabetes, and low blood pressure are disorders known to require special care when providers prescribe drugs. But any disease can change the effectiveness of a drug without warning. For example, a patient who is experiencing severe cancer pain needs stronger opiates to achieve a therapeutic effect.

Psychological Factors

The patient's mental state is an important factor in the success or failure of drug therapy. A patient with a positive attitude is likely to respond well to medication. A patient who is in a state of depression or despair may not respond to some drugs. Strong feelings such as worry, jealousy, anger, or fear may have a noticeable effect on drug action.

Sometimes a positive drug effect occurs simply because the patient has taken something that is supposed to make him or her "feel better." A patient with a positive attitude may feel better after taking a **placebo**, an inactive substance that has no pharmacological effect. The placebo effect relates to physiological changes related to emotions or beliefs. The action of the drug is not altered. For example, a patient may report pain relief after taking a simple oral preparation of sugar. Keep in mind that the use of a placebo is controversial and potentially unethical. A placebo should be administered cautiously.

As a member of the healthcare team, you can do much to create a positive attitude in the patient. One way is to review with the patient the important reasons for taking the medication. Another is to treat the patient in a cheerful and caring manner. Finally, your own positive, confident attitude toward the drugs you administer can influence the patient's response to medication.

Route of Administration

Drugs are absorbed, distributed, and metabolized differently when given by different routes (see Chapter 5). The route thus affects drug action. A drug acts most quickly when injected directly into the bloodstream. Drugs injected into or under the skin or into muscles require more time to take effect. Medications administered by mouth take the longest time to show their effects.

Time of Administration

Care must always be taken to give drugs at the time of day ordered by the provider. There are many time-related factors that influence drug action. Drugs taken orally are absorbed most quickly if the gastrointestinal tract is free of food. However, certain stomach-irritating drugs are taken with meals to avoid patient discomfort. When possible, drugs that make the patient sleepy are ordered to be taken at bedtime. Drugs with stimulating effects are given at times when they will not interfere with sleep. Normal bodily functions also vary with the time of day, thus affecting drug action.

Drug-Taking History

Drug action depends on whether a patient has previously taken doses of the same or another drug. Some drugs tend to collect in the body, producing a cumulative effect. In this case, later doses must be made smaller to avoid overmedicating the patient. Repeated doses of a drug may also make a patient less responsive to its effects. In that case, larger doses are required for the same effect.

Certain combinations of drugs can slow down or speed up effects, or they can cause unusual and sometimes dangerous reactions. This is why patients' medical histories and charts must include careful records of the drugs they have recently taken. Providers should also check medical histories to find out whether patients are allergic to particular drugs, such as penicillin. Patients should also be questioned about food allergies, because many medications have ingredients that are found in foods. One such example is shellfish. A patient who is allergic to shellfish may have potentially fatal results if given a contrast material, often iodine, before certain hospital procedures. The chart of a patient with an allergy must be clearly marked. This is usually done on the front of the chart with a brightly colored sticker, indicated on the patient with an allergy bracelet, and marked in the electronic health record (EHR) with a notification when a contraindicated drug is prescribed.

Drug combinations can be a problem for older adults. They often see several providers who may be unaware of one another and of the other drugs being prescribed. Each provider may prescribe what is needed in a patient's particular case, unaware of the medications other providers have prescribed. Multiple providers and multiple drugs can lead to serious drug interactions. When patients' providers all use the same EHR, transparency regarding all medications that each patient is prescribed is easier for providers to see. This can potentially eliminate drug interactions and adverse patient side effects because of drug interactions.

Table 2.2 Common Food and Drug Interactions

Foods That Affect Drug Absorption

- *Milk and milk products*—calcium decreases the absorption of antibiotics such as tetracycline.
- *Soda pop and fruit or vegetable juices*—high acid increases the stomach acid that may dissolve some drugs before they reach the intestines, therefore decreasing the absorption in the body.
- *Grapefruit juice*—affects the absorption of certain cholesterol medications, particularly statins, by increasing their effects.
- *Fatty foods*—increase the absorption of some drugs such as antifungals.
- *Green leafy vegetables*—decrease the effects of anticoagulants.
- *Salt substitutes*—increase the serum potassium and the effect of drugs used to treat hypertension and heart failure such as ramipril (*Altace*), lisinopril (*Zestril*), candesartan (*Atacand*), and valsartan (*Diovan*).
- *Licorice*—counteracts the effects of high blood pressure medications.

Table 2.3 Drug Effects on Nutritional Disorders

- Overuse of diuretics causes electrolyte loss, particularly potassium, putting the patient at high risk of cardiac rhythm problems.
- Use of diuretics such as *Lasix*, hydrochlorothiazide, and digitalis increase the risk of potassium loss.
- Excessive use of antacids such as *Gaviscon Regular Strength* and *Maalox Regular Strength* causes phosphate depletion which results in vitamin D deficiency such as osteomalacia.
- Use of oral contraceptives over a long period of time may result in folacin and vitamin C deficiencies if the woman's diet is deficient, too.
- An antihypertensive drug such as hydralazine may decrease the body's stores of vitamin B_6.

Environmental Conditions

Extremes of weather affect the action of drugs because body functions are influenced by heat and cold. Heat relaxes the blood vessels and speeds up the circulation, so drugs act faster. Cold slows their action by constricting the blood vessels and slowing the circulation. High altitude puts the body under stress because there is less oxygen in the air. This makes some drugs ineffective.

Food and Drug Interactions

Drug action is affected by food and drug interactions. These interactions can depend on the dose and the form in which the drug is taken. Refer to Table 2.2 for common food–drug interactions.

Drugs also affect nutritional status and the action of drugs. See Table 2.3 to understand these interactions.

DRUG EFFECTS [LO 2-3]

Drug action refers to the chemical changes the drug produces in cells and tissues. *Drug effect* is the combination of biological, physical, and psychological changes that take place in the body as a result of the drug action.

A drug is usually prescribed on the basis of its therapeutic effect. This is the desired effect, or the reason the drug is administered. However, most drugs have additional effects on the body that are not part of the goal of drug therapy. These are known as side effects. They may be either desirable or undesirable.

A provider must always take possible side effects into account when planning drug treatment. Side effects can be harmless, mildly annoying, or dangerous. Sometimes unpleasant side effects are tolerated because of the drug's therapeutic benefit. For example, morphine is administered for its painkilling effect, but it also has the side effects of respiratory depression, constipation, urine retention, possible addiction, and pruritus.

Many side effects can be controlled or lessened by substituting other drugs or using special procedures. For example, aspirin, when taken orally, is beneficial for the treatment of arthritis but tends to irritate the lining of the stomach and may cause bruising and bleeding. The side effect of an irritated stomach is controlled by giving the drug with milk or food. Diuretics can help ease water retention, but they may cause the body to excrete too much potassium. This situation can be corrected by giving a supplemental drug, potassium chloride, or by having the patient eat potassium-rich foods, such as bananas. Side effects are related to the actions of specific drugs. In later chapters you will learn which side effects accompany which drugs.

Drug effects are classified as either local or systemic. Some drugs affect mainly the area where they enter or are applied to the body: for example, eyedrops, sunburn creams, suppositories, and throat lozenges. These drugs are given for their **local** effects. Other drugs, such as pain medications, must travel through the bloodstream to affect cells or tissues in various parts of the body. These types of drugs are given for their **systemic** effects.

Proper administration of medications requires both knowledge of drug effects and observation of the results in the patient. The prescribed drug dosage indicates which drug, and how much of the drug, is needed to bring about the desired effect in a specific patient.

When you give medications, consider whether the drug is given for a local or a systemic effect. Then, while observing the patient's reaction, determine whether you are seeing the drug's therapeutic effect or a side effect. Your knowledge of drug effects is important to the work of the entire healthcare team—and is especially important to your patient.

ADVERSE REACTIONS [LO 2-4]

With proper administration, a drug usually has the desired effect—the patient feels better, bodily functions are restored, and side effects are under control. Occasionally, however, the body has an unexpected or dangerous response to a drug. These unexpected conditions are called *adverse reactions*. The most common adverse reactions are allergy, anaphylaxis, idiosyncrasies, tolerance, cumulative effect, overdose and toxicity, drug interactions (synergism, antagonism, and potentiation), and drug dependence. These adverse reactions are summarized, along with their causes, symptoms, and treatments, in **Table 2.4**. As a person giving medications, you are expected to be aware of possible reactions and notify your supervisor as soon as you notice any sign of an adverse reaction.

Drug Allergy

Drug **allergy** is an abnormal response that occurs because a person has developed **antibodies** against a particular drug. When a person takes the allergy-causing drug, called the **antigen**, the antibodies attack it. The reaction between antigen and antibodies causes damage to body tissues. The injured cells release a substance called **histamine**, which is responsible for the symptoms usually seen in allergic reactions.

Mild allergic symptoms can occur immediately after a drug is taken, or they can show up hours, days, or even weeks later. Severe allergic reactions, which can be fatal, usually begin within minutes of exposure and may require immediate emergency treatment.

The term *hypersensitivity* is often used synonymously with *allergy*. They are not the same, however, because there is not a precise definition of hypersensitivity, and it is frequently confused with other adverse reactions.

Anaphylaxis is an extreme hypersensitivity reaction to a previously encountered antigen. This reaction may be local or systemic. Systemic

Table 2.4 Adverse Effects of Drugs

Adverse Effect	Symptoms	Treatment	Potentiating Drugs
Idiosyncrasy	Opposite of expected effect	Stop medication	Genetically determined response to ordinary dose of any drug
Tolerance	Lessened effect	Increase dose or change medication	Opioid drug such as morphine or *Demerol*
Cumulation	Stronger effect	Stop medication	Alcohol (depends on patient's ability to properly excrete drug)
Toxicity	Diverse symptoms affecting multiple organs	Stop medication	Any drug given in excessive dose (e.g., central nervous system depressant)
Synergism	Stronger effect when more than one drug taken	Stop medication	Hydrochlorothiazide and enalapril (*Vasotec*) used for hypertension
Antagonism	Weaker effect when more than one drug taken	Stop medication	Tetracycline and antacid (decreased absorption)
Potentiation	Effect of one drug increases effect of another drug	Stop medication	Acetaminophen (*Tylenol*) and codeine
Interaction	Therapeutic or adverse effect on body	If therapeutic, continue medication If adverse effect, stop medication	Probenecid and Penicillin G Cimetidine (*Tagamet*) and theophylline; benzodiazepine antianxiety drugs and hypnotics; warfarin and some antiarrhythmics; calcium channel blockers
Physical dependence	Physiological need for drug	Substitute with similar drug and gradually withdraw	Opioid (e.g., as in case of cancer patient)
Psychological dependence	Psychological craving for drug	Stop medication	Benzodiazepines, narcotics, amphetamines

anaphylaxis is a generalized reaction characterized as a systemic condition that may be life threatening. Certain drugs, particularly penicillin, may cause a systemic anaphylaxis characterized by constriction of the bronchial muscle, edema of the pharynx and larynx, severe wheezing, and dyspnea (shortness of breath) that may lead to asphyxiation and death if emergency treatment is not implemented. Emergency treatment includes immediately establishing an airway and administering epinephrine, oxygen, and IV corticosteroids.

To avoid the problems of drug allergies and anaphylaxis, providers try to find out whether patients have a history of allergies, such as hay fever, asthma, or skin rashes. They also ask whether patients have shown unusual reactions to any drugs taken in the past.

Idiosyncrasy

Some people have abnormal or peculiar responses to certain drugs or have responses that are opposite of the expected effect. These abnormal effects, or **idiosyncrasies**, are thought to be caused by an abnormal metabolism of drugs as the result of an enzyme deficiency. Individuals who have an idiosyncratic response to a drug either overreact or underreact. Treatment for an idiosyncrasy is to stop medication.

Tolerance

Drug **tolerance** is the need for increasingly larger doses of a drug to produce the same physiological and/or psychological effects. The exact way in which

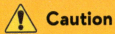
tolerance develops is unknown. It can occur in some people after repeated dosages of the same or a similar drug. Drugs that frequently produce tolerance are opiates such as oxycodone, nitrates, barbiturates, tobacco, and alcohol. For example, a cancer patient may require increasingly greater doses of an opiate to relieve pain.

Cumulative Effect

Cumulative effect occurs when the body cannot metabolize and excrete one dose of a drug completely before the next dose is given. With repeated doses, the drug starts to collect in the blood and body tissues. This can be dangerous because high concentrations of many drugs produce toxic effects. For example, cumulative toxicity occurs rapidly, as with ethyl alcohol, or slowly over time, as with lead. Treatment is to stop medication.

Overdose and Toxicity

Through error or poor judgment or as a result of attempted suicide, a patient may receive a drug overdose—a dose that is too large for his or her age, size, and/or physical condition. Also, some medications, such as over-the-counter (OTC) drugs, and herbal supplements may interact with a certain drug, increasing the chance of overdose. This can be dangerous because any drug can act like a poison if taken in too large a dose.

Toxicity refers to the drug's ability to poison the body. Emergency measures may be needed to keep the patient alive. There may be an antidote for the poison. An *antidote* is a drug that has the opposite effect and can reverse the overdose symptoms. A central nervous system depressant may cause toxicity if given in excessive doses.

Drug Interactions

Sometimes two or more drugs are given to a patient as part of drug therapy, or a patient may be taking an OTC medication at home for some other ailment. Whenever a patient is taking more than one drug, whether it is an over-the-counter drug or herbal supplement, the possibility of a drug interaction must be considered. Drug interaction occurs when one drug modifies the action of another drug.

Synergism.   When two drugs administered together produce a more powerful response than the effect of each drug given separately, this is called **synergism**. For example, a patient may be given two drugs for hypertension. Each drug lowers blood pressure in a different way. However, the combined effect of the two drugs lowers the blood pressure more effectively than either drug by itself. If an opioid analgesic is prescribed following some types of anesthetic, the dose of the opioid may be greatly decreased to as much as one-fourth the recommended dose because these drugs have a synergistic action on the central nervous system.

Potentiation. **Potentiation** refers to the administration of two drugs at the same time wherein one drug increases the effect of the other drug. Patients who take sedatives, for example, are advised to avoid drinking alcoholic beverages. Alcohol causes sedatives to have a much stronger, possibly fatal, effect.

Antagonism. A drug interaction in which two drugs inhibit or cancel each other's effect is called **antagonism**. Drugs such as *Maalox Regular Strength* and *Gaviscon Regular Strength* (antacids) and ferrous sulfate (an iron supplement) should not be given to patients who are on oral tetracycline, an antibiotic, because the antacid and the iron supplement work against the absorption of tetracycline through the intestines.

Food can also affect drug absorption and can interact with drugs. Food–drug interactions can occur, and you should be aware of them. One example is the interaction of monoamine oxidase (MAO) inhibitors with tyramine-containing foods such as alcohol, aged cheeses, beef and chicken livers, bananas, raisins, and avocados, to name a few.

There are many other ways in which drugs interact. Some of these interactions are detrimental, but not all are. In fact, providers sometimes make use of known drug interactions to control unwanted side effects or to increase the therapeutic effect of a particular drug. Probenecid is sometimes given with Penicillin G. Probenecid prolongs the action of penicillin and decreases excretion of the drug. This effect results in higher blood levels or allows a smaller dose of penicillin to be given.

It is unplanned drug interactions that are of concern in administering medications. Every member of the healthcare team must participate in observing the patient for possible drug interactions and take appropriate action when they occur.

Other Drug-Related Disorders

Some drugs, when administered over a period of time, can cause changes in body functioning or damage to certain organs. Bone marrow disease and a lower production of blood cells may result from fluorouracil therapy in cancer patients. Certain drugs may cause diseases of the liver and kidneys. Drugs can also have negative effects on behavior and emotions. Antianxiety drugs such as diazepam (*Valium*) have been known to disturb sleep and cause nightmares. Irritability and nervousness are common problems with many drugs.

Drug Dependence

Drug **dependence** is a strong psychological and/or physical need to take a certain drug. This need develops when a person takes a drug over a period of time. Usually the drug is prescribed to relieve pain or to control some physical or emotional problem. Eventually, some people find they cannot seem to get along without the drug. They keep taking it to avoid the discomfort they expect to feel if they stop.

In psychological or emotional drug dependence, a person has a drive or a craving to take a certain drug for pleasure or to relieve discomfort. There are no physical symptoms if the drug is taken away, but the person may feel anxious about not having the drug.

In physical drug dependence, the body grows so accustomed to the drug that it needs it to function. When the drug is taken away, the person develops **withdrawal symptoms** involving extreme physical discomfort and possibly death. Eventually, if no further dose of the drug is administered, the body returns to normal functioning. With physical dependence, the provider may substitute another, similar drug to ease the withdrawal symptoms and then gradually reduce the dosage of the substitute drug.

With both physical and psychological dependence, counseling may be needed to help the patient function without the drug. In the case of a dying or terminal patient who is in a great deal of pain, drug dependence is not a concern so that the patient can be as comfortable as possible.

DRUG DEPENDENCE OR DRUG ABUSE? [LO 2-5]

Drug dependence is a problem any healthcare worker may have to deal with in giving medications. The time may come when a patient asks for more pain medication, for example, and you may be worried that the patient is becoming too dependent on the drug. Is this drug abuse?

In this situation, your main responsibility is to consult the lead healthcare team member. The decision as to whether to medicate the patient further must be made jointly by the members of the healthcare team. Your own concerns may be eased, however, if you understand something about the difference between drug dependence and drug abuse.

Drug abuse refers to self-administration of a drug in chronically excessive quantities, resulting in a psychological or physical dependence. Feelings of euphoria or calmness or a heightened awareness of the senses (feeling "high") are some of the reasons people take these drugs. Some experts define drug abuse as taking any drug to the point where it interferes with health and daily living patterns. The most commonly abused drugs are alcohol; nicotine; anabolic steroids; barbiturates ("downers"), sedatives or hypnotics, and depressants; marijuana (pot, dope, grass); amphetamines and other stimulants ("uppers," "speed"); LSD and other hallucinogens; narcotics and opium; and cocaine.

Most of these commonly abused drugs are controlled substances. All of these drugs can create either physical or psychological dependence.

Drug abuse is part of a larger and more widespread problem—drug misuse. This is overuse or careless use of any drug, including alcohol. Drug misuse is most often a problem with people who take their own medications at home. Tranquilizers, stimulants, and painkilling drugs are frequently misused, as are common OTC drugs such as laxatives, acetaminophen, and aspirin. Nicotine and alcohol are widely misused, and both can create serious physical as well as psychological dependence.

Both drug abuse and drug misuse endanger people's health and well-being. This includes the medical staff as well as patients. As a healthcare worker, you must keep medicines locked up when not in use, administer only prescribed medications, and watch for signs of drug dependence and improper use of drugs.

Summary

Learning Outcome	Summary Points
2-1 Identify the basic drug actions and the body processes that affect drug actions.	• Basic drug actions: • Depressing • Stimulating • Destroying cells • Replacing substances • *Absorption* is the passage of a drug from the site of administration into the bloodstream. • *Distribution* is the transportation of a drug from the bloodstream to the body tissues and intended site of action. • *Metabolism* is a series of chemical reactions that inactivate a drug by converting it into a water-soluble compound to be excreted by the body. • *Excretion* is the body's way of removing the waste products of ordinary cell processes.

Learning Outcome	Summary Points
2-2 Identify the factors influencing drug action.	• Age • Size • Diet • Sex • Genetic factors • Pathological conditions • Psychological factors • Route of administration • Time of administration • Environmental conditions
2-3 Distinguish between systemic and local drug effects.	• *Systemic* drugs travel through the bloodstream to affect cells or tissues in various parts of the body (e.g., pain medications). • *Local* drugs are given for their local effect—they mainly affect the area where they enter or are applied to the body (e.g., suppositories).
2-4 Summarize the differences between the therapeutic effect, side effects, synergism, antagonism, and potentiation.	• The *therapeutic effect* is the desired effect of the drug, or the reason the drug is administered. • *Side effects* may be desirable or undesirable. They are effects on the body that are not part of the goal of drug therapy. • In *synergism,* two drugs taken together produce a stronger effect than the effect of either drug taken alone. Treatment is to decrease the dose of one of the medications or stop the treatment. • In *antagonism,* two drugs taken together inhibit or cancel each other's effect. Treatment is to decrease the dose of medication or stop the medication. • In *potentiation,* the effect of one drug increases the effect of another. Treatment is to stop the medication.
2-5 Explain the difference between psychological and physical drug dependence, and list commonly abused drugs.	• *Psychological* drug dependence occurs when a person has a drive or a craving to take a certain drug for pleasure or to relieve discomfort. • *Physical* dependence occurs when the body grows so accustomed to the drug that it needs the drug to function.

Chapter 2 Review

Complete each statement.

1. (LO 2-1) Pharmacokinetics is _____ .

2. (LO 2-1) The physical changes that occur because of the drug action are called the drug _____ .

3. (LO 2-1) Absorption is _____

_____ .

4. (LO 2-1) Distribution is _____

_____ .

5. (LO 2-1) Metabolism/biotransformation is _____
_____.

6. (LO 2-1) Excretion is _____
_____.

7. (LO 2-3) Drug effects that result from a drug circulating through the body are called _____
_____ effects.

8. (LO 2-3) Drug effects that are confined to the area where the drug was administered are called
_____ effects.

9. (LO 2-4) Drugs act by _____, _____, or
_____ the work of the cells.

10. (LO 2-1) Drugs also act by _____ substances that the body fails to produce.

11. (LO 2-1) Drug action is affected by four bodily processes: _____,
_____, _____,
and _____.

12. (LO 2-1) The organs that excrete waste are the _____,
_____, _____,
and _____.

13. (LO 2-3) Drugs used in therapy have two kinds of effects: _____ and _____.

14. (LO 2-4) Three symptoms of a drug allergy include _____, _____, and _____.

15. (LO 2-2) A placebo is _____
_____.

16. (LO 2-5) Drug abuse is _____
_____.

17. (LO 2-5) Drug misuse is _____
_____.

18. (LO 2-4) Idiosyncrasy is _____
_____.

19. (LO 2-5) Five groups of drugs that are often abused are _____, _____,
_____, _____, and _____.

20. (LO 2-5) If you suspect drug abuse, your obligation is to _____
_____.

21. (LO 2-4) Physical drug dependence is _____

_____.

22. (LO 2-4) Psychological drug dependence is _____

_____.

Answer the questions in the space provided.

23. (LO 2-4) What is an overdose? _____

_____

_____

24. (LO 2-4) What is the basis for treatment of drug overdose? _____

_____

_____

25. (LO 2-5) List four over-the-counter drugs that are commonly abused. _____

_____

_____

26. (LO 2-5) What two critical symptoms may occur when a patient takes an overdose of central nervous
system depressants? _____

_____

_____

27. (LO 2-5) What does alcohol do to a patient who has taken an overdose? _____

_____

_____

28. (LO 2-4) What is an antidote? _____

_____

_____

**The following is a list of patient characteristics. Place a check mark by those that you think might
influence drug action.**

_____ 29. (LO 2-2) Physical strength   _____ 34. (LO 2-2) Sex

_____ 30. (LO 2-2) Kidney disease   _____ 35. (LO 2-2) Diet

_____ 31. (LO 2-2) Hearing impairment   _____ 36. (LO 2-2) Popularity

_____ 32. (LO 2-2) Aging   _____ 37. (LO 2-2) Infancy

_____ 33. (LO 2-2) Genes   _____ 38. (LO 2-2) Anger

_____ 39. (LO 2-2) Obesity

_____ 40. (LO 2-2) Poor circulation

_____ 41. (LO 2-2) Nervousness

_____ 42. (LO 2-2) Height

_____ 43. (LO 2-2) Cheerful mood

_____ 44. (LO 2-2) Political affiliation

_____ 45. (LO 2-2) Drug-taking history

_____ 46. (LO 2-2) Hair color

_____ 47. (LO 2-2) Oral hygiene

Multiple Choice—Circle the correct letter.

48. (LO 2-2) Which condition relaxes the blood vessels and speeds up the circulation so that drugs act faster?

   a. Cold temperatures

   b. Heat

   c. High altitude

   d. Disease

49. (LO 2-3) A drug produces what type of effect when it has to travel through the bloodstream to affect cells or tissues in various parts of the body?

   a. Local

   b. Palliative

   c. Systemic

   d. Side

50. (LO 2-4) What is responsible for a drug allergy?

   a. Histamine

   b. Noncompliance with drug times

   c. Disease

   d. Gastrointestinal symptoms

51. (LO 2-4) Which of the following occurs when the body cannot metabolize and excrete one dose of a drug completely before the next dose is given?

   a. Cumulative effect

   b. Tolerance

   c. Toxicity

   d. Idiosyncrasy

52. (LO 2-4) As a healthcare worker, you know that drugs are generally detoxified by which organ?

   a. Gallbladder

   b. Pancreas

   c. Lungs

   d. Liver

Chapter 2 Case Studies

53. (LO 2-1) You have been assigned to administer insulin subcutaneously because of its absorption. What does absorption mean? How is a subcutaneous drug administered? Is it absorbed quickly or slowly? _____

_____

_____

_____

54. (LO 2-2) A patient asks you what things affect the excretion of drugs. What should you tell this patient? _____

_____

_____

_____

Critical Thinking

Select the term that best completes each sentence and write it in the blank.

antagonism	drug dependence	potentiation	cumulative effect	toxicity
drug allergy	drug interaction	tolerance	idiosyncrasy	

55. (LOs 2-4, 2-5) After taking several doses of medicine, Bill no longer seems to be affected by the drug. This may be a symptom of _____.

56. (LOs 2-4, 2-5) Mrs. Jones gets a stronger drug effect with each additional dose of her medication. She may be showing signs of _____.

57. (LOs 2-4, 2-5) Two drugs producing a greater effect than the sum of their individual effects is referred to as _____.

58. (LOs 2-4, 2-5) The provider has just canceled Ms. Williams's order for a narcotic pain medication. She has been taking the pain medication regularly since her hip operation. As the usual time for her medication approaches, Ms. Williams expresses the worry that she will not be able to sleep without her medication. You see this as a possible sign of _____.

59. (LOs 2-4, 2-5) A drug interaction wherein two drugs inhibit or cancel the action of the other is called _____.

60. (LOs 2-4, 2-5) Annie Peterson is reacting in an abnormal or peculiar way to her medication. You have never seen a person react this way to the medication she is taking. Drug allergy has been ruled out. Annie's response to the drug will probably be classified as a(n) _____.

61. (LOs 2-4, 2-5) An adverse reaction resulting from an antibody attacking an antigen is called a(n) _____.

62. (LOs 2-4, 2-5) You have recently given Mr. Smith a medication ordered by his provider. Mr. Smith is not reacting to the drug the way you expected. In talking with him, you discover that he has also been taking medication he brought with him from home. You suspect that his adverse reaction is due to a(n) _____.

63. (LOs 2-4, 2-5) Ms. Grimes seems very sleepy and confused after receiving her medication. You check her records and discover that someone misread the provider's order and gave Ms. Grimes a dose that was much too large. You notify the supervisor immediately because you think Ms. Grimes is showing signs of _____.

Applications

Obtain an electronic drug guide, a current copy of the *PDR*®, and a medical dictionary from your school, health facility, or clinic. Use them to answer the questions that follow.

64. Name the form printed in the drug guide or *PDR*® that the FDA and pharmaceutical manufacturers encourage healthcare professionals to fill out and send to the FDA's Division of Epidemiology and Surveillance.

_____

_____

_____

65. Where do you get this form? _____

_____

_____

66. What does VAERS signify? _____

_____

_____

_____

67. Why should the provider refer to the contraindication section of the *PDR*® or the manufacturer's package insert for each vaccine? _____

_____

_____

_____

chapter

3

MEASUREMENT AND DOSAGE CALCULATIONS

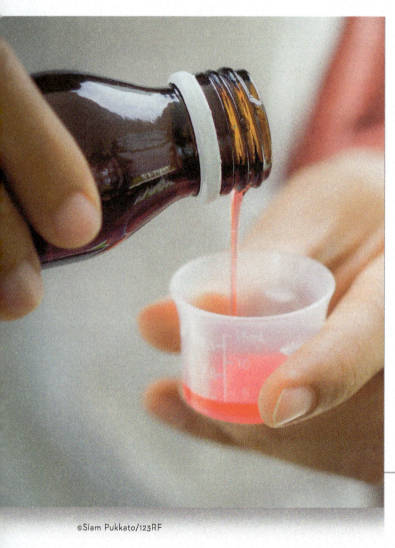

©Siam Pukkato/123RF

LEARNING OUTCOMES

3-1 Solve problems utilizing fractions and decimals.

3-2 Summarize the abbreviations and identify the most common equivalents among apothecary, metric, and household measures.

3-3 Solve Fahrenheit to Celsius temperature conversion and vice versa.

3-4 Calculate the number of tablets, capsules, and injectable medications to give when the available dose differs from the ordered dose.

3-5 Calculate a child's dose of medication.

3-6 Calculate drops per minute for IV therapy.

In this chapter you will learn several formulas used in measuring medication doses in pediatric and adult patients. In addition, you will learn how to calculate intravenous rates. You will learn how to solve simple dosage problems and how to convert doses from one system of measurement to another. You will also review fractions to help you brush up on your math skills.

apothecary system

Arabic numerals

body surface area (BSA)

Celsius

centimeter

convert

denominator

dosage range

Fahrenheit

fraction

grain

gram

household system

improper fraction

kilogram

liter

meter

metric system

milliliter

millimeter

minim

mixed number

nomogram

numerator

pound

proper fraction

Roman numerals

scored

MATH REVIEW: FRACTIONS [LO 3-1]

A **fraction** is a way of expressing an amount that is part of a whole, as shown in **Figure 3.1**. The more parts the whole is divided into, the smaller each part is, as you can see in **Figure 3.2**. The whole can be a set of anything; for example, nine squares or 100 milligrams (mg). **Figure 3.3** shows two sets that each make up a whole.

Figure 3.1

A fraction indicates an amount that is part of a whole.

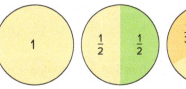 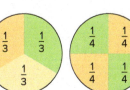 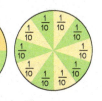

Figure 3.2

Dividing the whole into greater numbers of parts causes each part to become smaller.

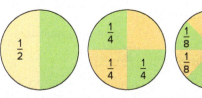 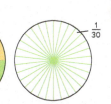

Figure 3.3

Whole sets and parts. The last item in each set is a whole plus part of another set.

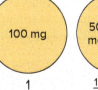 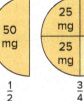 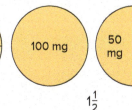

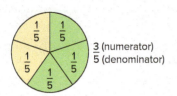

Figure 3.4

Expressing a fractional amount of a whole.

$\frac{3 \text{ (numerator)}}{5 \text{ (denominator)}}$

Figure 3.4 shows how to express a fractional amount of a whole. The top number of a fraction is the **numerator**. It is the number of parts you are taking of the whole. The bottom number of a fraction is the **denominator**. This number tells how many equal parts the whole is divided into.

A fraction is also a way of expressing a relationship between two numbers or quantities. For example, $\frac{3}{4}$ means 3 divided by 4, which can also be expressed as

$$3 \div 4 \quad \text{or} \quad 4\overline{)3} \quad \text{or} \quad 3:4$$

A relationship expressed as 350 mg/25 mg means the same as

$$350 \text{ mg} \div 25 \text{ mg} \quad \text{or} \quad 25 \text{ mg}\overline{)350 \text{ mg}} \quad \text{or} \quad 350 \text{ mg} : 25 \text{ mg}$$

An **improper fraction** is a fraction in which the value of the numerator is greater than or equal to the value of the denominator. The value of the improper fraction is greater than or equal to 1. **Figure 3.5** shows an example of an improper fraction.

$$\frac{4 \text{ (numerator)}}{3 \text{ (denominator)}} = \text{greater than 1}, \frac{4}{3} > 1$$

Figure 3.5

Improper fraction.

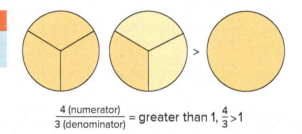

$\frac{4 \text{ (numerator)}}{3 \text{ (denominator)}} = \text{greater than 1}, \frac{4}{3} > 1$

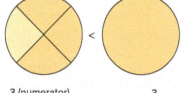

$\frac{3 \text{ (numerator)}}{4 \text{ (denominator)}} = \text{less than 1}, \frac{3}{4} < 1$

Figure 3.6

Proper fraction.

A **proper fraction** is a fraction in which the value of the numerator is less than the value of the denominator. The value of a proper fraction is less than 1. **Figure 3.6** shows an example of a proper fraction.

$$\frac{3 \text{ (numerator)}}{4 \text{ (denominator)}} = \text{less than 1}, \frac{3}{4} < 1$$

Simplifying Fractions

To make calculations easier, fractions may be reduced to their lowest terms. To reduce a fraction to its lowest terms, divide both the numerator and the denominator by the largest number that will go into both of them evenly. If no number can be evenly divided into both the numerator and the denominator, you cannot reduce the fraction, because it is already in its lowest terms. When you reduce a fraction, the amount stays the same, but the fraction is easier to work with (**Figure 3.7**).

Canceling is a way of showing that you have divided the top and bottom numbers of the fraction by the same number. For example, if you want to reduce $\frac{3}{15}$ to its lowest terms, you divide the top and bottom numbers by the largest number that will go into them evenly; in this case, 3. In the numerator, 3 goes into 3 once, so you cancel out the 3 and write 1. In the denominator, 3 goes into 15 five times, so you cancel out the 15 and write 5. Thus, after reducing to lowest terms, the fraction is $\frac{1}{5}$.

$$\frac{3}{15} \quad \frac{\overset{1}{\cancel{3}}}{\underset{5}{\cancel{15}}} \quad \frac{1}{5}$$

Figure 3.7

Reducing fractions to lowest terms.

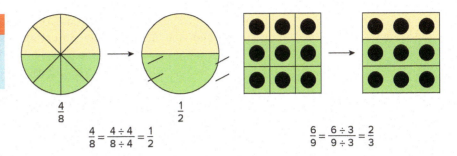

$$\frac{4}{8} \qquad \frac{1}{2}$$

$$\frac{4}{8} = \frac{4 \div 4}{8 \div 4} = \frac{1}{2} \qquad\qquad \frac{6}{9} = \frac{6 \div 3}{9 \div 3} = \frac{2}{3}$$

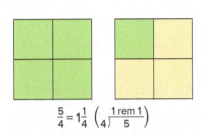

$$\frac{5}{4} = 1\frac{1}{4} \left(4\overline{)5}^{\;1 \text{ rem } 1} \right)$$

Figure 3.8

Changing an improper fraction to a mixed number.

You can also cancel units of measurement, as long as the same type of unit appears in both the numerator and the denominator.

$$\frac{18 \text{ mg}}{25 \text{ mg}} \quad \text{or} \quad \frac{3 \text{ gr}}{5 \text{ gr}} \quad \text{but not} \quad \frac{3 \text{ gr}}{50 \text{ mg}}$$

To simplify an improper fraction where the numerator is larger than the denominator, turn it into a **mixed number** (number written with both a whole number and a fraction). Improper fractions are changed to mixed numbers only in giving the final answer to a problem. During calculations, mixed numbers are awkward to work with and must be changed to improper fractions. Divide the numerator by the denominator. Express the remainder as a fraction with the same denominator (**Figure 3.8**).

Multiplying Fractions

To multiply a fraction by another fraction, multiply numerator by numerator and denominator by denominator.

$$\frac{3}{10} \times \frac{1}{10} = \frac{3 \times 1}{10 \times 10} = \frac{3}{100}$$

$$\frac{5}{8} \times \frac{2}{3} = \frac{5 \times 2}{8 \times 3} = \frac{10}{24}$$

Remember to reduce the answer to lowest terms.

$$\frac{\overset{5}{\cancel{10}}}{\underset{12}{\cancel{24}}} = \frac{5}{12} \text{ (top and bottom divided by 2)}$$

To multiply a fraction by a whole number, multiply the whole number by the numerator of the fraction. Express the whole number as a fraction by giving it the denominator 1. Then place the product over the denominator and simplify.

$$\frac{7}{9} \times 2 = \frac{7}{9} \times \frac{2}{1} = \frac{14}{9} = 1\frac{5}{9}$$

In multiplying fractions, you are allowed to cancel across the multiplication sign.

$$\frac{3}{\underset{1}{\cancel{4}}} \times \frac{\overset{1}{\cancel{4}}}{5} = \frac{3 \times 1}{1 \times 5} = \frac{3}{5}$$

$$\frac{\overset{4}{\cancel{8}}}{9} \times \frac{5}{\underset{7}{\cancel{14}}} = \frac{4 \times 5}{9 \times 7} = \frac{20}{63}$$

When you cancel, you divide the denominator of one fraction and the numerator of the opposite fraction by the same number. This makes it easier to work the problem because you are dealing with smaller numbers. In the same way, you can cancel identical units of measurement across the multiplication sign. This is an important step for certain formulas in dosage calculation.

$$2\,\text{tsp} \times \frac{5\ \text{mL}}{1\ \text{tsp}} = 10\ \text{mL}$$

$$\overset{0.5}{7.5}\ \text{gr} \times \frac{1\ \text{g}}{\underset{1}{15\ \text{gr}}} = 0.5\ \text{g}$$

Dividing Fractions

To divide fractions, invert (flip over) the divisor; then multiply the two fractions.

$$\frac{1}{2} \div \frac{2}{3} = \frac{1}{2} \times \frac{3}{2} = \frac{3}{4}$$

$$\frac{5}{8} \div \frac{5}{9} = \frac{\overset{1}{\cancel{5}}}{8} \times \frac{9}{\underset{1}{\cancel{5}}} = \frac{9}{8} = 1\frac{1}{8}$$

$$\frac{4}{5} \div 3 = \frac{4}{5} \times \frac{1}{3} = \frac{4}{15}$$

Decimal Fractions

When working with metric measures, fractions are expressed as decimals. The placement of numbers in relation to the decimal point shows that their values are multiples of 10 (**Figure 3.9**). Here are some examples of various whole numbers and fractions expressed as decimals.

$$1.0 = 1\frac{0}{10} = 1$$

$$0.75 = \frac{75}{100} = \frac{3}{4}$$

$$0.66 = \frac{66}{100} = \frac{2}{3}$$

$$0.5 = \frac{5}{10} = \frac{1}{2}$$

$$0.33 = \frac{33}{100} = \frac{1}{3}$$

$$0.25 = \frac{25}{100} = \frac{1}{4}$$

$$0.125 = \frac{125}{1000} = \frac{1}{8}$$

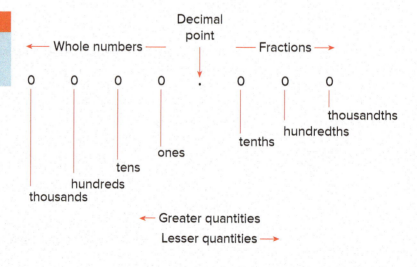

Figure 3.9

Number values in decimal fractions.

Any decimal fraction can be expressed as a regular or common fraction. In these examples, note the position of the final digit relative to the decimal point.

$$0.48 = \frac{48}{100} = \frac{\overset{12}{\cancel{48}}}{\underset{25}{\cancel{100}}} = \frac{12}{25}$$
hundredths

$$1.6 = 1\frac{6}{10} = 1\frac{\overset{3}{\cancel{6}}}{\underset{5}{\cancel{10}}} = 1\frac{3}{5}$$
tenths

Any common fraction can be changed to a decimal fraction by dividing the numerator by the denominator.

$$\frac{1}{3} = 3\overline{)1.00}^{\,0.333\ldots} = 0.33$$

$$\begin{array}{r} \underline{9} \\ 10 \\ \underline{9} \\ 1 \end{array}$$

To multiply decimal fractions, such as 1.5×0.35, set up the multiplication like a normal multiplication problem.

$$\begin{array}{r} 1.5 \\ \times\,0.35 \\ \hline 75 \\ \underline{45} \\ 0.525 \end{array}$$

To decide where the decimal goes, look at the original problem, and count the total number of places shown to the right of the decimal points in the two numbers; in this case, 3.

$$1.5 \times 0.35 = 0.525$$
$$\qquad 1 \qquad\quad 2 \qquad\quad 3$$

Then, starting from the last digit of the answer, count that many places to the left, and place the decimal directly after that digit. Placing the decimal point correctly is extremely important when calculating medications, because a misplaced decimal means a huge error in the dose.

To divide a decimal fraction, such as $30 \div 1.5$, arrange the numbers as in a regular division problem. If there is a decimal fraction in the divisor, move it to the right of the rightmost digit. Count the number of places you move it. Then move the decimal point in the dividend the same number of places to the right. Place the decimal point in the answer (quotient) directly above the decimal point in the dividend.

$$\text{divisor} \rightarrow 1.5\overline{)30.0}^{\,20.} \quad\leftarrow \text{quotient}$$
$$\leftarrow \text{dividend}$$

If the divisor is not a decimal fraction, the decimal point in the quotient is directly above the one in the dividend.

$$15\overline{)30.0}^{\,2.0}$$

SYSTEMS OF MEASUREMENT [LO 3-2]

Measurement has always been an important part of prescribing and administering medications, because different amounts of a drug give different effects. Some drugs are deadly poisons, but when given in tiny amounts, they can help relieve disorders. Other drugs are useless for therapy unless given in large amounts.

Most drugs have a certain **dosage range**, that is, different amounts that can produce therapeutic effects. Doctors prescribe an amount within the dosage range, depending on how strong an effect is needed and on the patient's age and physical condition. Doses below the dosage range will not produce the desired therapeutic effect. Doses above the dosage range can be harmful and possibly fatal.

To get the drug effects they want, providers and pharmacists try to make dosages exact by measuring drugs carefully. However, they have not always used the same units of measurement. There are different measurement systems, each having its own units of weight and volume.

Three different systems of measurement are used in the medical field. You should be familiar with the units of weight and volume in each system. Dosages on a medication order may be expressed in units ranging from milliliters (or cubic centimeters) to drops, teaspoons, drams, or minims. You need to know what each of these quantities means so that you can measure out the doses properly. In addition, you may be asked to **convert** (change) from one unit or system of measurement to another in the course of your daily routine. You need to know how to use conversion tables to convert from milligrams to grams, from milliliters to teaspoons, from grains to milligrams, and so forth.

The three systems of measurement used in ordering medications are the apothecary, metric, and household systems.

Apothecary System

Although the **apothecary system** of measurement is very old and infrequently used, it is worth reviewing here. Only a few medications are still available in the apothecary system. It is not as precise or convenient as the metric system and may be confused with it. As a result, it is being phased out.

The basic unit of weight in the apothecary system is the **grain** (gr). It was originally supposed to be the weight of one grain of wheat. The basic unit of volume is the **minim** (m). A minim is the space taken up by a quantity of water that weighs the same as a grain. The fluidram, fluid ounce, pint, quart, and gallon are all measurements derived from the minim. With the exception of the fluidram, the volume measurements are also considered household measurements.

Table 3.1 lists the units of weight and volume in the apothecary system. Note especially the abbreviations for these units. In the apothecary system, the abbreviation is placed before the number. You need to be able

---

Table 3.1   The Apothecary System

Weight (dry)	Volume (liquid)	Equivalents
grain (gr)	minim (m)	A minim of liquid weighs 1 grain
dram (dr or ℨ)	fluidram (dr or ℨ)	60 grains or 60 minims = 1 dram or fluidram
ounce (oz or ℥)	fluid ounce (oz or ℥)	8 drams or fluidrams = 1 ounce or fluid ounce
pound (lb)	pint (pt)	
ton (t)	quart (qt)	
	gallon (gal)	

Table 3.2 Lowercase Roman Numerals

1	i	9	ix
2	ii	10	x
3	iii	11	xi
4	iv	12	xii
5	v	13	xiii
6	vi	14	xiv
7	vii	15	xv
8	viii	$\left(\overline{ss} = \frac{1}{2}\right)$	

to recognize apothecary units on a medication order and write them on a medication chart.

In the apothecary system, dosage quantities are written in lowercase **Roman numerals** (Table 3.2). By convention the Roman numerals are written with a bar over them after the unit of measurement; for example, $\overline{ii}$ means 2 drams.

Fractions are expressed in **Arabic numerals** rather than decimals. For example, one-quarter grain is written $\frac{1}{4}$ gr, not 0.25 gr. Arabic numerals are usually written before the unit of measurement, though some people prefer to write them after the unit to avoid confusing grains with grams in the metric system. The only exception is the quantity $\frac{1}{2}$, for which the symbol $\overline{ss}$ is used with Roman numerals after the unit.

Here are some examples:

$$\overline{vii} = 7 \text{ fluid ounces}$$

$$\overline{iv} = 4 \text{ drams}$$

$$\text{gr } \overline{iss} = 1\tfrac{1}{2} \text{ grains}$$

$$5\tfrac{1}{4} \text{ dr} = 5\tfrac{1}{4} \text{ drams}$$

$$\text{gr } \tfrac{1}{150} = \text{grain } \tfrac{1}{150}$$

$$\text{gr } 15 = \text{grains } 15$$

$$30 \text{ min} = 30 \text{ minims}$$

Metric System

The **metric system** is a decimal system that is widely used in medicine. It is a simple, logical system of measurement based on units of 10.

The basic units of metric measurements are the meter, liter, and gram. The **meter** (m) is the unit of length; the **liter** (L), of volume; and the **gram** (g), of weight.

Prefixes added to the words *meter, gram,* and *liter* indicate smaller or larger units in the system (Table 3.3). All units are a result of either multiplying or

Table 3.3 Prefixes in the Metric System	
deca → × 10	deci → ÷ 10
hect → × 100	centi → ÷ 100
kilo → × 1000	milli → ÷ 1000
	micro → ÷ 1,000,000

dividing by 10, 100, or 1000. The **centimeter** (cm), for example, is 1/100th of a meter. A **millimeter** (mm) is 1/1000th of a meter. A kilometer (km) is 1000 meters.

In the metric system, units of length, weight, and volume are related to each other systematically. The unit of volume most often used in preparing liquid medications is the **milliliter** (mL), which is one-thousandth of a liter. One milliliter is the liquid contents of a cube measuring 1 centimeter on each side, or 1 cubic centimeter (cc). One liter is the liquid contents of a cube measuring 10 centimeters on a side, or 1000 cc. One gram is equal to the weight of 1 mL (or cc) of water. One liter contains 1000 mL of water, so it weighs 1000 g (1 kilogram). One **pound** is equivalent to 0.454 **kilogram** (kg). One kilogram is equivalent to 2.2 pounds.

Metric doses are always written in Arabic numerals. Fractions of metric doses are written as decimal fractions. For example, one-half gram is 0.5 g. In reading medication orders, pay special attention to where the decimal point is placed. The differences between 0.05 g, 0.5 g, and 5.0 g are huge when it comes to doses of medicine. A mistake could prove fatal.

Table 3.4 lists the basic units of volume and weight in the metric system and their equivalents. The bottom of the table shows how to change from milligrams to grams and vice versa. Note the instructions, because these are simple conversions you will probably often make on the job. The conversions are easy if you remember the hints shown in Table 3.4.

Household System

The **household system** of measurement is familiar to most of us because we have grown up using its basic units—drops, teaspoons, tablespoons, cups, pints, quarts, and gallons.

Table 3.4 The Metric System

Weight	Volume	Equivalents
microgram (mcg) milligram (mg) gram (g, Gm, gm) kilogram (kg)	milliliter (mL) cubic centimeter (cc) liter (L)	One milliliter (1 mL) is the same as 1 cubic centimeter (1 cc) 1000 milliliters = 1 liter = 1000 cubic centimeters 1000 micrograms = 1 milligram 1000 milligrams = 1 gram 1000 grams = 1 kilogram 100 milligrams = 0.1 gram 10 milligrams = 0.01 gram 1 kilogram = 2.2 pounds

Simple Conversions

From grams to milligrams

g × 1000 = mg

Hint: Move decimal point three places to the right

0.25 g = 250 mg

From milligrams to grams

mg ÷ 1000 g

Hint: Move decimal point three places to the left

500 mg = .500 g = 0.5 g

Table 3.5 The Household System

Weight (dry)	Volume (liquid)	Equivalents
ounce (oz)	drop (gtt); drops (gtt)	16 ounces = 1 pound
pound (lb)	teaspoon (t, tsp)	3 teaspoons = 1 tablespoon = $\frac{1}{2}$ ounce
ton (t)	tablespoon (T, tbsp)	16 tablespoons = 1 cup = 8 fluid ounces
	teacup (6 oz)	2 cups = 1 pint
	cup (c) or glass (8 oz)	2 pints = 1 quart
	pint (pt)	4 quarts = 1 gallon
	quart (qt)	
	gallon (gal)	

As a result of the changing insurance industry, the average length of hospital stays has shortened and the corresponding recovery at home has lengthened. Household utensils such as teaspoons and cups vary in size and should not be used when accuracy is important. For example, the average household teaspoon can hold 4 to 5 mL more than the standard 5 mL. Therefore, the healthcare professional working in a doctor's office or medical clinic should encourage patients to obtain accurate measuring utensils from a pharmacy or medical supply facility.

The basic units of the household system are listed in Table 3.5. All household doses are written in Arabic numerals.

TEMPERATURE SCALES [LO 3-3]

It is essential that you understand the importance of measuring the body temperature when caring for patients. A patient's body temperature represents the average temperature of the core body tissues and can alert healthcare providers to a variety of illnesses.

You may be required to convert a patient's temperature between the **Fahrenheit** (F) and **Celsius** (C) scales, although most hospitals and clinical facilities use electronic digital (Figure 3.10) or tympanic thermometers (Figure 3.11), many of which convert between the two scales. Some patients may have glass mercury thermometers in their home. Because of safety concerns related to mercury exposure, the healthcare team member may encourage the patient to purchase a digital thermometer. Glass mercury thermometers should be disposed of safely and in accordance with local ordinances (Figure 3.12).

The conversion between the Fahrenheit and Celsius scales is based on the difference between the freezing and boiling points of water on each scale. The Fahrenheit temperature scale has 32 degrees as the freezing point of water and 212 degrees as the boiling point of water. The Celsius temperature scale has 0 degrees as the freezing point of water and 100 degrees as the boiling point of water. There is a 180-degree difference between the freezing and boiling points on the Fahrenheit temperature scale and 100 degrees between the freezing and boiling points on the Celsius temperature scale. The Celsius degree is 180/100 or 1.8 the size of a Fahrenheit degree. Stated another way, one Fahrenheit degree is 100/180 or 5/9 the size of a Celsius degree.

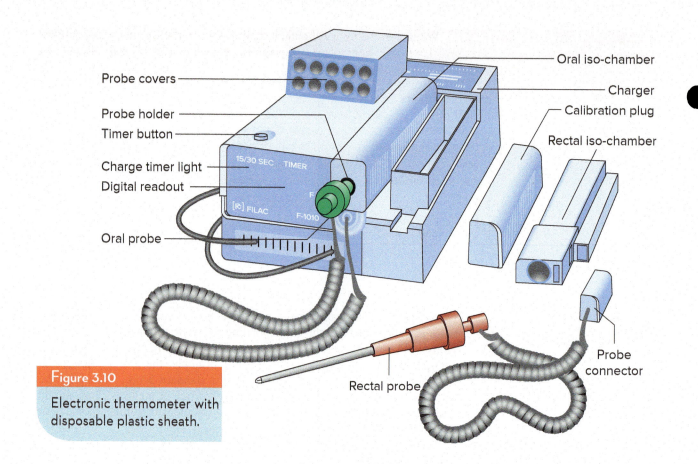

Probe covers

Probe holder

Timer button

Charge timer light

Digital readout

Oral probe

Oral iso-chamber

Charger

Calibration plug

Rectal iso-chamber

15/30 SEC   TIMER

F

[R] FILAC   F-1010

Rectal probe

Probe connector

Figure 3.10

Electronic thermometer with disposable plastic sheath.

Figure 3.11

Tympanic thermometer with disposable plastic sheath.

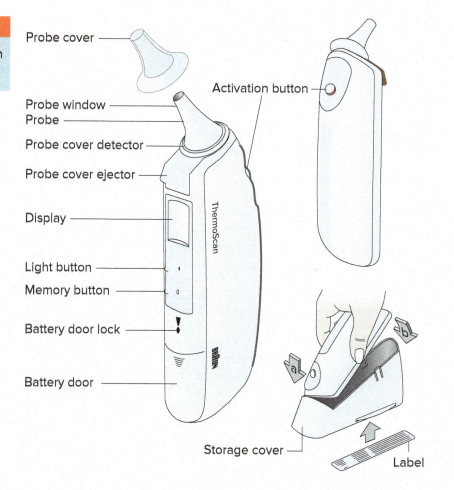

Probe cover

Probe window

Probe

Probe cover detector

Probe cover ejector

Display

Light button

Memory button

Battery door lock

Battery door

Activation button

ThermoScan

BRAUN

Storage cover

Label

When converting a Fahrenheit temperature to the Celsius scale, subtract 32 from the Fahrenheit temperature and then divide that number by 1.8 (Table 3.6).

To convert a Celsius temperature to the Fahrenheit scale, multiply the Celsius temperature by 1.8 and add 32 (Table 3.7).

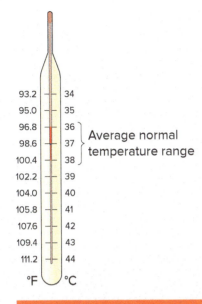

°F	°C
93.2	34
95.0	35
96.8	36
98.6	37
100.4	38
102.2	39
104.0	40
105.8	41
107.6	42
109.4	43
111.2	44

Average normal temperature range

Figure 3.12

Comparison of Fahrenheit and Celsius temperature scales.

Problem 1.

$$°C = \frac{98.6 - 32}{1.8}$$

$$°C = \frac{66.6}{1.8}$$

$$°C = 37°$$

Problem 2.

$$°F = 1.8 \times 37 + 32$$

$$°F = 66.6 + 32$$

$$°F = 98.6°$$

Table 3.6	Converting a Fahrenheit Temperature to the Celsius Scale
	$°C = \dfrac{°F - 32}{1.8}$

Table 3.7	Converting a Celsius Temperature to the Fahrenheit Scale
	$°F = 1.8 \times °C + 32$

CONVERTING AMONG MEASUREMENT SYSTEMS [LO 3-4]

From time to time you will find it necessary to change, or convert, from one system of measurement to another, in either the child or adult. The provider may write an order for milliliters that will have to be converted into teaspoons for a patient who will be taking the medicine at home. Conversions are usually performed by the pharmacist but other health workers should also know how to make simple conversions by referring to a conversion table. Table 3.8 shows the equivalents among measures in the apothecary, metric, and household systems. As you can see, the equivalents are not exact; they are only approximate. A 10 percent error usually occurs in making conversions. As the healthcare worker, it is important that these conversions be double-checked.

You can make most of the conversions you need if you know these basic equivalents:

$$1 \text{ mg} = \text{gr } \tfrac{1}{60}$$
$$60 \text{ mg} = \text{gr } 1$$
$$1 \text{ g} = \text{gr } 15$$

Table 3.8 Common Measurement System Equivalents

	Apothecary	Metric	Household
Liquid Volume	minim (m) 1 minims 15 fluidram (℥) 1 fluidrams 4 fluid ounce (℥) 1	0.06 mL (or cc) 1 mL 4–5 mL 15 mL 30 mL 180 mL 240 mL 500 mL 750 mL 1000 mL	1 drop (gt) 15 drops (gtt)[a] 1 teaspoon (60 gtt) 1 tablespoon 2 tablespoons (1 oz) 1 teacup (6 oz) 1 cup or glass (8 oz) 1 pint (16 oz) 1.5 pints (24 oz) 1 quart (32 oz)
Dry Weight	gr $\frac{1}{60}$ gr 1 gr $7\frac{1}{2}$ gr 15 gr 60 1 oz	1 mg 60 mg 500 mg (0.5 g) 1000 mg (1 g) 4 g 30 g 500 g 1000 g (1 kg)	 1 oz 1.1 lb 2.2 lb

[a]This figure varies; number of drops per milliliter depends on the substance being measured.

Table 3.9 Approximate Conversions between the Metric and Apothecary Systems

	Metric Amount	Apothecary Amount
	2 g (2000 mg) 1 g (1000 mg) 600 mg (0.6 g) 100 mg (0.1 g) 60 mg (0.06 g) 30 mg (0.03 g) 1 mg (0.001 g) 0.1 mg (0.0001 g)	gr 30 gr 15 gr 10 gr $1\frac{1}{2}$ gr 1 gr $\frac{1}{2}$ gr $\frac{1}{60}$ gr $\frac{1}{600}$
Approximation Formulas	grains × 60 = milligrams milligrams ÷ 60 = grains	grams × 15 = grains grains ÷ 15 = grams

If you can remember these, it is easy to work out other equivalents (Table 3.9). Figure 3.13 shows the relative sizes of containers you might use to measure out doses in the various systems.

DOSAGE CALCULATIONS [LO 3-4]

Calculating dosages is much easier today than it was in the past. In some healthcare facilities, pharmacists may do most of the calculations. They prepare the drug in a unit package that contains the correct amount of a drug for a single dose. In other facilities, you may have to make dosage calculations.

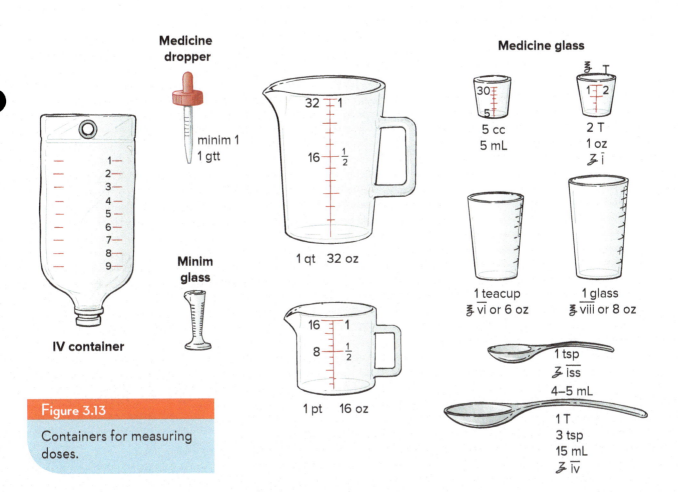

Medicine dropper

minim 1
1 gtt

Minim glass

IV container

1 qt   32 oz

1 pt   16 oz

Medicine glass

5 cc
5 mL

2 T
1 oz
℥ ī

1 teacup
℥ v̄i or 6 oz

1 glass
℥ v̄iii or 8 oz

1 tsp
℥ īss
4–5 mL

1 T
3 tsp
15 mL
℥ īv

Figure 3.13

Containers for measuring doses.

You must be able to perform all calculations correctly and with confidence. In medication administration, there is no room for error!

You will learn the formula to do all your calculations, figuring out the number of tablets, capsules, units, or milliliters you will administer. You will also use this formula to convert between different measurements.

$$\frac{D \text{ (desired)}}{H \text{ (on hand)}} = \frac{X \text{ (what you are solving for)}}{V \text{ (vehicle)}}$$

When setting up your problem, you need to label all parts of the problem, such as *mg* or *tablet,* to avoid confusion or error.

With this formula, you will set up a fraction that you will simply reduce as you solve your problems. You should also keep several calculation guidelines (**Table 3.10**) in mind when solving all your problems.

Problem 3. The provider orders 100 mg of a drug to be given orally two times a day (bid). The available dose of the drug is 50-mg tablets. You need to determine how many tablets to administer.

$$\frac{D}{H} = \frac{X}{V}$$
$$\frac{100 \text{ mg}}{50 \text{ mg}} = \frac{X}{1}$$
$$50X = 100$$
$$100 \div 50 = 2$$
$$X = 2 \text{ tablets}$$

You would be correct to administer 2 tablets.

Table 3.10 Calculation Guidelines

1. All numbers less than 1 must be documented with a zero before the decimal point. This is called a leading zero.
    Example: 0.75 mg
2. A math problem answer must always be labeled with the appropriate unit of measure.
    Example: 60 mL
3. All weights must be rounded to the tenth place.
    Example: 44.2 kg
4. Round medications to the hundredth place.
    Example: 1.25 mg
5. If the last number in rounding is less than 5, round down.
    Example: 4.32 = 4.3
6. If the last number in rounding is greater than 5, round up.
    Example: 2.38 = 2.4

Problem 4. The provider orders 250 mg of a drug to be administered orally daily. The available dose of the drug is 100-mg tablets. You need to figure out how many tablets to administer.

$$\frac{D}{H} = \frac{X}{V}$$

$$\frac{250 \text{ mg}}{100 \text{ mg}} = \frac{X}{1 \text{ tablet}}$$

$$100X = 250$$

$$250 \div 100 = 2\frac{1}{2}$$

$$X = 2\frac{1}{2} \text{ tablets}$$

Notice that this answer contains a fraction of a tablet. When determining if this is possible, consider whether the tablet is **scored**. When the tablet is scored, the surface is bisected by a groove to allow for breakage into halves (**Figure 3.14**). You may administer half a tablet if the tablet is scored. You should never divide an unscored tablet. This is a very unsafe and dangerous practice. It may result in either underdosing or overdosing the patient.

Problem 5. The provider orders 0.5 mg of a drug to be administered orally daily. The available dose of the drug is 0.25-mg tablets. Figure out how many tablets to administer.

$$\frac{D}{H} = \frac{X}{V}$$

$$\frac{0.5 \text{ mg}}{0.25 \text{ mg}} = \frac{X}{1 \text{ tablet}}$$

$$0.25X = 0.5$$

$$0.5 \div 0.25 = 2$$

$$X = 2 \text{ tablets}$$

You will administer 2 tablets.

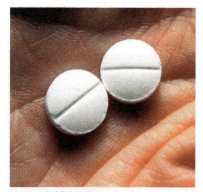

©Ingram Publishing/SuperStock

Figure 3.14

Scored tablets.

Problem 6. The provider orders 100 mg of a drug to be administered intramuscularly. The available dose of the drug is 50 mg/mL. You will need to determine how many milliliters to administer.

$$\frac{D}{H} = \frac{X}{V}$$

$$\frac{100 \text{ mg}}{50 \text{ mg}} = \frac{X}{1 \text{ mL}}$$

$$50X = 100 \qquad \text{or} \qquad$$

$$100 \div 50 = 2$$

$$X = 2 \text{ mL}$$

$$\frac{\cancel{100 \text{ mg}}}{\cancel{50 \text{ mg}}} = \frac{X}{1 \text{ mL}}$$

$$\frac{2}{1} = \frac{X}{1 \text{ mL}}$$

$$1X = 2$$

$$X = 2 \text{ mL}$$

You should administer 2 mL intramuscularly to the patient.

> ⚠ **Caution**   Correct Formula
>
> Don't assume the V (vehicle) is 1. It may be more than 1, and that makes the difference between administering a correct dose, underdosing, or overdosing the patient.

Problem 7. The provider orders 100 mg of an elixir. Available is 125 mg per 5 mL. You need to figure out how many milliliters to administer. In this case, the vehicle is 5.

$$\frac{D}{H} = \frac{X}{V}$$

$$\frac{100 \text{ mg}}{125 \text{ mg}} = \frac{X}{5 \text{ mL}}$$

$$\frac{4}{5} = \frac{X}{5 \text{ mL}}$$

$$5X = 20$$

$$5X = 4$$

Remember to reduce terms before attempting to solve the problem. Working with smaller terms is much easier and reduces the chance of error.

$$X = 4 \text{ mL}$$

You will administer 4 mL of the elixir.

Problem 8. The provider orders 300,000 units of an antibiotic to be administered intramuscularly. The available dose of the drug is 100,000 units per mL. You need to determine how many milliliters to administer.

$$\frac{D}{H} = \frac{X}{V}$$

$$\frac{300,000 \text{ units}}{100,000 \text{ units}} = \frac{X}{1 \text{ mL}}$$

$$\frac{3}{1} = \frac{X}{1}$$

$$1X = 3$$

$$3 \div 1 = 3$$

$$X = 3 \text{ mL}$$

You should draw up 3 mL to administer intramuscularly to the patient.

Dosage Calculations with Conversions

The healthcare provider may order a dose of a drug in another form from that which is available. As a result of this, you will need to convert from one unit of measurement to another.

Problem 9. (Grams to milligrams) The provider orders 0.5 g of a drug to be given daily. You need to know how many milligrams you will administer.

First, identify the appropriate conversion.

1 g is equivalent to 1000 mg.

Then set up the conversion.

$$0.5 \text{ g} \times \frac{1000 \text{ mg}}{1 \text{ g}}$$

$$0.5 \times 1000 = 500 \text{ mg}$$

The decimal point moves three points to the right when changing grams to milligrams. You would be correct to administer 500 mg to the patient.

(Milligrams to grams) The provider orders 500 mg of a drug to be given daily. You need to know how many grams you will administer.

First, identify the conversion.

1000 milligrams is equivalent to 1 gram.

Then set up the conversion.

$$500 \text{ mg} \div 1000 \text{ g} = 0.5 \text{ g}$$

The decimal moves three places to the left when changing milligrams to grams.

You would be correct to administer 0.5 g to the patient.

Remember to convert the larger unit to the smaller unit or into the terms of the available dose. After identifying the appropriate conversion between units of measurement, you should use the same drug dosage formula to calculate the problem.

Problem 10. The provider orders 500 mcg of a drug to be administered orally. The available dose is 0.25 mg. You need to determine how many tablets to give.

First, identify the conversion.

1 milligram is equivalent to 1000 micrograms.

Then set up the problem.

$$\frac{D}{H} = \frac{X}{V}$$

$$\frac{500 \text{ mcg}}{250 \text{ mcg}} = \frac{X}{1 \text{ tablet}} \qquad \text{or} \qquad \frac{500 \text{ mcg}}{250 \text{ mcg}} = \frac{X}{1 \text{ tablet}}$$

$$250X = 500 \qquad\qquad\qquad \frac{2}{1} = \frac{X}{1 \text{ tablet}}$$

$$500 \div 250 = 2 \qquad\qquad\qquad 1X = 2$$

$$X = 2 \text{ tablets} \qquad\qquad\qquad X = 2 \text{ tablets}$$

You should administer 2 tablets to the patient.

Problem 11. The provider orders 6 tsp of an elixir orally daily. You need to determine how many tablespoons you should administer.

First, identify the conversion.

3 teaspoons is equivalent to 1 tablespoon.

Then set up the conversion.

$$6 \text{ tsp} \times \frac{1 \text{ T}}{3 \text{ tsp}}$$
$$\frac{6}{3} = 2$$

You would administer 2 tablespoons of the elixir to the patient.

Think about it—it makes much more sense to administer 2 tablespoons to a patient instead of 6 teaspoons.

Weight Calculations

You will need to be able to convert between kilograms and pounds to do many calculations. Remember that 1 kilogram is equivalent to 2.2 pounds. When converting pounds to kilograms, round the kilogram weight to one decimal place (tenth).

Problem 12. The provider orders a drug to be administered to a child weighing 60 lb. You will need to convert the child's weight to kilograms.

$$1 \text{ kilogram (kg)} = 2.2 \text{ pounds}$$
$$60 \text{ lb} \div 2.2 \text{ kg} = 27.2 \text{ kg}$$

Problem 13. You need to administer an ordered drug to an adult weighing 44 kg. Before working the problem, you will need to convert the weight to pounds.

$$1 \text{ kilogram (kg)} = 2.2 \text{ pounds}$$
$$44 \text{ kg} \times 2.2 \text{ lb} = 96.8 \text{ lb}$$

PEDIATRIC DOSES [LO 3-5]

Pediatric doses of drugs are based on children's unique characteristics and constantly changing small bodies. Because of these facts you must consider body weight, height, age, body surface, and the general overall condition of the child. There are several methods of calculating pediatric doses that are widely used today. One method is based on body weight and another is based on **body surface area (BSA)**. In most pediatric situations, the body weight method is the most commonly used. Generally, the body surface area is used only in the critical care and oncology environments. In addition to learning how to calculate pediatric medications according to body weight and surface area, you will be asked to determine if a medication dose is within the safe range.

When administering medications to children, it is important to understand that numerically, pediatric doses are smaller than adult doses but may be proportionally larger per kilogram of body weight as compared to an adult dose. Infants less than one year of age have a larger percentage of water in the body than children of a larger body size and may necessitate a higher dose of some drugs because they have a decreased ability to absorb water-soluble drugs. Likewise, children from 1 to 12 years of age metabolize drugs faster than adults and may also require a higher dose. Because the bodies of infants and children are constantly changing, they have immature physiological responses to absorption, distribution, metabolism, and excretion. Special care must be taken to prevent overdoses and toxic reactions.

Frequently, children or adolescents from 13 to 18 years of age are incorrectly thought of as adults. This is a very dangerous assumption because their bodies are still immature and have unpredictable growth and hormonal spurts. Pediatric calculation methods should still be used for them. Although administration of any drug is a serious matter and safety cannot be stressed enough, the risks are even greater in the pediatric population.

Pediatric Dose Calculation Methods and Examples

Body Weight. The provider may order a drug for a child in pounds or kilograms, so it is essential that you be able to convert kilograms to pounds: 1 kilogram (kg) equals 2.2 pounds (lb).

> *Problem 14.* The provider orders phenytoin (*Dilantin*) for a 44-lb child. The appropriate dose is 10 mg/kg/24 hours. How much *Dilantin* should you give in 4 divided doses?
>
> **Helpful hint:** First remember to convert pounds to kilograms.

$$44 \text{ lb} = 20 \text{ kg}$$

Therefore, 10 mg × 20 kg = 200 mg per 24 hours.

200 mg/day divided by 4 doses = 50 mg/dose

Body Surface Area (BSA) Using Formulas. Body surface area is generally reserved for critical care and oncology pediatric calculations.

BSA Formula Using Metric Measurements. To calculate BSA in m^2 based on the metric measurement of height and weight:

$$\text{BSA (m}^2) = \sqrt{\frac{\text{ht (cm)} \times \text{wt (kg)}}{3600}}$$

Problem 15. Calculate the body surface area for a child who is 75 cm tall and weighs 10.9 kg.

$$\text{BSA (m}^2) = \sqrt{\frac{75 \times 10.9}{3600}} = \sqrt{\frac{817.5}{3600}} = \sqrt{0.227} = 0.476 \text{ m}^2 = 0.48 \text{ m}^2$$

BSA Formula Using Household Measurements. To calculate BSA in m^2 based on the household measurement of height and weight:

$$\text{BSA (m}^2) = \sqrt{\frac{\text{ht (inches)} \times \text{wt (lbs)}}{3131}}$$

Problem 16. Calculate the body surface area for a child who is 30 inches tall and weighs 15 lb.

$$\text{BSA (m}^2) = \sqrt{\frac{30 \times 15}{3131}} = \sqrt{\frac{450}{3131}} = \sqrt{0.1437} = 0.379 \text{ m}^2 = 0.38 \text{ m}^2$$

Body Surface Area Using a Nomogram. A **nomogram** is a graphic device showing the relationship between numerical values designed for healthcare providers in pediatrics to estimate the body surface area of a child according to height and weight (Figure 3.15).

To determine body surface area using a nomogram, draw a straight line from the child's height and weight. The intersection of the line with the surface area is the estimated BSA (m^2).

Figure 3.15

Pediatric nomogram.

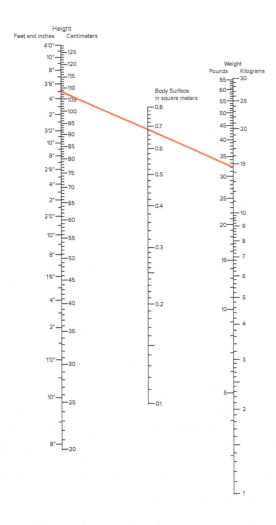

Height
Feet and Inches   Centimeters

Body Surface
in square meters

Weight
Pounds   Kilograms

Problem 17. Calculate the body surface area using a nomogram for a child who is 41 inches tall and weighs 32 lb.

$$BSA = 0.65 \text{ m}^2$$

Safe Dose Range.   After a provider orders a medication, the package may have a safe range, and you will need to determine if the ordered dose is within the safe range.

Problem 18. The provider orders cephalexin (*Keflex*) 150 mg oral suspension every 6 hours. The child weighs 22 kg. The drug package insert states that the recommended dose is 25 to 50 mg/kg/day in 4 divided doses. Is the ordered dose within the safe range for this drug?

Step 1: Determine the safe range for this child.

$$25 \text{ mg} \times 22 \text{ kg} = 550 \text{ mg/day}$$
$$50 \text{ mg} \times 22 \text{ kg} = 1100 \text{ mg/day}$$

The safe range of *Keflex* for a child weighing 22 kg is 550 to 1100 mg daily.

The actual dose ordered is 150 mg every 6 hours. You may figure out if this is a safe dose in one of two ways.

Step 2: Multiply the actual dose by 4 ($150 \times 4 = 600$ mg). Since 600 mg is within the range of 550 to 1100 mg, this is a safe dose.

Step 3: Divide the dose ranges by 4 to determine the range for the individual doses.

$$550 \text{ mg divided by 4 doses} = 138 \text{ mg}$$
$$1100 \text{ mg divided by 4 doses} = 275 \text{ mg}$$

A dose of 150 mg falls between the recommended range of 138 to 275 mg per dose for this child and is a safe dose.

CALCULATING INTRAVENOUS (IV) FLOW RATE [LO 3-6]

Another important formula is one that is used with parenteral, or intravenous (IV), therapy. We will work with one simple formula to calculate the rate for the IV solution the provider orders for your patient. In addition to manual calculations of IV flow rates, there are IV pumps and controllers that calculate drip rates. Using them is an advanced skill and will not be discussed here. To administer an IV solution to your patient, you will need to know the type and amount or total volume of the IV fluid, the length of time over which it is to be given, the calibration of the tubing, and the flow rate or drop factor per minute.

Dextrose 5% in water (D5W) 1000 mL in 8 hours is an example of the type and volume of IV fluid to be given in a specific time frame. The volume, or 1000 mL, is expressed in milliliters. The time frame will be given in either hours or minutes. The calibration of the tubing (drop factor) is expressed in gtt per mL. The drop factor permits you to figure out the rate per minute that you will deliver. The drop factor is generally 15 or 16 drops per mL for an adult patient and 60 microdrops per mL for a pediatric patient. The drop factor is identified on the package containing the tubing.

$$\frac{V \text{ (volume) in mL}}{T \text{ (time) in hours}} \times \frac{\text{calibration or drop factor}}{60 \text{ min}} = \text{rate (gtt/min)}$$

Problem 19. The provider orders 1000 mL of dextrose 5% in water (D5W) to be administered in 8 hours. The drop factor is 15 drops per mL. You should regulate the IV to deliver _____ gtt per minute.

$$\frac{1000 \text{ mL}}{8 \text{ hours}} = 125 \text{ mL/hour}$$

$$\frac{125 \text{ mL}}{60 \text{ min}} \times 15 \text{ (drop factor)} = 31 \text{ gtt/min}$$

Problem 20. The provider orders an IV medication for your patient. It comes in 80 mL and is to be administered in 60 minutes. The drop factor is 60 drops per mL. You should regulate the IV to deliver _____ gtt per minute.

$$\frac{80 \text{ mL}}{60 \text{ min}} \times 60 \text{ (drop factor)} = 80 \text{ gtt/min}$$

When in Doubt

As one who gives medications, you share in the healthcare team's responsibility for making sure that the patient gets the correct dose. To meet this responsibility, you must learn all you can about dosage calculation and conversions among measurement systems. If you study hard and do the practice exercises until you have mastered them, you will be prepared to handle most routine dosage questions. It is safe practice, however, to have your supervisor check all calculations.

Healthcare for Today and Tomorrow | Combination Drugs

Combination drugs such as *Percocet* and *Vicodin* have long been popular pain relievers. Because additional strengths are increasingly becoming available, it is recommended that the prescriber specify both amounts of the combination drugs. Simply relying on the name of the drug is no longer acceptable. For example, oxycodone (*Percocet*) comes in combination with acetaminophen, and you will see an order such as *Percocet* 2.5 mg/325 mg, which is 2.5 mg of oxycodone and 325 mg of acetaminophen. Similarly, hydrocodone (*Vicodin*) comes in different strengths. For example, *Vicodin* comes in 5 mg of hydrocodone and 500 mg of acetaminophen as well as 7.5 mg/750 mg and 10 mg/600 mg.

 Legal and Ethical Issues | Pediatric Metric Weights

If you receive an order without a metric weight for a pediatric patient, it is your responsibility to ask the prescriber for clarification. Fatal errors can and often do happen if a child is given the usual adult dose. For example, if a small child receives 1.5 mL of digoxin (usual adult concentration 0.25 mg/mL) instead of 0.1 mg/mL (pediatric concentration), the child may die. This kind of error can be prevented if the metric weight for the dose is included in the original order. If a prescriber orders the digoxin by volume and fails to include the pediatric concentration based on weight, immediately contact the prescriber for the pediatric metric weight.

Summary

Learning Outcome	Summary Points
3-1 Solve problems utilizing fractions and decimals.	• A *fraction* is a way of expressing an amount that is part of a whole. • A *decimal* point shows that the numbers' values are multiples of 10.
3-2 Summarize the abbreviations and identify the most common equivalents among apothecary, metric, and household measures.	• *Apothecary system:* The basic unit of weight is the grain and the basic unit of volume is the minim. 60 grains or 60 minims is equivalent to a dram. • *Metric system:* The basic units of metric measurements are the meter, liter, and gram; 1 milliliter is the same as 1 cubic centimeter, and 1 kilogram equals 2.2 pounds. • *Household system:* The basic units of household measurements are drops, teaspoons, tablespoons, cups, pints, quarts, and gallons; 16 ounces equal 1 pound, and 4 quarts equal 1 gallon. • To convert *grams to milligrams*, multiply by 1000 or move the decimal point three places to the right. • To convert *milligrams to grams*, divide by 1000 or move the decimal point three places to the left. • The average teaspoon holds 4 to 5 mL more than the standard 5 mL.

Learning Outcome	Summary Points
3-3 Solve Fahrenheit to Celsius temperature conversion and vice versa.	• To convert *a Fahrenheit temperature to the Celsius scale,* subtract 32 from the Fahrenheit temperature and divide by 1.8. • To convert *a Celsius temperature to the Fahrenheit scale,* multiply the Celsius temperature by 1.8 and add 32.
3-4 Calculate the number of tablets, capsules, and injectable medications to give when the available dose differs from the ordered dose.	• The formula method for converting between different measurements is: $$\frac{D \text{ (desired)}}{H \text{ (on hand)}} = \frac{X \text{ (what you are solving for)}}{V \text{ (vehicle)}}$$ • Calculate the adult's dose of medication using the D-over-H formula.
3-5 Calculate a child's dose of medication.	• The two methods for calculating pediatric doses are body weight and body surface area (BSA).
3-6 Calculate drops per minute for IV therapy.	• The formula for calculating intravenous (IV) flow rate is: $$\frac{V \text{ (volume) in mL}}{T \text{ (time) in hours}} \times \frac{\text{calibration or drop factor}}{60 \text{ min/hr}}$$ $$= \text{rate (gtt/min)}$$

Chapter 3 Review

Define each of the terms listed.

1. (LO 3-2) Dosage range _____

    _____

    _____

2. (LO 3-2) Grain _____

    _____

    _____

3. (LO 3-2) Metric system _____

    _____

    _____

4. (LO 3-2) Minim _____

    _____

    _____

5. (LO 3-2) Liter _____

_____

_____

6. (LO 3-2) Meter _____

_____

_____

7. (LO 3-1) Fraction _____

_____

_____

8. (LO 3-2) Centimeter _____

_____

_____

9. (LO 3-2) Milliliter _____

_____

_____

10. (LO 3-1) Denominator _____

_____

_____

11. (LO 3-1) Improper fraction _____

_____

_____

Match the fraction as either a proper fraction or an improper fraction (LO 3-1).

_____ 12. $\frac{3}{4}$ a. Proper fraction

_____ 13. $\frac{5}{8}$ b. Improper fraction

_____ 14. $\frac{9}{5}$

_____ 15. $\frac{2}{3}$

_____ 16. $\frac{6}{4}$

Write abbreviations for these units of measurement.

17. (LO 3-2) Minim _____   19. (LO 3-2) Dram _____

18. (LO 3-2) Grain _____   20. (LO 3-2) Fluidram _____

21. (LO 3-2) Ounce _____

22. (LO 3-2) Drop _____

23. (LO 3-2) Pint _____

24. (LO 3-2) Tablespoon _____

25. (LO 3-2) Pound _____

26. (LO 3-2) Milligram _____

27. (LO 3-2) Milliliter _____

28. (LO 3-2) Liter _____

29. (LO 3-2) Gram _____

Practice decoding abbreviations. The following dosage orders are given using Roman numerals and abbreviations for the apothecary system of measurement. Write them out in full, using Arabic numerals (LO 3-2).

30. ℥ $\overline{\text{iv}}$ _____

31. gr $\overline{\text{iss}}$ _____

32. m $\overline{\text{ii}}$ _____

33. ℥ $\overline{\text{ix}}$ _____

Fill in the blanks. Refer to Tables 3.4, 3.8, and 3.9 if necessary.

34. (LO 3-2) A grain weighs the same as _____ minim(s) of liquid.

35. (LO 3-2) One minim is the same as _____ drop(s).

36. (LO 3-2) One milliliter is approximately equivalent to _____ drop(s).

37. (LO 3-2) Grains fifteen is _____ gram(s).

38. (LO 3-2) Grain one is _____ milligram(s).

39. (LO 3-2) One gram is equal to _____ milligrams.

40. (LO 3-3) One milliliter is the same as _____ cubic centimeter(s).

41. (LO 3-2) One-half of a gram equals _____ milligram(s).

42. (LO 3-2) One liter (1000 mL) is about _____ quart(s).

Reduce these fractions to the lowest terms (LO 3-1).

43. $\frac{4}{8}$ = _____

44. $\frac{3}{9}$ = _____

45. $\frac{24}{32}$ = _____

46. $\frac{21}{28}$ = _____

47. $\frac{250}{1000}$ = _____

48. $\frac{25}{45}$ = _____

Change these improper fractions to mixed numbers (LO 3-1).

49. $\frac{8}{3}$ = _____

50. $\frac{5}{2}$ = _____

51. $\frac{17}{12}$ = _____

52. $\frac{55}{20}$ = _____

53. $\frac{18}{4}$ = _____

54. $\frac{68}{3}$ = _____

55. $\frac{350}{100}$ = _____

56. $\frac{27}{5}$ = _____

Multiply these fractions and reduce them to the lowest terms (LO 3-1).

57. $\frac{3}{10} \times \frac{1}{10} =$ _____

58. $2 \times \frac{5}{8} =$ _____

59. $250 \text{ mg} \times 1 \text{ gr}/60 \text{ mg} =$ _____

60. $\frac{5}{8} \times \frac{2}{3} =$ _____

61. $\frac{5}{4} \times \frac{7}{6} =$ _____

62. $3 \text{ gr} \times 60 \text{ mg}/1 \text{ gr} =$ _____

Divide these fractions and reduce them to the lowest terms (LO 3-1).

63. $\frac{1}{2} \div \frac{2}{3} =$ _____

64. $\frac{1}{60} \div 3 =$ _____

65. $\frac{5}{8} \div \frac{5}{9} =$ _____

66. $1 \div \frac{1}{600} =$ _____

Write these fractions as decimals (LO 3-1).

67. $\frac{1}{2} =$ _____

68. $\frac{1}{4} =$ _____

69. $\frac{3}{4} =$ _____

70. $\frac{25}{100} =$ _____

71. $\frac{23}{1000} =$ _____

72. $\frac{1}{3} =$ _____

73. $\frac{2}{3} =$ _____

74. $\frac{6}{10} =$ _____

75. $\frac{89}{100} =$ _____

76. $3\frac{3}{4} =$ _____

Change these decimals to fractions and reduce them to the lowest terms (LO 3-1).

77. $0.75 =$ _____

78. $1.5 =$ _____

79. $0.005 =$ _____

80. $0.2 =$ _____

81. $5.66 =$ _____

82. $0.375 =$ _____

Multiply or divide these decimals as directed (LO 3-1).

83. $1.5 \times 3 =$ _____

84. $1.5 \times 0.03 =$ _____

85. $7.5 \div 25 =$ _____

86. $1.5 \times 0.3 =$ _____

87. $2.75 \times 0.1 =$ _____

88. $7.5 \div 2.5 =$ _____

Convert from grams to milligrams or from milligrams to grams as directed (LO 3-2).

89. $0.1 \text{ g} =$ _____ mg

90. $0.03 \text{ g} =$ _____ mg

91. $325 \text{ mg} =$ _____ g

92. $3000 \text{ mg} =$ _____ g

93. $2.5 \text{ g} =$ _____ mg

94. $0.125 \text{ g} =$ _____ mg

95. $1200 \text{ mg} =$ _____ g

96. $5 \text{ mg} =$ _____ g

Convert these Fahrenheit temperatures to Celsius (LO 3-3).

97. $97.4°\text{F} =$ _____ °C

98. $99°\text{F} =$ _____ °C

99. $100°\text{F} =$ _____ °C

100. $101.8°\text{F} =$ _____ °C

101. $102°\text{F} =$ _____ °C

102. $104°\text{F} =$ _____ °C

Convert these Celsius temperatures to Fahrenheit (LO 3-3).

103. 35.4°C = _____ °F

104. 37.4°C = _____ °F

105. 39.2°C = _____ °F

106. 40°C = _____ °F

107. 41°C = _____ °F

108. 42°C = _____ °F

Convert these pounds to kilograms (LO 3-5).

109. 150 lb = _____ kg

110. 86 lb = _____ kg

111. 109 lb = _____ kg

112. 234 lb = _____ kg

113. 45 lb = _____ kg

114. 8 lb = _____ kg

Convert these kilograms to pounds (LO 3-5).

115. 16 kg = _____ lb

116. 32 kg = _____ lb

117. 80 kg = _____ lb

118. 5 kg = _____ lb

119. 94 kg = _____ lb

Multiple Choice—Circle the correct letter.

120. (LO 3-3) Which of the following is a calculation guideline to consider when performing a calculation?
   a. Label the math problem only when it is necessary.
   b. All weights must be rounded to the hundredth place.
   c. Round down when the last number is less than 5.
   d. All numbers greater than 1 must be documented with a zero before the decimal point.

121. (LO 3-3) Which of the following is important when converting temperatures between the Fahrenheit and Celsius scales?
   a. Consider the difference between the freezing and boiling temperatures of water.
   b. The freezing temperature of water is 42 degrees.
   c. The boiling temperature of water is 180 degrees.
   d. The Fahrenheit degree is 212/100.

122. (LO 3-2) Which of the following is a step in the conversion process used in the metric system?
   a. Move the decimal point two places to the left for converting grams to milligrams.
   b. mg ÷ 500 g.
   c. Move the decimal point three places to the left for converting milligrams to grams.
   d. g × 500 = mg.

123. (LO 3-2) For use of the metric system, which principle is correct?
   a. One pound is equivalent to 0.728 kilogram.
   b. Metric doses are written in lowercase Roman numerals.
   c. The centimeter is 1/1000th of a meter.
   d. One milliliter is the same as 1 cubic centimeter.

124. (LO 3-2) Which system of measurement is very old and, although still used, is used infrequently?

    a. Apothecary system

    b. Weight measurements

    c. Metric system

    d. Household system

Chapter 3 Case Studies

125. (LO 3-3) You first calculate a problem before giving a medication to a patient. What are the calculation guidelines you must consider before correctly performing this calculation? _____

_____

_____

_____

126. (LO 3-3) You are preparing to give a medication and assume that the vehicle (V) is 1. You perform your calculation and show it to your supervisor before administering the medication. The supervisor tells you that you are about to make a very serious medication error that could be deadly. In reviewing your practices, what do you determine that you are doing wrong? What should you do to correct this problem? _____

_____

_____

_____

Critical Thinking

Solve these problems (LO 3-4).

127. 0.1 mg = gr _____

128. gr $\frac{1}{60}$ = _____ mg

129. 4 mg = gr _____

130. 150 mg = gr _____

131. 0.5 mg = gr _____

132. gr 5 = _____ mg

133. 1 g = gr _____

134. gr $7\frac{1}{2}$ = _____ g

Drug Calculations—Fill in the blank with the answer.

135. (LO 3-4) Meperidine (*Demerol*) 50 mg IM has been ordered. Available is 100 mg per mL. You will give _____ mL to the patient.

136. (LO 3-4) The provider orders heparin 8000 units to be given subcutaneously. On hand is heparin 10,000 units/mL. You should draw up _____ milliliters to deliver 8000 units.

137. (LO 3-4) The provider orders ibuprofen 0.6 g p.o. bid. Available are 600-mg tablets. You will give the patient _____ tablet(s).

138. (LO 3-4) The provider orders hydroxyzine (*Vistaril*) 12.5 mg p.o. bid. Available are 25-mg tablets that are scored. You give _____ tablets to the patient.

139. (LO 3-4) Penicillin G procaine 450,000 units has been ordered to be given IM. Available is 300,000 units per mL. You will give the patient _____ mL.

140. (LO 3-4) You are to prepare imipramine (*Tofranil*) 20 mg for IM injection. Available is 25 mg per 2 mL. You will give _____ mL to the patient.

141. (LO 3-4) Hydromorphone (*Dilaudid*) 3 mg is ordered IM. Available is 4 mg per 1 mL. You will give _____ mL to the patient.

142. (LO 3-4) The provider orders heparin 3000 units to be administered subcutaneously. Available is 10,000 units per mL. You will give the patient _____ mL.

143. (LO 3-4) The provider orders neomycin 400 mg IM. Available is 500 mg per 2.5 mL. You will give _____ mL to the patient.

144. (LO 3-4) Furosemide (*Lasix*) 15 mg has been ordered IM. Available is 10 mg/mL. You will give _____ mL to the patient.

145. (LO 3-4) The provider orders acetaminophen (*Tylenol*) elixir 600 mg/10 mL every 4 hours for a temperature greater than 101°F or 38.3°C. Available is 120 mg per 5 mL. You will give _____ mL to the patient.

146. (LO 3-4) The provider orders methocarbamol (*Robaxin*) 1.5 g p.o. stat. Available are *Robaxin* 750-mg tablets. You give the patient _____ tablets.

147. (LO 3-4) Heparin 6000 units subcutaneously has been ordered. The available heparin is 10,000 units/mL. You will administer _____ mL of heparin subcutaneously to the patient.

148. (LO 3-4) The provider orders cefoxitin sodium 0.75 g IM every 12 hours. The vial of *cefoxitin* contains 5 grams of powder. The instructions are to add 13.2 mL of sterile water to the vial; 3 mL = 1 g. You administer _____ milliliters of the solution to contain the prescribed dose.

149. (LO 3-4) The provider orders meperidine (*Demerol*) 75 mg IM every 4 hours for pain. Available *Demerol* is 100 mg per 2 mL. You give the patient _____ mL.

150. (LO 3-4) The provider orders meperidine (*Demerol*) 60 mg and hydroxyzine (*Vistaril*) 25 mg IM prn. Available is *Demerol* 100 mg/2 mL and *Vistaril* 25 mg/mL. You should administer a total volume of _____ milliliters of *Demerol* and *Vistaril* in one dose to the patient. Can you mix the *Demerol* and *Vistaril* in one syringe? Hint: Look at a compatibility chart in the medication room or in many drug books to determine if *Demerol* and *Vistaril* may be mixed.

151. (LO 3-4) You are to prepare amoxicillin 500 mg p.o. bid from a 250-mg per 5-mL suspension. You should give the patient _____ mL.

152. (LO 3-4) The provider orders 0.3 mg of atropine to be given IM. Available is 0.3 mg per mL. You should give _____ mL to the patient.

153. (LO 3-4) The provider orders potassium 10 mEq p.o. qid. You have available potassium 20 mEq per 15 mL. You will give the patient _____ mL.

154. (LO 3-4) The provider orders hydroxyzine (*Vistaril*) 100 mg p.o. prn. Available are 50-mg tablets. You give _____ tablets to the patient.

155. (LO 3-4) You are to administer furosemide (*Lasix*) 15 mg IM. Available is 20 mg/2 mL. You give the patient _____ mL.

156. (LO 3-4) The provider orders acetaminophen (*Tylenol*) 650 mg p.o. prn. Available are 325-mg tablets. You will give the patient _____ tablets.

157. (LO 3-4) The provider orders neomycin 0.75 g p.o. qid. Available are 500-mg tablets. You will give the patient _____ tablets.

158. (LO 3-4) The provider orders 0.2 mg of cyanocobalamin (vitamin B_{12}) IM daily. Available is 100 mcg in 1 mL. You are to administer _____ mL.

159. (LO 3-4) The provider orders tolbutamide 250 mg p.o. Available are 0.5-g tablets. You give _____ tablets to the patient.

160. (LO 3-4) The provider orders heparin 5000 units subcutaneously. Available is 10,000 units per mL. You will give _____ mL to the patient.

161. (LO 3-4) The provider orders meclizine 50 mg p.o. prn. Available are 25-mg tablets. You will give the patient _____ tablets.

162. (LO 3-4) The provider orders ceftazidime (*Fortaz*) 0.25 g to be given IM. Available is 500 mg/mL. You will give _____ mL to the patient.

163. (LO 3-4) The provider orders meperidine (*Demerol*) 35 mg IM every 4 hours for pain. Available is *Demerol* 100 mg per mL. You will give the patient _____ mL.

164. (LO 3-4) The provider orders Penicillin G 800,000 units IM daily. Available is 1,000,000 units per 2 mL. You will give _____ mL to the patient.

165. (LO 3-4) The provider orders codeine 60 mg every 4 hours for pain. Available is 30 mg per tablet. You will give the patient _____ tablets.

166. (LO 3-4) The provider orders levothyroxine 0.1 mg p.o. daily. Available are 50-mcg tablets. You will give the patient _____ tablets.

167. (LO 3-4) The provider orders nitroglycerin 0.6 mg sublingually prn for chest pain. Available are 0.3-mg tablets. You will give the patient _____ tablets.

168. (LO 3-4) The provider orders diazepam (*Valium*) 2.5 mg p.o. prn. Available are 5-mg tablets. You will give the patient _____ tablet.

Practice Problems for Pediatric Patients

169. (LO 3-4) Morphine sulfate 10 mg subcutaneously has been ordered every 4 hours. The child weighs 35.5 kg. The package insert states the recommended maximum dose of morphine sulfate is 0.1 to 0.2 mg/kg/dose. What is the safe range for this child? Is this dose within the safe dose range?

_____

170. (LO 3-5) The provider orders 20 mg/kg/24 hours of a drug to be given orally to a child weighing 22 kg. How much should you give every 12 hours? _____

171. (LO 3-4) The provider orders furosemide (*Lasix*) 2 mg/kg/24 hours orally for a child weighing 26 kg. How much should you give in 4 equally divided doses? How much should you give in a 24-hour period?

_____

172. (LO 3-4) The provider orders clindamycin (*Cleocin*) 75 mg orally four times a day. The child weighs 9 kg. The package insert states the recommended dose should not exceed 25 mg/kg/day. How much should you give in each dose? _____

173. (LO 3-5) The provider orders phenobarbital IV for a child weighing 56 kg. The recommended dose is between 1 and 3 mg. How much should you give every 6 hours? _____

_____

174. (LO 3-5) An oral antibiotic has been ordered for a client weighing 20 kg. The usual recommended dose is 50 mg/kg/day in 4 equally divided doses. How much should you give in each dose? _____

_____

175. (LO 3-5) The provider orders 40 mg of a drug to be administered orally to a child weighing 18 kg. The package insert states that the dose range is between 6 and 7.5 mg/kg/day. What is the safe dose range for 24 hours? What is the safe dose range in 4 divided doses? _____

_____

176. (LO 3-5) The provider orders penicillin 500 mg orally to a child weighing 20 kg. The recommended safe dose range is 25 to 50 mg/kg/day. What is the dose range? Is this within the safe dose range?

_____

177. (LO 3-5) The provider orders a drug to be administered orally to a child weighing 20 kg. The recommended dose is 10 mg/kg/day. How much should you give every 6 hours? _____

_____

178. (LO 3-5) Calculate the body surface area for a child who is 27 inches tall and weighs 17 lb.

_____

179. (LO 3-5) Calculate the body surface area for a child who is 93 cm tall and weighs 17 kg.

_____

Practice Problems for Intravenous Calculations—Fill in the blank with the answer.

180. (LO 3-6) The provider orders 1000 mL of D5W to infuse in 4 hours. You are using an infusion set with a drop factor of 15 gtt per mL. You should regulate the IV tubing to deliver _____ gtt per minute.

181. (LO 3-6) The provider orders 200 mL of normal saline 0.9% to run in 2 hours. You are using an IV set that delivers 15 gtt per mL. You will regulate the IV to deliver _____ gtt per minute.

182. (LO 3-6) The provider orders 1000 mL of normal saline 0.45% to run in 6 hours. The IV set delivers 15 gtt per mL. You will administer _____ gtt per minute to the patient.

183. (LO 3-6) The provider orders 1000 mL of D5NS to infuse in 24 hours. You are using an IV set that delivers 15 gtt per mL. You will regulate the IV to deliver _____ gtt per minute.

ADMINISTERING PARENTERAL MEDICATIONS

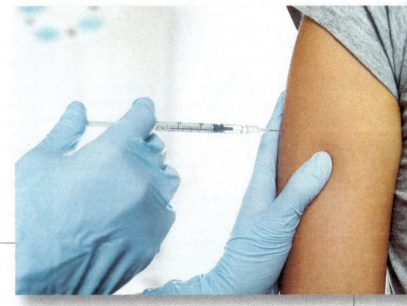

LEARNING OUTCOMES

4-1 Describe the major routes, sites, and procedures of injectable medications.

4-2 Use Standard Precautions.

4-3 Identify the parts of a syringe needle and the sizes of needles while identifying doses.

4-4 Draw up medications from vials and ampules, and reconstitute medications.

4-5 Identify the most common injection sites for intradermal, subcutaneous, and intramuscular administration.

4-6 Identify the various types of intravenous solutions, indications, advantages, disadvantages, and signs and symptoms of complications.

In this chapter you will learn how to give medications accurately and safely by the parenteral route and to protect yourself using Standard Precautions. You will also learn how to handle injection equipment and how to prepare medications for injection. You will learn to locate the proper sites of injections and follow specific injection procedures. In addition, you will learn the basic principles of intravenous therapy including the types of solutions, uses, advantages, disadvantages, and complications.

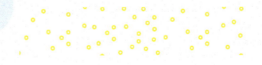

abscess	hub	reconstituting
acromion process	iliac crest	sciatic nerve
aqueous	induration	shaft
aspirate	intravenous therapy	sloughing
barrel	lumen	Standard Precautions
flange	necrosis	syringe
gauge (G)	needle cover	tracking
gluteal arteries	plunger	viscous
greater trochanter	precipitate	Z-track

ORIENTATION TO THE PARENTERAL ROUTE [LO 4-1]

Parenteral administration is the method of giving drugs by injection using a needle and syringe. It is used when other routes would be ineffective or impractical. Because injection puts medication into direct contact with body tissues that contain many blood vessels and capillaries, absorption is more rapid by this route than by the oral, rectal, or topical routes. It is thus a valuable route in emergencies. Certain drugs that can be destroyed by digestive enzymes are given by the parenteral route so that they remain effective. Injections are also given when patients cannot take oral medications because of difficulty swallowing, nausea or vomiting, intestinal obstructions, or unconsciousness.

Parenteral drugs can be administered by four different routes:

- Intradermal (ID)
- Subcutaneous (subcut)
- Intramuscular (IM)
- Intravenous (IV)

The parenteral route involves breaking through the skin's protective covering, which increases the risk of infection. The rapid absorption that occurs with injection means that the dose must be exact; reactions to an overdose can set in very rapidly and may require emergency treatment. Injections that are done improperly can stretch and injure tissues or hit bones, nerves, and blood vessels, causing pain and possibly serious damage. Table 4.1 lists the safe practices for Medical Injections from the Centers for Disease Control and Prevention (CDC).

Because of the dangers of injury, underdose, overdose, and infection, special training and certification are required for people who give medications parenterally. State laws regulate which categories of healthcare workers are permitted to give injections and what type of certification they must have. If you are not permitted to give injections, never administer drugs parenterally.

Table 4.1 Safe Practices for Medical Injections from CDC (Centers for Disease Control and Prevention)

1. Never administer medications from the same syringe to more than one patient, even if the needle is changed or you are injecting through an intervening length of IV tubing.
2. Do not enter a medication vial, bag, or bottle with a used syringe or needle.
3. Never use medications packaged as single dose or single use for more than one patient. This includes ampules, bags, and bottles of intravenous solutions.
4. Always use aseptic technique when preparing and administering medications.

Table 4.2 Standard Precautions for Medical Injection Safety

Employer: Protect Healthcare Worker	Worker: Use Appropriate Barrier Precautions	Worker: Prevent Needlestick Injuries
Explain activities that expose workers to blood-borne pathogens.	Wear gloves to reduce blood contamination of skin surface.	Do not break, bend, or remove needles by hand from syringes.
Develop standard operating procedures to prevent worker exposure.	Wash hands/skin immediately when exposed.	Do not recap used needles.
Provide initial and ongoing education on Standard Precautions.	Change and discard punctured or torn gloves.	Place uncapped disposable needles in a rigid, puncture-resistant container.
Follow up on worker compliance with guidelines.	Wear masks, gowns, and eye/face shields to protect mucous membranes when there is a risk of exposure to blood or body fluid.	Place these containers as close to the work area as possible.
Redesign the workplace and modify the workplace environment.	Do not work if you have dermatitis or exudative lesions.	Transport contaminated equipment to the appropriate waste area.
Provide appropriate personal protective equipment (PPE) including masks, gowns, gloves, and eye/face shields.	If you are pregnant, *do not* risk exposing the fetus to blood-borne pathogens by lack of caution.	Use safety syringes with an automatic retractable needle when possible.

STANDARD PRECAUTIONS [LO 4-2]

Under **Standard Precautions**, all patients are considered potentially infectious with blood-borne pathogens. Examples are hepatitis B virus (HBV) and human immunodeficiency virus (HIV), the virus that causes acquired immune deficiency syndrome (AIDS). Healthcare workers are exposed to these pathogens primarily through mucous membranes, nonintact skin, and needlesticks. Standard Precautions apply to infections caused by blood, body fluids, nonintact skin, and mucous membranes. Standard Precautions combine the features of both Universal Precautions and Body Substance Isolation.

Blood is the most important vehicle for transmission of pathogens. Other body fluids that can be involved are cerebrospinal (CSF), synovial, pleural, peritoneal, and amniotic fluids; semen; vaginal secretions; and human breast milk. Gloves should be worn for all contact with body fluids, mucous membranes, and nonintact skin. Use extreme caution in handling contaminated needles and other sharp instruments. To prevent needlesticks, used needles should not be recapped, bent, broken, or removed from disposable syringes. Table 4.2 lists the standard blood and body fluid precautions.

EQUIPMENT [LO 4-3]

Syringes

Five types of **syringes** (Figure 4.1) are used for injecting medications:

- Standard hypodermic syringe
- Insulin syringe
- Tuberculin syringe
- Prefilled syringe
- Tubex/Carpuject syringe (must have a prefilled cartridge to use)

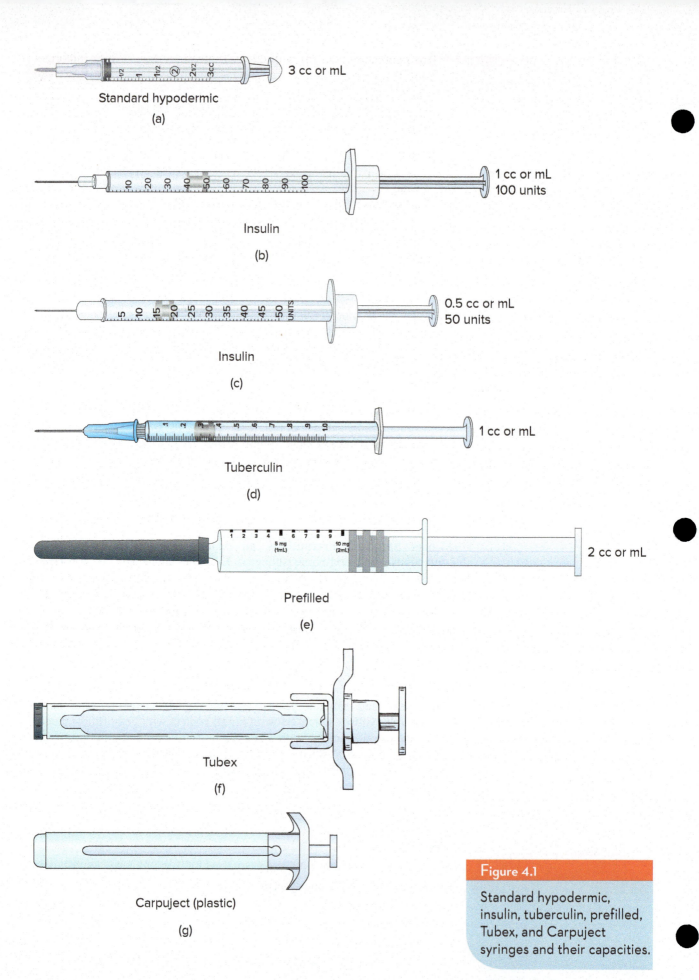

3 cc or mL

Standard hypodermic

(a)

1 cc or mL
100 units

Insulin

(b)

0.5 cc or mL
50 units

Insulin

(c)

1 cc or mL

Tuberculin

(d)

2 cc or mL

Prefilled

(e)

Tubex

(f)

Carpuject (plastic)

(g)

It is calibrated (marked) with different measurements so it is important to consider the measurement of the syringe. This may consist of cubic centimeters (cc), milliliters (mL), or minims (m).

The insulin syringe, as its name implies, is used for subcutaneous injection of insulin and is calibrated in units (U). Most insulin is available as U100, indicating that each milliliter contains U100 of insulin. A U100 syringe must be used for U100 insulin. When a patient takes a smaller dose, insulin syringes with larger black lines are marked for 25, 30, or 50 U and are also used for U100 insulin.

The tuberculin syringe is designed for intradermal injection of very small amounts of substances in tests for tuberculosis and allergies. It is calibrated in hundredths of cubic centimeters and less frequently in minims.

Syringes are sized according to the volume of liquid they can hold. The most common size of the standard syringe is 3 cc or milliliters (mL). Larger syringes of 5 to 50 cc are also available. These are usually used not for injections but for adding fluids to intravenous flasks, for irrigating wounds, and for removing fluids from body cavities.

Syringes are made of disposable plastic or glass. They are packaged either separately or together with needles of appropriate sizes. Syringes with preattached needles should never have the needle removed. Syringes and needles are packaged in peel-open paper wrappers. Syringes may be empty or prefilled with specific doses of medication. Prefilled glass cartridges are available for use with a special metal or plastic holder and plunger called a Tubex or Carpuject syringe.

The two main parts of a syringe are the **barrel** and the **plunger**. The barrel is a hollow cylinder that holds the medication. The plunger fits snugly in this cylinder and is used to change the pressure within. Pulling the plunger back lowers the air pressure inside the barrel, allowing air or medication to be pulled in from outside. Pushing in the plunger increases the pressure inside the barrel and forces air or medication out.

The barrel, plunger, and other parts of a syringe are identified in Figure 4.2. Obtain sample syringes from your instructor and locate these parts.

Needles

Needles for injection are made of stainless steel and are available in various sizes for different purposes. They come packaged with a protective **needle cover**, or sheath, that keeps them from becoming contaminated. To understand how parts of the needle are labeled, see Figure 4.2. The tip of the needle, the point, breaks through

Figure 4.2

Parts of the syringe and needle.

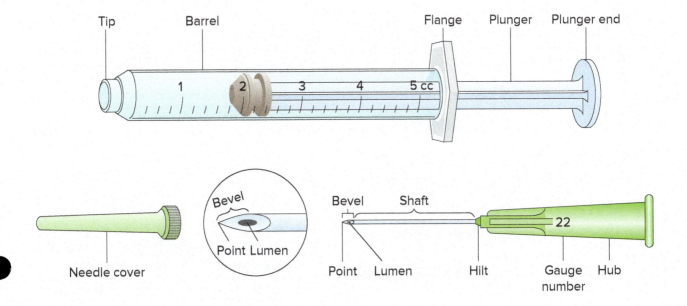

the skin layers. The bevel or slanted portion of the needle tip spreads the tissues apart so that the needle can enter smoothly. The longer the bevel, the sharper the needle and the more easily it passes through tissues, thus minimizing the discomfort of subcutaneous and intramuscular injections. The **shaft** (stem or cannula) is the long part of the needle. It is embedded in the **hub**, which attaches to the syringe.

Needles are sized according to their length and gauge. The length of a needle is the distance from the point to the hub—in other words, the length of the shaft. The **gauge (G)** is the diameter of the **lumen**, the hollow part inside the needle through which medication passes. Needle lengths vary from $\frac{1}{4}$ inch to 5 inches. In general, the shorter lengths ($\frac{1}{4}$ to $\frac{5}{8}$ inch) are used for subcutaneous and intradermal injections, and the longer lengths (1 to $1\frac{1}{2}$ inches) are used for intramuscular injections. The longest needles (e.g., 5 inches) are often used for other purposes, such as withdrawing fluids from body cavities.

The choice of needle length depends in part on the patient's age and body fat. Babies and small children require shorter needles to reach the proper tissues. People with heavy fat deposits require longer needles to reach their muscles (e.g., 2 inches). If a patient is obese or very thin and you are unsure what needle size to use, check with your supervisor.

The most common needles used are 19, 20, 21, 23, and 25 G (Figure 4.3). The smaller the gauge, the larger the needle diameter. Which gauge to use depends on how thick the medication is. Liquids that are thin and watery are described as **aqueous**, and those that are thick and sticky are described as **viscous**. Penicillin and other oil-based solutions are viscous, whereas most other medications are aqueous. Ordinary gauges (22G to 25G) are used for aqueous medications, but lower-numbered gauges (18G to 20G) must be used with viscous medications, which could easily clog a thinner needle. Package inserts for viscous medications may suggest the proper gauge to use.

The paper packages on disposable needles are labeled by both length and gauge. Always be certain you are using the proper length and gauge of needle for the route and medication.

Figure 4.3

Diagram of the most common needles used.

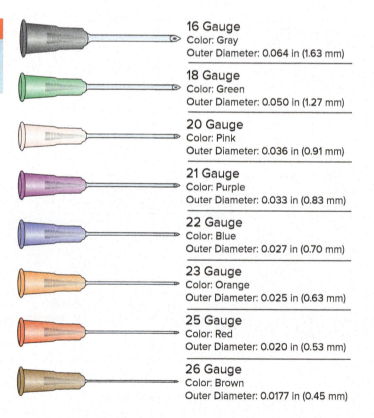

16 Gauge
Color: Gray
Outer Diameter: 0.064 in (1.63 mm)

18 Gauge
Color: Green
Outer Diameter: 0.050 in (1.27 mm)

20 Gauge
Color: Pink
Outer Diameter: 0.036 in (0.91 mm)

21 Gauge
Color: Purple
Outer Diameter: 0.033 in (0.83 mm)

22 Gauge
Color: Blue
Outer Diameter: 0.027 in (0.70 mm)

23 Gauge
Color: Orange
Outer Diameter: 0.025 in (0.63 mm)

25 Gauge
Color: Red
Outer Diameter: 0.020 in (0.53 mm)

26 Gauge
Color: Brown
Outer Diameter: 0.0177 in (0.45 mm)

Keeping Injection Equipment Sterile

Because an injection breaks the skin that protects the body from microbes, it is vital to maintain asepsis when handling needles, syringes, and injectable medications. The parts of a needle and syringe that must be protected from contamination are the inside of the needle cover, the needle point and shaft, the inside and outside of the hub, the syringe tip, the inside of the syringe barrel, and the plunger. The only parts you may safely touch with your hands are the outside of the needle cover, the outside of the barrel, the **flange** (the flared part of the barrel), and the plunger end.

Disposable needles and syringes are presterilized and packaged in paper wrappers or plastic containers. To open these, peel back the paper or remove the cover and slide out the contents from that end. If the needle and syringe are packaged separately, attach them as follows: Hold the needle cover and twist or press the hub onto the syringe tip, depending on the type of connection. After use, disposable equipment must be discarded in special puncture-resistant containers located within the working area. Contaminated materials should be disposed of properly.

Needleless Systems

Needleless systems are now available at many facilities to decrease the risk of needlesticks. Needlesticks are the most common route of exposure to blood-borne diseases. "Safety syringes" are equipped with a plastic guard or shield that automatically slips over the needle as it is taken out of the skin (**Figure 4.4**).

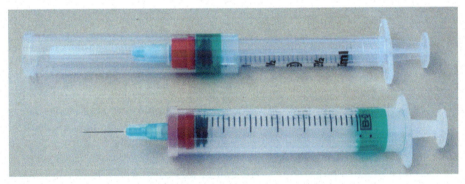

(a)

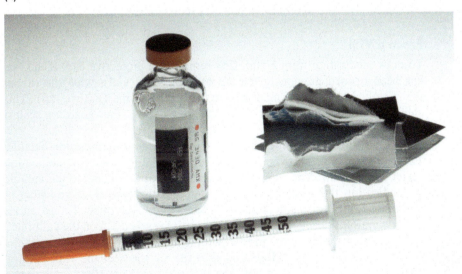

(b)

> **Figure 4.4**
>
> Safety syringes:
> (a) All syringes should have a safety mechanism. A protective sheath is pushed over the needle after use.
> (b) This 50-unit insulin safety syringe has a shield that covers the needle, minimizing needlestick injuries.

(a) ©McGraw-Hill Education/Mark Dierker, photographer; (b) ©Creatas/PunchStock

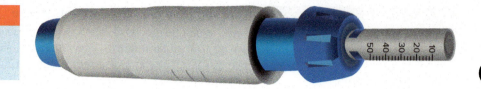

Figure 4.5

Needleless jet injector system.

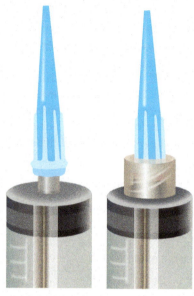

Luer Slip   **Luer Lock**

Figure 4.6

Needleless Luer Slip and Luer Lock systems.

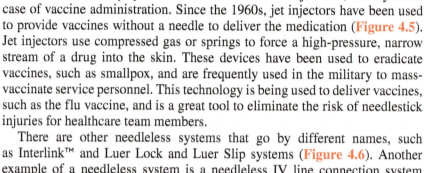

Needleless delivery systems are also available for injections, usually in the case of vaccine administration. Since the 1960s, jet injectors have been used to provide vaccines without a needle to deliver the medication (**Figure 4.5**). Jet injectors use compressed gas or springs to force a high-pressure, narrow stream of a drug into the skin. These devices have been used to eradicate vaccines, such as smallpox, and are frequently used in the military to mass-vaccinate service personnel. This technology is being used to deliver vaccines, such as the flu vaccine, and is a great tool to eliminate the risk of needlestick injuries for healthcare team members.

There are other needleless systems that go by different names, such as Interlink™ and Luer Lock and Luer Slip systems (**Figure 4.6**). Another example of a needleless system is a needleless IV line connection system called a lever lock (**Figure 4.7**). While slightly different, these all reduce needles in the healthcare setting to minimize needlesticks from contaminated needles.

DRAWING UP MEDICATIONS [LO 4-4]

When you are ready to fill a syringe with medication, attach the proper needle, if necessary, and remove the needle cover by pulling it straight off. The proper method for filling a syringe depends on whether the medication is contained in an ampule or a vial. Recall that an ampule is a single-dose glass container with a bulb that can be broken off at the neck. A vial is a small bottle with a rubber stopper through which a needle can be inserted. A vial can contain either a single dose or multiple doses. An example of a single-dose vial is heparin. Insulin is an example of a multiple-dose vial. Remember to check the vial or ampule label against the medication administration record as you set up the parenteral medications.

The practice procedures at the end of this chapter will help you learn to draw up medications smoothly, accurately, and without contaminating the equipment. Be sure to observe Standard Precautions.

From a Vial

To draw medication from a vial, first remove the protective cap. If the vial has been opened previously (e.g., a multiple-dose vial), wipe the rubber seal firmly in a circular motion with an alcohol wipe (**Figure 4.8**). This cleans the surface through which the needle will pass, thus guarding against contamination.

The air pressure inside the vial is less than the pressure outside. Therefore some air must be injected into the vial to make the medication easier to withdraw. You should inject an amount of air equal to the volume of medication that you are withdrawing. In other words, if you plan to withdraw 1.5 mL of medication, then you should first inject 1.5 mL of air into the vial. Pull back the stopper to the point marked 1.5 on the calibrated syringe. Insert the tip of the needle, with the bevel pointing up, through the center of the rubber seal. Inject air into the air space of the vial, holding on to the plunger. You may hold the vial right side up, tilted, or inverted as you inject the air. Hold the vial securely and do not touch the rubber stopper.

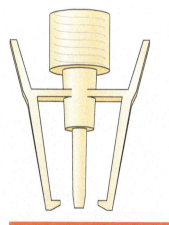

Figure 4.7

Needleless lever lock system.

Figure 4.8

To draw medication from a vial, (1) cleanse the seal; (2) inject air; and (3) withdraw the measured dose.

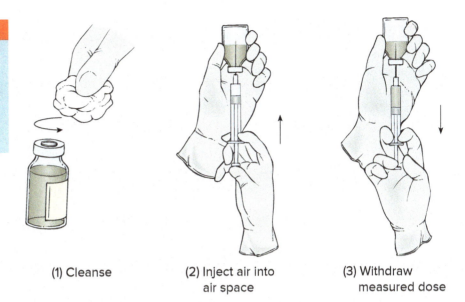

(1) Cleanse   (2) Inject air into air space   (3) Withdraw measured dose

Next, invert the vial and place the needle into the medication. Inverting the vial allows the fluid to accumulate in the lower half of the vial. Hold the vial between the thumb and middle fingers of your nondominant hand. Grasp the end of the syringe barrel and plunger with the thumb and forefinger of the dominant hand. Keep the needle below the surface of the liquid to avoid taking in air. Air pressure will fill the syringe slowly with the medication, but you may need to gently pull back on the plunger to withdraw the desired volume.

Before taking the needle out of the vial, check for air bubbles in the syringe. Air bubbles keep you from measuring an accurate dose. The tiny bubbles that often collect on the rubber tip of the plunger are no problem. However, if you see larger bubbles in the barrel, hold the syringe straight up at a 90-degree angle and tap it sharply with your finger. This will cause the bubbles to collect and join together at the tip of the syringe. Force the bubbles out by pushing in slightly on the plunger, and then withdraw more medication.

When you have drawn up the medication, replace the needle cover with a scoop technique and assemble the remaining items you need for giving the injection: the medication administration record and an antiseptic wipe. As long as the needle cover is on, you may place the needle and syringe on a tray or cart without risking contamination.

From an Ampule

Although ampules are not used as much as they once were for IM injections since the PCP pump gained in popularity, they are still used and will be discussed here.

To withdraw medication from an ampule, first inspect the ampule to see if there is any medication in the top portion. If so, tap the top with the tip of your finger to send the medication back into the bottom portion. The scoring line of the ampule is usually marked with a colored band. Most ampules are prescored. Then place a small gauze pad or alcohol swab around the ampule neck to protect your fingers from getting cut when you break the ampule (Figure 4.9). After covering the ampule neck, quickly snap it away from you to prevent shattering the glass toward your face or fingers.

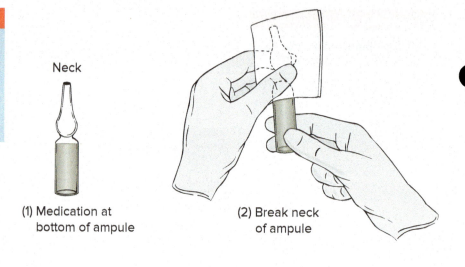

Figure 4.9

Withdrawing medication from an ampule is similar to withdrawing from a vial, except that it is not necessary to inject air.

Neck

(1) Medication at bottom of ampule

(2) Break neck of ampule

or

(3) Insert needle in ampule and withdraw medication through a filter needle

Because the air pressure is the same on the outside and inside of the opened ampule, there is no need to inject air before withdrawing the medication. Add a filter needle (Figure 4.10) to the syringe before withdrawing. Insert the needle into the ampule while holding the ampule on a flat surface in a tilted or upright position. As you pull back on the plunger, keep the needle submerged in the medication at all times. Do not allow the needle tip or shaft to touch the rim of the ampule. Some people prefer to invert the ampule while withdrawing the medication. This makes it easier to draw up all the medication without getting air bubbles.

No matter which hand position you use, be certain not to touch anything except the outside of the ampule, the outside of the syringe barrel, the flange, and the end of the plunger.

Next, check for air bubbles. If air bubbles are aspirated, do not expel air into the ampule. The air pressure may force fluid out of the ampule and medication may be lost. Remove the filter needle, hold the syringe upright, tap the side of the syringe to force the bubbles to rise toward the needle, draw back on the plunger, and push the plunger upward to expel air. Replace the filter needle with the appropriate gauge needle to administer the medication. If the syringe contains excess fluid, hold the syringe vertically with the needle tip up over a sink and slowly eject the excess. Replace the needle cover, and assemble the remaining items you need for giving the injection (e.g., medication administration record, antiseptic wipe).

Figure 4.10

Filter needle.

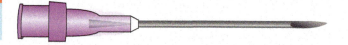

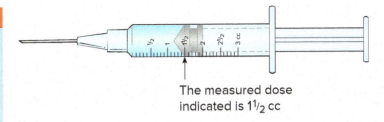

The measured dose
indicated is 1$\frac{1}{2}$ cc

Figure 4.11

To withdraw a measured dose, line up the top ring of the rubber plunger with the desired dose. Note the plunger is rounded toward the tip of the syringe. Pay careful attention to measure to the point of the plunger flush with the measurement.

Measuring Doses Accurately

To get an accurate dose, pay close attention to the calibrations on the particular syringe you are using. On a 3-cc or -mL syringe, each mark represents two-tenths of a milliliter. Count the number of marks between labeled units of measurement. If there are 10, then each mark measures off one-tenth of the unit. If there are five marks, then each mark measures two-tenths of the unit. Figure 4.11 shows how to read the calibrations when withdrawing a measured dose of medication. The top ring of the rubber plunger should be lined up with the desired dosage.

Reconstituting Powdered Drugs

Certain drugs, such as antibiotics, are stored in their powdered form because they quickly lose freshness and effectiveness when in liquid form. These powders come packaged in vials and must be **reconstituted** before injection. In other words, liquid must be added to make a solution or suspension.

Drug powders are reconstituted using sterile water or saline solution for injection. To find out how much sterile water or saline solution to add, read the directions on the vial label or package insert. Then fill a syringe with the proper measured amount of fluid and inject it into the vial. If you must inject a large amount of fluid into the vial, withdraw some air as you proceed so that pressure does not build up. After adding the fluid, gently roll the vial between your hands to dissolve or disperse the medication completely. Do not shake the vial.

Although you may reconstitute a multidose vial, most reconstituted medications come in single-dose vials.

Mixing Two Medications in a Syringe

When a patient is to receive more than one medication by injection, it saves discomfort for the patient if both medications can be given in the same injection. However, not all drugs can be mixed with others in the same syringe. Some drugs, when mixed together, form a **precipitate**, or granules, that cloud the liquid or settle to the bottom. Other drugs may change color when mixed. Either change can signal loss of effectiveness. Even with no visible change, the medications may still react to cancel each other's effects. Consult a pharmacist, the *PDR*®, or a drug reference book if you are unsure whether two medications may be mixed.

When premixed unit doses are not available and you wish to mix two drugs that can be mixed, use the following procedure. Inject air in both vials equal to the amount of drug to be withdrawn from the vial. Measure the first drug accurately and eliminate air bubbles in the syringe. Then withdraw the second drug. The total amount of liquid in the syringe should be the same as the two individual doses added together (Figure 4.12). If more than one medication is ordered, change to a fresh needle after withdrawing the first dose to avoid getting any of the first medication in the second vial.

When mixing different types of insulin in a syringe, withdraw the fast-acting or clear insulin first and then the long-acting type. Note that most insulin syringe needles are attached so when mixing insulin from clear to cloudy, the needle will not be changed.

Figure 4.12

To mix two drugs in one dose, inject air into both vials, then withdraw the first medication, change needles, and withdraw the second medication.

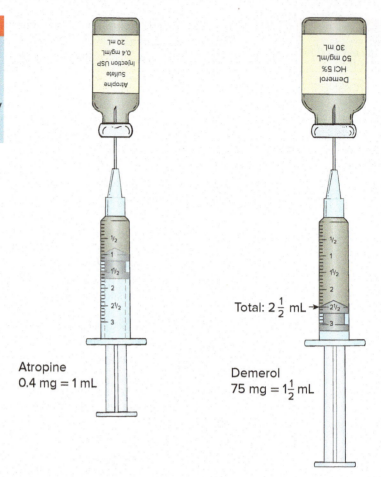

Atropine
0.4 mg = 1 mL

Total: 2½ mL →

Demerol
75 mg = 1½ mL

COMMON INJECTION SITES [LO 4-5]

The exact location for an injection depends on whether it is to be subcutaneous, intramuscular, or intradermal. The provider orders the route, but it may be up to you to decide exactly where to administer it. There are several options for each parenteral route. The specific site to choose depends on the patient's build (thin, fat, heavily muscled), the patient's age (infant, young child, average adult, older adult), and the sites of other recent injections.

Intradermal Sites

Intradermal injections are usually administered into the skin on the inner surface of the lower arm (Figure 4.13). In special cases (e.g., allergy tests),

Figure 4.13

Intradermal sites and injection technique.

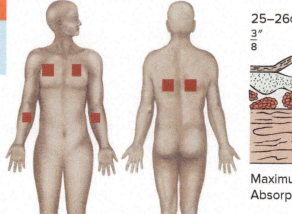

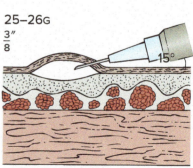

25–26G
3/8″

15°

Maximum dose: 0.3 mL
Absorption: Slow

they may also be given in the upper chest area and on the upper back below the shoulder blades.

Very small amounts of medication are given by this route—usually 0.1 to 0.2 mL—so a tuberculin syringe is used with a 25G to 26G, $\frac{3}{8}$-inch needle. The needle, with the bevel pointing up, should be held at a 5- to 15-degree angle to the skin. It should pass just below the epidermis into the dermis and be inserted to a depth of $\frac{1}{16}$ to $\frac{1}{8}$ inch (you will be able to see the needle point through the skin). As the medication is injected, you should see a small bleb or blister form under the skin. If no bleb forms, withdraw the needle slightly, as you may have gone too deeply into the skin. If medication leaks out around the needle as you push the plunger, insert the needle a bit more deeply. After injecting the medicine, withdraw the needle and gently apply an alcohol swab. Do not massage the injection site. Massaging the site may disperse medication into underlying tissue and alter the test results.

Intradermal injections are used to determine exposure to tuberculosis. About 48 to 72 hours after intradermal injection of tuberculin, the area is checked for **induration** (hardening of tissue caused by inflammation or edema) and erythema (reddening). This procedure is usually called "reading a diagnostic skin test." Induration with erythema is measured to determine exposure to tuberculosis; erythema without hardness rules out tuberculosis. An area less than 5 mm in diameter is a negative reaction. A site that is 5 to 9 mm is read as doubtful, and another test must be done. An area of 10 mm or more is a positive reaction. A similar test is used for histoplasmosis, so it is important to read the directions that come with the medication carefully.

Subcutaneous Sites

The sites for subcutaneous injection are the fatty tissues on the outer upper arm, the front of the thigh, the abdomen, and the upper back below the shoulder blades (Figure 4.14). The most common of these sites are the arm and the thigh, with 1 inch of fatty tissue. These sites may be difficult to find on an older adult, so be cautious in choosing an area. Most medication given subcutaneously is absorbed slowly because of the lesser vascularity of this tissue compared to muscle tissue.

Not more than 0.5 to 1 mL of water-soluble medication may be given subcutaneously. A 2- to 3-mL syringe may be used. The most common needle size for an average adult is 25G, $\frac{5}{8}$ inch. The needle is inserted at a 45- to 90-degree angle, through the epidermis and the dermis, into the subcutaneous tissue. In an obese person, it may be desirable to use a 1-inch needle at a 90-degree angle. Check with your supervisor as to which angle is preferred for specific cases in your health facility. Do

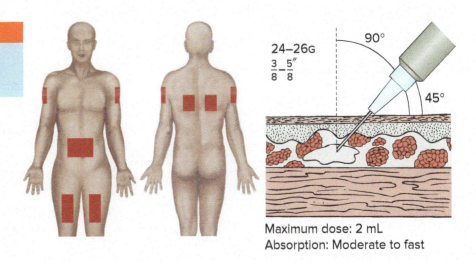

Figure 4.14

Subcutaneous sites and injection technique.

24–26G $\frac{3}{8} - \frac{5}{8}''$ 90°   45°

Maximum dose: 2 mL
Absorption: Moderate to fast

not massage the site after an injection of heparin or insulin. Massaging after heparin causes bleeding, and massaging after insulin may increase absorption of insulin.

Intramuscular Sites

The intramuscular route places the needle deep into body tissues where there are nerve bundles, large blood vessels, and bones. Therefore, it is especially important to locate the sites properly. The danger of causing tissue damage is less when the medicine enters deep muscle, but there is a risk of inadvertently injecting medicine into a blood vessel. You should locate the sites by touch, using certain prominent bones as landmarks. Advantages of the intramuscular route are as follows:

- A larger amount of medication may be injected—up to 3 mL.
- The muscles can absorb more medication than can other tissues.
- Absorption is quite rapid because muscles are well supplied with capillaries.
- The route is appropriate for oily medications that do not come in oral form.
- It can be used with uncooperative patients and with those who cannot swallow to get a rapid effect from a drug, and to avoid loss of drug effects.

Intramuscular injections must be made only into the thickest parts of large, healthy muscles. There are four possible sites (Figure 4.15):

- The dorsogluteal sites, both above and to the outside of the buttock area
- The ventrogluteal sites, both above and to the outside of the buttock area
- The deltoid site of the upper arm
- The vastus lateralis muscle of the thigh

In the two sites near the buttock area, the aim is to inject into large muscle masses that are as far away as possible from the **sciatic nerve**, the largest nerve in the body, and the **gluteal arteries**, which supply the muscles of the buttock area. Piercing the sciatic nerve could cause pain and possibly paralysis so care should be taken when administering in the dorsogluteal site. The dorsogluteal or posterior gluteal site is the most commonly used intramuscular site in average-sized adults. Two ways of locating the dorsogluteal site are shown in Figure 4.16.

One method is to draw imaginary lines dividing one side of the lower back and buttock area into quarters. The injection is given in the upper outer corner of the upper outer quarter. The other method is to draw an imaginary line between the **greater trochanter** (head of the femur where the leg joins the hip) and the posterior superior iliac crest. The injection is given above and to

Figure 4.15

Intramuscular sites and injection technique.

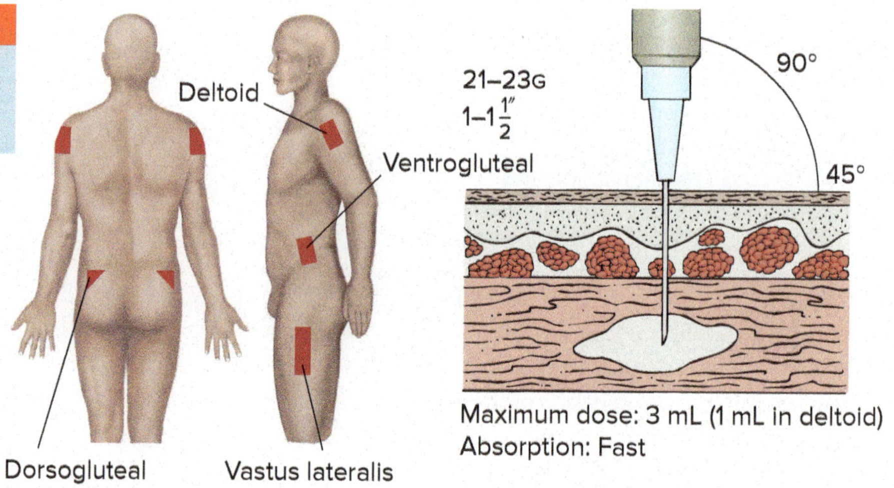

Deltoid

Ventrogluteal

21–23G
1–1$\frac{1}{2}$"

90°

45°

Dorsogluteal

Vastus lateralis

Maximum dose: 3 mL (1 mL in deltoid)
Absorption: Fast

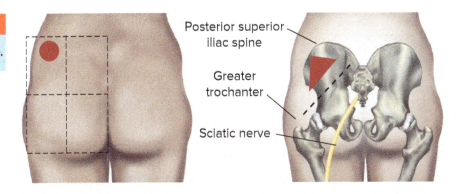

Figure 4.16

Locating the dorsogluteal site.

Posterior superior iliac spine

Greater trochanter

Sciatic nerve

the outside of this line. Study Figure 4.16 carefully and then practice locating the dorsogluteal site on a classmate or friend.

When you use the dorsogluteal site, the patient may lie in a prone position (on the stomach), with the toes pointed inward, or in a side-lying position with the upper leg flexed at the hip and knees.

The ventrogluteal site is close to the dorsogluteal site and is usually approached from a side-lying position. The site can be located by placing the palm of your hand on the patient's greater trochanter and then feeling for two spots on the hip bone, the **iliac crest**, or highest point, and the anterior superior iliac spine. The V formed by touching these spots with your index and third fingers identifies the correct placement of the ventrogluteal injection (Figure 4.17). This site is especially useful when a large amount of medication is to be injected into a patient who must lie flat on his or her back.

The deltoid site is in the deltoid muscle of the outer upper arm, 1 to 2 inches below the spot where the arm and shoulder join (the **acromion process**). This is a small site, and it may not have much muscle even in a well-developed body. The maximum amount to inject into the deltoid is 1 mL, and a shorter needle (1 inch maximum) is used.

The vastus lateralis site is on the outer upper thigh, in the middle third of the area between the knee and the greater trochanter. This is the preferred site for infants and children, because their buttock (gluteal) muscles are not well enough developed to safely receive dorsogluteal or ventrogluteal injections.

For intramuscular injections, the needle should be long enough to pass through the subcutaneous tissue and deep into muscle tissue. A 21G to 23G, 1- to $1\frac{1}{2}$-inch needle is usually used, with a 2- to 3-mL syringe. An 18G to 20G needle may be used for viscous medication. The needle is inserted at a 90-degree angle.

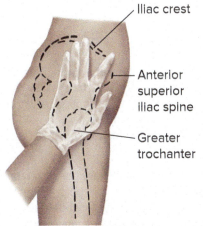

Iliac crest

Anterior superior iliac spine

Greater trochanter

Figure 4.17

Locating the ventrogluteal site.

Pediatric Considerations · Intramuscular Injections

The vastus lateralis is the preferred site for intramuscular injections for infants and children. The deltoid muscle and dorsogluteal sites should never be used for an injection in an infant and only as a last resort in a child.

Older Adult Considerations · Intramuscular Injections

The muscle tissue may be degenerated in older adult, nonmobile, or emaciated patients and should be used with extreme caution.

General Procedure for Injections

Although the various types of injections require different sites, needle sizes, and angles of penetration, certain steps and principles (i.e., Standard Precautions) are common to all. With these general directions in mind, you will be prepared to practice the step-by-step procedures for intradermal, subcutaneous, and intramuscular injections at the end of the chapter (Practice Procedures 4.3, 4.4, and 4.5). All procedures are described for a right-handed person. If you are left-handed, simply reverse the positions.

Step 1. *Locate and inspect the injection site.* Use the provider's ordered route and the site rotation plan, if any, to determine where to give an injection. Find the proper injection site using anatomical landmarks. Remove clothing or sheets as necessary to get a full view of the physical landmarks that enable you to locate the proper sites. If the injection is intramuscular, choose only healthy, heavy muscles that are free of tenderness. Inspect the skin carefully for signs of rash, redness, lumps, hair, or birthmarks. Rash or redness may be signs of reactions to previous injections given in that area. Do not proceed with the injection if there has been a reaction, but chart the appearance of the skin and consult the nurse in charge. Hardness in the skin or underlying muscle suggests that a previous injection was poorly absorbed or caused tissue damage. The next injection should be given at least 1 inch away or in another site.

Step 2. *Disinfect the skin.* Use an antiseptic wipe (e.g., alcohol) to cleanse the skin so that microorganisms do not enter the body at the injection site. Cleanse the skin in a circular motion. Using an antiseptic swab, start at the center and rotate outward in a circular motion for 2 inches. Allow the antiseptic to air dry. This is especially important with alcohol, because it can sting if it enters body tissues. Save the antiseptic wipe and hold it between the third and fourth fingers of the nondominant hand. You will use it later when you are ready to withdraw the needle.

Step 3. *Stretch and firm the skin.* With your left hand, hold the skin taut. Use your thumb and middle finger to stretch the skin and push it down. Alternately, when the site is on the arm, grasp the tissue from behind the arm and pull down and back. For the subcutaneous route, spread the skin tightly over the injection site, which allows the needle to penetrate more easily than through loose skin, or pinch the skin. Pinching the skin elevates the subcutaneous tissue and may desensitize the area.

Step 4. *Insert the needle at the proper angle.* Use the correct angle of insertion for the route, site, and needle size. With your right hand, hold the needle and syringe at the correct angle in relation to the skin surface (15, 45, or 90 degrees). The bevel should be facing up. Then insert the needle quickly and smoothly with a firm thrust.

Step 5. *Release the skin and change the hand position.* Lift your left hand so that the skin is no longer stretched or pinched. Move this hand over to the lower end of the syringe barrel so that your right hand can operate the plunger. Do not release the syringe from your right hand until your left hand is holding it steady. Any sideward movement of the needle at this step could damage underlying tissues.

Step 6. *Aspirate.* While the needle is fully inserted, pull back slightly on the plunger. This is called **aspirating**. It is a safety check to make sure that the needle has not entered a blood vessel. If it is not in a vessel, you will feel some resistance on the plunger and you will not see blood in the syringe. You may then proceed with the injection. If the needle has entered a vessel, however, blood will become visible in the syringe as you pull the plunger. If this happens, remove the needle, discard the medication and syringe, and repeat the procedure. Aspirating is important because medications ordered for subcutaneous and intramuscular injections must not be injected intravenously. If this were to happen accidentally, it could cause serious harm. There are two cases in which you should not aspirate: (1) intradermal injections, because the needle does not penetrate deep enough to contact large vessels, and (2) anticoagulant injections (e.g., heparin), because aspirating could lead to uncontrolled bleeding. Some facilities are no longer requiring injections to include aspiration. Check with your facility protocol or supervisor regarding the need to aspirate.

Step 7. *Inject the medication slowly.* Still holding the syringe with your left hand, change your right-hand position to push in the plunger. This forces the medication out of the syringe and into the body tissues. It must be injected slowly to avoid overstretching and injuring the tissues. Be sure to inject all the medication by pushing in the plunger fully.

Step 8. *Firm the skin and remove the needle.* The skin must once again be firmed so that the needle does not pull the skin as it is withdrawn. Hold the antiseptic wipe (which you tucked between your fingers in Step 2) near the needle and press gently on the skin. Pull the needle out quickly at the same angle at which it was inserted. This technique reduces pain and prevents tissue damage.

Step 9. *Remove and discard equipment.* Never recap the needle. Engage the safety device to cover the needle. Always observe standard blood and body fluid precautions. Do not break the needle. Dispose of the contaminated syringe and needle in a puncture-resistant waste container in the working area.

Step 10. *Chart the medication.* Include the specific parenteral route (intradermal, subcutaneous, or intramuscular), and note the location of the injection (right or left arm, right or left dorsogluteal site, etc.). Some facilities may require the gauge to be included in the documentation.

Step 11. *Observe the patient for expected and adverse reactions.* Try to remain with the patient for at least 1 minute; then check frequently to see how the patient is feeling. The length of observation time depends on the drug. In certain cases, you may have to stay near the patient for a certain time (e.g., 20 minutes the first time a person is injected with penicillin). Be alert for the call button of a patient who has recently received an injection. One aim of observation is to see whether the drug is working—whether an analgesic, for example, is successfully relieving pain. The other aim is to detect unexpected side effects and adverse reactions.

Parenteral medications work very quickly compared to oral, rectal, and topical medications, so reactions can occur within minutes of the injection. Systemic adverse reactions may occur as a result of overdose or allergy. These require immediate medical treatment, so you should notify the supervisor immediately if they occur.

Local reactions result from irritation of the tissues where the drug was injected. Redness, rash, and the appearance of a lump have already been mentioned as signs of drug sensitivity, tissue irritation, poor absorption, and extravasation. More serious local reactions can result in severe tissue damage—for example, death of tissue (**necrosis**), shedding of skin (**sloughing**), and formation of pus inside the tissues (**abscess**). These conditions require special treatment by a provider. Your duty is to chart and report any unusual signs of inflammation or irritation that appear in the injection area.

This general procedure includes specific steps required for parenteral administration. In addition to following these steps, you must follow the other basic rules for administering medications, such as identifying the patient, explaining the procedure, assisting the patient into a comfortable position both before and after the injection, and observing Standard Precautions.

Special Instructions for Injections

Site Rotation. Some people must have injections several times a day—for example, penicillin for a systemic infection. If all these injections were to be given in the same site, the tissues might be damaged and scar tissue might form, making further injections difficult. For these reasons, injection sites must be rotated according to some pattern (site rotation) that allows the medical staff to keep track of whether and where the last injection was given. Most health facilities adopt a rotation plan such as that shown in Figure 4.18. This method gives them a systematic way to administer regular injections without damaging body tissues. Site rotation is used with subcutaneous (except insulin) and intramuscular injections. Rotating injection sites for insulin is no longer recommended. Human insulin is the most widely used type of insulin prescribed for patients and carries a low risk for hypertrophy. Human insulin is also most cost-effective and carries a lower incidence of an allergic reaction. As a result, patients can select one anatomical area such as the abdomen and systematically rotate sites within that area. Rotating the sites within one anatomical area decreases the variability of the absorption of the insulin from day to day, thus allowing patients more success at maintaining their blood sugar levels. Intradermal medications are not usually given over many days.

Prevention of Tracking. As a needle is withdrawn after an injection, it leaves a small channel or track where the needle was inserted. **Tracking** is the leaking of medication into the channel. Medication that did not clear the needle may leak into the track as the needle is pulled out. Alternatively, the pressure of the medication in the tissue where it was injected may force some of the medication to back up into the track. In either case, tracking is not desirable, because the medication may irritate or stain other tissue layers. Penicillin, for example, causes a burning pain if it contacts subcutaneous tissue, and iron dextran can cause stains. There are several ways to prevent tracking:

- Inject very slowly and wait at least 10 seconds before withdrawing the needle.
- Avoid massaging the injection site, as this increases the pressure on the medication.
- Advise patients to wear loose-fitting clothing and to avoid heavy exercise.
- Use an air bubble, or use the Z-track method.

Use of an Air Bubble. Some health facilities recommend the use of an air bubble to prevent tracking in intramuscular injections. In this method, a small

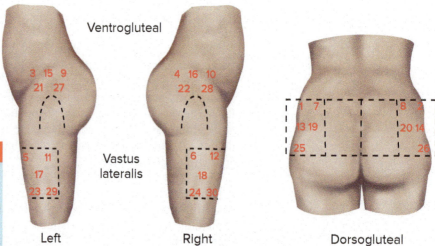

Figure 4.18

Site rotation plan for IM injections with location of injections numbered in order of administration.

amount of air (0.2 mL) is taken into the syringe after the correct dose is measured. When the medication is injected, the air bubble leaves the syringe last. Make sure the air bubble is closest to the plunger so it enters the patient last. It serves to clear the needle of all medication so that none can leak out as the needle is withdrawn. The air bubble also provides a space into which the medication can flow and thus lessens the pressure on surrounding tissues. Finally, the bubble seals off the needle track to block leakage. Ask your supervisor if this is the preferred procedure for intramuscular injections in your facility.

Z-Track Intramuscular Injection. The **Z-track** method of intramuscular medication injection may be used to minimize irritation by sealing the medicine in muscle tissue to prevent discoloration (Figure 4.19). A large, deeper muscle, such as the ventrogluteal, should be selected. After drawing up the medication, put a new needle on the syringe so that no medication remains in the needle shaft. After cleansing the injection site with alcohol, pull the skin and subcutaneous tissues 1 to $1\frac{1}{2}$ inches to the side. Hold the prepared site taut and insert the needle deep into the muscle. After aspirating for blood, slowly administer the medication. The needle should remain inserted for 10 seconds to promote even distribution of the medicine. Release the skin after withdrawing the needle. This technique leaves a zigzag pattern that seals the needle track, preventing the medicine from escaping into surrounding tissues. The Z-track method is primarily required when injecting iron dextran.

Your Attitude toward Injections. No matter how skillful you are at giving injections, they are bound to cause fear and discomfort in some patients. This is where psychological factors come into play. You need to explain how and why you are giving the medication, as always. But more than ever, your attitudes toward the procedure and the patient are crucial.

Your attitude toward the patient is important in getting the patient to cooperate in the procedure. Be a good listener, and let patients know that you care about their concerns. A relaxed patient who has confidence in you will feel less discomfort than a tense, anxious patient.

Where the procedure itself is concerned, you can be only as confident as the amount of supervised practice you put into learning how to give injections. Practice must, of course, include some feedback on how well you performed the procedure. When you really understand what you are doing, your confidence will show. The key, then, is to study carefully the theoretical information about injections and then practice the injection procedures until you can perform them with 100 percent accuracy. Remember that performing injections is a learned motor skill and takes practice to obtain expertise.

Figure 4.19

The Z-track method of injection prevents medication from backing up into other tissue layers.

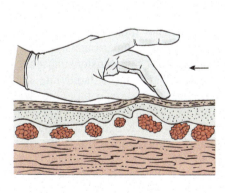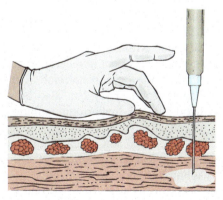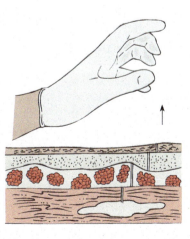

PRINCIPLES OF INTRAVENOUS THERAPY [LO 4-6]

Intravenous therapy is the administration of fluids, electrolytes, medications, blood, or even nutrients through a vein. Although the administration of intravenous therapy is generally reserved for the nurse, various health occupations recommend their graduates become familiar with the basic principles of intravenous therapy. This ensures the understanding of the purpose and use of the various intravenous solutions, as well as the advantages, disadvantages, and complications. It is through this understanding that the allied health professional may educate the patient as well as alert the nurse to potential complications.

Classifications of Intravenous Solutions

The five classifications of intravenous solutions are crystalloids, colloids, hydrating solutions, hypertonic-hyperosmolar preparations, and blood or blood components. *Crystalloids* are generally electrolytes such as isotonic, hypotonic, or hypertonic solutions that have the ability to form crystals or are capable of crystallization.

Colloid solutions commonly used consist of albumin, dextran, plasmanate, ethoxylated amylopectin (*Hetastarch*), and artificial blood substitute. These solutions are gluelike substances that cannot form a true solution because their molecules do not dissolve but remain uniformly suspended and have a cloudy appearance. They raise the colloid osmotic pressure and are often called plasma or volume expanders.

Hydrating solutions are administered for the purpose of supplying supplemental calories or nutrients, or for providing free water for rehydration or maintenance while promoting effective renal output. Glucose solutions such as dextrose 5% in water and dextrose 5% in 0.45% normal saline (NaCl) are commonly used.

Hypertonic-hyperosmolar preparations (parenteral nutrition) are mixtures of partial or complete nourishment that are administered to patients who are unable to ingest or use sufficient calories and nutrients to sustain metabolic functions. The three major nutrients in parenteral nutrition are amino acids, dextrose, and fat emulsions. Parenteral preparations are strictly administered by a registered nurse.

Blood or blood components are life-sustaining constituents such as whole blood, packed red blood cells, or modified blood products such as platelets, plasma, coagulation factor concentrates, and blood product volume expanders. The administration of blood is a high-level skill reserved for the registered nurse under a strict protocol.

Isotonic, Hypotonic, and Hypertonic Solutions

Isotonic, hypotonic, and hypertonic solutions are administered based on their tonicity such as the addition of glucose or electrolytes.

Isotonic solutions have the same tonicity as the body. They remain constant within the intravascular space because their osmotic pressure is equal between intracellular and extracellular compartments. Because of this, they are beneficial in the treatment of hypotension caused by hypovolemia. They can also be administered at a more rapid rate than hypotonic or hypertonic solutions because they are compatible with plasma. The most common isotonic solutions used are dextrose 5% in water (D5W), 0.9% NaCl, 0.2% dextrose in 0.9% NaCl, Ringer's solution, and lactated Ringer's solution. Other isotonic solutions are multiple electrolyte solutions, alkalinizing fluids, acidifying fluids, 5% mannitol in 0.45%

NaCl, and plasma volume expanders. It must be noted that D5W is isotonic when administered but becomes hypotonic when infused because dextrose is rapidly metabolized.

Hypotonic solutions cause a lower serum osmolarity by shifting fluid out of the blood and into the cells and interstitial spaces. They are used to hydrate the intracellular and interstitial compartments and lower the sodium levels. The rate must be carefully monitored to prevent water intoxication and circulatory depletion. Because of the risk of circulatory depletion, they should not be administered to patients who are hypotensive to avoid lowering the blood pressure further. The most common hypotonic solution is 0.45% NaCl.

Hypertonic solutions cause fluids to be pulled out of the intracellular and interstitial compartments into the blood vessels, thus raising serum osmolarity. They greatly expand the intravascular compartment in the presence of a serious saline depletion. The rate of administration must be carefully monitored to prevent circulatory overload. Examples of hypertonic solutions include dextrose 10% in water, 2.225% NaCl, dextrose 5% in 0.45% NaCl, dextrose 5% in 0.9% NaCl, dextrose 5% in Ringer's solution, dextrose 5% in lactated Ringer's solution, and a variety of electrolyte solutions.

Table 4.3 is a summary of commonly used isotonic, hypotonic, and hypertonic solutions and their uses.

Purposes and Indications of Intravenous Therapy

Although administering fluids, medications, blood, and nutrition supplementation by the intravenous route carries potential risks, there are times when it is often the route of choice because oral or other parenteral routes are not appropriate. Intravenous fluids may be administered for fluid volume maintenance and replacement therapy. They may be ordered when the patient is not allowed to have oral fluids or for a short period of time during a minor surgical procedure or during a diagnostic test. Fluid volume replacement may be ordered when the patient has suffered a loss of blood, body water, electrolytes, and nutrients such as occurs during major surgery or prolonged illnesses involving vomiting and diarrhea. Medications that need to be administered fast, as in a life-threatening situation or during chemotherapy, will be administered intravenously. The intravenous route of medication provides direct access to the venous system, and the most rapid action often occurs within minutes. Blood and blood products are administered during some surgical procedures, because of medical conditions, or after trauma. When the body is unable to take oral nutrition and a negative nitrogen balance exists, nutrition may need to be supplied intravenously.

Advantages and Disadvantages

While the advantages of intravenous therapy may outweigh the disadvantages, there are some situations when intravenous therapy may pose problems. In some older patients or in patients who are debilitated, the venous route may be difficult to access, causing several attempts to stick a vein. With repeated venous sticks, the patient may feel discomfort. Not only may the patient have some discomfort from an IV catheter being in place, but the patient has to maneuver the IV tubing while in bed or ambulating. Certain medications such as potassium chloride are also irritating to the vein. Although the intravenous route provides the fastest absorption of a drug and may be an advantage, it also has disadvantages. The patient may have an almost instantaneous adverse reaction, which can place the patient in a potentially fatal situation arising from an incorrect drug dose or overdose.

Table 4.3 Summary of Commonly Used Isotonic, Hypotonic, and Hypertonic Solutions and Their Uses

Solution	Composition	Indications	Considerations
Isotonic Solutions			
0.9% NaCl	154 mEq Na+ 154 mEq Cl–	Intravascular volume expander Blood transfusions Hypercalemia Fluid replacement in diabetic ketoacidosis	Administer cautiously because it may cause intravascular volume overload and pulmonary edema in clients with heart and renal failure
D5W	50 g dextrose	Replacement of water losses in dehydration Hypernatremia Diluent for medication administration	Initially isotonic but becomes hypotonic because glucose is metabolized
Lactated Ringer's	130 mEq Na+ 4 mEq K+ 3 mEq Ca++ 109 mEq Cl– 28 mEq lactate	Burns Gastrointestinal fluid losses, especially below pylorus Dehydration Hypovolemia	Similar to serum except it does not contain magnesium Contraindicated in renal failure and liver disease Do not administer if pH is >7.5
Hypotonic Solutions			
0.45% NaCl	77 mEq Na+ 77 mEQ Cl–	Hypertonic dehydration Replacement of gastric fluid loss due to nasogastric suctioning or vomiting Diabetic ketoacidosis after NaCl infusion if blood glucose is still >250 mg/dL	May cause increased intracranial pressure if admin-istered too quickly
Hypertonic Solutions			
D5 in 0.45% NaCl	77 mEq Na+ 77 mEq Cl– 50 g dextrose	Diabetic ketoacidosis when the glucose falls below 250 mg/dL Provide free water, sodium, and chloride replacement	Becomes hypotonic once glucose is metabolized
D5 in 0.9% NaCl	154 mEq Na+ 154 mEq Cl– 50 g dextrose	Hypotonic dehydration Syndrome of inappropriate antidiuretic hormone (SIADH) Addisonian crisis	Administer cautiously in clients with heart or renal failure
D10%	100 g dextrose	Free water replacement Calories	Monitor for hyperglycemia May dilute plasma electrolytes and lead to imbalances Monitor for water excess May stimulate overproduction of insulin

Risks and Complications

As a result of the break in the skin that occurs with intravenous therapy, the body's first line of defense is interrupted. This is compounded by a direct access to the circulatory system and the rapid action of both fluids and medications. It is essential that when caring for a patient on IV therapy, you monitor your patient and alert the nurse to potential complications (Table 4.4).

Table 4.4 Complications of Intravenous Therapy

Complication	Causes	Symptoms
Local infiltration	Dislodging of the IV needle from the vein	Edema at the IV site No blood return when the IV bag is lowered below the heart Discomfort at the IV site Significant slowing or complete stoppage of the flow
Pyrogenic reaction	Pyrogenic substance in the IV tubing, solution, or needle	Abrupt temperature elevation from 100° to 106°F Severe chills usually occurring 30 minutes after the start of the infusion Backache, headache General malaise Nausea and vomiting Vascular collapse with hypotension and cyanosis if reaction is severe
Speed shock	Too-rapid administration of solution containing drugs	Syncope Shock
Thrombophlebitis	Clot formation in an inflamed vein Irritating solution to the vein, such as potassium chloride	Pain along the course of the vein Redness and edema at the IV site (red tract) If severe reaction occurs, fever, malaise, and tachycardia
Circulatory overload	Excessive administration of IV fluid especially to patients with cardiac decompensation	Venous distention Dyspnea Tachycardia Hypertension Coughing Pulmonary edema Cyanosis Rales
Air embolism	Entrance of air into the vein (as little as 10 mL may be fatal)	Cyanosis Hypotension Weak rapid pulse Elevated central venous pressure Unconsciousness
Phlebitis	Administration of irritating fluid Prolonged use of the same vein	Redness Warmth Discomfort along the vein

Practice Procedure 4.1 (LO 4-4)

DRAWING UP MEDICATION FROM A VIAL

Demonstrate how to correctly draw up medication from a vial.

Equipment

Medication order (e.g., regular insulin 5 U subcutaneous)

Medication administration record, patient chart

Variety of syringes and needles with covers

Vial of medication (e.g., 100 U regular insulin in a multiple-dose vial); check the expiration date

Vials of sterile water for injection (for practice)

Antiseptic wipes or sponges

Sterile gauze

Procedure

1. Read the medication order and assemble the equipment. Check for the "seven rights" (discussed in detail in Chapter 5). Read the vial label by holding it next to the medication administration record or provider's order.

2. Wash your hands.

3. Select the proper-sized needle and syringe for the medication and the route (e.g., for subcutaneous injection of insulin, U100 insulin syringe and 25G, $\frac{5}{8}$-inch needle). If necessary, attach the needle to the syringe.

4. Check the vial label against the medication administration record a second time.

5. Remove the metal or plastic cap from the vial of insulin. If the vial has been opened previously, clean the rubber stopper by applying an antiseptic wipe in a circular motion.

6. Remove the needle cover (pull it straight off).

7. Inject air into the vial as follows:
   - Hold the syringe pointed upward at eye level. Pull back the plunger to take in a quantity of air equal to the ordered dose of medication (5 U in our insulin example).
   - Place the vial on a flat surface. Take care not to touch the rubber stopper.
   - Insert the needle through the center of the rubber stopper of the vial. Inject the air into the vial's air space by pushing in the plunger.

8. Invert the vial and withdraw the medication: Hold the vial and the syringe steady. Pull back on the plunger to withdraw the measured dose of medication. Measure accurately. Keep the tip of the needle below the surface of the liquid; otherwise, air will enter the syringe.

9. Check the syringe for air bubbles. Remove them by tapping sharply on the syringe. If you are using an air bubble to prevent tracking, add 0.2 mL of air to the syringe after measuring the dose accurately and expelling air bubbles.

10. Remove the needle from the vial. Replace the sterile needle cover.

11. Check the vial label against the medication administration record a third time.

12. Place the filled needle and syringe on a medicine tray or cart, with an antiseptic wipe and the medication administration record. The dose is now ready for injection.

13. Return multiple-dose vials of insulin to the proper storage area (cabinet or refrigerator). Dispose of unused medication in a single-dose vial according to your agency's procedure. (Remember, disposal of a controlled substance must be witnessed and the proper forms signed.)

Practice Procedure 4.2 (LO 4-4)

DRAWING UP MEDICATION FROM AN AMPULE

Demonstrate how to correctly draw up medication from an ampule.

Equipment

Medication order (e.g., *Vistaril,* 25 mg IM stat)

Medication administration record, patient chart

Variety of syringes and needles with covers

Ampule of medication (e.g., 1-mL ampule of *Vistaril* containing 100 mg/mL); check the expiration date

Ampules of sterile water for injection (for practice)

Sterile gauze

Antiseptic wipes or sponges

Procedure

1. Read the medication order and assemble the equipment. Check for the "seven rights." Read the ampule label by holding it next to the medication administration record or provider's order.

2. Wash your hands.

3. Select the proper-sized needle and syringe for the medication and the route (e.g., 3-mL standard hypodermic syringe and 22G, $1\frac{1}{2}$-inch needle for intramuscular injection of *Vistaril*). If necessary, attach the needle to the syringe.

4. Check the ampule label against the medication administration record a second time.

5. Tap down any medication in the top of the ampule.

6. Place a small gauze pad around the neck of the ampule to protect your fingers from broken glass.

7. Snap the neck of the ampule quickly and firmly away from you.

8. Withdraw the medication. Insert the needle into the open end of the broken ampule. Check your agency policy to see if a filter needle is to be used for drawing up the medication. Do not let the needle touch the rim of the ampule; this contaminates the needle. The needle should be kept below the fluid level to prevent drawing up air. The ampule may be tipped to allow the fluid to accumulate in one corner of the ampule to facilitate drawing up all the medicine. Pull back on the plunger and remove a measured dose of medication. The ampule may be held right side up on a flat surface or inverted. Measure accurately. (If using the sample order of *Vistaril,* draw up 1.0 mL of the drug.)

9. Check the syringe for air bubbles. Remove them by tapping sharply on the syringe. Draw back on the plunger and then slowly push the plunger upward to expel air. Be careful not to eject any of the medicine.

10. If the syringe contains too much medicine, hold the syringe vertically with the needle tip up and slanted toward the sink. Slowly eject the excess medicine into the sink. Place the syringe vertically and recheck the dose.

11. If you used a filter needle, change the needle to the appropriate size. Replace the needle cover.

12. Check the ampule label against the medicine administration record a third time.

13. Place the filled needle and syringe on a medicine tray or cart with an antiseptic wipe and the medication administration record. The dose is now ready for injection.

14. Discard the unused portion of the ampule according to your agency's procedure. Most facilities require broken ampules to be placed in the sharps container.

Practice Procedure 4.3 (LO 4-5)

ADMINISTERING AN INTRADERMAL INJECTION

Demonstrate the safe administration of an intradermal injection.

Equipment

Medication order for an intradermal preparation (e.g., Mantoux test for tuberculosis)

Medication administration record

Vial or ampule of medication for intradermal injection; check the expiration date

Sterile needle, 26G, $\frac{3}{8}$ inch with cover

Sterile tuberculin syringe

Sterile antiseptic wipes, gloves

Medicine tray

Puncture-resistant container for disposal of contaminated materials

Plastic arm for practice injections

Procedure

1. Read the medication order and check for the "seven rights."

2. Assemble equipment and prepare the injection. Use sterile technique and measure accurately.

3. Identify the patient, following agency policy. Explain what you are going to do. Wear gloves.

4. Assist the patient into a comfortable position that allows access to the injection site (lower inner arm, upper back, or upper chest).

5. Inspect the injection site. Inject only into healthy skin free of rash, redness, or lumps.

6. Cleanse the site with an antiseptic wipe and allow it to dry.

7. With the nondominant hand, spread the skin over the site with forefinger or thumb.

8. With the dominant hand, hold the needle at a 5- to 15-degree angle to the skin surface. Insert the needle slowly until resistance is felt. Advance the needle to a depth of $\frac{1}{8}$ inch below the skin. The needle tip can be seen under the skin. Do not aspirate.

9. Inject the medication slowly and fully. It is normal to feel resistance. If you do not meet resistance, the needle is too deep and you should remove the needle and restart the procedure. You should see a small blister or bleb, approximately 6 mm or $\frac{1}{2}$ inch, form just under the skin while injecting medication. The bleb means the medication is deposited in the dermis.

10. Withdraw the needle and apply an alcohol swab or gauze to support the tissues. There is some evidence that discomfort may arise with alcohol, and a dry gauze may be preferred. Do not massage the tissues. Massaging the tissues may cause the medicine to disperse into underlying tissues and alter the test results.

11. Dispose of the uncapped syringe in a puncture-resistant and leakproof container.

12. Remove gloves.

13. Stay with the patient and observe for allergic reaction. A severe allergic reaction is characterized by wheezing, shortness of breath, tightness or swelling in the mouth and throat, and circulatory collapse.

14. Chart the medication.

15. Draw a circle around the perimeter of the injection site with a pencil and return in 48 to 72 hours after the injection to evaluate the patient's response to the medication.

Practice Procedure 4.4 (LO 4-5)

ADMINISTERING A SUBCUTANEOUS INJECTION

Demonstrate the safe administration of a subcutaneous injection.

Equipment

Medication order for a subcutaneous preparation

Medication administration record

Vial or ampule of medication prepared for subcutaneous injection; check the expiration date

Sterile needle, 25G, $\frac{5}{8}$ inch or 27G, $\frac{1}{2}$ to 1 inch with cover

Sterile antiseptic wipes, gloves

Medicine tray

Puncture-resistant container for disposal of contaminated materials

Plastic mannequin or arm for practice injections

Procedure

1. Read the medication order and check for the "seven rights."

2. Assemble equipment and prepare the injection. Use sterile technique and measure accurately.

3. Identify the patient following agency policy. Explain what you are going to do. Wear gloves.

4. Assist the patient into a comfortable position that allows access to the injection site (outer upper arm, upper back, anterior thigh).

5. Inspect the injection site. If rash or redness is present, chart and report to your supervisor and do not give the injection. If lumps are present, inject at least 1 inch away or choose another site.

6. Cleanse the site with an antiseptic wipe and allow it to dry. Secure the wipe between your third and fourth fingers for later use.

7. With the nondominant hand, spread the skin tightly or pinch the skin and subcutaneous tissue between the thumb and finger. For an obese patient, pinch the skin at the site and insert the needle at a 90-degree angle. Obese patients have a fatty layer of tissue above subcutaneous tissue.

8. With the dominant hand, insert the needle at a 45-degree angle to the skin, bevel side up. Insert the needle quickly and smoothly.

9. Use the dominant hand to stabilize the syringe. Be careful not to move the needle from side to side.

10. Aspirate by pulling back on the plunger. If no blood appears, proceed with the injection. If blood appears, prepare a new injection with fresh equipment and move to another site. *Never* aspirate with anticoagulants such as heparin.

11. Inject the medication slowly. Push the plunger all the way in to inject the full dose.

12. Withdraw the needle quickly, firming the skin with the antiseptic wipe held near the needle. Pull out the needle at the same angle (45 or 90 degrees) at which it was inserted.

13. Do not massage the site after injecting insulin or heparin. Massaging the site after heparin causes bleeding and after insulin increases absorption of the insulin.

14. Dispose of the uncapped syringe in a puncture-proof container.

15. Chart the medication: name, dosage, route, site, and time.

16. Observe the patient frequently (or as ordered) to be sure that the medication is working and there are no adverse reactions. Subcutaneous injections usually take 30 minutes or more to absorb. Instruct the patient in any necessary self-care, and advise the patient to rest quietly for at least a few minutes.

Practice Procedure 4.5 (LO 4-5)

ADMINISTERING AN INTRAMUSCULAR INJECTION

Demonstrate the safe administration of an intramuscular injection.

Note: This procedure is for use on the average adult.

Equipment

Medication order for aqueous intramuscular preparation

Medication administration record

Vial or ampule of medication prepared for intramuscular injection; check the expiration date

Sterile needle, 22G, $1\frac{1}{2}$ inches with cover (1-inch size for the deltoid site)

Sterile syringe, size $2\frac{1}{2}$ to 3 mL

Sterile antiseptic wipes, gloves

Medicine tray

Puncture-resistant container for disposal of contaminated materials

Plastic mannequin for practice injections and standard injection procedure

Procedure

1. Read the medication order and check for the "seven rights."

2. Assemble equipment and prepare the injection. Add a 0.2-mL air bubble to the syringe after measuring the medication if this method is used in your health facility.

3. Identify the patient following health facility policy. Explain what you are going to do. Wear gloves.

4. Assist the patient into a comfortable position that allows access to the injection site (dorsogluteal, ventrogluteal, deltoid, or vastus lateralis).

5. Inspect the injection site for signs of redness, rash, or lumps. If rash or redness is present, chart and report to your supervisor and do not give the injection. If a lump is present, make the injection at least 1 inch away or choose another site.

6. Cleanse the site with an antiseptic wipe. Start cleansing at the center of the site and rotate outward in a circular motion for up to 2 inches.

7. With the nondominant hand, spread the skin taut between two fingers.

8. With the dominant hand, hold the needle at a 90-degree angle to the skin, bevel side up. Insert the needle quickly and smoothly, with a firm thrust.

9. Release the taut skin and use this hand to steady the inserted needle and syringe. Be careful not to move the needle from side to side.

10. Aspirate, using your free hand to pull back on the plunger. If no blood appears, proceed with the injection. If blood appears, prepare a new injection with fresh equipment and move to another site.

11. Inject the medication slowly. Push the plunger all the way in to inject the full dose.

12. Withdraw the needle quickly, firming the skin with the antiseptic wipe held near the needle. Pull out at the same 90-degree angle at which the needle entered.

13. Do not massage the injection site. Massaging the injection site causes underlying tissue damage.

14. Dispose of the uncapped syringe in a puncture-resistant container.

15. Remove gloves.

16. Chart the medication.

17. Return to the patient in 10 to 30 minutes to evaluate the effects of the medication.

Summary

Learning Outcome	Summary Points
4-1 Describe the major routes, sites, and procedures of injectable medications.	• *Intradermal (ID):* administered into the skin. • *Subcutaneous (subcut):* administered into the fatty tissues. • *Intramuscular (IM):* administered deep into the body tissues. • *Intravenous (IV):* administered through a vein.
4-2 Use Standard Precautions.	• Under Standard Precautions, all patients are considered potentially infectious with blood-borne pathogens. Precautions apply to infections caused by blood, body fluids, nonintact skin, and mucous membranes.

Learning Outcome	Summary Points
4-3 Identify the parts of a syringe needle and the sizes of needles while identifying doses.	• The *parts of a syringe* include the barrel and plunger. • *The parts of the needle* are the bevel, point, lumen, shaft, hilt, gauge number, and hub. • Insulin syringes come in U25, U30, U50, or U100. The most common standard syringe is the 3 cc or mL; 5-cc to 50-cc syringes are also available. The most common needles used are 19, 20, 21, 23, and 25 gauge.
4-4 Draw up medications from vials and ampules, and reconstitute medications.	• When administering a medication *from a vial,* inject measured air into the vial and then invert the vial and withdraw the desired amount of medicine. • When drawing up a medication *from an ampule,* place a small gauze around the neck of the ampule and snap the neck of the ampule. Withdraw the desired amount of medication. No air is added to an ampule. • Liquid is added to a powder in a vial and reconstituted into a solution or suspension.
4-5 Identify the most common injection sites for intradermal, subcutaneous, and intramuscular administration.	• *Intradermal* injections are administered in the skin on the inner surface of the lower arm, in the upper chest area, and on the back between the shoulder blades. • The sites for *subcutaneous* injection are the outer upper arm, the front of the thigh, the abdomen, and the upper back below the shoulder blades. • Four *intramuscular* sites include the dorsogluteal sites, ventrogluteal sites, deltoid site, and vastus lateralis. • For an *intradermal* injection, spread the skin over the site with the forefinger or thumb. Hold the needle at a 5- to 15-degree angle to the skin surface with the dominant hand. Insert the needle slowly until resistance is felt. Advance the needle to a depth of $\frac{1}{8}$ inch below the skin. Avoid aspirating and watch for a bleb. • For a *subcutaneous* injection, with the nondominant hand, spread the skin tightly or pinch the skin between the thumb and the finger. With the dominant hand, insert the needle at a 45-degree angle to the skin, bevel side up. After inserting the needle, aspirate and inject the medicine. • For an *intramuscular* injection, with the nondominant hand, spread the skin taut between two fingers. With the dominant hand, hold the needle at a 90-degree angle to the skin, bevel side up. Insert the needle with a firm thrust. Aspirate and then inject the medicine slowly.
4-6 Identify the various types of intravenous solutions, indications, advantages, disadvantages, and signs and symptoms of complications.	• *Crystalloids* are electrolytes such as isotonic, hypotonic, or hypertonic solutions. • *Isotonic solutions* remain constant within the intravascular space and are administered in hypotension. • *Hypotonic solutions* lower serum osmolarity and are used for hydration. • *Hypertonic solutions* raise serum osmolarity and are used for saline replacement. • *Colloid solutions* consist of albumin, dextran, plasmanate, ethoxylated amylopectin (*Hetastarch*), and artificial blood substitute. • *Hydrating solutions* supply supplemental calories or nutrients. • *Hypertonic-hyperosmolar preparations* are given to patients unable to ingest calories to meet metabolic needs. • *Blood components* are life-sustaining constituents. • *D5W* is an isotonic intravenous solution used to replace water losses in dehydration, for hypernatremia, or as a diluent for medication administration. • *0.45% NaCl* is a hypertonic solution used in ketoacidosis. It also provides free water, sodium, and chloride replacement.

- *Advantages of intravenous therapy:*
  1. Provides the fastest route of absorption.
- *Disadvantages of intravenous therapy:*
  1. Discomfort for the patient from the repeated sticks and certain medications.
  2. May cause an instantaneous reaction that could be fatal.
- Signs and symptoms of complications of intravenous therapy:
  - *Local infiltration:* edema at the IV site, no blood when the IV bag is lowered below the heart, discomfort at the site, slowing or stoppage of the flow.
  - *Pyrogenic reaction:* temperature elevation, severe chills 30 minutes after starting the IV, backache, headache, malaise, nausea, vomiting.
  - *Speed shock:* syncope, shock.
  - *Thrombophlebitis:* pain along the course of the vein, redness and edema at the IV site; with severe reaction: fever, malaise, and tachycardia.
  - *Circulatory overload:* venous distention, dyspnea, tachycardia, hypertension, coughing, pulmonary edema, cyanosis, rales.
  - *Air embolism:* cyanosis, hypotension, weak rapid pulse, unconsciousness.
  - *Phlebitis:* redness, warmth, discomfort along the vein.

Chapter 4 Review

Define each of the terms listed.

1. (LO 4-2) Standard Precautions _____

2. (LO 4-5) Aspirate _____

3. (LO 4-3) Viscous _____

4. (LO 4-3) Aqueous _____

5. (LO 4-6) Intravenous therapy _____

Answer the questions in the space provided.

6. (LO 4-3) Identify the parts of a syringe and needle on the drawings.

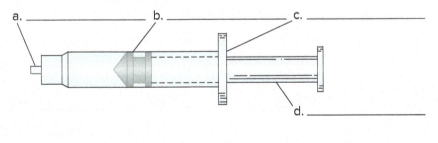

a. _____ b. _____ c. _____

d. _____

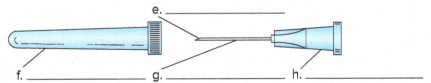

e. _____

f. _____ g. _____ h. _____

7. (LO 4-3) These syringes are filled with measured amounts of medication. Tell the exact dose in each.

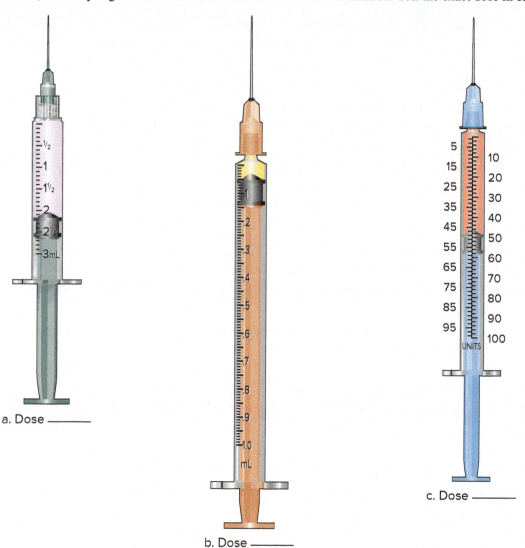

a. Dose _____

b. Dose _____

c. Dose _____

8. (LO 4-3) In question 7, name the type of syringe shown in each case.

a. _____ c. _____

b. _____

9. (LO 4-5) Summarize what you have learned about parenteral routes and equipment by filling in the blanks in the table.

	Intradermal	Subcutaneous	Intramuscular
a. Injected into (name tissue layer)	_____	_____	_____
b. Type of syringe	_____	_____	_____
		or _____	
c. Needle length	_____	_____	_____
d. Needle gauge	_____	_____	_____
			_____
e. Angle of entry	_____	_____	_____

10. (LO 4-1) List at least three reasons that a provider might order a drug to be given by the parenteral route.

_____

_____

_____

11. (LO 4-5) What does it mean to aspirate before injecting medication? Why is this done?

_____

_____

12. (LO 4-5) What should you do if you see blood in the syringe when you aspirate?

_____

_____

13. (LO 4-6) List five classifications of intravenous solutions.

_____

_____

_____

_____

_____

14. (LO 4-6) Name two indications for intravenous therapy.

_____

_____

15. (LO 4-6) List three symptoms of a phlebitis.

_____

_____

_____

Match sites of injection to routes of injection.

16. _____ (LO 4-5) Anterior thigh, upper outer arm, abdomen, upper back under shoulder blades

17. _____ (LO 4-5) Vastus lateralis, deltoid, dorsogluteal, ventrogluteal

18. _____ (LO 4-5) Inner lower arm, upper chest, upper back under shoulder blades

19. _____ (LO 4-6) Veins of arms and legs

a. intramuscular

b. intravenous

c. intradermal

d. subcutaneou

Complete the statements by filling in the blanks.

20. (LO 4-5) Injections in the buttock area must be placed very carefully to avoid the gluteal arteries and

the _____ nerve.

21. (LO 4-5) When you are holding the needle and syringe at the proper angle to the skin, the bevel should be

facing _____ (*down* or *up*).

22. (LO 4-4) Before drawing up a measured amount of medication from a vial, inject an equal amount of

_____ into the vial.

23. (LO 4-4) The neck of an ampule must be _____ before use.

24. (LO 4-4) After reconstituting a powdered drug in a multiple-dose vial, write the _____,

_____, and _____ on the label.

25. (LO 4-6) Hypertonic solutions cause fluids to be pulled out of the _____ and

_____ compartments into the blood vessels, raising serum osmolarity.

Place a T in the blank if the statement is true. Place an F in the blank if the statement is false.

_____ 26. (LO 4-6) The most common hypertonic intravenous solution is 0.45% NaCl.

_____ 27. (LO 4-6) Potassium chloride is a medication that may be irritating to the vein when infused intravenously.

_____ 28. (LO 4-3) Dispose of injection equipment into a puncture-resistant container.

_____ 29. (LO 4-6) Lactated Ringer's solution is administered with burns and gastrointestinal losses.

_____ 30. (LO 4-6) Circulatory overload occurs when too much of an IV solution is administered.

Multiple Choice—Circle the correct letter.

31. (LO 4-6) A patient with an intravenous solution has edema at the IV site. What complication of IV therapy do you suspect?
   a. Speed shock
   b. Air embolism
   c. Pyrogenic reaction
   d. Local infiltration

32. (LO 4-6) 0.45% NaCl has been hung for which of the following conditions?
   a. Hypotonic dehydration
   b. Calorie replacement
   c. Gastric fluid loss due to nasogastric suctioning or vomiting
   d. Hypernatremia

33. (LO 4-5) What drug must you administer by Z-track intramuscular injection?
   a. Iron dextran
   b. Meperidine (*Demerol*)
   c. Enoxaparin (*Lovenox*)
   d. Cobalamin (vitamin B_{12})

34. (LO 4-5) It is critical that you do what after the administration of penicillin?
   a. Administer an increased fluid intake
   b. Take the patient's blood pressure
   c. Observe and stay with the patient
   d. Massage the area where the drug was administered

35. (LO 4-6) A patient develops redness and edema at the IV site. You should report this as which of the following?
   a. Circulatory overload
   b. Thrombophlebitis
   c. Air embolism
   d. Local infiltration

Chapter 4 Case Studies

36. (LO 4-4) You have been assigned to administer a reconstituted powdered drug. Why are reconstituted drugs stored in powder form? What should you reconstitute the powdered drug with? After adding fluid to the vial, what must you do? _____

_____

_____

_____

37. (LO 4-6) You are caring for a patient who has an intravenous solution that you determine has infiltrated. What is the cause of an infiltration? What are the symptoms of an infiltration? What should you do when you discover an IV has infiltrated? What is the usual treatment? _____

_____

_____

_____

Critical Thinking

Answer the following questions in the spaces provided.

38. (LO 4-5) Review the 11 general steps in any injection procedure. Then write them here (from memory, if possible).

_____

_____

_____

_____

_____

_____

39. (LO 4-1) List the local reactions that can occur following injections.

_____

_____

40. (LO 4-5) What should you do if the injection site you have chosen is covered with a rash?

_____

_____

41. (LO 4-5) How do practice and attitude affect your ability to give injections?

_____

_____

42. (LO 4-6) What should you do when your patient spikes a temperature of 102°F and complains of severe chills after an IV is started? _____

_____

_____

Applications

Obtain an electronic drug guide, a current copy of the *PDR*®, or a drug reference book. Use it to answer the questions that follow about a broad-spectrum antibiotic.

43. What is the generic name of *Fortaz*? _____

44. Name two strains of bacteria that this drug can affect. _____

_____

_____

45. Give the usage and indications of this drug. _____

_____

_____

_____

_____

46. When is *Fortaz* contraindicated? _____

_____

_____

MEDICATION THERAPY

LEARNING OUTCOMES

5-1 Describe the various forms of medication, ranging from liquids to solids, and their abbreviations.

5-2 Describe the routes for administering medications.

5-3 Describe the routes of administration of medication and their abbreviations, administration times including use of the military clock, types of drug orders, and general medical terms.

5-4 Carry out setting up medications following proper procedures.

5-5 Explain the rules for giving medications, identifying parts of a medication label, and utilizing single-dose packaging.

5-6 Describe the problem-oriented medical record and the subjective-objective-assessment-plan method of charting and how the medication record is used to communicate a medication order.

5-7 Carry out accurate, complete, and organized charting.

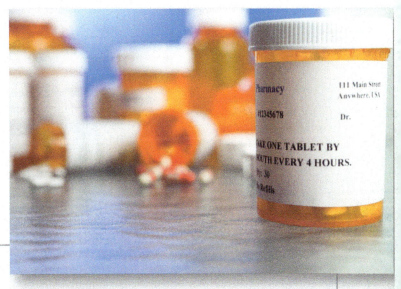

©fstop123/Getty Images

In this chapter you will learn about various forms of medications and the routes by which they are administered. You will learn how to translate medication orders so that you can give medications in the proper form at the correct time and by the right route. You will learn how to do the routine tasks involved in giving medications: how to order, store, and dispose of drugs; how to keep track of medication orders; how to set up medications; and how to chart medications after giving them. You will learn how to read and interpret medication labels. You will also learn how to give drugs safely by following the basic rules of medication administration.

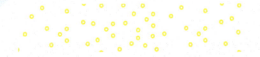

active ingredient

automated medication dispensing
system

computerized order

controlled substances

enteric-coated

expiration date

facsimile order

incident report

infusion

inhalation

insertion

instillation

irrigation

medication administration record
(MAR)

outpatient

pharmacy requisition form

PRN order

phone order

problem-intervention-evaluation
(PIE)

problem-oriented medical record
(POMR)

routine order

standing order

stat order

subjective-objective-assessment-
plan (SOAP)

verbal order

FORMS OF MEDICATION [LO 5-1]

Drugs are mixed with various ingredients to make them suitable for patients. There are ingredients to make oral medicines taste good. Older adults as well as young patients take these medications more easily. There are ingredients to thin out a drug mixture so that the dosage can be controlled. Other ingredients allow drugs to be applied on the skin or placed into body parts, such as the eyes, ears, or rectum. These combinations of drugs with various ingredients are called drug preparations or products.

Different forms of drugs are appropriate for different routes of administration, so it is important to use the correct form. Failure to administer the drug in the correct form results in medication error. Using an incorrect form can also cause damage to body cells. Therefore, you need to learn about the various drug preparations and their uses. Medication forms are classified as liquids, semiliquids, semisolids, and solids. **Table 5.1** lists medication forms and their abbreviations.

Liquids and Semiliquids

Many drugs are administered in liquid form. They may be given by mouth, rubbed onto the skin, or dropped into eyes, ears, or other parts of the body. Liquid preparations are useful because they allow rapid absorption of the drug. Liquid oral medicines are especially convenient for children and older adult patients who have trouble swallowing solid capsules or tablets.

Some drugs are soluble, or able to dissolve in liquids, and others are not. When **active ingredients** are mixed with water, alcohol, or both, the resulting preparations are either solutions or suspensions. In solutions, the drug is completely dissolved in alcohol or water. In suspensions, the drug is incapable of completely dissolving, and tiny particles or droplets of the drug are held, or suspended, throughout the liquid.

If suspensions are left standing for a while, particles settle to the bottom of the bottle (oils rise to the top). The clear liquid portion is then visible. This situation is normal and can be corrected by shaking the bottle well before giving the medication (**Figure 5.1**). Solutions, on the other hand, rarely separate when left standing. If they do, it is because they have been stored improperly or are past the **expiration date** for safe usage. Separated solutions must be discarded.

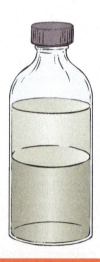

Figure 5.1

A medication that is in the form of a suspension should be shaken before administering.

Table 5.1 Medication Forms and Abbreviations

Classification	Forms	Abbreviations	Examples
Liquid	Solution Syrup Fluidextract Spirits Elixir Fluid	soln. syr. fld. ext. sp. elix. fl.	Normal saline *Robitussin AC* cough syrup Vanilla extract Spirits of peppermint *Dexamethasone* elixir IV solutions
Semiliquid	Tincture	tinct., tr.	Tincture of iodine
Solid	Capsule Tablet	cap., caps. tab.	*Amoxicillin* *Lanoxin*
Semisolid	Suppository Ointment	supp. oint.	*Ducolax Suppository* *Petroleum jelly*
Suspension	Emulsion Magma Gel Liniment Lotion Aerosol	no abbreviations	Cod liver oil Milk of magnesia *Gelusil* *BenGay Greaseless* *Caladryl Clear* *Proventil HFA*

Within the broad categories of solutions and suspensions, there are several specific liquid forms of medication. Tinctures, fluidextracts, elixirs, spirits, and syrups are all types of solutions. Emulsions, magmas, gels, and lotions are types of suspensions.

Solutions

Tinctures, fluidextracts, elixirs, and spirits are highly concentrated forms of drugs. They contain much higher amounts of drug per unit of liquid than do other liquid forms. Therefore, the dose is smaller. These preparations must be measured carefully, using a dropper or a medicine glass. The medicine may be added to water, juice, or another solution suggested by the provider. The patient then drinks this mixture. These mixtures should never be injected.

 Caution Solutions with Alcohol

Tinctures, fluidextracts, elixirs, and spirits contain alcohol. Do not administer them to a diagnosed alcoholic or a patient with diabetes. Storage is important with these alcohol solutions. They must be kept tightly stoppered so that the alcohol cannot evaporate. Store them in a dark place, as stated on the labels. Otherwise, the drug may separate from the alcohol. If this should happen, do not use the preparation. Order another preparation from the pharmacy.

Tinctures. Tinctures are solutions made with alcohol or alcohol with water. The active ingredients make up 10 to 20 percent of the solution. Tinctures are potent drugs. Examples are tincture of iodine, a strong antiseptic; belladonna tincture, an anticholinergic used to decrease intestinal motility; and camphorated opium tincture, commonly known as paregoric, an antidiarrheal.

Fluidextracts. Fluidextracts are alcohol extracts from plant sources. They are the most concentrated and potent of any liquid preparation. An example is Vanilla extract fluidextract, used as a laxative.

Elixirs. Elixirs are solutions of alcohol and water containing 10 to 20 percent of a drug. Elixirs have special added ingredients to make them sweet-tasting and pleasant-smelling. Because they have a sweet taste, they are better tolerated by children and older adults. Phenobarbital elixir, an anticonvulsant, and diphenhydramine (*Benadryl Allergy*) elixir, an antihistamine, are examples.

Spirits. Spirits are alcohol solutions of volatile oils, or oils that evaporate. An example is peppermint spirit, used to remove excess gas from the gastrointestinal tract. Spirits contain 5 to 20 percent active ingredients.

Syrups. Syrups are heavy solutions of water and sugar, usually with a flavoring added to disguise the unpleasant taste of the drug. They may be as much as 85 percent sugar. They are mixed with a very small amount of a drug. Examples include cough syrups, such as guaifenesin (*Robitussin AC*).

Suspensions

Emulsions, magmas, and gels are given in small amounts because they contain large portions of active drug ingredients, the ingredients that produce the therapeutic effects. Suspensions must be shaken before use.

Emulsions. Emulsions are suspensions of oils and fats in water with an emulsifying agent. Cod liver oil (a laxative) is an example. Emulsions separate into layers with time and need to be shaken before use.

Magmas. A magma contains heavy particles mixed with water that forms a milky liquid. Magmas must be shaken prior to administration. Milk of magnesia (a laxative) is a familiar example of a magma.

Gels. Gels are similar to magmas, but they contain finer particles. An example is *Gelusil* (an antacid).

Liniments. Liniments are liquid suspensions. They are rubbed onto the skin to promote absorption. For example, *BenGay Greaseless* applied to the skin produces a feeling of heat to the area to relieve pain and swelling.

Lotions. Lotions are suspensions of drugs in a water base for external use. Lotions are patted onto the skin rather than rubbed in. They may be protective, emollient (soothing and softening to overcome dryness), astringent (vasoconstricting), or antipruritic (to relieve itching). Lotions tend to settle out and must be shaken before use. *Caladryl Clear* lotion is a common example used for its protective, astringent, and antipruritic effects for poison ivy.

Aerosols. Aerosol medications are commonly delivered by oral inhalers that allow for rapid absorption into the bloodstream (Figure 5.2). An example is albuterol (*Proventil HFA*), a bronchodilator used in the treatment of obstructive airway disease such as asthma.

Solids and Semisolids

Solid forms of drugs are widely used in drug treatment. Except for powders, there is no mixing, shaking, and measuring to be done, as there is with many liquids. The solid forms are also a convenient way to take unpleasant-tasting or irritating drugs.

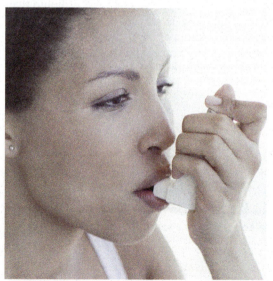

©Sam Edwards/age fotostock

Figure 5.2

Oral inhaler.

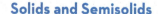

Ointments. Ointments are drugs mixed in lanolin, a fine oil taken from the skin of sheep, or in petrolatum, a jelly made from petroleum. They are usually applied to skin surfaces, but some ointments can be placed into the eyes. Eye ointments must always bear the label "Sterile—for ophthalmic use."

Pastes. Pastes are semisolid preparations that are thicker and absorbed more slowly than ointments. They are used for skin protection. An example is zinc oxide paste.

Powders. Powders are fine, dry particles of drugs. They may be dissolved in liquids or used as is, depending on the provider's orders. Powders have both internal and external uses. An example is *GoLytely*, which is mixed with water or juice and swallowed as a bowel evacuant.

Tablets. Tablets are drug powders that have been pressed or molded into small disks. They are designed to be swallowed with a drink of water. Tablets come in a variety of sizes, shapes, and weights. Some have colored coatings and flavorings and are stamped or printed with the name of the manufacturer. Tablets may be scored, which allows for breakage into halves.

Capsules. A capsule is a gelatin sheath that contains one dose of medication. The drug inside the capsule can be either a powder, an oil, or a liquid. When the capsule is swallowed, the gelatin quickly dissolves and releases the medicine into the stomach.

Caplets. Caplets are identical to capsules in size and shape but have the consistency of a tablet.

Sustained-Release Tablets and Capsules. These medication forms contain several doses of a drug. The doses have special coatings that dissolve at different rates so that medicine is released into the stomach gradually. Some doses are released immediately. Others are released up to 12 hours later. Sustained-release tablets and capsules allow drug effects to continue at the same level over a long period. *Delayed release* and *timed release* are other terms used to describe these products. An example is diltiazem (*Cardizem SR*), a calcium channel blocker used in the treatment of chest pain and high blood pressure. See **Figure 5.3**.

Enteric-Coated Tablets and Capsules. These are tablets and capsules with a special coating that keeps them from dissolving in the acid secretions of the stomach. They do not dissolve until they reach the alkaline secretions of the intestine. The **enteric coating** prevents an irritating drug from upsetting the stomach. It also prevents the stomach juices from interacting with the drug to change its effect. An example is *Ecotrin,* a nonnarcotic analgesic used for pain, an antipyretic used for fever, and a nonsteroidal anti-inflammatory used in the treatment of arthritis. See **Figure 5.4**.

Troches and Lozenges. Troches and lozenges are tablets designed to dissolve in the mouth rather than be swallowed. They may be flat, round, or rectangular and are used for their local effects. They contain a high concentration of a drug in a sugar base that comes into contact with the mouth and throat as they dissolve. They can help relieve pain or soothe irritation in those areas.

Suppositories. Suppositories are drugs mixed with a firm base, such as cocoa butter, that melts at body temperature. The drug mixture is molded into a shape suitable for insertion into the vagina, urethra, or rectum. After insertion, the suppository dissolves against the warm mucous membranes of these openings and releases the drug. The active ingredients take effect locally or are absorbed into the bloodstream for systemic effects. An example of a vaginal suppository is miconazole nitrate (*Monistat 7*), an antifungal used for vaginal fungal infection. An example of a rectal suppository is bisacodyl (*Dulcolax Suppository*), a laxative used for relief of constipation.

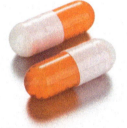

©MirageC/Getty Images

Figure 5.3

Sustained-release capsule; often called a spansule.

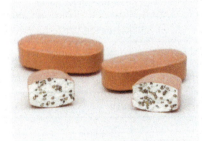

©Pornthip Chukitkosol/Shutterstock

Figure 5.4

Enteric-coated tablet. The tablet has been split for visualization only. Enteric-coated tablets should never be split when given to patients.

Caution Sustained-Release Tablets and Capsules

Never crush, open, or empty a sustained-release tablet or capsule into food or liquid. Using sustained-release medication in this way can cause the patient to receive an overdose.

 Patient Education Enteric-Coated Tablets

- Explain what signs to watch for to know if the drug is taking effect, because some patients' intestines are not able to dissolve a tablet's enteric coating.

- Do not crush or mix enteric-coated tablets and capsules into food or liquid, because this would destroy the enteric coating and cause the medication to be released in the stomach instead of the intestine.

ROUTES OF ADMINISTRATION [LO 5-2]

Drugs can be administered to patients through several methods or routes. Each route has its advantages and disadvantages. The route chosen depends on the type of medication, the dosage form, and the desired effects. Table 5.2 lists routes of administration and their abbreviations.

Oral

Oral administration means that a drug is given by mouth and swallowed, either alone or with a glass of liquid. The drug is then absorbed into the bloodstream through the lining of the stomach and intestine.

Oral administration is the easiest, safest, and most economical way for a patient to take medicine. However, it is also the slowest way for a drug to

Route	Meaning	Abbreviations
Buccal	Inside the cheek	buc
Intradermal	Into the skin	ID
Intramuscular	Into the muscle	IM
Intravenous	Into the vein	IV
Oral	By mouth	PO, p.o.
Rectal	By rectum	R
Subcutaneous	Under the skin (into fatty layer)	subcut
Sublingual	Under the tongue	subling, subl, SL
Topical	On the skin	No abbreviation
Vaginal	By vagina	vag

Table 5.2 Routes of Administration

reach the cells of the body. The drug can be broken down by enzymes in the digestive system. Its absorption can be affected by the presence of food. Irritating medicines may cause nausea and stomach discomfort. Nevertheless, the oral route is well accepted and often used in drug therapy. Oral medications are usually in liquid, tablet, or capsule form.

Sublingual

Sublingual administration means placing a drug under the tongue, where it dissolves in the patient's saliva. It is quickly absorbed through the mucous membrane that makes up the lining of the mouth. The patient is not permitted to drink or eat until all the medication is dissolved.

Compared to the oral route, the sublingual route has the advantage of faster absorption. It also yields a higher concentration of the drug in the blood, because the drug does not pass through the digestive system first. This is a convenient route as long as drugs are not irritating or bad-tasting.

Medications for sublingual administration are in the form of tablets. They are usually given for their systemic effects. Nitroglycerin, a drug that dilates heart vessels, is often administered sublingually.

Buccal

Buccal administration is similar to sublingual administration, except that the medication is placed in the mouth next to the cheek. The drug is absorbed through the mucous membrane that lines the inside of the cheek. Buccal medications are in the form of tablets. They should not be swallowed, and no food or drink is permitted until after they dissolve. Teach patients to alternate cheeks with each dose to avoid mucosal irritation. Clotrimazole oropharyngeal is indicated to treat oral candiasis and is administered buccally.

Topical

Topical administration is the method of applying a drug directly to the skin or mucous membrane, usually for a local effect. Medications such as nitroglycerin or estrogen may also be applied by disk or patch. The disk or patch contains the medicine, which is released into the skin. This route of administration has systemic effects. Drugs for topical use are often designed to soothe irritated tissues or to prevent or cure local infections. They are in the form of creams, liniments, lotions, ointments, and liquids. Liquids may be sprayed, swabbed, or painted onto the desired surfaces. Other forms are rubbed or patted on or held against the skin surface with a bandage. Absorption through the skin is slow, whereas absorption through mucous membranes is rapid.

Topical medications can be dropped into the eyes, ears, and nose (**instillation**), and they can be inserted into the vagina, urinary bladder, and rectum (**insertion**). Any of these areas may also be rinsed with water containing drugs (**irrigation**). These applications are easy to perform, but correct procedure must be followed to avoid damaging the tissue.

Rectal

Inserting medication into the rectum in the form of a suppository is called rectal administration. Enemas are also administered into the rectum. Absorption through the lining of the rectum is slow and irregular. However, this may be the best route when a patient cannot take medications orally. For example, a vomiting patient or an unconscious patient may require rectal administration.

Vaginal

The vaginal route of administration requires inserting a cream, foam, tablet, or suppository into the vagina. Medications inserted vaginally are usually given for their local effects, as in the treatment of a vaginal infection with miconazole (*Monistat 7*).

Inhalation

In **inhalation** administration, medicine is sprayed or inhaled into the nose, throat, and lungs. The drug is absorbed through the mucous membranes in the nose and throat or through the tiny air sacs that fill the lungs. Drugs to be inhaled are in the form of gases or fine droplets (sprays, mists, steam, etc.).

The lungs contain a large surface area, so there is good absorption. However, it is hard to regulate the dose. The inhalation method is not suitable for drugs that might irritate the lungs.

Inhalation is widely used for rapid treatment of asthma symptoms. An example of an inhalation drug is *Proventil HFA*. Special devices, such as inhalers, nebulizers, and atomizers, make inhalation therapy relatively convenient. Because microorganisms can easily enter the body through the lining of the lungs, the equipment used for inhalation therapy must be very clean.

Parenteral

Parenteral administration involves injecting a drug into the body with a needle and syringe. This method gives much more rapid absorption and distribution than oral administration. The dosage can also be carefully controlled. The parenteral route is especially useful in emergencies, when a drug effect is needed immediately.

There are several disadvantages to the parenteral route. All injection equipment and medicines must be sterile, or free of microorganisms. The method is expensive, sometimes painful, and awkward for patients to administer to themselves. Except for the intravenous route, there is the danger of injecting a drug incorrectly into a vein, which could cause serious harm and even death.

 Caution Laws for Administering Medications

Parenteral administration requires special training, special safety precautions, and special equipment. State regulations allow only certain licensed healthcare workers to administer medications parenterally: for example, nurses and nurse practitioners.

Medicine for injection must be in liquid form. Often it must be prepared as a suspension of a powder in distilled water.

The parenteral route is divided into four main categories, according to the location of the injection.

In intradermal administration, a small amount of medicine is injected just beneath the outer layer of skin. The dose is usually less than 0.3 mL. The injected drug forms a small bubble (bleb) under the skin. Intradermal injections are used in tuberculin tests, allergy tests, and vaccinations. The drug is absorbed slowly with this type of injection.

In the subcutaneous route, medication is injected into a layer of fatty tissue that lies right below the skin. This is called the subcutaneous (under the skin) tissue. The dose is approximately 1 to 2 mL. Insulin, hormones, and local anesthetics are among the medications administered by subcutaneous injection.

Figure 5.5

(a) IM injection sites;
(b) locating the ventrogluteal
site; (c) two ways to locate
the dorsogluteal site.

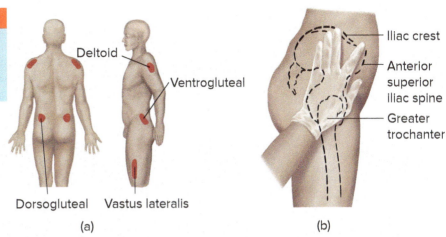

Deltoid

Ventrogluteal

Dorsogluteal   Vastus lateralis

(a)

Iliac crest

Anterior
superior
iliac spine

Greater
trochanter

(b)

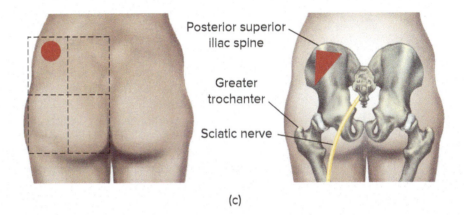

Posterior superior
iliac spine

Greater
trochanter

Sciatic nerve

(c)

Intramuscular administration is the injection of a drug deep into muscle
and administered at a 90-degree angle. Extreme caution must be used by
giving intramuscular injection in the dorsogluteal site. Improper site selection
can result in damage to the sciatica nerve or injection into the superior gluteal
artery or vein. Because the muscles are well supplied with blood, absorption
from the muscles is faster than absorption from the skin layers. Muscles can
also absorb a greater amount of fluid without discomfort to the patient; the
usual dose is 1 to 3 mL. The common sites for intramuscular administration
include dorsogluteal, vastus lateralis, ventrogluteal, and deltoid muscles
(Figure 5.5). Intramuscular injection is also preferred for substances that can
irritate the skin layers. Penicillin is often injected intramuscularly. The danger
of causing tissue damage is lessened because the injection is entering deep
into the muscle. There is, however, a risk of injecting the drug directly into
a vein. For example, if penicillin were injected into a vein, it could cause
serious side effects or prove fatal. During intramuscular administration, care
must be taken to inject only large, healthy muscles and to avoid injecting into
nerves, bones, and blood vessels.

Intravenous injection is a method for placing a sterile drug solution directly
into a vein. It is the most desirable route when a fast-acting medication is
needed quickly, as in emergency situations. However, introducing a drug
directly into a vein is the most dangerous method of administering drugs,
because there is no time to correct an error.

Intravenous injection differs from intravenous infusion, or IV drip, mainly
in speed of action. **Infusion** is the insertion of a tube or a needle into a vein
through which fluids are slowly added to the bloodstream over a period of
time. Infusion is used often in nursing care to keep the body's fluid level in
balance. Drugs can be added to IV fluids for a continuous drug effect. Or they

can be injected into the IV tube that leads into the vein, which is almost the same as injecting directly into the vein. This is called IV push.

Although there are other methods for administering drugs by the intravenous route, all drugs administered intravenously are administered only by a registered nurse, provider, or specially trained individual such as a paramedic.

Intracardiac, intra-arterial, intrathecal or intraspinal, and intraosseous are types of injections that only providers are permitted to perform. These methods are for injecting a drug into the heart muscle, into an artery, into the spinal spaces, or into a bone, respectively.

THE MEDICATION ORDER [LO 5-3]

When a provider tells a nurse or another healthcare worker which drug or drugs to administer to a patient, the provider is giving a medication order. It may be expressed in writing or verbally. It is preferable to give medication orders in writing. Ideally, orders should not be given verbally because of the possibility of error. When an order must be given verbally, as in an emergency situation, it should be written down and signed by the provider within 24 hours. Written orders are stated in a special book for doctors' orders or on a provider's order sheet in a patient's chart (Figure 5.6).

A prescription blank is used to write medication orders for patients who are being discharged from the hospital or who are seeing the provider in a medical office or clinic (Figure 5.7). These patients are called **outpatients**.

Providers are not the only healthcare professionals allowed to prescribe medicines. In many states, nurse practitioners, pharmacists, and provider assistants are permitted to prescribe. They prescribe drugs under the direct supervision of a provider with whom they work.

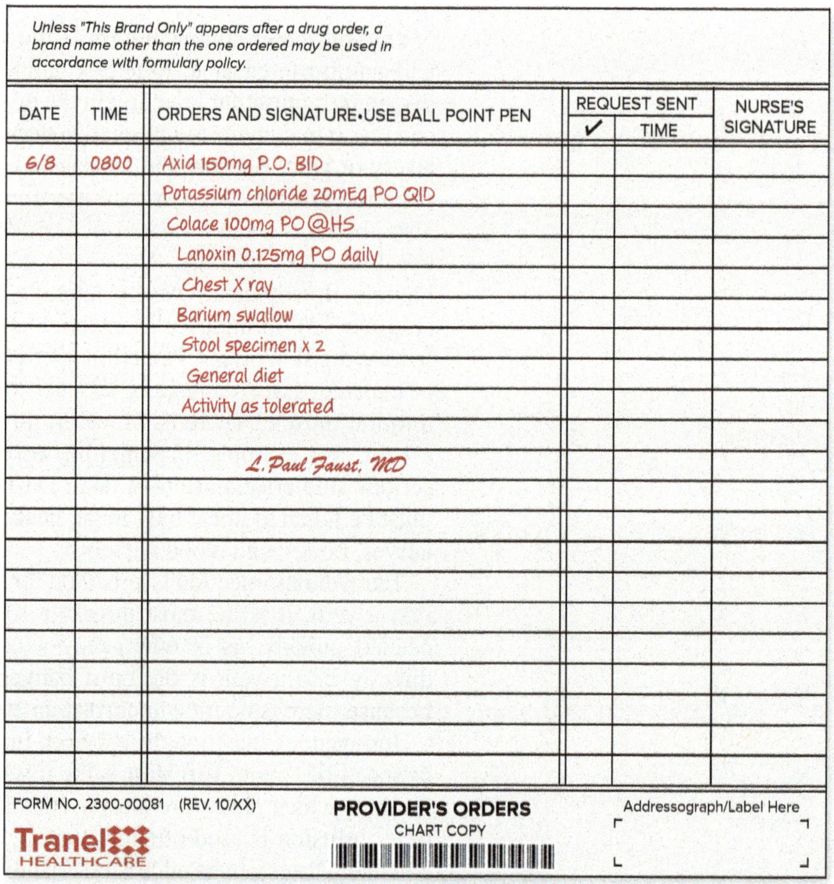

Figure 5.6

Provider's order sheet.

Unless "This Brand Only" appears after a drug order, a brand name other than the one ordered may be used in accordance with formulary policy.

DATE	TIME	ORDERS AND SIGNATURE•USE BALL POINT PEN	REQUEST SENT ✔	TIME	NURSE'S SIGNATURE
6/8	0800	Axid 150mg P.O. BID			
		Potassium chloride 20mEq PO QID			
		Colace 100mg PO @HS			
		Lanoxin 0.125mg PO daily			
		Chest X ray			
		Barium swallow			
		Stool specimen x 2			
		General diet			
		Activity as tolerated			
		L. Paul Faust, MD			

FORM NO. 2300-00081 (REV. 10/XX) **PROVIDER'S ORDERS** CHART COPY Addressograph/Label Here

Tranel HEALTHCARE

Figure 5.7

An outpatient prescription blank.

Tranel ▨
HEALTHCARE   1014862

JAHN MEMORIAL HOSPITAL   JAHN MEMORIAL HOSPITAL WEST

PATIENT'S
NAME _____ DATE _____

ADDRESS _____ AGE _____

℞

LABEL _____   ☐ GENERIC AND/OR EQUIVALENT ALLOWED.

REFILL _____

_____ _____ M.D.
Provider's Signature   (Print Provider's Name)

DEA NO. _____ ADDRESS _____
Form No. 01805308 (Rev. 2/XX)

Who is allowed to take down verbal orders differs according to each health facility's policies. Ask about your health facility's specific policies regarding the writing and receiving of medication orders. No medication is ever given without an order.

The medication order includes several important pieces of information. You, the healthcare worker, must read and understand all this information so that you may correctly prepare and administer the medication. The basic parts of a medication order include the patient's name, date, drug name, dosage, route of administration, time and frequency, provider's signature, quantity and number of refills, and, when the prescription is for a controlled substance, the provider's DEA number.

- *Patient's full name.* For proper identification, the patient's first and last names are needed. The patient's admission number is included in some health facilities. The patient's age should be included, especially if the dosage should be checked (e.g., for children and older adult patients).

- *Date of the order.* The day, month, and year are included. Often the time of day is also shown. This practice helps avoid confusion when the staff changes shifts. Most health facilities currently use military time, a 24-hour system, to avoid confusing a.m. and p.m. times that occur in the 12-hour system. For example, 9:15 a.m. would be written as 0915 hours, and 5:45 p.m. would be written as 1745 hours. **Figure 5.8** illustrates military time. In the figure, a.m. hours are numbered in the inner circle and p.m. hours in the outer circle. Using military time, the day begins at 0001 (12:01 a.m.) and ends at 2400 hours (12:00 midnight). The number of the hour is used with zeros as appropriate to indicate both hours and minutes; for example, 0600 (6 a.m.) and 2300 (11:00 p.m.).

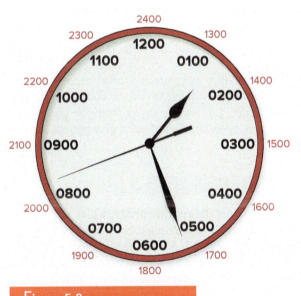

Figure 5.8

Military time—a 24-hour system.

- *Name of the drug.* On a prescription blank, the drug name is preceded by "Rx," which means "take thou." The drug's generic name or brand name is written out. For reasons of cost, it is becoming more common for providers to order drugs by their generic names. There may be a special line on the prescription blank for writing in the generic name or for indicating "may substitute generic drug." If a drug name is not familiar to you, consult a drug reference such as the *USP Drug Information for the Health Care Professional* or the *PDR®*.

- *Dosage.* This includes the amount of the drug and the strength of the preparation (e.g., two 100-mg tablets as opposed to 50-mg or 250-mg tablets).

- *Route of administration.* The specified route is important because some medicines can be given by several different routes. If no special route is ordered, notify your supervisor so that the provider may be called to identify the correct route of administration. Never assume that a medication is administered by a certain route. Accuracy is essential.

- *Time and frequency.* Both the time to administer the drug and how often must be clearly stated (e.g., BID for 10 days).

- *Provider's signature.* Without the signature of the provider, the medication order is not legal. When a nurse or another staff member must take an order by phone, the nurse signs the order, and the provider co-signs it within 24 hours. When a provider prescribes drugs for clinic outpatients or private patients, the medication order also includes the number of refills and the quantity.

- *Number of refills and quantity.* Some drugs, especially Schedule II drugs, may not be refilled without another prescription. For other drugs, the order may show a certain number of refills, ranging from no refills to PRN (as needed). No prescription or refill is good for more than 1 year. The medication label shows the number of refills following the Latin word *repetatur,* meaning "repeat." Outpatient prescriptions must specify the quantity of the drug to be dispensed to the patient (e.g., 30 tabs).

- *Provider's DEA number.* This registration number from the Drug Enforcement Administration is required on all prescriptions for controlled substances.

State laws and health facility policies regulate who may carry out the routine responsibilities in medication administration. Check the policy manual of your health facility to find out who may calculate and measure doses; set up and administer medications; transcribe medication orders; count and handle controlled substances; order, reorder, and receive drugs from the pharmacy; observe patients and chart progress; report to the provider; give patients health instruction; and so on.

TYPES OF DRUG ORDERS [LO 5-3]

The most common type of drug order is the **routine order**, which means that the ordered drug is administered until a discontinuation order is written or until a specified termination date is reached. Some agencies use automatic stop dates, which are a means to force the provider to reevaluate a patient's medication schedule and either continue current medications or change them, based on the patient's condition.

Another type of order is the **standing order**, which outlines a specific condition in which a drug is to be administered. Standing orders are written and signed by the provider in charge of a patient's care before the drugs are needed. They are frequently used in critical care units, where a patient's condition changes rapidly and immediate action is required, such as administration of a certain drug for an irregular heartbeat. Standing orders are also used in long-term care facilities where a provider is not readily available; for example, "Give *Tylenol* 500 mg PO q 4 hrs for temperature of 101°F or above."

A **PRN order** is an order written by the provider for a drug to be given when a patient needs it. The majority of drugs written as PRN orders are pain medications; for example, "*Demerol* 75 mg IM q 3–4 hrs for incisional pain." A single (one-time) order is an order to be given only once at a specified time. These orders are frequently written for preoperative drugs or drugs to be given before diagnostic procedures. An example is "*Valium* 10 mg PO at 0700." A **stat order** is a single order that is administered immediately. Stat orders are usually written for emergencies when a patient's condition suddenly changes; for example, "Give amiodarone 150 mg IV over 10 minutes stat."

A **verbal order** is one expressed orally and not written down. It may be a frequent way of giving a medication order in the provider's office. It is essential that you write down exactly what is said. It is also safe practice to repeat what is heard for confirmation of the order.

A **phone order** is a type of verbal order that is communicated over the phone. It is essential that you know your responsibility in transmitting this kind of order. In some states, only the provider may give a phone order. In other states, a designated and qualified person may call in a provider's order to a pharmacist.

A **facsimile order** is an order transmitted using a facsimile (fax) machine. It may be sent by the provider or a designated individual whose name and title must be included. The fax machine used to transmit prescriptions must be placed in the pharmacy.

A **computerized order** transmitted via computer is becoming the routine replacement for handwritten orders in the inpatient setting. Computerized orders are innovative because they have the ability to cross-reference lab data with drug orders, such as international normalized ratio value with warfarin (*Coumadin*) and provide pop-up reminders regarding lab results and drug dosages. They can also verify drugs that look or sound alike and have drug alerts for drugs that are easily confused. Computerized orders are also helpful because they assist with dosage calculations and eliminate confusing abbreviations. Computerization of drug orders promotes medication safety at the point of administration. Laptop computers and bar-code scanners may be supplied on medication carts. Some facilities have installed computers either inside or adjacent to patients' rooms, allowing easy access to the medication administration record. Drug references are frequently also accessible on the computer. The bar-code scanning device allows scanning of the bar code on the patient's identification nameband followed by the bar code on the medication. The software may automatically chart the drug, dose, and time given. An alarm may also sound if the wrong drug or the right drug is about to be administered.

QUESTIONING A MEDICATION ORDER [LO 5-3]

You will occasionally have questions about a medication order. Perhaps you cannot read the prescriber's handwriting. The prescribed dosage may seem unusually high. You may find that a patient does not tolerate a certain drug well. Or the patient may have trouble taking the drug by the prescribed route. When these situations arise, it is your duty to check the order with the provider or supervisor. In no case should you give a medication unless the orders are clearly written.

It is also important to know your agency's policies concerning which staff members are allowed to carry out which procedures. You should not be asked to carry out any procedure that is against agency policy; for example, to administer an adjusted medication dose without a new medication order.

Table 5.3 Abbreviations for Times of Administration

Abbreviations	Meaning	Abbreviations	Meaning
a.c.	Before meals	PRN, prn	As necessary
ad lib.	As desired	q.h.	Every hour
AM, a.m.	Morning	q2h, q.2h.	Every two hours
BID, bid	Twice a day	q3h, q.3h.	Every three hours
h., hr.	Hourly	q4h, q.4h.	Every four hours
n., noc.	Night	QID, qid	Four times a day
p.c.	After meals	stat	Immediately
PM, p.m.	After noon	TID, tid	Three times a day

Table 5.4 Abbreviations of Medical Terms

Abbreviations	Meaning	Abbreviations	Meaning
a̅	Before	ophth., op.	Ophthalmic
c̄.	With	p̄.	After
°C	Degrees Celsius (Centigrade)	per	By means of
c/o	Complains of	pH	Hydrogen concentration (acidity and alkalinity)
DC, d/c	Discontinue	PO, p.o.	By mouth
dil.	Dilute	q.	Every
°F	Degrees Fahrenheit	®	Registered product name
♀	Female	Rx	Take
♂	Male	s̄.	Without
NKA	No known allergies	sig.	Label
n.p.o.	Nothing by mouth		

STANDARD MEDICAL ABBREVIATIONS [LO 5-3]

Abbreviations are a shorthand form used to write medication orders. They are a quick, convenient way to summarize instructions on what drug to give and how to give it. Certain standard abbreviations are familiar to most people in the medical field. Tables 5.3 and 5.4 show some abbreviations commonly used in writing medication orders. You must memorize standard medical abbreviations to enable you to read and understand any medication order that you are expected to carry out. At some time, you may also have to translate a prescription into simple language for a patient's family. In addition to being aware of the approved abbreviations, you need to be aware of abbreviations that are prone to error in interpretation. See Table 5.5 for examples.

Table 5.5 Abbreviations That Are Prone to Error in Interpretation

Abbreviations	Current Recommendations
AD	Right ear
AS	Left ear
AU	Both ears
h.s.	Bedtime
MS4	Morphine sulfate
MgSO4	Magnesium sulfate
OD	Right eye
OS	Left eye
OU	Both eyes
Os	By mouth, PO, orally
q.d., QD	Daily
q.o.d., QOD	Every other day
SC, SQ, subq	Subcut, subcutaneously

There is often variation in the style of drug orders. You may find abbreviations capitalized on some orders and not capitalized on others. You may also find differences in punctuation. The use of capital letters and periods is inconsistent in the profession. Check to see if your agency has its own list of approved abbreviations and follow that list.

ORDERING DRUGS FROM THE PHARMACY [LO 5-3]

After a provider writes a medication order for a patient, the proper drugs must be obtained. The way this is done depends on the type of facility in which you work. Most hospitals have a pharmacy within the building. They may also have satellite or minipharmacies on each unit.

Hospital and long-term care facility pharmacy requests can be made in several ways. Although most hospitals transmit orders via computer, long-term care facilities generally use a paper method of sending orders to a pharmacy. The provider's order sheet has a second page that makes a carbon copy of the medication order. This second page can be torn out and sent to the pharmacy. It tells the pharmacist which drugs, and in which form, to send back to the floor for the patient.

If a copy of the provider's order sheet cannot be used, the nurse must write out the drug orders on a **pharmacy requisition form** (Figure 5.9). This is sent to the pharmacist, and the orders are filled from it. There may be more than one drug order on each requisition form. When filling out a pharmacy requisition form, be sure to copy all the information correctly from the provider's order and to fill in every item on the form.

Using the provider's order sheet for ordering drugs is safer than using a requisition form, because no copying is required. There is less chance of a medication error. When and if there is an error, it is much easier to find the

Figure 5.9

Pharmacy requisition form.

Tranel▧▧
HEALTHCARE

JAHN MEMORIAL HOSPITAL   JAHN MEMORIAL HOSPITAL WEST

NURSING/PHARMACY COMMUNICATION SLIP
(Addressograph space)

MEDICATION AS ORDERED/DOSES NEEDED/TIME REQUIRED:
1. _____
2. _____
3. _____

REASON FOR REQUEST:
( ) TRANSFERRED TO _____
( ) GOING ON PASS – NEED DOSES
( ) NEW ALLERGY_____
( ) RECEIVED W/O MEDS FROM_____
( ) MEDS DAMAGED / DROPPED
( ) PRN/REFILL MEDS:
   ( ) NEED 24–HR SUPPLY (AROUND–THE–CLOCK)
   ( ) RETURN TO PAR LEVEL (UP TO 2 DOSES)
( ) OFF UNIT – NEED MAKE-UP DOSE(S)
( ) MEDS LOST / NOT RECEIVED
( ) OTHER _____
NURSE SIGNATURE: _____
PHARMACY WILL NOT DISPENSE FROM YELLOW COPY
WHITE COPY–PHARMACY   YELLOW COPY–CASSETTE

847–0003–10–91

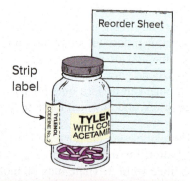

Figure 5.10

To reorder drugs, remove the strip label from the container and affix it to the reorder sheet.

source. State laws have helped to establish this single-entry ordering system wherein the order goes from the provider directly to the pharmacy.

In a hospital, drugs are requested every day as soon as they are ordered. The pharmacy usually sends up enough of each drug to last 8 hours. At some facilities the pharmacist or pharmacy technician checks the medicine supplies of the unit PRN. In some hospitals, drug orders are entered into a computer, either by the provider or by a nurse or unit clerk following the provider's verbal or written orders. In some facilities, drugs are reordered by sending the empty containers to the pharmacy along with appropriate requisition forms.

Some long-term care facilities have their own pharmacies, but most do not. They must order drugs from an outside pharmacy. The ordering system is somewhat different from that used in hospitals. Drugs can be ordered using either a carbon copy of the provider's order sheet or a pharmacy requisition form. These forms are sent to the pharmacy at a certain time each day. The drugs are prepared at the pharmacy and sent back within 24 hours. When they come in, they are checked by comparing the delivery ticket with the provider's orders.

Reorders are listed on a special reorder sheet. To make up the list, part of the original drug label called the strip label is pulled off each container and pasted onto the reorder form (**Figure 5.10**). The form then goes to the outside pharmacy where the orders are filled.

Most drugs for long-term care patients are ordered for an indefinite period. In other words, they are standing orders. For that reason, drugs are ordered in large batches and are reordered only every 30 to 90 days.

DRUG PACKAGING [LO 5-3]

The pharmacy supplies drugs in one of two forms: single-dose packages or multiple-dose packages such as vials.

Single or Unit Dose

In single-dose or unit-dose packaging, each dose of medication is individually wrapped or bottled and supplied for a 24-hour period. Single-dose ampules, vials, and prefilled syringes are supplied for most parenteral medications. Each single-dose package contains the proper dose for one administration. It is labeled with the drug name, strength, expiration date, and sometimes the patient's name.

Unit-dose packaging provides the safest and most convenient means of administering medicines. The drugs require little handling and no special preparation before being taken to the patient. Unused doses can be returned to the pharmacy for credit if the pharmacy sends them up for individual patients. In hospitals, a dose that is not used can be returned to the computerized dispensing system. The individual wrappings ensure that the drugs will not become contaminated in handling.

Multiple Dose

Some drugs, such as insulin, are sent from the pharmacy in multiple-dose bottles or vials. A vial is a small, vacuum-sealed container with a rubber seal at the top that must be punctured with a needle before administering a dose. Today, liquid medications such as cough syrups or antacids often come in unit-dose packages, but many long-term care facilities may use multiple-dose bottles. The person who is to administer the drug must measure and pour out single doses of liquid medications from a bottle. Because these drugs require more handling, there is more chance for error than with unit-dose packages. Unused drugs from multiple-dose containers cannot be credited to the patient's account. Therefore multiple-dose drugs are less used.

STORAGE AND DISPOSAL OF DRUGS [LO 5-3]

Medicine Room

All medications are stored in a computerized dispensing system, a medication room, a portable medicine cart, or an individual storage unit adjacent to the patient's room.

The medication room contains a sink, a refrigerator, and storage cabinets. The refrigerator is necessary because some drugs must be stored in a cool place so as not to lose their effectiveness. Drugs that need refrigeration are labeled. Among them are certain antibiotics and tetanus vaccine.

If a computerized dispensing system is not used, there is a special cabinet in the medicine room for controlled substances. It is kept locked so that the use of these restricted drugs can be monitored. A lead healthcare team member keeps the narcotics keys throughout the shift.

Another cabinet may hold stock supply drugs, or drugs commonly used by many patients. Some stock supply drugs are also kept in the refrigerator. Drugs such as aspirin, *Tylenol,* milk of magnesia, and *Maalox Regular Strength* most commonly are for single dose. If a facility has stock emergency drugs, they are generally kept in a separate cabinet from other stock drugs. Stock supply drugs are declining in use because of the potential for medication errors caused by the large assortment of stock medications to choose from. Other problems include financial loss resulting from misplaced or forgotten charges,

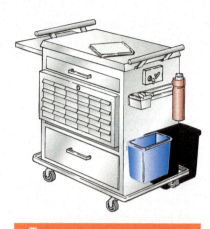

Medicine cart.

expired drugs, the need for frequent inventorying of the drugs, and lack of available storage space. The stock supply system thus costs more and is less safe for the patient. The national trend is currently the unit-dose system.

Cabinets in the medicine room should be kept closed. Drugs that are for external use only are always kept in separate cabinets or compartments. Keep the medicine room and refrigerator clean and tidy at all times. This is vital in helping to prevent medication errors.

Medicine Cart

For convenience, doses of routine drugs are often stored in a medicine cart. Currently, medicine carts are popular in long-term care and assisted living facilities. There may be more than one medication cart, depending on the size of the unit or facility. Each medication cart covers a set number of rooms. In some facilities, medication carts may be kept in the halls near the rooms they serve. They may be kept locked when not in use. The carts have drawers marked off for different patients. A 24-hour supply of unit-dose packages is kept in each patient's drawer. When it is time to administer a dose, the cart can be wheeled from room to room. The medications are then dispensed right out of the drawers. The pharmacist or pharmacy technician refills each patient's drawer at a designated time of day. A limited number of PRN medications are also placed in each patient's drawer (Figure 5.11).

A special locked drawer in the cart contains the Schedule II, III, and IV drugs. The healthcare worker unlocks this drawer only when a dose of a controlled substance is needed. The drawer is relocked immediately, before giving the medication to the patient.

A folder or chart on top of the medicine cart contains each patient's medication administration record, which tells which drugs are to be administered at which times.

Automated Medication Dispensing Systems

Automated medication dispensing systems, such as the Pyxis® MedStation™ system, are designed to make medication management simpler and safer. They are configured to meet the needs of specific facilities, such as hospital patient care units, long-term care facilities, and surgical centers. Each medication is dispensed in accordance with federal, state, and hospital guidelines. Some of the key advantages include increased patient safety, the timely administration of medications, reporting functions, and secure access, either through encrypted passwords or through fingerprint scanning recognition systems. An additional advantage is that the automation of medication delivery reduces manual administrative tasks, allowing nursing and pharmacy staff to focus more on patient care (Figure 5.12).

How the System Works. Each station communicates with the Pyxis® MedStation™ main computer, called the console, located in the central pharmacy. It is connected to several of the hospital's information systems to automate the flow of data. It gets patient information from the admission, discharge, transfer (ADT) system, and it captures information on medication use and sends that to billing. If you have an electronic charting system, it may send the information there, too. The Pyxis® MedStation™ system is most commonly set up in profile mode, which means that it is linked to the pharmacy information system's patient medication profile. This mode allows you to see the list of medications that have been ordered by a provider and verified by a pharmacist.

Components of the Stations. Each station is equipped with the Pyxis® BioID fingerprint identification system, which is a security system that will physically verify your identity before granting you access to the station. You also use a station touch screen and keyboard. The station has a printer that allows you to print numerous activity reports and transaction receipts. There

Figure 5.12

Pyxis® MedStation™ system.

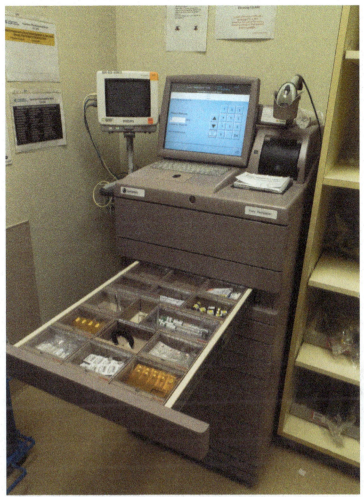

©BARRY SLAVEN/Science Source

is also plenty of space where you can lay your medication administration record or supplies while you're removing medications from the station.

There are four different drawer types available with the Pyxis® MedStation™ system. Each drawer offers different levels of capacity and security. Your hospital will determine which drawers it wants to use in order to maximize safety and ensure availability of medications when and where they are needed. Drawer types include Pyxis CUBIE® drawers filled with Pyxis CUBIE® pockets, Pyxis® MiniDrawers, Pyxis® Carousel drawers, and Pyxis® Matrix drawers. The system has a station tutorial that allows you to learn the basics of using the station. It also has a return bin that lets you securely return medications that are removed from the station and not used. Another couple of useful features that you will likely use are the Lexi-Comp Drug Reference database, which provides up-to-date drug reference information right at the station, and the Lexi-Comp patient education leaflets, which you can use to educate your patients about the medications they have been prescribed.

In summary, the Pyxis® MedStation™ system improves the efficiency of the medication use process, thus helping to save you time and support your efforts to provide safe, high-quality patient care.

Disposing of Unused Drugs

If an automated medication dispensing system (Pyxis®) is not used, never return unused doses of medications to stock supply bottles. Discard the unused doses in the proper manner. Each health facility has its own policy regarding drug disposal. Usually the drugs must be returned to the pharmacy. In some cases, they must go to a certain person or to a storage area. They are then held until there is a batch of drugs to return to the pharmacy. Disposal of controlled substances must be witnessed by another staff member. The amount wasted must then be documented on the narcotic sign-out sheet.

KEEPING TRACK OF MEDICATION ORDERS [LO 5-3]

Whenever more than one patient is being cared for, it is necessary to keep track of which patient is to get which medicine at what time. In a unit of 20 patients, some of whom are to receive several drugs, careful preparation is needed to keep their medications straight. Medical facilities and long-term care facilities have various ways of handling this problem. One common method is use of the medication administration record.

Medication Administration Record

The **medication administration record (MAR)** is a convenient way to document all the drugs administered to a patient every day. It is especially helpful when several drugs must be given at different times. The name of each drug is written once on a patient's MAR (**Figure 5.13**). Routine medications are usually written at the top of the medication administration record and PRN medications at the bottom or on a separate form. The amount, strength, and route are recorded.

If a drug is to be given regularly, a complete schedule is written for all administration times. Then, each time a dose is administered, the healthcare worker checks off the time it was given and initials the sheet. Never sign off on a drug before actually giving it. The full name of each person who

Figure 5.13

Medication administration record showing routine medications at the top of the form and PRN medications at the bottom of the form.

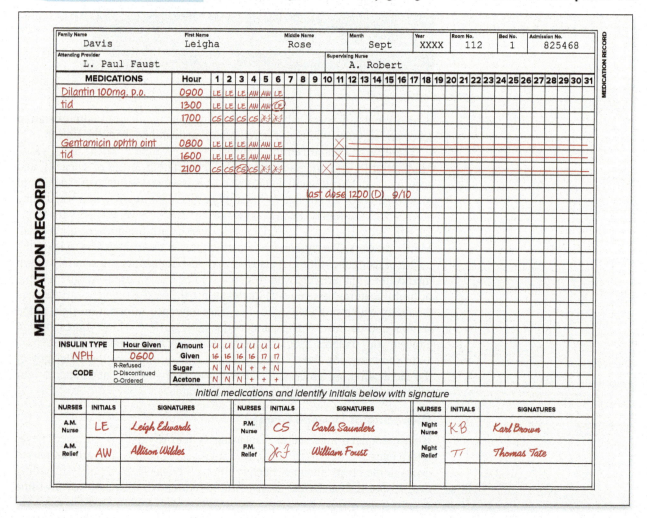

dispenses medications is listed generally at the bottom of the sheet so that initials can be identified, if necessary.

The MAR is prepared by the clerk, pharmacist, or other healthcare worker as drugs are ordered. The nurse then checks the form against the provider's order and signs it. The current day's MARs for all patients are kept in a special folder or chart on the medicine cart or in the medication room. The MARs from previous days are placed in the individual patients' charts. Documentation is computerized when computerized records are used.

Self-Terminating Orders

Self-terminating or automatic stop orders mean that a drug is to be given only until a certain date or time. When this type of order is copied from the provider's order sheet, the nurse or clerk makes a special note or mark on the medication administration record. This notation shows the date and time after which the drug should no longer be given. In **Figure 5.14**, the order for *Gentamycin* shows such a note. When that time comes, the nurse or clerk notifies the patient's provider that the order has terminated. If the provider decides the patient should continue receiving the drug, a new order is written. Automatic stop orders usually cover antibiotics, narcotics, corticosteroids, anticoagulants, and barbiturates.

Figure 5.14

Medication administration record showing a self-terminating drug order.

UNIT-DOSE MEDICATION RECORD

START STOP	RN OK	MEDICATIONS AND DOSE	RTE	SCHEDULE	DATE 8/6/xx	DATE 8/7/xx	DATE 8/8/xx	DATE 8/9/xx
8/5		Dilantin 100mg.	pO	tid	AC AC SJ 0900–1300–1700	AC AC SJ 0900–1300–1700	AC AC SJ 0900–1300–1700	AC AC SJ 0900–1300–1700
8/6		Lanoxin 0.125 mg	pO	q.d.	AC 1000	AC 1000	SJ 1000	SJ 1000
8/5 8/7		Gentamicin ophth. oint.	Op	tid	AC 0800, 1600, 2100	AC AC 0900–1200 (Disc)		
8/6		Prochlorperazine 10mg prn for nausea	IM	q.4h.	AC AC 1000 1600	AC SJ 1400 1800		
8/6		Nembutal 120mg prn	pO	h.s.	SJ 2000			

SCHEDULED DRUGS

PRN

06-0535-2-2-77

Signatures
Andrew Carlton
Sandy Jinke

Controlled Substances

Controlled substances are drugs whose use is restricted. This group of drugs includes narcotics, stimulants, and depressants. Because of legal restrictions, these medications must be counted or measured at the beginning of each shift when drugs are manually dispensed. As the shift changes, the person coming off duty and the person coming on duty count the narcotics together. They record the quantity of each controlled substance on the narcotics form. They then sign a special form so that there is a record of who counted the drugs on each shift. If the count is found to be incorrect at a later shift, the error can be traced to the proper personnel. When drugs are dispensed by the automated medication dispensing system, the controlled substances count is done each time a controlled substance is taken.

Controlled substances are packaged in either single doses or multiple doses. For example, *Demerol* 50 mg for injection is packaged in a box of 10 prefilled syringes. Oral narcotics such as *Percodan* may come in single-dose packages in a box of 25. The packages are given a special seal at the pharmacy.

Each time a controlled substance is administered from the stock supply, the healthcare worker must sign a proof-of-use record, such as the one shown in **Figure 5.15**. Each health facility has its own form for this purpose. The form

Figure 5.15

Administering controlled substances requires documentation on a proof-of-use record.

NARCOTIC/BARBITURATE PROOF-OF-USE RECORD — Tranel HEALTHCARE — JAHN MEMORIAL HOSPITAL WEST

CHECK ONE:
- ☐ DO NOT REISSUE
- ☑ REISSUE
- ☐ MED DISCONTINUED
- ☐ PAT. DISCHARGED
- ☐ OTHER

RETURNED BY: _Adam Gray, Pharm. Aid_ DATE: _8/11_
RECEIVED BY: _L. Peters, R.N_ DATE: _8/11_

ALL PREPS LOST, DESTROYED OR UNACCOUNTED FOR MUST BE EXPLAINED.

NO	DATE	TIME	PATIENT	BED	AM'T mgs	PROVIDER	ADMIN. BY	AMOUNT & WITNESS
25	8/11	1600	Cindy Gregory	921	100 mg	C. Adams	D. Fox	
24	8/12	0800	Shawn Jones	912	75 mg	L. Faust	J. Stan	25 mg/C. Smith
23	8/14	1400	Robby Hibet	924	100 mg	P. David	T. Smith	
22	8/19	1300	Rosalia Little	916	100 mg	L. Faust	T. Smith	
21	8/21	0630	Ken Peters	910	50 mg	J. Francis	D. Fox	50 mg/K. Frank
20								
19								
18								
17								
16								
15								
14								
13								
12								
11								
10								
9								
8								
7								
6								
5								
4								
3								
2								
1								

USE LINES BELOW FOR CORRECTION OF ERRORS WHEN APPLICABLE

ISSUED TO:
Unit D
UNIT OR PATIENT NAME & BED NO.
ISSUED BY: _N. Nelson, R.PH_
RECEIVED BY: _Adam Gray, Pharm. Aid_

SERIAL NO. _425_ NO. ISSUED _25_ DATE _8/11_

DRUG NAME	STRENGTH	FORM	SIZE
Demerol	100 mg	ampuls	2mL

usually shows the number of doses sent to the unit's stock supply from the pharmacy. As each dose is used, the date, time, patient, room number, amount given, provider, and person administering the dose must be recorded. If a dose less than the prepared individual dose is given, the amount actually given is noted. The unused portion must be destroyed in front of a witness, who must also sign the form.

Many healthcare facilities use the computer-controlled dispensing system for dispensing narcotics. After the designated healthcare member enters the security code and the patient's identification number, the specified drug is delivered—for example, *Demerol* 100 mg IM q4h for Mrs. Decoda, Room 412B.

SETTING UP MEDICATIONS [LO 5-4]

Medications are ordered by the provider, requested from the pharmacy, and stored in the proper area. Now comes the time when you, the giver of medications, must be most alert—setting up medications. Setting up medications means taking information from the computer and medication administration record and preparing an actual dose of medication for a patient. You will be setting up several drugs at a time, and you must be aware of all of the possibilities for error. Here are some guidelines to help you prepare a medicine tray or drug cart for your rounds.

1. **Clear your mind of everything except getting the medications set up properly.** Do not try to carry on a conversation with someone while you work; the task at hand needs your full attention.

2. **Before handling any medications, think about cleanliness.** Microorganisms can be transmitted to patients on tablets and other medications, so follow aseptic procedure (discussed in Chapter 7). Wash your hands before touching any drug product. Never touch the drugs; put them directly into paper or plastic medicine cups. Never give a pill that has fallen on the floor; throw it away. Do not cough or sneeze on the medications. Keep unit doses sealed until you are ready to give them.

3. **Setting up is the time when you need to decide whether you must calculate a dose.** You will notice whether the pharmacist's order is in a unit of measurement different from that of the provider's order. At this point you will utilize the skills you learned in Chapter 3. Use the appropriate conversion tables and have your work checked if you have any doubts at all. If you need to divide a tablet, use a pill cutter (**Figure 5.16**). Place the pill in the pill cutter form and close the lid. The

Figure 5.16
Pill cutter.

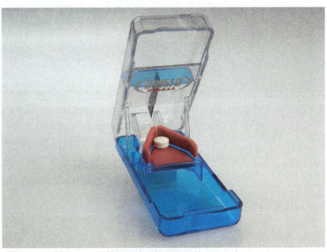

©McGraw-Hill Education/Christopher Kerrigan, photographer

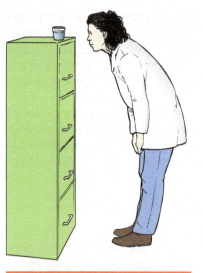

Figure 5.17

Medication should be measured at eye level on a stable surface.

pill form holds the pill firmly in place. As you close the lid, a knife in the top lid divides the pill in half. If a pill cutter is not available, use a knife edge to press down hard on the scored part of the tablet to make a quick, clean break, or cover the pill in a tissue and hold it with the fingers to break it.

4. **When you pour liquid medication from a bottle, pour it from the side away from the label.** Remove the cap from the bottle and place it upside down to prevent contamination. Hold the bottle with the label against the palm of the hand while pouring to prevent liquid from running down the bottle and destroying the label. Place the medication cup on a surface at eye level to ensure accuracy of the dose (**Figure 5.17**). Do not hold the cup at eye level, because it is difficult to make sure the cup is level and not tipped.

5. **If preparing a unit-dose tablet, place the packaged tablet directly into the medicine cup.** Never open the package until administering the medication to the patient.

6. **Decide whether the medication is to be mixed with a liquid or food.** Drugs are sometimes mixed with a soft, palatable food such as applesauce or fluid such as juice to hide their taste. Tablets may be crushed and capsules opened and mixed to make them easier for a patient to swallow. Check a drug reference book to make sure the medication can be crushed. Never crush enteric-coated or sustained-action medications.

THE SEVEN RIGHTS: RULES FOR GIVING MEDICATIONS [LO 5-4]

The rules, or "seven rights," for giving medications are the same no matter who is giving them. The seven rights of medication administration are:

- Right drug
- Right dose
- Right patient
- Right route
- Right time
- Right technique
- Right documentation

It is imperative that you administer the right drug and dose, by the correct route, at the correct time, using the appropriate technique, and document your actions.

Right Drug

Give only medicine that you have prepared yourself. Never give any medication that someone else has prepared. Give drugs only from labeled containers. Keep unit-dose packages wrapped until you are ready to administer the drug to the patient so that the label stays with the medication. When administering drugs, compare the label three times with the unit-dose recording form:

1. **Compare before taking it from the shelf or drawer where it is stored.**

2. **Compare as you remove the ordered amount of the drug from the container.**

3. **Compare before you place the drug in a medication cup.**

If a patient refuses medication that has been removed from its package, throw it away. If a single-unit dose package is unopened, you may return it to the patient's drawer or automated medication dispensing system.

Be aware of the different names for the same drug—the generic name and the brand name. For example, furosemide is the generic name for a common diuretic. *Lasix* is the brand name. Also be aware that very different drugs can have similar names. Alprazolam and lorazepam, for example, might be mistaken for each other, but one is for diabetes and the other is for a stuffy nose. You should carefully note the spelling of a drug's name and be sure to verify an order if the handwriting is unclear.

Know the abbreviations for the different dosage forms.

Recheck any medicine that the patient feels is wrong. Be sure the label corresponds to the name of the drug that appears on the computer or is written on the medication administration record.

Right Dose

Medication errors are significantly reduced by the unit-dose system, because the medications are already in the correct dose. When calculations are required to achieve a correct dose, have another member of the healthcare team check them. Many facilities require the healthcare worker who sets up insulin or anticoagulants to check them with another worker.

Know the correct dosage symbols and abbreviations. Use properly marked measuring containers: medicine glasses marked with metric or apothecary units, and a medicine dropper, if drops are ordered.

Be sure that the amount the patient receives matches the amount stated on the provider's order. Stay with each patient until he or she takes the medicine.

Help weak patients take medication to be sure they get the full amount.

Correctly divide or crush a tablet, as previously discussed.

Right Patient

An essential step to safe medication administration is to give the right medication to the right patient. Always identify the patient. Make absolutely certain that you know who the patient is. Read the identification wristband that all hospital patients wear. Avoid calling a patient by name, because a confused patient may respond to someone else's name. Ask patients their names, reassuring them that it is routine procedure to have them state their name.

Check the patient's name against the name on the medication administration record each time you administer medication.

Right Route

Always document the route on the medication administration record. Package inserts, drug references, and the patient chart reveal information about the right route. Call the nurse in charge if you still have questions after checking these references. The provider should be contacted if the route is not specified on the medication order. Know the correct abbreviations for the routes. (Refer to Table 5.2.)

Be aware of factors or changes in the patient's condition that can affect the route of administration. For example, the rectal or parenteral routes are the preferred routes instead of the oral route for a patient who is vomiting. Ask the provider to write a different order when changes such as this arise.

Right Time

Know the correct abbreviations for times of administration. (Refer to Table 5.3.) Check the medication administration record for the correct time to give a medication. All routine medications should be given within 30 minutes of the scheduled time.

Never leave a drug at the patient's bedside. To make sure all medications are taken, observe while the patient takes the medication.

Organize your work time at the beginning of each shift so that you can get medications to each patient on schedule. Review all of the day's nursing activities and your own duties. Plan accordingly, taking into account the times when patients are to receive medications.

Check whether an oral drug should be taken on an empty stomach or with food. Drugs to be taken on an empty stomach should be given 1 hour before meals or 2 hours afterward. Drugs given after meals should be given within 30 minutes of the ordered time. Drugs such as insulin must be given exactly as ordered before a meal. Administer medications that cause sleepiness at bedtime. Administer diuretics, or water pills, in the early part of the day.

Right Technique

To be a safe and competent practitioner, you must always use the appropriate technique when administering a medication. If you are not familiar with one of the various methods of medication administration, you should review the technique before giving the medicine.

Right Documentation

Summarizing that medication administration to a patient was done correctly can be done only through documentation. The right dose of the right drug must be documented for the right patient at the right time. Not only is documenting the correct medication administration essential, but going back and assessing the patient for any reaction to the medication is important. With the exception of an intravenous medication that acts almost immediately and within minutes, generally reassessing a patient in 30 minutes is a good guideline to follow. In addition to documenting medication administration, you must also document a medication that the patient refuses. The reason the patient refused the medication must be given.

READING AND UNDERSTANDING A MEDICATION LABEL [LO 5-5]

Before you can set up and administer a medication, you need to understand the information that appears on the drug label, such as the trade or brand name, generic name, form of the drug, dosage strength, route of administration, precaution or warning label, storage requirement, the National Drug Code (NDC) numbers, and the expiration date, lot number, or batch number (Figure 5.18).

Every drug has a generic name that is listed in the *United States Pharmacopeia (USP)* and the *National Formulary (NF)*. When "USP" appears on the label, this indicates that the name of the drug is recorded with the United States Pharmacopeia. In addition to their generic names, many drugs have trade

Figure 5.18

Locating information on medication label.

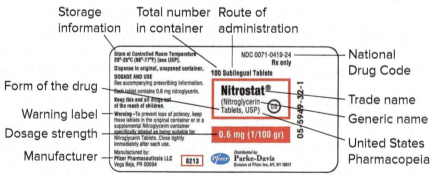

Source: Pfizer, Inc.

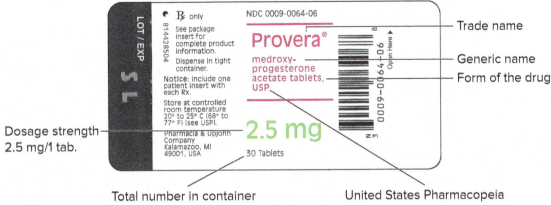

Trade name

Generic name

Form of the drug

Dosage strength
2.5 mg/1 tab.

Total number in container

United States Pharmacopeia

Source: Pfizer, Inc.

Figure 5.19

Form of drug.

names listed. The trade or brand name is the property of the drug company that manufactures the drug. A registered trademark appearing in the upper right corner of a drug label indicates that the name of the drug has been registered with the U.S. Patent and Trademark Office. It is important that you understand a drug has only one generic name but may have several brand names. For example, the generic drug levothyroxine sodium is also sold under the brand names of *Levoxyl, Synthroid,* and *Unithroid.* Although many generic drugs have brand names, some drugs such as heparin sodium have no brand name.

The manufacturer of a drug may supply a drug in several forms such as oral, injectable, topical, inhalant, drops, spray, mist, or rectal. For example, morphine sulfate is produced to be administered orally, rectally, and as an injectable including intramuscular, subcutaneous, intravenous, intrathecal, and epidural.

The amount of drug present in the type of medication such as oral or liquid is listed on the drug label. Generally the drug is listed in grams, milligrams, micrograms, and grains. Liquid drugs are listed in milliliters, and special drugs such as heparin and insulin are listed in units.

Assume that the dose of a solid medication is in one tablet, capsule, or gelcap unless stated otherwise. For example, *Provera* 2.5 mg is in one tablet (**Figure 5.19**).

The dose of a liquid medication is the amount of the drug in a quantity of solution. In *Tigan,* the dose of a drug is 100 mg in 1 milliliter (mL) (**Figure 5.20**).

In the case of liquid medications, don't assume that the medication is always delivered in 1 mL. Assuming the amount of solution the medication is in is 1 mL may result in an incorrect calculation and medication error. Look at the drug label for amoxicillin and notice that the dose amount is 250 mg in 5 mL.

The final dose of medication you may encounter is in units. Look at the *Novolin R* insulin label to find that the available dose is 100 units per 1 mL and the calculated amount is the units. Again, be careful to read the medication label correctly to prevent a medication error.

Pay attention to how the medication is to be given. For example, all tablets are not meant to be swallowed. *Nitrostat* tablets are to be administered sublingually, under the tongue (**Figure 5.21**). The *Singulair* tablets are to be chewed (**Figure 5.22**). Some oral medications such as *Proventil HFA* may be administered by oral inhalation (**Figure 5.23**).

Figure 5.20

Dosage strength.

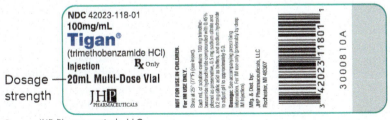

Dosage strength

Source: JHP Pharmaceuticals, LLC.

Figure 5.21
Sublingual administration.

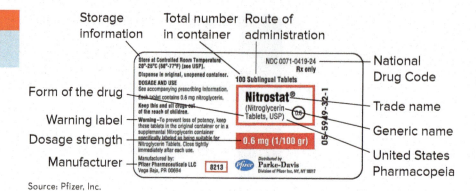

Storage information — Total number in container — Route of administration

National Drug Code

Form of the drug

Trade name

Warning label

Generic name

Dosage strength

United States Pharmacopeia

Manufacturer

Source: Pfizer, Inc.

Figure 5.22
Chewable tablets for oral administration.

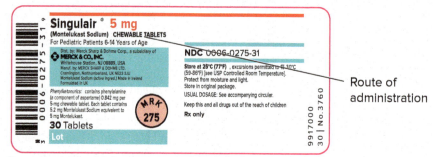

Route of administration

Source: Merck Sharp & Dohme Corp., a subsidiary of Merck & Co., Inc., Whitehouse Station, New Jersey, USA.

Figure 5.23
Inhalation administration.

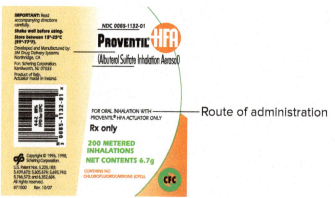

Route of administration

Source: Merck Sharp & Dohme Corp., a subsidiary of Merck & Co., Inc., Whitehouse Station, New Jersey, USA.

Figure 5.24
Intramuscular (IM) administration.

Route of administration

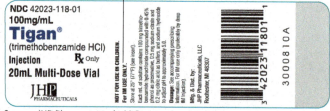

Source: JHP Pharmaceuticals, LLC.

Likewise, you cannot assume that all injectable medications are administered by the same route. For example, *Tigan* is administered intramuscularly (IM) (**Figure 5.24**) and *Diprivan* is administered intravenously (IV).

The precaution and warning label outline information that assists you to administer a drug safely. The warning label on *Nitrostat* states, "To prevent loss of potency, keep these tablets in the original container. . . . Close tightly after each use." See Figure 5.18. The warning label on a narcotic such as *Lortab* indicates that the drug may be habit-forming. Other labels may include information such as "Keep out of reach of children" and "Not safe for pregnant women."

If a certain drug has specific storage requirements, they will be listed on the medication label. For example, *Proventil HFA* should be stored between 15° and 25°C (59° and 77°F). See Figure 5.23. Other storage requirements may include statements regarding exposure to light and the length of time a drug will be potent after being opened.

The National Drug Code (NDC) number such as 0071-0419-24 that appears on the *Nitrostat* label identifies the manufacturer, the product, and the size of the container. See Figure 5.18.

Each drug has both an expiration date, abbreviated EXP, and a lot or batch number on the container. The expiration date is the date after which the drug should no longer be used. Drugs are produced in batches known as lots that specifically identify where and when a drug was produced, enabling a manufacturer to trace a problem to a particular batch and thus facilitating a drug recall. Contamination, unexpected side effects, or suspected tampering are potential reasons a certain batch may need to be recalled.

CHARTING MEDICATIONS [LO 5-6]

Whenever a patient receives some form of treatment, such as medication, a record is kept of that treatment. Special problems or circumstances are also recorded, such as new symptoms, the patient's own statements, laboratory tests performed, and so on. All the events in the course of a patient's treatment are written in the patient chart or medical record, which is a permanent record of care received.

The chart is important because it is a form of communication among the patient, provider, and other members of the healthcare team. The patient chart is also a legal document. It is the official record of the care a patient receives. The patient or the patient's family may question the quality of treatment. The health facility can evaluate quality by referring to the chart. In the event of a lawsuit, the chart can be used in court to decide whether the patient received competent or incompetent care. The chart is taken as proof of the care the patient received.

Researchers may also use the chart to study certain diseases or drugs. The chart may serve as a teaching tool for medical and nursing students. Or it may be used to gather facts and figures about the overall performance of a health facility.

For all these reasons, it is important to learn how to write the necessary information on a patient chart. This is called charting, or documenting. All documentation and reports become part of the patient's medical record and must be factual, accurate, complete, current, organized, and confidential.

First, you should know that not all charts look alike. Different health facilities have their own forms for keeping records. The traditional patient chart consists of a collection of different forms. Individual staff members chart the problems for which they are responsible and the treatment or care they give. Other team members refer to these specific reports as needed.

The traditional patient chart contains the provider's order sheet. The patient's provider, or in the case of verbal or phone orders, a registered nurse, fills it out. It contains orders for tests, procedures, and drugs to treat the patient's condition. The provider also fills out a patient history sheet, describing the patient's medical problems in more detail. Various other forms are used to record such things as laboratory tests, x-rays, reports of specialists, and the patient's progress. Two forms you will deal with in administering medications are the medication administration record and the nurses' notes.

Medication Administration Record

You have learned what the medication administration record (MAR) is. Now you will learn how to chart after administering a medication. You must include these facts on the MAR:

- Name of the drug.
- Strength and/or amount of the drug.
- Times at which the drug is given.
- Route by which the drug is given.
- Initials and signature of the health worker who administers the drug.

For routine medications, most of this information is written or printed from the computer ahead of time. You need chart only your initials each time you administer a drug.

In case a dose of medicine is not given at a scheduled time, you should record both the time for the missed dose and the time the medication was administered. Usually this is done by circling the skipped time on the medication administration record. You should also explain why the drug was not given, either on the nurses' notes or MAR or on both, depending on facility policy. Some reasons that you may not be able to give a drug on time are that the patient may be having an x-ray taken, abnormal laboratory results may have been reported, or there may have been a rise or fall in the patient's pulse, respiration, or blood pressure.

If the medication administration record has a section for PRN medications, chart the time and reason for administration and your initials. Many facilities also require documentation of PRN medications in the nurses' notes.

Nurses' Notes

The traditional form known as nurses' notes is called by several names, including progress notes and nurses' progress notes. The nurse uses these notes to chart observations of the patient and the nursing care provided (Figure 5.25). Stat medications, and sometimes PRN medications, are also charted on the nurses' notes.

The following information must be charted in the nurses' notes each time a stat or a PRN medication is given:

- Name of the drug.
- Strength and/or amount of the drug administered.

Figure 5.25

Nurses' notes.

NURSES' NOTES

Tranel HEALTHCARE
JAHN MEMORIAL HOSPITAL WEST

Family Name	First Name	Attending Provider	Room No.	Hosp. No.
Frederick	Lindsey	Dr. Jones	125	25-859

Date	Time	REMARKS - TREATMENT	Nurses' Signature
8/1	0100	Demerol 100 mg given IM for c/o severe right knee pain	A. Kasal, LPN
8/1	1800	Refused Motrin 400 mg P.O. Pt states "it upsets my stomach." Supervisor notified.	L. Smith, Med Aid
8/2	1015	Procardia 10 mg. given PO stat for B/P $^{196}/_{104}$	T. Stewart, LPN Student

- Route.
- Time of administration.
- Results of checking vital signs (blood pressure, temperature, respiration, pulse) if required for specific drugs.
- Any special information regarding the drug or the patient (e.g., problems in getting the patient to take the drug, unusual reactions).
- Signature (first initial and last name) and title of the person who administers the drug.

In addition to providing a record of stat and PRN medications, the form includes other information. Whenever you do not give a medication or notice something unusual with any medication, chart it on the nurses' notes. You should also make a note on the nurses' notes anytime a scheduled medication is not given. The second entry in Figure 5.25 shows a case like this.

THE PROBLEM-ORIENTED MEDICAL RECORD (POMR) [LO 5-6]

One method of documenting used in some hospitals is called the **problem-oriented medical record (POMR)**. In this system the chart is organized according to a numbered list of problems or diagnoses (**Figure 5.26**). All health team members chart on the same form. They chart their observations, plans of action, treatments, and results, with a number telling which particular problem they are working on. The list of problems includes any social and

Figure 5.26

The POMR (problem-oriented medical record) shown at the top and the SOAP (subjective-objective-assessment-plan) notes shown at the bottom allow members of the healthcare team to chart what they do for the patient's individual problems.

Tranel HEALTHCARE
Patient Record

7209
347841-6 m 28-447
WELSH, KELVIN
DR. JAMIE THOMAS
1 - PROT 5/6/20

ALLERGIES	BLOOD TYPE
Penicillin	AB+

PROBLEM NUMBER	DATE	PROBLEM DESCRIPTION	DATE RESOLVED
#1	3/25	Diabetes mellitus, insulin-controlled	
#2	3/25	Midline abdominal incision	
#3	3/25	Wife seriously ill	

Progress Notes

PROBLEM NO. & DESCRIPTION	SUBJECTIVE(S)-OBJECTIVE(O)-ASSESSMENT(A)-PLAN(P)
#2 - Incision	S: Complains of incisional pain ————————————
	O: Generalized redness around incision line;
	sm. amt. greenish drainage; T 101.4° F —————————
	A: Possible wound infection ————————————————
	P: Obtain culture; notify Dr. Paul ————————————
	———————————————— M. Ryan, LPN

psychological factors in the patient's life that may have an effect on treatment. The POMR is designed to make sure that all members of the healthcare team are aware of what the others are doing and planning for the patient. In this way, the patient receives coordinated care.

Where the POMR is in use, patient progress is often charted by **subjective-objective-assessment-plan (SOAP)** or **problem-intervention-evaluation (PIE)** notes. These are ways to organize information for charting. When you want to make an entry using SOAP, include the following:

- *Subjective data:* the patient's complaints and feelings in his or her own words.
- *Objective data:* your own observations or measurements (e.g., blood pressure, appetite).
- *Assessment:* an interpretation of the patient's condition.
- *Plan:* specific orders, such as treatments, diagnostic tests, medications, or patient education, that will help the patient's current problem.

To make an entry using PIE, include the following:

- *Problem:* a problem pertinent to the patient.
- *Intervention:* your actions to address the problem.
- *Evaluation:* your assessment of interventions and the patient's response to therapy.

Another method is charting by exception. It is designed to decrease the amount of time spent charting. With this method, the healthcare team establishes normal assessment findings and standardized interventions for each patient. Then, a team member has only to write a note when a patient's condition does not meet the standardization.

Charting in Long-Term Care Facilities

The forms used for charting in a long-term care facility are different from those used on a hospital unit. Any drugs administered are charted on a patient history sheet or on the nurses' notes. Again, all important information must be charted: drug name, strength and/or amount, route, time of administration, your signature and title, and any other notes about the patient or the drug.

PRINCIPLES OF CHARTING [LO 5-7]

Because the chart is a record of a patient's treatment, it must record only facts. You must write only things you did or saw or heard the patient say. Your own conclusions and opinions about a patient's behavior are not to be charted. The only exception to this rule is in the SOAP method of charting, which calls for your assessment of the patient's problem. In this case, it is clear that you are stating your own conclusions.

All charted information must be factual. Why are facts better than opinions in charting? Let us take an example. If you found Mrs. Smith in her room crying, you would not write on the chart "seems depressed about upcoming operation." Instead, you would write "was crying," since there could be many reasons why Mrs. Smith is crying. Suppose that Mr. Jones gagged on a tablet this morning. If you wrote "doesn't like medicine" on the chart (your opinion of the situation), your information would be misleading. Perhaps a physical problem caused Mr. Jones to have trouble swallowing. The chart shows the problem more clearly if you write simply "difficulty noted in swallowing tablet." Avoid terms like "appear" or "seems," which can lead you to draw assumptions without objective data to support them.

Another important feature of charting is that it is a summary of events. It must be accurate, complete, current, and organized. For example, "incision to chest not healing" is not accurate, complete, or based on facts. It allows for assumptions that are not legally sound in healthcare. Instead, chart "generalized redness noted length of chest incision and warm to touch." Use abbreviations when appropriate. They allow you to say a great deal in a small space. Learn them well and use them carefully so that others can understand your notes. It is also useful to learn the proper medical terms for symptoms and body functions. Most people in the healthcare field understand them, and they are a kind of shorthand for complicated explanations. Be careful of similar spellings of words with very different meanings that would be confusing; for example, *dram* and *gram.*

Charting is not difficult, but it requires some practice. Your own charting will be appropriate if you follow a few simple rules:

- Before you begin, make sure you have the right chart.
- Chart medications directly from a medication administration record. If one is not used, chart directly from the patient chart.
- Chart only after you give a drug, never before.
- Be specific. Do not write "Gave *Demerol* for pain in the evening." Instead, write "[date], *Demerol* 100 mg given IM in right upper outer quadrant of gluteus maximus for c/o sharp pain in left arm."
- Document the effect of PRN medication 30 minutes after you give the drug.
- Record events in the order they occur.
- Mark D/C, for discontinued, after the last dose of a drug is given, or cross out the remaining scheduled times, as required by your agency. The provider will have specified the day and time of the last dose.
- Do not leave gaps or skip lines. If a note does not fill up a complete line, draw a straight line to fill the gap. Put your signature at the right-hand side directly after the note. (Refer to the nurses' notes in Figure 5.25.)
- If you make an error, do not erase it. Draw one line through the mistake. It should still be visible; do not black it out. Initial it, and write the word *error* on the line. Then rechart the information correctly.
- Never use ditto marks.
- Write only in ink, never in pencil. Only ink ensures a permanent record. Most agencies require you to use a certain color ink. Black ink is the most widely used, but check the policy at your agency. Always print or write legibly when charting. You may print or you may write neatly in longhand.
- Always use proper abbreviations and symbols. Many agencies have lists of the abbreviations they prefer. Check with your agency.
- Consult the nurse in charge when in doubt about a charting rule.

The patient chart is kept strictly confidential. Do your part to make sure that only authorized people see the chart or discuss its contents. Never discuss a patient with another healthcare worker in a public setting, such as the elevator or cafeteria. This is a breach of confidentiality for which you could be held legally responsible.

Computer Charting

Although little changed in the process of documentation until the late 20th century, charting forms have changed over time to meet the changing needs of healthcare. Computerized technology is not new, but many healthcare professionals are challenged by the necessary skills to address this technology. You may ask yourself whether you need to become versed in computer charting if your facility still maintains traditional paper files. The answer is a simple yes. Becoming familiar with computer charting makes you proactive and increases your marketability. If you lack computer experience, most facilities will provide on-site training, or you may take a computer course at a local college.

Computers in healthcare made their first appearance in the late 1960s and early 1970s. Initially used for accounting systems, their usage spread to laboratory, radiology, pharmacy, and nursing applications. A lot of time and effort has gone into the development of computerized charting forms. Initially, point-of-care documentation was developed to permit the taking of vital signs and the recording of intake and output on a keyboard at the bedside. Documenting patient care was also possible. All entries were time-stamped and electronically signed through the healthcare facility's secure log-on code. In paper charting, the user needed to write a date and time for each entry. In computer charting, the date and time appear when the user makes an entry. Systems designed in the late 1980s and 1990s allowed for measurement and documentation and for graphing temperature, pulse, and blood pressure using bar-code technology.

Not until recently have computer systems been able to network to other clinical systems. It is important to understand that computers are not automatic. They must be told what to do. Although computers are routinely customized to the needs of each facility, you will still be prompted to enter an authorization code, along with a password and signature. Most computers provide menus containing words or phrases for recording notations. In addition to these basic functions, software generally allows for manipulating a sequence of words to develop a narrative note.

Computerized charting is here to stay, and it is just a matter of time before it becomes the primary method for maintaining patient records and eventually turns handwritten charts into a thing of the past. Becoming proficient at using the computer is an excellent goal to set for yourself. Once the skills are learned, you may decide you prefer the electronic to the paper chart. Computerization also advances the healthcare profession as a whole while increasing the quality of care to patients. There are numerous advantages to computer charting (Table 5.6).

Reporting Medication Errors

Medication errors are serious and can be fatal to a patient. A medication error occurs when you violate one or more of the "seven rights":

- Give the wrong drug.
- Give the wrong dose.
- Give a drug to the wrong patient.
- Give the drug by the wrong route.

Table 5.6 Advantages of Computer Charting

- Produces legible charts
- Saves time
- Avoids repetition and misspellings
- Provides consistency
- Enables easy storage of charts on hard drive or diskette
- Increases confidentiality (A chart may be quickly put out of sight by using "File Save" to close it if someone walks in or by using a screen saver.)
- Increases confidence and job satisfaction
- Provides easily retrievable, reviewed, and amended files to healthcare personnel in remote locations
- Increases patient care time and decreases time spent documenting
- Is in compliance with institutional policies and The Joint Commission (formerly the Joint Commission on Accreditation of Healthcare Organizations (JCAHO) standards)
- Produces uniform and precise records
- Increases communication between departments
- Increases continuity of care
- Reduces inefficiencies

- Give the drug at the wrong time.
- Give the drug by the wrong technique.
- Document the drug incorrectly.

Any of these seven situations must be reported immediately to the nurse in charge. You must also complete an **incident report** or a medication error form, or an event report form (Figure 5.27). The incident report is an objective, factual account of what took place. The incident report does not become part of the chart. Agencies use incident reports to monitor the frequency of medication errors so as to take corrective measures to prevent them in the future. The incident report is signed by the health worker who made the error and by the lead healthcare team member. Many health facilities require that the provider be notified and the patient seen after the medication error. The provider's orders for further patient care must be followed carefully. It is your legal duty to report an error. Not reporting an error can seriously harm your patient and your future in the healthcare field.

As a final step, review the events that led to the error. Medication errors can be prevented by carefully reading medication labels. Pay attention to the name and dose of the medication and to the name of the patient. Some drugs have similar names (e.g., *Keflex* and *Keppra*). Have all your calculations checked by another health team member. Many errors occur as the result of incorrect placement of the decimal point. If a medication order is illegible, notify your supervisor so that the provider can be called for clarification.

Figure 5.27

Any medication error requires completion of an incident report.

INCIDENT REPORT

JAHN MEMORIAL HOSPITAL	JAHN MEMORIAL HOSPITAL WEST	JAHN SENIOR CARE	OTHER

NAME: AGE _____ SEX _____   DIAGNOSIS:

MR#:   ADM. DATE: PT. LOCATION:

USE THIS FORM TO REPORT:
1) ANY IDENTIFIED HAZARD: A CONDITION THAT MIGHT CAUSE AN INJURY.
2) AN INJURY OR DEATH THAT IS UNEXPECTED, AND IS MORE RELATED TO CARE, OR LACK OF CARE, THAN TO THE PATIENT'S UNDERLYING CONDITION.
****DO NOT MAKE COPIES OF THIS REPORT.****

DETAILS OF THE EVENT

Date: Time: _____am/pm   Location of Incident:

DESCRIPTION OF HAZARD OR DESCRIPTION OF INJURY AND SURROUNDING CIRCUMSTANCES:

_____

_____

_____

_____

_____

Persons involved (Name, Title):

Address/Phone#/Ext.:

CORRECTIVE ACTION TAKEN IN RESPONSE TO THIS INCIDENT:

_____

_____

Name of provider who examined the patient:

Treatment for injury:

Names of witnesses (Use back of form if space needed):

Address/Phone #/Ext. of witnesses:

Name/Title and Signature of person submitting this report:

_____

Date/Time report written:

Signature of supervisor:

_____

TRANSCRIBING MEDICATION ORDERS

Demonstrate how to transcribe a medication order.

Equipment

Provider's order sheet with drugs ordered

Medication administration record

Procedure

1. Read the medication orders on the provider's order sheet.

2. Transcribe each medication order exactly as it appears on the provider's order sheet. Use proper medical terms and abbreviations. Be sure to record all necessary information, including:
   - Name of patient, room number, and bed number.
   - Name of drug.
   - Route.
   - Dosage (strength and frequency of administration).
   - Time(s) of administration.
   - Special administration or nursing instructions, if any.

3. Following the provider's order sheet, transcribe each order onto a medication administration record. Include the same information as in Step 2.

4. Check off each order as you finish transcribing it onto the medication administration record.

5. Sign or initial the provider's orders after each set of orders is transcribed.

   Show your work to your instructor.

Practice Procedure 5.2 (LO 5-3)

COUNTING CONTROLLED SUBSTANCES IF AN AUTOMATED MEDICATION SYSTEM IS NOT USED

Demonstrate how to count controlled substances if an automated system is not used.
In a laboratory setting, practice this procedure with a partner. Pretend that one of you is going off duty and the other is coming on duty.

Equipment

Controlled substance folder with the forms used by your health facility (sign-in/out form, proof-of-use records for several drugs)

Locked box, cabinet, or drawer, and keys

Sample containers of controlled substances (divided containers, unit-dose packages, etc.)

Procedure

1. The person coming on duty obtains the key to the controlled-substance storage area from the person going off duty. (Some areas have double doors and require two keys.)

2. Unlock the controlled-substance cabinet, box, or drawer in the medicine room. Remove the containers.

3. Count the amount of medicine in each container.

   - *Divided containers (tablets or capsules).* Look for the slot that has the last tablet or capsule in it. The number of this slot is the number of tablets left.

   - *Unit-dose packages.* Unit doses are numbered. The package with the highest number tells how many doses are left.

4. As you count each drug, write the quantity on the appropriate form. Each drug has a form to accompany it. If the form is a proof-of-use record, check that your count matches the amount of drug shown as still available. Different facilities have different ways of verification. Sign your name where requested.

5. If your count differs from the number shown in the records, do a recount. If there is still a difference, look at the other forms to locate the source of error. Notify the nurse in charge if you cannot find the source of error.

6. Correct errors on your forms according to the policy of your health facility.

7. Sign any of the forms required by your health facility (sign-in/out, key count, etc.).

8. Return medications to the lockbox, and close and lock the doors. Return the controlled-substance folder to the place where it is kept.

9. The person who has just come on duty keeps the key(s) for use in administering controlled substances during the next shift.

Show your work to your instructor.

Practice Procedure 5.3 (LO 5-3)

RECORDING THE USE OF CONTROLLED SUBSTANCES

Demonstrate how to record the use of controlled substances.

Equipment

Locked storage area (box, cabinet, or drawer) and keys

Medication administration record

Proof-of-use records for several controlled substances

Sample containers of controlled substances (unit dose)

Procedure

1. Unlock the storage area and read the medication orders. Follow Steps 2 through 7 for one medication at a time.

2. Read the label as you remove a container from the storage area.

3. Choose the proof-of-use form that goes with that drug. Fill out the form, giving the date of administration, time of administration, patient's full name, room and bed number, amount of medication taken from the container, patient's provider, name of the person giving the medication, and amount of medication given to the patient.

4. Have someone act as a witness if you must discard some of the medication. You may have to discard medication if:

   - You must give a smaller amount than the smallest unit-dose size.
   - You suspect that a drug is contaminated, or you contaminate the drug when setting it up.

   The witness should sign the proof-of-use record and state how much of the drug was destroyed.

5. Set up the medication as you would any other. Be sure to read the label again as you open the container.

6. Replace the container in the storage area. Read the label one last time as you do so.

7. Repeat these steps for the remaining controlled substances.

8. Lock the storage area and replace the controlled-substance folder. Keep the keys in your pocket for use on duty.

Show your work to your instructor or the lead healthcare team member.

Practice Procedure 5.4 (LO 5-3)

DISPENSING UNIT-DOSE MEDICATIONS FROM A CART IF AN AUTOMATED DISPENSING SYSTEM IS NOT USED

Demonstrate how to dispense unit-dose medications if an automated dispensing system is not used.

Equipment

Folder with medication administration records

Medicine cart, drawers labeled with names of patients

Unit doses of medicine placed in appropriate drawers of medicine cart

Medicine cart supplies (water, cups, spoons, etc.)

Procedure

1. Open the folder to the first patient's medication administration record.

2. Go to that patient's room and identify the patient by:
   - Checking the name on the wristband or on the bed.
   - Asking the patient his or her name. (Never use this method as the only way to identify a patient.)
   - Asking personnel to help you identify any patient who seems confused or who does not have a wristband.

3. Open the appropriate patient's drawer, identify the right medication, and give it to the patient, following these steps:
   - Read the medication administration record, and identify the medication.
   - Read the label of the unit-dose package, and compare it with the medication administration record.
   - Read the label of the unit-dose package as you give it to the patient.
   - Read the label of the unit-dose package as you discard it.

4. Chart administration of each drug on the medication administration record.

5. Make the patient comfortable.

6. Go to the next patient's room. This should be the patient whose medication administration record is next in the medication folder.

Show your work to your instructor.

FILLING OUT AN INCIDENT REPORT FORM OR EVENT REPORT FORM

Demonstrate how to fill out an incident report form or event report form.

Equipment

Incident report form

Written or oral summary of an actual or made-up medication error (a tape recording or a written story)

Procedure

1. Read or listen to the report of a medication error.
2. Record all information requested on the appropriate incident/accident form. Usually this includes:
   - Patient's name, room number, and bed.
   - Date, time, and location of the incident.
   - Name of the provider or supervisor who was notified of the incident.
   - Nature of the incident or accident and injuries received.
   - Diagram of the location of the injury on the body.
   - Date and time of this report.
   - Your signature.
3. Obtain signatures of all persons involved as required on the form.

   Show your work to your instructor or the lead healthcare team member.

Summary

Learning Outcome	Summary Points
5-1 Describe the various forms of medication, ranging from liquids to solids, and their abbreviations.	• Forms of medications are *solutions,* such as tinctures, elixirs, spirits, and syrups; *suspensions,* such as emulsions and lotions; and *solids and semisolids,* which include ointments, tablets, and capsules. Proper use of medication forms is critical to patient safety.
5-2 Describe the routes for administering medications.	• Oral • Sublingual • Buccal • Topical • Rectal • Vaginal • Inhalation • Parenteral • State regulations allow only certain licensed healthcare workers to administer parenteral medications.
5-3 Describe the routes of administration of medication and their abbreviations, administration times including use of the military clock, types of drug orders, and general medical terms.	• It is critical to be familiar with the abbreviations for medication routes, administration times, types of drug orders, and general medical terms to safely administer medications. • The military clock is a 24-hour system that is used to avoid confusing the a.m. and p.m. times that occur in the 12-hour system.

Learning Outcome	Summary Points
5-4 Carry out setting up medications following proper procedures.	• Appropriately identify the patient according to agency policy. • Read the medication administration record, and identify the medication. • Read the label of the unit-dose package, and compare it with the medication administration record. • Read the label of the unit-dose package as you give the medication to the patient. • Read the label of the unit-dose package as you discard it. • Chart the medicine on the MAR. • The MAR documents all drugs administered to a patient every day.

5-5 Explain the rules for giving medications, identifying parts of a medication label, and utilizing single-dose packaging.	• The "seven rights" or rules are:
	  Right drug
	  Right dose
	  Right patient
	  Right route
	  Right time
	  Right technique
	  Right documentation
	• Parts of a medication order are: patient's name, date, drug name, dosage, route of administration, time and frequency, provider's signature, quantity and number of refills, and provider's DEA number (if prescription is for a controlled substance).
	• The parts of a medication label are: trade name, generic name, form of the drug, dose strength, route of administration, precaution or warning label, expiration date, lot number, and batch number.
	• Single-dose medication is also called a unit dose.
	• Each dose of medication is individually wrapped or bottled and supplied for a 24-hour period.

5-6 Describe the problem-oriented medical record and the subjective-objective-assessment-plan method of charting and how the medication record is used to communicate a medication order.	• *Problem-oriented medical record (POMR):* The chart is organized according to a numbered list of problems or diagnoses. • *Subjective-objective-assessment-plan (SOAP) method:* The chart organizes content according to subjective data, objective data, assessment, and plan.
5-7 Carry out accurate, complete, and organized charting.	• A patient's chart must contain only the facts and serve as a summary of events.

Chapter 5 Review

Define each of the terms listed.

1. (LO 5-1) Active ingredient _____

   _____

2. (LO 5-1) Irrigation _____

   _____

3. (LO 5-1) Inhalation _____

_____

4. (LO 5-1) Instillation _____

_____

5. (LO 5-3) Outpatient _____

_____

6. (LO 5-3) Provider's order sheet _____

_____

7. (LO 5-3) Routine order _____

_____

8. (LO 5-3) Standing order _____

_____

9. (LO 5-3) PRN order _____

_____

10. (LO 5-3) Stat order _____

_____

Match the forms of medication to their descriptions.

_____ 11. (LO 5-1) Heavy sugar and water solution with flavoring

_____ 12. (LO 5-1) Alcohol mixed with a volatile oil

_____ 13. (LO 5-1) 10 to 20 percent drug solution in alcohol and/or water

_____ 14. (LO 5-1) Highly concentrated alcohol solution

_____ 15. (LO 5-1) Sweetened, alcoholic, and aromatic preparation

_____ 16. (LO 5-1) Oils and fats suspended in water

_____ 17. (LO 5-1) Mixture of heavy particles with water; looks like milk

_____ 18. (LO 5-1) Thick mixture of fine particles with water

_____ 19. (LO 5-1) A soothing or counterirritant preparation for external use, designed to be patted on

_____ 20. (LO 5-1) Gelatin sheath that contains 1 dose of medication

_____ 21. (LO 5-1) A topical or ophthalmic preparation in a base of lanolin or petrolatum

a. ointment

b. gel

c. emulsion

d. fluidextract

e. spirit

f. syrup

g. tincture

h. elixir

i. magma

j. capsule

k. lotion

Match the abbreviation to the proper route.

_____ 22. (LO 5-1) Under the tongue

_____ 23. (LO 5-1) Under the skin

_____ 24. (LO 5-1) Into the skin

_____ 25. (LO 5-1) Into the muscle

_____ 26. (LO 5-1) Into the vein

_____ 27. (LO 5-1) By mouth

_____ 28. (LO 5-1) Inside the cheek

a. buc

b. PO

c. ID

d. IV

e. subl

f. subcut

g. IM

Match the appropriate abbreviation to each phrase.

_____ 29. (LO 5-2) Drop

_____ 30. (LO 5-2) Medications given as necessary

_____ 31. (LO 5-2) Administration times

_____ 32. (LO 5-2) Before or after meals

_____ 33. (LO 5-2) Discontinue

_____ 34. (LO 5-2) Immediate, one-time order

_____ 35. (LO 5-2) Nothing by mouth

_____ 36. (LO 5-2) Chemical symbols

a. stat

b. BID, QID, q4h, h.s., a.m.

c. a.c., p.c.

d. HCl, NaCl, H_2O

e. ad lib., PRN

f. DC, d/c

g. NPO

h. gt

Write the term that the abbreviation stands for.

37. (LO 5-1) Ext. _____

38. (LO 5-1) Syr. _____

39. (LO 5-1) Tinct. _____

40. (LO 5-1) Supp. _____

41. (LO 5-1) Sp. _____

42. (LO 5-1) Fld. ext. _____

43. (LO 5-1) Cap. _____

44. (LO 5-1) Elix. _____

45. (LO 5-1) Tab. _____

46. (LO 5-1) Soln. _____

47. (LO 5-1) Susp. _____

Describe the solid forms.

48. (LO 5-1) Troche _____

_____

49. (LO 5-1) Suppository _____

_____

50. (LO 5-1) Sustained-release capsule _____

_____

51. (LO 5-1) Scored tablet _____

_____

Fill in the blanks with the word or phrase that best completes each statement.

52. (LO 5-1) Because of their high drug concentrations, spirits, tinctures, and fluidextracts must be measured with a(n) _____.

53. (LO 5-1) To prevent alcohol solutions from separating, store them in _____.

54. (LO 5-1) Bottles containing tinctures, fluidextracts, elixirs, and spirits are kept tightly closed so that the _____ cannot evaporate.

55. (LO 5-1) All suspensions must be _____ before use.

56. (LO 5-1) When a drug dissolves in water or alcohol, the result is called a(n) _____.

57. (LO 5-1) When a drug does not dissolve in liquid, the preparation is called a(n) _____.

58. (LO 5-1) _____ -coated capsules and tablets prevent stomach irritation by dissolving only when they reach the intestine.

59. (LO 5-1) Liquid suspensions for external application to the skin to relieve pain and swelling are known as _____.

60. (LO 5-1) Suppositories may be inserted into the _____, the _____, or the _____.

61. (LO 5-1) A diagnosed alcoholic should not be given any _____ solutions.

62. (LO 5-1) Sustained-release capsules are also called _____.

63. (LO 5-1) Oral medicines are made to taste good to help _____ as well as _____ take them.

64. (LO 5-1) Elixirs of phenobarbital or *Benadryl Allergy* are _____ to help children and older adults take them better.

65. (LO 5-1) In sublingual and buccal administrations, no _____ is permitted until the medication is dissolved.

66. (LO 5-1) Applying local medications to the skin or the mucous membranes is known as the
_____ route.

67. (LO 5-1) Injecting medications into the body with a needle and syringe is known as the
_____ route.

68. (LO 5-1) Parenteral medications and equipment must be _____; otherwise, there is
danger of infection.

Convert from the military time clock to the regular clock and vice versa.

	Regular Clock	Military Clock
69. (LO 5-3)	7:00 a.m.	_____
70. (LO 5-3)	_____	1100 hours
71. (LO 5-3)	_____	1330 hours
72. (LO 5-3)	2:00 p.m.	_____
73. (LO 5-3)	_____	2000 hours

Answer the questions in the space provided.

74. (LO 5-4) What should you do if you have a question about a medication order? _____

_____

75. (LO 5-3) What members of the health team, in addition to providers, are allowed to prescribe medications
in some states? _____

_____

76. (LO 5-1) What is the important rule to remember when administering delayed-release tablets and
capsules? Why is this rule important? _____

_____

_____

77. (LO 5-4) List seven items of information that must be included on any written medication order. _____

_____

_____

_____

_____

_____

_____

Translate these providers' orders. Use your knowledge of medical abbreviations to give their meanings.

78. (LO 5-1) *Vicodin PO* q4h prn for pain _____

_____

_____

79. (LO 5-1) Phenobarbital elix. 1 tsp (20 mg) at bedtime _____

_____

_____

80. (LO 5-1) *Keflex* 250 mg caps q6h po _____

_____

_____

81. (LO 5-1) *Lotrimin AF* cream bid × 2 weeks _____

_____

_____

82. (LO 5-1) Bacitracin ophth. oint. in the right eye tid for conjunctivitis _____

_____

_____

83. (LO 5-1) Propantheline tabs. 15 mg a.c. _____

_____

_____

84. (LO 5-1) Heparin 5000 units IV stat _____

_____

_____

85. (LO 5-1) Acetaminophen 120 mg R supp. qid _____

_____

_____

Match the medical forms to their descriptions.

_____ 86. (LO 5-4) Form for charting medications administered on a regular schedule

_____ 87. (LO 5-4) One form used to chart care given by all health team members

_____ 88. (LO 5-4) Provider's orders for an outpatient

_____ 89. (LO 5-4) Describes the patient's medical problems in more detail

_____ 90. (LO 5-6) Used to record medication errors

a. POMR

b. prescription blank

c. incident report form

d. patient history sheet

e. medication administration record

Answer the questions in the space provided.

91. (LO 5-4) How many doses of medication are contained in a unit-dose package? _____

_____

92. (LO 5-6) What does PIE charting stand for? _____

_____

93. (LO 5-3) What must be counted or measured at the beginning of each shift? _____

_____

94. (LO 5-3) List two examples of controlled substances. _____

_____

95. (LO 5-3) Where should controlled substances be stored? _____

_____

96. (LO 5-4) List two advantages of single-dose packaging. _____

_____

97. (LO 5-3) Where should drugs labeled "For external use only" be kept? _____

_____

98. (LO 5-1) How can you best make a clean break when dividing a scored tablet? _____

_____

99. (LO 5-4) List the seven rights of medication administration. _____

_____

_____

_____

_____

_____

100. (LO 5-2) List two rules for giving the correct medication. _____

_____

_____

101. (LO 5-6) List three reasons why the patient chart is an important document. _____

_____

_____

_____

102. (LO 5-6) What is the SOAP system of charting? _____

_____

_____

103. (LO 5-6) On a medication administration record, how would you show that a dose of medicine was not given when scheduled? (Check the procedure in your own health facility.) _____

_____

_____

_____

104. (LO 5-6) How would you show that you gave a dose of medicine? (Check the procedure in your own health facility.) _____

_____

_____

Drug Calculations—Fill in the blank with the answer.

105. (LO 5-3) The provider orders clozapine (*Clozaril*) 50 mg orally bid. Using the medication label for *Clozaril*, you should administer _____ tablets to your patient.

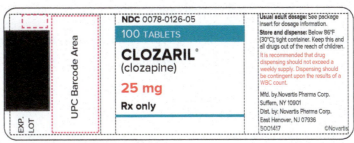

Source: 2013 Novartis International AG.

106. (LO 5-3) The provider orders erythromycin (*Ery-Tab*) 500 mg orally daily. Using the medication label for *Ery-Tab*, prepare to administer _____ tablets to your patient.

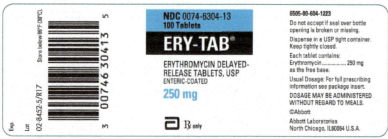

Source: Abbott Laboratories.

107. (LO 5-3) The provider orders trimethobenzamide (*Tigan*) 200 mg to be administered intramuscularly. Using the medication label for *Tigan*, administer _____ mL to your patient.

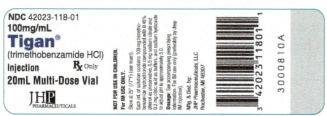

Source: JHP Pharmaceuticals, LLC.

Multiple Choice—Circle the correct letter.

108. (LO 5-3) Which is a correct abbreviation to use in medication administration?

    a. AD

    b. OS

    c. q. d.

    d. p.c.

109. (LO 5-3) Which abbreviation is defined correctly?

    a. PRN—permission required and necessary

    b. NKA—necessary knowledge acquired

    c. n.p.o.—nothing by mouth

    d. c/o—comments offered

110. (LO 5-4) Which is the most common type of drug order to follow?

    a. Routine order

    b. Standing order

    c. PRN order

    d. Verbal order

111. (LO 5-1) You administer which of the following types of medications for a patient with asthma?

    a. Liniment

    b. Aerosol

    c. Magma

    d. Syrup

112. (LO 5-4) Which principle is a step in the setup of medications?

    a. Open unit dose before reaching the patient

    b. Pour a liquid medication toward the side of the medication label

    c. Determine if medication is to be mixed with food

    d. Wipe off pill that fell on the floor before administering

Chapter 5 Case Studies

113. (LO 5-4) While checking morning vital signs you discover that a patient's temperature is 102°F. The patient complains of a general not-feeling-well sensation. You review the medication administration record to see if there is anything that should be administered to the patient. There is an order for *Tylenol* 500 mg PO q4h for temperature 101° or above. What kind of order is this? What should you do?

_____

_____

_____

114. (LO 5-6) You just finished administering medications to a patient, and you discover that you gave the wrong dose of the medication. What should you do? Should any forms be completed? Will this form become part of the permanent chart?

_____

_____

_____

Critical Thinking

Show how you would chart the following events in the nurses' notes. Be sure to include all of the required information. Remember that only facts are to be charted, not assumptions or opinions.

Mr. Schwartz is undergoing treatment for a blood clot in the leg. He has been taking *Coumadin,* an anticoagulant, for several days. He is also taking *Diuril,* a diuretic, to reduce the swelling in his leg. The provider has confined Mr. Schwartz to bed. This is because any movement of the leg might cause the clot to break off and travel in the bloodstream, which could be dangerous.

115. (LO 5-6) At 0800 on October 5 you give Mr. Schwartz two 5-mg tablets of *Coumadin* to swallow with a glass of water. You chart it on the medication administration record. As you refill the water pitcher, Mr. Schwartz asks if you happen to have something for an upset stomach. He says his stomach hurts the way it did when he had an ulcer 20 years ago. Because the anticoagulant can cause internal bleeding (e.g., from an old ulcer), you have been alert for signs of this side effect. You notify your supervisor, who asks the provider to order a test for internal bleeding. The test results are negative. The supervisor then directs you to give Mr. Schwartz 2 tsp of *Maalox Regular Strength* to calm his stomach.

_____

_____

_____

116. (LO 5-6) It is 1200 hours and time for Mr. Schwartz's next dose of *Diuril*. Mr. Schwartz complains again about his upset stomach, but this time he tells you it is worse right after he takes the *Diuril*. You skip this dose of *Diuril* and notify the supervisor. The supervisor tells you to continue giving the *Diuril* but to keep an eye out for signs of internal bleeding.

_____

_____

_____

117. (LO 5-6) It is 2000 hours the next evening and time to give Mr. Schwartz a laxative. The laxative (*Dulcolax Suppository*) has been ordered by the provider because bedridden patients often develop constipation, which can lead to impaction (blocking of the intestine). Straining during a bowel movement might cause the blood clot to break off and become an embolism (a traveling clot). Mr. Schwartz tells you that he has been having regular bowel movements and doesn't want the laxative. He asks why he needs it when he has been in bed for only 2 days. You explain that it is preventive medicine to avoid the problems of impaction and embolism. Mr. Schwartz becomes tearful and tells you that he is afraid he will die. He refuses the laxative. You then notify the supervisor. After consulting with the provider, the supervisor instructs you to give Mr. Schwartz 10 mg of diazepam intramuscularly right away. Diazepam is a tranquilizer that will ease Mr. Schwartz's anxiety so that he can relax.

_____

_____

_____

Applications

Obtain an electronic drug guide and a current copy of the *PDR*® from your school, health facility, or clinic. Use it to answer the questions that follow.

118. What is the name of the section where the listing of unit-dose systems is given? _____

_____

119. In this section, locate the drug spironolactone (*Aldactone*). How is this drug supplied as a unit dose?

_____

_____

120. In the same section, locate diazepam (*Valium*). What information does the manufacturer give about unit-dose systems? _____

_____

VITAMINS, MINERALS, AND HERBS

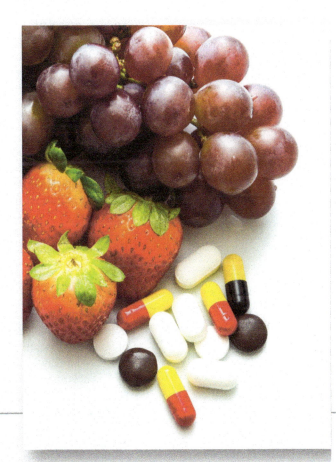

©Cesar Okada/iStock/Getty Images

In this chapter you will learn about vitamins and minerals and their importance in the diet for normal growth and development. You will also learn the functions, food sources, recommended daily requirement, and symptoms of deficiency or excess for each. You will be able to identify the conditions in which appropriate supplementation is necessary. You will also learn about the growing interest in herbs and the potential dangers of some herbal remedies.

anions

cations

electrolytes

fat-soluble vitamins

homeostasis

hypervitaminosis

hypovitaminosis

inorganic

ions

macrominerals

microminerals

minerals

organic

recommended daily allowance (RDA)

vitamins

water-soluble vitamins

INTRODUCTION TO MYPLATE [LO 6-1]

Food is essential to life, and the food selections we make are important in maintaining health and preventing disease. Today, with a growing interest in health promotion and disease prevention, this interest has led to an awareness of the connection between nutrition and the onset of disease. Vitamins and minerals have a significant role in controlling many of the body's functions. An individual who consumes a well-balanced diet should have no need for supplementation. The United States Department of Agriculture (USDA) developed MyPlate to assist in food buying and preparation (**Figure 6.1**). It is based on a diet of 2000 calories per day. If an individual follows the guidelines set by the USDA in Choose MyPlate, the recommended daily allowance (RDA) requirements for vitamins and minerals will be met. However, there are certain conditions in which supplementation may be necessary. A daily diet consisting of less than 1200 calories, increased physical activity, pregnancy, illness, and medication interaction may require vitamin supplementation. Based on the RDA for vitamins and minerals, children will require less.

RECOMMENDED DAILY ALLOWANCE [LO 6-2]

An individual's vitamin needs depend on age, sex, weight, level of activity, and overall state of health. The **recommended daily allowance (RDA)** is the level of intake for essential nutrients considered to be adequate to meet the nutritional needs of healthy individuals. The RDA is published by the National Academy of Science and revised approximately every five years. It provides the only available and reliable recommendation for nutrients. The RDA for each nutrient is expressed in international units, or IUs. It is important to understand that the RDA includes not only the amount of food one eats but also the amount present in supplementation. It is essential to teach patients this fact to prevent toxicity caused by taking unnecessary megadoses. Reading food labels began in the United States in 1994 to provide an at-a-glance method of determining how food fits into the diet. The label provides information regarding serving size, calories, nutrients, and daily values (**Figure 6.2**). Always remind patients that the RDA for vitamins and minerals is based on the average, normal, healthy adult.

VITAMINS [LO 6-2]

Vitamins are **organic,** or carbon-containing, substances that are necessary for metabolism and normal growth and development. They must be supplied through the diet because they are either not made in the body or made in insufficient quantity. Avitaminosis is a condition that results from a deficiency or lack of vitamin absorption in the diet. It is also known as **hypovitaminosis.** A decreased intake of vitamins may occur because of an inadequate diet

Figure 6.1

MyPlate (U.S. Dept. of Agriculture).

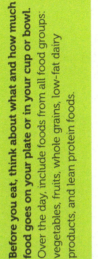

Before you eat, think about what and how much food goes on your plate or in your cup or bowl. Over the day, include foods from all food groups: vegetables, fruits, whole grains, low-fat dairy products, and lean protein foods.

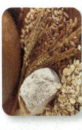

Make at least half your grains whole.

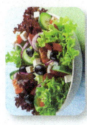

Make half your plate fruits and vegetables.

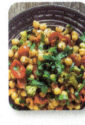

Vary your protein food choices.

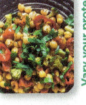

Switch to skim or 1% milk.

What's on your plate?

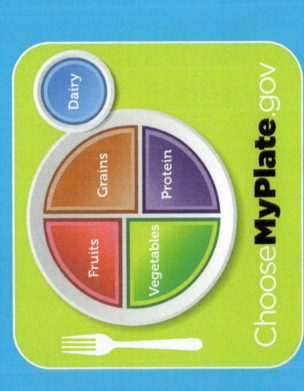

Choose**MyPlate**.gov

Figure 6.1 (Continued)

MyPlate (U.S. Dept. of Agriculture).

Vegetables	Fruits	Grains	Dairy	Protein Foods
Eat more red, orange, and dark-green veggies like tomatoes, sweet potatoes, and broccoli in main dishes.	Use fruits as snacks, salads, and desserts. At breakfast, top your cereal with bananas or strawberries; add blueberries to pancakes.	Substitute whole-grain choices for refined-grain breads, bagels, rolls, breakfast cereals, crackers, rice, and pasta.	Choose skim (fat-free) or 1% (low-fat) milk. They have the same amount of calcium and other essential nutrients as whole milk, but less fat and calories.	Eat a variety of foods from the protein food group each week, such as seafood, beans and peas, and nuts as well as lean meats, poultry, and eggs.
Add beans or peas to salads (kidney or chickpeas), soups (split peas or lentils), and side dishes (pinto or baked beans), or serve as a main dish.	Buy fruits that are dried, frozen, and canned (in water or 100% juice), as well as fresh fruits.	Check the ingredients list on product labels for the words "whole" or "whole grain" before the grain ingredient name.	Top fruit salads and baked potatoes with low-fat yogurt.	Twice a week, make seafood the protein on your plate.
Fresh, frozen, and canned vegetables all count. Choose "reduced sodium" or "no-salt-added" canned veggies.	Select 100% fruit juice when choosing juices.	Choose products that name a whole grain first on the ingredients list.	If you are lactose intolerant, try lactose-free milk or fortified soymilk (soy beverage).	Choose lean meats and ground beef that are at least 90% lean.
				Trim or drain fat from meat and remove skin from poultry to cut fat and calories.

For a 2,000-calorie daily food plan, you need the amounts below from each food group.
To find amounts personalized for you, go to ChooseMyPlate.gov.

Eat 2½ cups every day	Eat 2 cups every day	Eat 6 ounces every day	Get 3 cups every day	Eat 5½ ounces every day
What counts as a cup? 1 cup of raw or cooked vegetables or vegetable juice; 2 cups of leafy salad greens	What counts as a cup? 1 cup of raw or cooked fruit or 100% fruit juice; ½ cup dried fruit	What counts as an ounce? 1 slice of bread; ½ cup of cooked rice, cereal, or pasta; 1 ounce of ready-to-eat cereal	What counts as a cup? 1 cup of milk, yogurt, or fortified soymilk; 1½ ounces natural or 2 ounces processed cheese	What counts as an ounce? 1 ounce of lean meat, poultry, or fish; 1 egg; 1 Tbsp peanut butter; ½ ounce nuts or seeds; ¼ cup beans or peas

Cut back on sodium and empty calories from solid fats and added sugars

Look out for salt (sodium) in foods you buy. Compare sodium in foods and choose those with a lower number.

Drink water instead of sugary drinks. Eat sugary desserts less often.

Make foods that are high in solid fats—such as cakes, cookies, ice cream, pizza, cheese, sausages, and hot dogs—occasional choices, not every day foods.

Limit empty calories to less than 260 per day, based on a 2,000 calorie diet.

Be physically active your way

Pick activities you like and do each for at least 10 minutes at a time. Every bit adds up, and health benefits increase as you spend more time being active.

Children and adolescents: get 60 minutes or more a day.

Adults: get 2 hours and 30 minutes or more a week of activity that requires moderate effort, such as brisk walking.

USDA U.S. Department of Agriculture • Center for Nutrition Policy and Promotion
August 2011
CNPP 25
USDA is an equal opportunity provider and employer.

Sources: Pizza: ©Don Farrall/Getty Images, Soda: ©amnatn/Shutterstock, Fried Food: ©Hannamariah/Shutterstock.com

Figure 6.2

Nutrition labels show the percent daily values of recommended daily allowance (RDA).

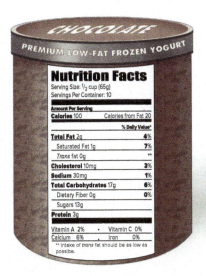
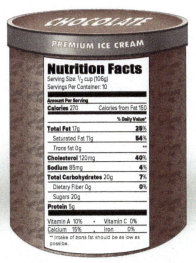

resulting from cultural, religious, or personal practices, fad diets, alcoholism, poverty, or lack of available food. In the United States, avitaminosis most likely results from alcoholism or fad diets. However, hypovitaminosis related to inadequate food accessibility is more of a problem than many realize. Vitamins may also be adversely affected in the processing, storage, and preparation of food. Foods that are used quickly and have not been exposed to air or the heat and water used in cooking have the highest vitamin content. Vitamins are classified as being either **fat soluble** (A, D, E, and K) or **water soluble** (B complex and C). Understanding vitamins' individual functions, food sources, RDA, and symptoms of deficiency and excess is important to determining if a need for supplementation exists.

Fat-Soluble Vitamins

Fat-soluble vitamins consist of the A, D, E, and K vitamins and are less widely distributed in nature. They are found mostly in fortified milk, whole milk products, green leafy vegetables, yellow fruits and vegetables, fish, liver oil, and sunlight (Table 6.1). Because they are not soluble in water, they are not easily eliminated from the body. A deficiency would take many months to develop. Vitamin deficiencies are rare in most developed countries. When present, a deficiency involves several vitamins. In the United States, the RDA can be met by eating a diet from foods found in Choose MyPlate. When vitamin deficiencies occur, they are usually found in people addicted to alcohol or drugs, those who are poor or homeless, people with poor dietary patterns, and those who have a poor intake due to a chronic or serious disease. Toxicity can also occur over time when there is a consistent intake of megadoses of synthetic vitamins. A condition called **hypervitaminosis** results from taking large doses of vitamins over a period of time.

Water-Soluble Vitamins

Water-soluble vitamins are widely found in plant and animal food sources (Table 6.2). They consist of the B complex and C vitamins. Because they cannot be stored in the body, they must be supplied through daily food intake. Some of them can be destroyed by cooking. Because these vitamins are water soluble, they are eliminated from the body in sweat and urine. Although water-soluble vitamins cannot be stored in the body, recent evidence proves that individuals who take megadoses or excessively large quantities of riboflavin (B_2), niacin, and vitamin C can develop a toxicity. Water-soluble vitamins act as catalysts in protein, fat, and carbohydrate metabolism. When the body contains a sufficient supply of the vitamins to assist in protein, fat, and carbohydrate metabolism, additional amounts can be toxic.

Table 6.1 Fat-Soluble Vitamins

Vitamin	Functions	Sources	RDA	Symptoms of Deficiency	Symptoms of Excess
Vitamin A (retinol)	Helps form and maintain skin and mucous membranes, bone growth, development of teeth, vision, immune functions	Whole milk; whole milk products; eggs; yellow and green leafy vegetables; yellow fruits; liver; liver oil; fish	5000 IU	Night blindness; rough skin; dry mucous membranes; lack of bone growth; susceptibility to infection	*Mild:* nausea; vomiting; abdominal pain *Severe:* growth retardation; damage to liver and spleen; hair loss
Vitamin D (cholecalciferol)	Maintains healthy bones and teeth	Sunlight; fortified milk and dairy products; fish; liver oil	600 IU	Rickets (in children); retarded growth; bowed legs; protruding abdomen; osteomalacia (in adults); bone softening; bone fragility; muscle twitching and spasms	*Mild:* anorexia; nausea; weight loss *Severe:* calcium drawn from bony tissues and deposited in soft tissues, blood vessels, and kidneys
Vitamin E (tocopherol)	Prevents oxidation of fatty acids	Vegetable oils; green leafy vegetables; milk; eggs; cereal; wheat germ	30 IU	Breakdown of red blood cells	Increased bleeding; intestinal upset; headache; tiredness
Vitamin K (phytonadione)	Helps form prothrombin (for blood clotting)	Green leafy vegetables, dairy products, cauliflower, soybeans, liver, peas, potatoes, and tomatoes; manufactured in intestinal tract	80 mg	Hemorrhage in newborns; increased clotting time in adults	Anemia and jaundice in newborns; blood clot and vomiting in adults

A megadose refers to the administration of high doses of a vitamin, usually 10 to 20 times the RDA. If a serious vitamin deficiency exists, it can involve one or even several vitamins. Caution must be used to avoid toxicity. For example, vitamin C increases the renal excretion of uric acid and may cause formation of kidney stones in susceptible people taking megadoses. Taken in large doses, vitamins are classified as drugs rather than nutrients and may cause toxic effects. The fat-soluble vitamins are stored and may accumulate to toxic levels. Because vitamins are bought without a prescription, fat-soluble vitamins, which cannot be eliminated, may cause serious health problems.

 Caution Megadoses

Never take megadoses of any vitamin unless under the supervision of a provider.

Table 6.2 Water-Soluble Vitamins

Vitamin	Functions	Sources	RDA	Symptoms of Deficiency	Symptoms of Excess
Vitamin B$_1$ (thiamine)	Is necessary for normal nerve conduction and heart function	Pork; fish; poultry; eggs; whole grains; pasta; yeast; wheat germ	1.5 mg	Tingling in extremities; muscle weakness; numbness; mental confusion; disturbances in heart rate; beriberi (rare)	Rapid heart rate; difficulty sleeping; headaches
Vitamin B$_2$ (riboflavin)	Metabolizes proteins, carbohydrates, and fats; aids in growth	Liver; whole grains; dark vegetables; milk	1.7 mg	Cracks at corners of mouth; sore tongue; sensitivity to light	Rare; symptoms of excess vitamin B (riboflavin) are rare but can include kidney stones
Niacin	Helps utilize protein; breaks down fat	Meat; poultry; tuna; whole grains; cereals; liver	20 mg	Pellagra; skin disorders, esp. when exposed to sun; diarrhea; confusion	Flushing; headache; nausea; itching; diarrhea
Vitamin B$_6$ (pyridoxine)	Metabolizes proteins, carbohydrates, and fats; helps form red blood cells	Most food groups; liver; whole grains; green beans; potatoes; nuts	2 mg	Cracks at corners of mouth; anemia; skin lesions	Bloating; headache; fatigue
Folic acid B9	Helps form body proteins and genetic material; helps form red blood cells; essential for a healthy pregnancy and needed to prevent neural tube defects	Most food groups; liver, kidneys; green leafy vegetables; whole grains	400 µg	Anemia; fatigue; sore tongue	May obscure existence of pernicious anemia (vitamin B$_{12}$ deficiency); diarrhea; irritability
Vitamin B$_{12}$ (cyanocobalamin)	Helps build genetic material; helps form red blood cells; is necessary for normal functioning of nervous system	Liver; kidneys; meat; fish; eggs; milk	6 µg	Pernicious anemia; degeneration of peripheral nerves	None reported
Pantothenic acid	Metabolizes proteins, carbohydrates, and fats; helps form hormones	Meats; whole grains; nuts	10 mg	None reported	None reported
Biotin	Helps form fatty acids; metabolizes protein	Kidney liver; egg yolks; dark green vegetables; green beans	0.3 mg	None reported	None reported
Vitamin C (ascorbic acid)	Maintains healthy bones, teeth, and blood vessels; helps form collagen	Citrus fruits; strawberries; melon; dark green vegetables	60 mg	Scurvy; wounds that will not heal; bleeding gums; bruising; loose teeth	Kidney stones; urinary tract infection; when megadose discontinued, deficiency symptoms may appear briefly until body adapts

MINERALS [LO 6-3]

Minerals are **inorganic** elements (they do not contain carbon) essential to the body for health and growth. They serve many important functions in the body. Among these are the formation of bones and teeth, regulation of body fluids and hormone production, muscle contraction, and metabolism of nutrients in foods. Minerals are classified as **macrominerals,** minerals with a daily requirement of 100 mg or more, and **microminerals,** minerals with a daily requirement of less than 100 mg. Calcium, phosphorus, magnesium, sodium, potassium, chloride, and sulfur are examples of macrominerals (Table 6.3). Microminerals, also known as trace minerals, include iron, manganese, copper, iodine, zinc, cobalt, fluoride, and selenium (Table 6.4). Although minerals are essential to good health, they can be harmful in excess. Excessive amounts of minerals can pose a risk for children, older adults, pregnant women, and individuals with a poor diet or with certain diseases. Their functions, food sources, RDA, and symptoms of deficiency and excess are essential in determining the need for supplementation.

Minerals are found in both plant and animal foods. Unlike vitamins, minerals are not damaged by heat or light, but some are lost in cooking excessively in water. It is important to educate patients about the appropriate use of vitamins and minerals.

 Patient Education Vitamins and Minerals

- Avoid taking vitamin or mineral supplementation without the direction of a provider.
- The best way to avoid vitamin or mineral deficiency is through a well-balanced diet.
- Choose MyPlate outlines the basic food requirements.
- Megadoses of vitamins can be dangerous.

 Pediatric Considerations Vitamins and Minerals

- Children may need vitamin supplements if deficiencies exist.
- Dosages of vitamin supplements should not exceed the recommended dose.
- Avoid accidental overdose because of attractive packaging and taste. Keep out of reach of children, because they may mistake the drugs, which come shaped like animals or action characters, for candy.
- The FDA regulates supplements for children under the age of 4 years but not those for older children.
- Liquid preparations are available for infants and young children. Chewable tablets are available for older children.
- Preterm infants may need more vitamin supplements than term infants because of their faster growth rate.
- A vitamin-mineral supplement may be prescribed for children who eat poorly.
- Avoid accidental overdose of iron-containing medications and supplements because death can occur.

Table 6.3 Macrominerals

Macromineral	Functions	Sources	RDA	Symptoms of Deficiency	Symptoms of Excess
Calcium	Forms bones and teeth; aids in blood clotting and transmission of nerve impulses	Milk; milk products; green leafy vegetables; sardines; clams; oysters; egg yolk	1000 mg for adults 19–50 years of age; 1000 mg for males and 1200 mg for females over 51 years of age	Hypocalcemia; stunted growth in children; osteoporosis in adults; pathological fractures; tingling in fingers; tetany; convulsions	Hypercalcemia; relaxed skeletal muscles; kidney stones; cardiac irregularities
Sodium	Maintains acid-base balance; controls body's fluid balance; regulates heart, muscle, and nerve activity	Most foods; meats; sardines; milk; eggs; cereal	500 mg	Hyponatremia; muscle cramps; depression; decreased appetite; weakness	Hypernatremia; confusion; fluid retention
Potassium	Chief cation in the intracellular fluid; maintains acid-base balance; maintains body's fluid balance; aids in nerve impulse conduction and muscle irritability; regulates heart rate	Cereals; meats; legumes; fresh vegetables (potatoes); dried peas; fresh fruits (bananas, oranges, prunes, raisins)	2000 mEq	Hypokalemia; muscle weakness; thirst; cardiac abnormalities; arrhythmias; confusion; dizziness	Hyperkalemia; confusion; cardiac abnormalities; weakness; decreased blood pressure
Magnesium	Maintains electrical activity in nerves and muscles; regulates body temperature; aids in fat metabolism and protein synthesis	Whole grains; nuts; legumes; green vegetables; seafood; meats	400 mg	Hypomagnesemia; neuromuscular irritability (tetany); failure to grow; behavioral disturbances; weakness; confusion	Hypermagnesemia; diarrhea; lethargy; cardiac and respiratory disturbances
Phosphorus	Energy from foods; forms bones and teeth; regulates acid-base balance; metabolizes proteins, carbohydrates, and fats	Milk and milk products; eggs; meat; fish; poultry; grains; legumes; nuts	700 mg	Hypophosphatemia; bone demineralization; bone pain; pathological fractures	Hyperphos-phatemia; calcium loss

Table 6.4 Microminerals

Micromineral	Functions	Sources	RDA	Symptoms of Deficiency	Symptoms of Excess
Iron	Forms hemoglobin; aids in synthesis of vitamins	Liver; lean meats; legumes; whole grains; dark green vegetables; eggs; cereals; potatoes	18 mg for females 19–50 years of age; 8 mg for adult males and females over 51 years of age	Anemia; weakness; dizziness; pallor; lowered resistance to infection; fatigue; anorexia; spoon-shaped nails	Nausea; vomiting; black stools; abdominal pain; toxicity (hemochromatosis)
Iodine	Is a component of thyroid hormone; is important in development and functioning of thyroid gland; helps prevent goiter; formation of thyroxine (T4) and triiodothyronine (T3)	Iodized salt; seafood; food additives	150 μg	Cretinism (decrease in stature, mental capacity, and muscle coordination) in infants; decreased thyroid function in adults; simple goiter	Toxic goiter; myxedema
Zinc	Aids in enzyme activity involved in digestion; helps in wound healing and immune response; growth	Meats; liver; oysters; poultry; legumes	12–15 mg	Decreased wound healing; failure to grow; decrease in taste and smell; anorexia; skin lesions	Fever; nausea; vomiting; diarrhea; interference with calcium absorption; muscle pain and weakness
Copper	Helps form red blood cells; aids in enzyme activity involved in digestion; helps the central nervous system function properly	Liver; kidneys; shellfish; nuts; raisins; dried peas	1.5–3.0 mg	Anemia; bone demineralization	Headache; dizziness; gastrointestinal upset

 Older Adult Considerations Vitamins and Minerals

- Older adults are at risk of poor nutrition and of deficiencies of vitamins and minerals.
- Vitamin requirements for older adults are the same as those for younger adults.
- Deficiencies of vitamins A, D, and B₁₂ and of folic acid, riboflavin, and thiamine are common.
- A daily multivitamin is recommended.

- Use caution when giving fat-soluble vitamins A and D because of toxicity.
- Deficiencies of the minerals calcium and iron are common in older adults.
- Because of older adults' decreased renal function, retention of magnesium and potassium may occur.

ELECTROLYTES [LO 6-4]

Water makes up 45 to 75 percent of total body weight, depending on an individual's percentage of body fat. Infants and children have a greater percentage of water content than the average adult. Within the body's water content are **electrolytes,** or solutions that carry an electrical charge. Macrominerals such as calcium, potassium, sodium, and magnesium are electrolytes. **Ions** are particles that release an electrical charge. Some ions, **cations,** have a positive electrical charge, while others, **anions,** have a negative charge. There must be an equal number of cations and anions in all of the body's fluids to maintain **homeostasis,** or a state of fluid balance.

HERBS [LO 6-5]

Long before the advent of modern medicine, even before the discovery of vitamins and minerals, people relied on herbs to cure their ills. Many cultures still believe that a simple herb can cure or prevent health problems. Today, there is an explosion of interest in "natural" products, which has dramatically increased the use of herbal remedies. This "back-to-nature" phenomenon developed because of warnings about food preservatives and additives or products that are said to be carcinogenic, or cancer-causing. The emphasis on *natural* and *nature* has generated a multimillion-dollar enterprise. There has been a great increase in the number of health food stores selling natural organic vegetables, vitamins, and cosmetics. While these products once appealed only to certain cultural or ethnic groups, today they appeal to the general population. Because the manufacturing of herbs as pharmaceuticals is not regulated by the FDA, patients may consider them natural and safe for use regardless of their conditions. This is not always the case, and herbs may have deterimental effects for patients.

Several familiar and much-needed medications come from plant sources. Digitalis (*Lanoxin*), used in the treatment of heart disease, comes from the foxglove plant. Vincristine and vinblastine, made from the periwinkle plant, are common antineoplastic agents frequently used in the treatment of Hodgkin's disease, leukemia, and breast and testicular cancer.

A summary of the common herbs is found in Table 6.5. As a healthcare team member in a provider's office, clinic, or hospital, you are in a position to question patients about the use of herbal remedies and inform them about those that can be harmful (Table 6.6). However, all too often healthcare professionals are not asking such questions and patients are not volunteering this information. Obtaining a complete list of the herbs that a patient is using is essential in identifying potential herb interactions with prescription medications or excessive bleeding that may occur in surgery. Patients especially at risk for drug–herb interactions include those taking prescription drugs such as anticoagulants, hypoglycemics, antidepressants, sedative-hypnotics, and certain cardiac and respiratory medications such as digoxin and theophylline.

 Healthcare for Today and Tomorrow   Echinacea

Current research indicates that echinacea is promoted in the United States for prevention and treatment of the common cold. Although this herb is promoted in Europe for topical wound healing and for intravenous stimulation of the immune system, research does not yet support these uses in the United States. Website: www.herbs.org (Herb Research Foundation).

Table 6.5 Common Herbs

Common Name	Effects	Possible Uses	Prescription Drug Interactions
Aloe vera	Is an anti-inflammatory; accelerates wound healing	Minor burns; wound healing	*DiaBeta*, topical corticosteroids
Astragalus	Stimulates immune system	Cancer	None known
Bilberry	Improves circulation in eyes; is a mild anti-inflammatory	Myopia; retinal problems; gastrointestinal disorders	None known
Cat's claw	Stimulates immune system; is an antioxidant and anti-inflammatory; lowers blood pressure	Cancer; gastrointestinal disorders; infection; hypertension	None known
Chamomile	Is an anti-inflammatory, antispasmodic, and anti-infective	Inflammatory gastrointestinal disorders; respiratory and skin disorders	Chemotherapy, cisplatin, cyclophosphamide, docetaxel, fluroruracil methotrexate, paclitaxel
Cranberry	May have anti-infective properties (Use sugar-free cranberry juice with diabetes mellitus.)	Prophylaxis only; not treatment for urinary tract infections or for kidney stones	None known
Dong quai	Is an antispasmodic and mild sedative; aids in vaso-dilation; provides estrogen	Menstrual cramps and disorders	Heparin, *Coumadin*
Echinacea	Stimulates immune system; is an anti-inflammatory and anti-infective	Common cold; upper respiratory infections	Chemotherapy, cisplatin, cyclophosamide, docetaxel, fluroruracil, methotrexate, paclitaxel
Feverfew	Is an anti-inflammatory; aids in vasodilation	Arthritis; migraine headaches; relief of pain	Avoid taking with anticoagulants (increases bleeding); avoid aspirin (increases antiplatelet effect)
Garlic	Lowers lipid level; is an anti-infective; inhibits aggregation of platelets; anti-inflammatory properties	Elevated cholesterol level; infections; diabetes mellitus; hypertension	Chlorzoxazone, *Persantine*, *Coumadin*
Ginger	Is an antiemetic	Nausea and vomiting; motion sickness	None known
Ginkgo biloba	Improves memory; increases blood flow; is an antioxidant	Dementia; Alzheimer's disease; peripheral vascular disease	Aspirin, *Celexa*, cyclosporine, *Prozac*, fluvoxamine, *Amaryl*, *Glucotrol*, *DiaBeta*, haloperidol, heparin, *Glucophage*, *Paxil*, *Prandin*, *Zoloft*, thiazide diuretics, trazodone, *Coumadin*
Ginseng	Increases physical endurance; relieves stress	Fatigue; anxiety	*Coumadin*; headache with *Nardil*; may reduce blood sugar in Type 2 diabetes

Table 6.5 *(continued)*

Common Name	Effects	Possible Uses	Prescription Drug Interactions
Goldenseal	Is an anti-inflammatory, anti-infective, and laxative	Gastrointestinal and respiratory disorders; infection of mouth and lungs	*Vibramycin*, tetracyline
Hawthorn	Increases oxygenation through heart; is a peripheral vasodilator	Angina pectoris; coronary artery disease	Digoxin
Milk thistle	Promotes the growth of liver cells; protects the liver from damage	Liver disorders	*Tylenol*, chemotherapy, cisplatin, fluoruracil, methotrexate, paclitaxel, general anesthetics, nitrous oxide, *Haldol, Mevacor, Flagyl, Pravachol*
St. John's wort	Inhibits uptake of serotonin, norepinephrine, and dopamine; is an anti-infective	Mild depression; infections	Benzodiazepines, chemotherapy, cyclosporine, digoxin, *Allegra Allergy*, fluvoxamine, *Crixivan, Serzone*, oral contraceptives, *Paxil, Nardil, Zoloft*, theophylline, trazodone, tricyclic antidepressants, venlafaxine, *Coumadin*
Valerian	Is a minor tranquilizer and central nervous system depressant; decreases restlessness in sleep	Anxiety; sleep disorders	Sedative effects of barbiturates, opiates, benzodiazepines

Table 6.6 Unsafe Herbs

Common Name	Proposed Uses	Harmful Features
Borage	Diuretic; antidiarrheal	Contains toxic chemicals
Calamus	Fever reduction; digestive aid	Contains certain carcinogenic agents
Chaparral	Anticancer	Is toxic to liver
Coltsfoot	Antitussive	Contains toxic chemicals
Comfrey	Wound healing	Contains toxic chemicals; may cause veno-occlusive disease
Ephedra	Central nervous system stimulation; anorectic; bronchodilator; cardiac tissue stimulation	Extremely dangerous for patients with hypertension, diabetes mellitus, or thyroid disease
Germander	Anorectic	Is toxic to liver
Life root	Menstrual flow stimulation	Is toxic to liver
Pokeroot	Anticancer; antirheumatic	Is fatal in children
Sassafras	Stimulant; antispasmodic; antirheumatic	Contains carcinogenic agents

Representative Drugs for Vitamin and Mineral Deficiencies

Category, Name,[a] and Route	Uses and Diseases	Actions	Usual Dose[b] and Special Instructions	Side Effects and Adverse Reactions
Fat-Soluble Vitamins				
vitamin D Oral, IM	Rickets; hypocalcemia; malabsorption	Promotes absorption and utilization of calcium	Initially, 12,000 IU PO or IM daily; increased up to 500,000 IU daily	Rare; seen only with vitamin D toxicity
vitamin K (*AquaMEPHYTON*) PO, subcut, IM	Hypoprothrombinemia	Formation of prothrombin	25 mg PO daily	Rare; flushing, taste alterations, redness at injection site
Water-Soluble Vitamins				
thiamine hydrochloride (vitamin B_1) Oral, IM, IV	Beriberi; malabsorption syndrome; anemia; polyneuritis	Combines with ATP enzyme necessary for carbohydrate metabolism	*Beriberi:* 10–500 mg IM TID for 2 weeks, followed by 5–100 mg for 1 month *Anemia and polyneuritis:* 100 mg PO daily *Crisis state:* 500 mg–1 g IV	Rare; skin rash, itching, wheezing after IV administration
riboflavin (vitamin B_2) Oral	Malnutrition; malabsorption	Converted into two coenzymes necessary for normal tissue respiration	50 mg PO daily	Rare; bright yellow urine with high doses
cyanocobalamin (vitamin B_{12}) Oral, subcut, IM	Malabsorption; pernicious anemia; strict vegetarianism	Necessary for red blood cells, protein, fat, and carbohydrate metabolism	30–100 µg subcut or IM daily for 5–10 days; monthly maintenance dose 100–200 µg IM	Rare; itching
vitamin C (ascorbic acid) Subcut, IM, IV	Poor nutritional habits; delayed wound healing	Promotes tissue repair and wound healing	200–500 mg	Rare

Representative Drugs for Vitamin and Mineral Deficiencies (*continued*)

Category, Name,[a] and Route	Uses and Diseases	Actions	Usual Dose[b] and Special Instructions	Side Effects and Adverse Reactions
Macrominerals				
calcium carbonate (*Tums, Tums Extra*) Oral	Hypocalcemia; osteoporosis	Replaces and maintains calcium	250–650 mg PO daily	Constipation; cardiac changes if calcium level goes too high
potassium chloride (*Micro-K*) Oral	Hypokalemia; diuretic use; vomiting; diarrhea; starvation diet	Replaces and maintains potassium	40–100 mEq PO TID or QID	Cardiac changes if potassium level goes too high
Microminerals				
iron (ferrous sulfate) Oral, IM	Iron-deficiency anemia	Formation of red blood cells	325 mg PO TID or QID, 50–100 mg IM daily	Constipation; black stools; nausea

[a]*Trade names given in parentheses are examples only. Check current drug references for a complete listing of available products.*

[b]*Average adult doses are listed. However, dosages are determined by a provider and vary with the purpose of the therapy and the particular patient. The doses presented in this text are for general information only.*

Summary

Learning Outcome	Summary Points
6-1 Explain the food groupings according to Choose MyPlate.	• The food groups in MyPlate are grains, vegetables, fruits, milk, and meat and beans.
6-2 Distinguish between the fat-soluble and water-soluble vitamins, and the various vitamins.	• *Vitamins* are classified as being either fat soluble (A, D, E, and K) or water soluble (B complex and C). • *Fat-soluble vitamins* are less widely distributed in nature. Table 6.1 lists the functions of and RDA for fat-soluble vitamins. • *Water-soluble vitamins* are found mostly in plant and animal sources. Table 6.2 lists the functions of and RDA for water-soluble vitamins. • Vitamin C, ascorbic acid (water soluble), maintains healthy bones, teeth, and blood vessels and helps form collagen. • Vitamins A, D, E, and K are found in milk products, green leafy vegetables, yellow fruits and vegetables, fish, and sunlight. • Vitamin K (fat soluble) helps form prothrombin (for blood clotting); deficiency results in hemorrhage in newborns and increased clotting time in adults. • The *B complex and C vitamins* are found in most plant and animal foods. • The RDA for fat-soluble vitamin A is 5000 IU. • The RDA for water-soluble folic acid is 400 μg. • Fat-soluble *folic acid* deficiency causes anemia, fatigue, and sore tongue. • It is critical to assess patients for vitamin deficiencies as described in Tables 6.1 and 6.2. A deficiency may indicate a need for supplementation. • Hypervitaminosis may result from taking large doses of vitamins over a period of time. Toxicity may occur over time from consistent megadoses.

Learning Outcome	Summary Points
6-3 List the various minerals, their functions, food sources, and the recommended daily allowances.	• *Macrominerals* are minerals with a daily requirement of 100 mg or more. They include calcium, sodium, potassium, magnesium, and phosphorus. • *Microminerals* are minerals with a daily requirement of less than 100 mg. They include iron, iodine, zinc, and copper. • Table 6.3 lists the functions of, RDA, and symptoms of deficiency and excess for macrominerals. • Table 6.4 lists the functions of, RDA, and symptoms of deficiency and excess for microminerals. • *Minerals* are found in both plant and animal foods. • The RDA for potassium is 2000 mEq. • The RDA for iodine is 150 µg. • It is critical to assess patients for mineral deficiencies as described in Tables 6.3 and 6.4. A deficiency may indicate a need for supplementation. • A deficiency in the macromineral *calcium* results in hypocalcemia, stunted growth in children, osteoporosis, tetany, and convulsions. • A deficiency in the micromineral *iron* causes anemia, weakness, dizziness, pallor, and fatigue. • An excess of *sodium* results in hypernatremia, confusion, and fluid retention. • An excess of copper causes headache, dizziness, and gastrointestinal upset. • Correctly performing calculations for minerals enhances patient safety.
6-4 Explain the importance of water and electrolytes.	• *Electrolytes* include macrominerals such as calcium, potassium, sodium, and magnesium. • *Water* is also essential and makes up 45 to 75 percent of total body weight, depending on an individual's percentage of body fat.
6-5 Identify herbal supplements, their uses, their potential dangers.	• *Aloe vera* is taken for minor burns and wound healing. • *Bilberry* is taken for eye problems and gastrointestinal disorders. • *Cat's claw* is taken for cancer, infection, hypertension, and gastrointestinal disorders. • *Astragalus* is taken for cancer. • *Chaparral, germander,* and *life root* may be toxic to the liver. • *Pokeroot* may be fatal in children. • *Coltsfoot* contains toxic chemicals. • *Calamus* contains certain carcinogenic agents.

Chapter 6 Review

Match the medical terms to their definitions.

_____ 1. (LO 6-2) Inorganic elements essential to the body   a. homeostasis

_____ 2. (LO 6-2) Condition resulting from a diet lacking in vitamins   b. vitamins

_____ 3. (LO 6-2) Organic substances essential for normal metabolism   c. ion

_____ 4. (LO 6-4) State of fluid balance within the body   d. minerals

_____ 5. (LO 6-4) Particle that carries an electrical charge   e. hypovitaminosis

Complete the statements by filling in the blanks.

6. (LO 6-1) The level of intake for essential nutrients considered to be adequate to meet the nutritional needs of healthy individuals is called _____.

7. (LO 6-3) Another name for microminerals is _____.

8. (LO 6-1) MyPlate was developed by the _____ to assist in the buying and preparation of food.

Answer the questions in the space provided.

9. (LO 6-2) Name the water-soluble vitamins. _____

_____

_____

_____

10. (LO 6-2) List at least five food sources for fat-soluble vitamins. _____

_____

_____

_____

11. (LO 6-2) Name the fat-soluble vitamins. _____

_____

_____

12. (LO 6-3) Both a deficiency and an excess of which mineral cause cardiac abnormalities? _____

_____

_____

_____

Match each vitamin to its function.

_____ 13. (LO 6-2) Nerve conduction

_____ 14. (LO 6-2) Formation of collagen

_____ 15. (LO 6-2) Maintenance of healthy bones and teeth

_____ 16. (LO 6-2) Formation of prothrombin for blood clotting

a. vitamin K

b. vitamin D

c. vitamin C

d. vitamin B_1

Match each mineral to its function.

_____ 17. (LO 6-3) Formation of hemoglobin

_____ 18. (LO 6-3) Development of the thyroid gland

_____ 19. (LO 6-3) Control of fluid balance in the body

_____ 20. (LO 6-3) Formation of bones and teeth

a. iodine

b. calcium

c. iron

d. sodium

Match each herb to its use.

_____ 21. (LO 6-5) Improves circulation in the eye   a. ginger

_____ 22. (LO 6-5) Is an antiemetic   b. ginseng

_____ 23. (LO 6-5) Improves memory   c. bilberry

_____ 24. (LO 6-5) Increases physical endurance   d. ginkgo biloba

Drug Calculations—Fill in the blank with the answer.

25. (LO 6-3) The provider orders cyanocobalamin (vitamin B$_{12}$) 30 µg subcutaneously daily. Available is 100 µg/mL. Prepare to administer _____ mL to your patient.

26. (LO 6-3) The provider orders phytonadione (vitamin K) 0.5 mg intramuscularly daily. Available is 2 mg/mL. You will administer _____ mL to your patient.

27. (LO 6-4) The provider orders potassium chloride 40 mEq orally bid. Available are 10-mEq tablets. You will give _____ tablets to your patient.

28. (LO 6-3) The provider orders ferrous sulfate 325 mg orally daily. Available are 325-mg tablets. You will give _____ tablets to your patient.

29. (LO 6-3) The provider orders calcium carbonate 650 mg orally daily. Available are 1250-mg tablets. Prepare to give _____ tablets to your patient.

Multiple Choice—Circle the correct letter.

30. (LO 6-5) Which of the following unsafe herbs is fatal to children?

    a. Germander   c. Pokeroot
    b. Comfrey   d. Calamus

31. (LO 6-5) Name two prescription drugs that interact with milk thistle.

    a. Heparin, _Coumadin_   c. _Allegra Allergy, Zoloft_
    b. _Tylenol, Haldol_   d. _Parafon Forte DSC, Persantine_

32. (LO 6-3) A patient taking iron complains of which three symptoms of an iron deficiency?

    a. Fatigue, weakness, dizziness   c. Bruising, loose teeth, wounds that will not heal
    b. Decrease in taste and smell, thirst,   d. Cracks in the corner of the mouth, sore tongue,
       confusion   diarrhea

33. (LO 6-1) A patient asks you how many servings of milk are required daily according to MyPlate. What response should you give?

    a. 2 cups   c. 4 cups
    b. $2\frac{1}{2}$ cups   d. 3 cups

34. (LO 6-2) Which foods are rich in tocopherol (vitamin E)?

    a. Green leafy vegetables, eggs, milk

    b. Pork, pasta, liver

    c. Chicken, yellow fruits, fish

    d. Potatoes, nuts, meat

Chapter 6 Case Studies

35. (LO 6-5) You are caring for a patient who appears with jaundice and complains of itching. After you take her medication history, the patient tells you that she is on an antihypertensive, an antibiotic, calcium, potassium, dong quai, and life root. You determine what medication, supplement, or herb to be responsible? Why? What should you do? _____

_____

_____

_____

36. (LO 6-3) A 55-year-old patient asks you how much calcium she needs in a day and what foods are high in calcium? What should you tell her? _____

_____

_____

_____

Critical Thinking

From this list, choose the vitamin or mineral you would give to each patient described, and explain why.

    vitamin C   calcium   vitamin B_1 vitamin A   iodine

37. (LO 6-3) Mrs. Smith is admitted to the hospital with tingling and numbness of the extremities.

_____

38. (LO 6-2) Mr. Jones is diagnosed with scurvy and is experiencing bleeding gums, bruising, and a wound that does not heal.

_____

39. (LO 6-2) Mr. Adib comes to the provider's office complaining of rough, dry skin and night blindness.

_____

40. (LO 6-3) Mrs. Peterson is shrinking in height, and she sustained a broken hip without having fallen.

_____

41. (LO 6-3) Mrs. Gomez has been diagnosed with decreased thyroid function.

_____

Applications

Obtain an electronic drug guide and a current copy of a drug reference book or the *PDR*® and use it to answer the following questions.

42. Look up *potassium chloride* and list all its trade names. _____

_____

_____

43. From the dosage section, summarize the information referring to child and adult dosages for potassium chloride.

_____

_____

_____

ANTIBIOTICS, ANTIFUNGALS, AND ANTIVIRALS

LEARNING OUTCOMES

7-1 Distinguish between the external and internal immune systems.

7-2 Explain why drug resistance, hypersensitivity, and superinfection are important concerns in antibiotic drug therapy.

7-3 Identify the most common types and uses of antibiotics.

7-4 Describe the antifungal and antiviral drugs and infectious diseases.

7-5 Describe the correct procedure for administering a medication to a patient in isolation.

7-6 Describe the primary ways a healthcare worker can be exposed to hepatitis B virus and human immunodeficiency virus.

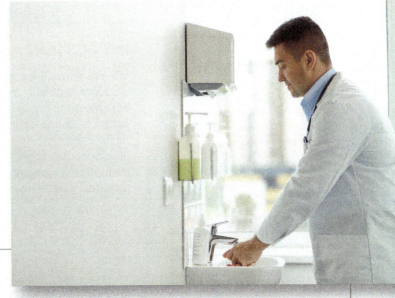

©Syda Productions/Shutterstock

In this chapter you will learn how an infection develops. You will learn how infection affects the body and how drugs are used to treat it. You will also learn how healthcare workers can stop the spread of infection.

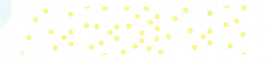

Key Terms

aerobic	culture and sensitivity test	mycoses
anaerobic	Gram stain	nosocomial
anaphylaxis	hypersensitivity	penicillinase
antibody	immune	photosensitivity
aseptic	immunization	resistance
autoclave	infectious diseases	Standard Precautions
bactericidal	inoculation	superinfection
bacteriostatic	leukocytes	Universal Precautions
Clostridium difficile	microorganisms	

INFECTION AND IMMUNITY [LO 7-1]

We are surrounded by tiny, one-celled plants and animals—called germs or, more properly, **microorganisms** or microbes. They are in the air we breathe, on the food we eat, and on the things we touch. Many of them are harmless. Some are even beneficial; for example, certain bacteria that live in the intestine help create important vitamins out of the waste products of digestion. But some microorganisms produce infection and disease. These harmful microorganisms—known as pathogens—include bacteria, fungi, protozoa, rickettsiae, and viruses (**Figure 7.1**).

Figure 7.1

Pathogens produce infection and disease.

Bacteria

Cocci (round)

Bacilli (rods)

Spiral (spirochetes and spirilla)

Fungi

Viruses

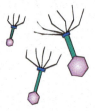

Protozoa

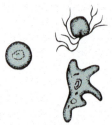

Rickettsiae

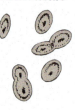

Infection is an invasion by pathogens that reproduce, multiply, and cause disease. For an infection to develop, certain conditions must be present in the environment:

- Food
- Oxygen (presence or absence)
- Moisture
- Heat
- A pH of 5 to 8 (slightly alkaline)
- Darkness

Microorganisms require some type of nutrition. Some thrive on organic matter, such as *Clostridium perfringens,* which causes gangrene. Others, such as *Escherichia coli,* receive nourishment from undigested food in the colon. **Aerobic** bacteria grow in the presence of oxygen, whereas **anaerobic** bacteria can survive without oxygen. For example, an infection deep within the body, such as in a joint, grows without oxygen. Moisture is necessary for most pathogens to survive. A few pathogens, such as botulism and tetanus, can survive without water. Some pathogens can even survive exposure to extreme temperatures. Pathogens also require an alkaline and dark environment to flourish.

Infectious diseases—those caused by direct or indirect spread of pathogens from one person to another—have distinct sets of symptoms that help in diagnosis. Fever, chills, headache, nausea, vomiting, diarrhea, and pus formation at the infection site are some of the signs that may indicate an infection.

The Immune System

The immune system has two parts: external and internal.

External Immune System. The external immune system protects against infection because of normally functioning defenses. The most important of these is the skin. It provides a tough physical barrier to microorganisms. Some natural conditions of the skin that prevent most microorganisms from growing on the skin are relative dryness, low moisture, low pH (acidity), and salinity. When the skin barrier is damaged, as when it is cut or burned, microorganisms can enter the body and cause infection. Natural openings such as the eyes, nose, and mouth are protected by tears, saliva, and nasal secretions that contain lysozyme, which breaks down bacterial cell walls.

Internal Immune System. The internal immune system is made up of microscopic substances whose specialized function is to fight infection. Certain cells, called neutrophils, surround and digest the microorganisms. **Leukocytes**, also called white blood cells, produce antibodies, which are proteins that help destroy microorganisms as they enter the body.

Antibodies. The immune system helps fight germs by producing substances to combat them. **Antibodies** are proteins that either destroy or stop the growth of certain types of microorganisms. Antibodies are carried in the bloodstream and can readily move to the site of entry.

Specific antibodies act against specific microorganisms. When an unfamiliar microorganism enters the body, proteins in the blood are stimulated to produce a special antibody to act against it. The next time that same microorganism enters the body, the antibody "remembers" it and proceeds to destroy it. Antibodies make the body **immune** to a great many infections.

Immunity can be either temporary or permanent, depending on the type of antibody. People who, for some reason, cannot form antibodies are at risk because they cannot defend themselves against the microorganisms to which we are all constantly exposed.

Sometimes, despite all these defenses, microorganisms can multiply and spread in the body, and the result is infection. The infection can be local, such as in a cut or a surgical wound, or it can be systemic and affect the whole body, as in measles.

Immunization

Because of the pioneering work of Edward Jenner, Jonas Salk, and others we are able to prevent many deadly or debilitating infectious diseases that in the past affected many lives. **Immunization** protects against measles, mumps, rubella (MMR), and hepatitis B, polio, tetanus, diphtheria, pertussis (whooping cough), chickenpox (varicella), and meningitis. Through immunization, we are able to stimulate the body to produce antibodies against disease-producing microorganisms. Antibodies are produced by placing a small amount of dead or weak disease germs into the body, a process called **inoculation** or vaccination. Because the microorganisms are not at full strength, they do not cause full-blown disease, but they provide enough material to stimulate the body to manufacture the necessary antibodies. Thus, when living microorganisms come along, the antibodies are already there to fight them off. Immunization has been so successful that diseases that used to kill thousands of people during sweeping epidemics, such as polio and yellow fever, are now rare.

Reemerging and New Disease. In recent years there has been a reemergence of some vaccine preventable illnesses such as measles and mumps due to parents' misconceptions and fears, and choosing to not allow their babies to receive the MMR vaccine. At the root of these fears is the belief that the MMR immunization is the cause of the increased incidence of autism. This theory has since been scientifically disproven but the fear continues to persist.

Scientific research must be ongoing to prevent mass epidemics and death related to newly discovered and reemerging diseases. The mutation of organisms that once were effectively killed by antibiotics has led to ongoing need for newer drugs to halt the proliferation of mutated harmful organisms.

A very important role for healthcare workers is to educate their patients to take all the prescribed anti-infective medications as ordered. Some medications must be taken every four hours and others once a day. The length of time for taking anti-infective medication also varies for different drugs from one day to several days or even weeks. Stopping after a person feels better in about three days does not mean that the infectious organisms have all been destroyed.

Practitioners, too, must be resilient to the demands of their patients and refuse to order antibiotics at the first signs of an infection that may have specific causes other than bacterial and for which the drug is ineffective. An example is treating the common cold—which is a virus—with an antibacterial. This is ineffective and contraindicated. Over-prescription or inappropriate prescription of antibiotics for infections without isolation and identification of the infecting organism has contributed to mutations of organisms causing illness and the patient's immune system not building up antibodies to fight a future reinfection.

An area of current research and public concern is the use of antibiotics in animal feed that enters the human body when the meat is ingested. Urbanization of the world's population and access to very remote areas has led to the discovery of previously unknown or very confined illnesses. International travel has increased for both business and recreational purposes and travelers are exposed to disease-causing organisms for which their bodies have no defense. They may have already returned to their own home before symptoms of illness appear and they have already exposed fellow travelers, their families, their coworkers, and their communities resulting in an urgent need to identify the cause of the illness and how to fight it. The arsenal of infection control measures include development of new immunizations for diseases such as avian flu, West Nile disease, Zika, and Ebola.

Patients at Risk

Most individuals can fight off infection successfully. If they are in good health, their natural defenses prevent the spread of microorganisms, so there are few disease symptoms. Even when a disease develops, generally healthy people are able to survive while the infection runs its course. It is the people who are *not* healthy who are at greatest risk. Age, nutritional status, stress, medical condition, or an actual medical treatment may predispose an individual to infection.

Patients with surgical wounds or with lowered resistance because of other conditions, such as acquired immune deficiency syndrome (AIDS), are especially prone to infections. Weakened patients have a harder time recovering quickly and avoiding complications. The very young and older adults also have less resistance to infection.

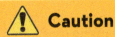 **Caution** Risk Factors for Infection in the Older Adult Patient

- Thin, less elastic skin
- Decreased sensitivity
- Decreased saliva production
- Less ability to perform oral hygiene
- Decreased secretion of stomach acid
- Decreased cough reflex

- Decreased hormone production
- Weakened muscular structures
- Poor nutrition
- Use of corticosteroids or cytotoxin drugs
- Residency in a long-term care facility

Hospitals and other healthcare facilities have large numbers of at-risk patients located in one place. A **nosocomial** infection is an infection that occurs in a hospital or long-term care facility. Once started, an infection can spread rapidly through such settings. For this reason, medical personnel must be especially concerned with avoiding the spread of pathogens. They are trained in **aseptic** (pathogen-free) techniques of caring for patients. Medical personnel also learn to perform hand hygiene through hand-washing with soap and water or with alcohol hand rub before and after caring for each patient. They learn to sterilize equipment, change bed linens frequently, use Standard Precautions when potentially coming into contact with bodily fluids, and place patients with certain diseases into isolation.

Staph (staphylococcal) infections are a common danger for hospitalized patients. People who develop such infections must be kept in isolation. No one may enter or leave these patients' rooms without special precautions against spreading staph pathogens. Practice Procedure 7.1 at the end of this chapter shows you how to prepare to administer medications to a patient in isolation.

The term **Standard Precautions** refers to the primary strategies for prevention of infections. The term applies to infections transmitted by blood, body fluids, nonintact skin, and mucous membranes of infected persons. Standard Precautions combine the major features of the categories of Universal Precautions and Body Substance Isolation (see later in this chapter). Standard Precautions provide protection for the healthcare worker as directed by the Occupational Safety and Health Administration (OSHA) and the Centers for Disease Control and Prevention (CDC). Standard Precautions apply in the care of all patients, not just in hospitals but "in all care settings," such as long-term care facilities, clinics, providers' offices, and home health, regardless of their diagnosis or presumed infection status. They reduce the transmission of microorganisms in both recognized and unrecognized infections in patients. The CDC developed guidelines for isolation precautions, both Standard Precautions and Transmission-Based Precautions. Transmission-Based Precautions are used for patients who are known to be infected or suspected to be infected with a pathogen that is epidemiologically significant and can be transmitted by air, droplet, or contact with contaminated surfaces.

ANTIBIOTIC DRUGS [LO 7-2]

The discovery of so-called miracle drugs—antibiotics—changed the practice of medicine radically. Antibiotics are drugs that destroy microorganisms. The major classifications of antibiotics are penicillins, cephalosporins, tetracyclines, macrolides, aminoglycosides, sulfonamides, and quinolones. (See Table 7.1.)

Antibiotics kill microorganisms either directly (indicated by the suffix -*cidal,* as in *bactericidal*) or by keeping them from growing (suffix -*static,* as in *bacteriostatic*). Some interfere with cell wall production in the microorganisms. Others inhibit protein synthesis. Still others mix up the chemical messages for producing nucleic acid, a major substance in cell growth. Some act better on rapidly multiplying pathogens, whereas others are more effective with slow-growing organisms.

Administration Considerations

Before prescribing antibiotics for specific ailments, a provider must consider three points.

- *Condition of the patient's defense system.* The provider must note whether the patient's immune system is functioning properly. Some antibiotics kill microorganisms directly and others slow the growth or reproduction of microorganisms. Both types depend on the body's natural defenses (leukocytes and antibodies) for help in eliminating an infection.

- *Type of infection and its cause.* What organism is causing the infection is important. Some infectious diseases have distinct symptoms, but many have similar symptoms. When in doubt, an attempt must be made to identify the bacteria. The identity of the pathogen determines the choice of a specific antibiotic. Specific identification of bacteria requires a **Gram stain** and culture with chemical testing.

  When placed on a microscope slide along with a stain, some microbes turn blue and others turn red. The blue-staining microbes are called Gram-positive microbes; the red-staining ones, Gram-negative microbes. There are different shapes of microbes, including slender, straight rods or spherical cocci. The shape and color help identify the correct antibiotic to administer. For example, vancomycin is effective against most Gram-positive microbes, and tobramycin is effective against most Gram-negative microbes.

- *Type of drug and its effects.* The provider must consider the type of antibiotic because antibiotics have varying degrees of effectiveness and

Table 7.1 Antibiotics, Antifungals, and Antivirals

Antibiotics

Penicillins
  amoxicillin
  amoxicillin/clavulanate (*Augmentin*)
  ampicillin
  ampicillin/sulbactam (*Unasyn*)
  dicloxacillin
  nafcillin
  oxacillin
  penicillin VK
  piperacillin/tazobactam (*Zosyn*)

Quinolones
  ciprofloxacin (*Cipro*)
  enoxacin (*Penetrex*)
  gemifloxacin (*Factive*)
  levofloxacin (*Levaquin*)
  moxifloxacin (*Avelox*)
  ofloxacin

Cephalosporins
  cefaclor
  cefazolin
  cefixime (*Suprax*)
  cefotaxime
  cefotetan (*Cefotan*)
  cefoxitin
  ceftaroline (*Teflaro*)
  ceftazidime (*Fortaz, Tazicef*)
  ceftriaxone

  cefuroxime (*Zinacef*)
  cefuroxime axetil
  cefadroxil
  cephalexin (*Keflex*)

Sulfonamides
  sulfadiazine
  sulfamethoxazole/trimethoprim (*Bactrim, Septra*)

Aminoglycosides
  amikacin
  gentamicin
  kanamycin
  neomycin
  streptomycin
  tobramycin (*Tobrex*)

Macrolides
  azithromycin (*Zithromax*)
  clarithromycin (*Biaxin*)
  erythromycin
  fidaxomicin (*Dificid*)

Tetracyclines
  doxycycline (*Vibramycin*)
  minocycline (*Minocin*)
  tetracycline hydrochloride
  tigecycline (*Tygacil*)

Miscellaneous Antibiotics
  aztreonam (*Azactam*)
  chloramphenicol

  imipenem/cilastatin (*Primaxin*)
  metronidazole (*Flagyl*)
  spectinomycin
  rifaximin (*Xifaxan*)
  vancomycin (*Vancocin*)

Antifungals
  amphotericin B
  clotrimazole (*Lotrimin AF*)
  fluconazole (*Diflucan*)
  flucytosine (*Ancobon*)
  griseofulvin
  ketoconazole (*Nizoral AD*)
  miconazole (*Monistat-7* and *Monistat-Derm*)
  nystatin
  sertaconazole (*Ertaczo*)
  terbinafine
  terconazole (*Terazol 7*)

Antivirals
  acyclovir (*Zovirax*)
  amantadine
  didanosine (ddI) (*Videx*)
  foscarnet (*Foscavir*)
  ganciclovir (*Cytovene*)
  oseltamivir (*Tamiflu*)
  ribavirin (*Virazole*)
  zanamivir (*Relenza*)
  zidovudine (AZT) (*Retrovir*)

varying side effects. Although the initial antibiotic selection may be made by the provider's examination of the patient and the Gram stain, the antibiotic may be changed following a **culture and sensitivity test**. A sample of fluid (e.g., pus obtained from a throat scraping) is taken from an infected person and used to start a culture of bacteria in the laboratory. Then pieces of paper saturated with samples of different antibiotics are placed on the culture. The results show which drugs kill the bacteria and which drugs are resistant to the bacteria. The provider chooses the drug that bacteria is sensitive to and will have the fewest side effects for the particular patient (**Figure 7.2**).

Sometimes it is hard to isolate the microorganism that is causing an illness. In these situations a provider may prescribe a broad-spectrum antibiotic. This type of antibiotic destroys a wide variety of microorganisms. The cephalosporins are one group of broad-spectrum antibiotics. In contrast, narrow-spectrum antibiotics are effective against only a few types of pathogens.

Providers try to choose the antibiotic that is most effective against a particular bacterium and that causes the fewest side effects for the patient.

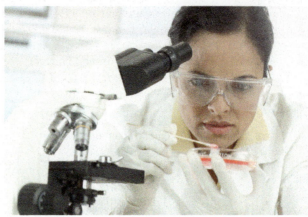

©JGI/Blend Images LLC

If the disease-producing organism can be identified, a narrow-spectrum drug is usually a better choice than a broad-spectrum drug. Pathogens are able to develop **resistance** to antibiotics. After exposure to a certain antibiotic for a particular period of time, a specific pathogen may no longer be sensitive to its action. Once this happens, it is of no benefit to continue giving that antibiotic to the patient. (Note that the *bacteria,* not an individual, become resistant to an antibiotic.) Use of broad-spectrum antibiotics gives more types of organisms a chance to develop resistance. Because of resistance, the overuse of antibiotics is now recognized as an important public health problem. The results of overuse are seen in hospitals where certain strains of resistant bacteria have appeared, causing hospital-acquired or nosocomial infections.

Another problem a provider considers in prescribing antibiotics is drug **hypersensitivity**. Hypersensitivity can occur in reaction to all antibiotics. It is an altered state of reactivity in which the body reacts with an exaggerated immune response. Some antibiotics may cause a minor rash, which the patient may easily tolerate. Other antibiotics can cause an anaphylactic reaction, which is a serious medical emergency.

The provider weighs the benefits of the drug against the dangers of not giving the drug. Usually the provider has several drugs to choose among, with a varying range of side effects. A more dangerous drug is chosen only when a less dangerous one has failed to stop an infection, when the patient has become hypersensitive to the drug, or when the bacteria have become resistant to it.

Superinfection is a secondary infection that occurs while an antibiotic is destroying the first infection. Most antibiotics decrease or destroy normal flora in the gastrointestinal tract. Approximately 2 percent of patients contract superinfections. Patients are at higher risk of developing superinfections if they are taking more than one antibiotic or a broad-spectrum antibiotic. When a superinfection occurs, the drug should be changed to another drug to which the organism is sensitive.

Schedules

Timing is important in antibiotic therapy. Pathogens may be present long after symptoms disappear. The provider must order the antimicrobial drug in the appropriate dose and for the specified period of time. It is important for patients to take the drug until they have finished all the doses. An antimicrobial drug often fails because the dose is too small or the drug is taken too briefly. Antimicrobial drugs should not be discontinued until the patient has been fever-free and feeling well for 48 to 72 hours. Follow-up cultures should be done to determine if the drug was effective.

Time of day is also important, because doses of antimicrobials must be scheduled around mealtimes. Oral antimicrobials can cause gastric irritation.

Giving them on a full stomach or with milk can help soothe irritation. On the other hand, some are made less effective when food or milk is present in the stomach. It is important to find out if oral antimicrobials should be given with food or milk or on an empty stomach. An instruction to "give between meals" means that the drug is to be given at least 1 hour before or 2 hours after meals, when the stomach is assumed to be empty.

MAJOR TYPES OF ANTIBIOTICS [LO 7-3]

An antibiotic is a substance with the ability to destroy life. It is produced by a microorganism and has **bactericidal** activity or **bacteriostatic** activity on other microorganisms.

Penicillins

Penicillin consists of a group of natural and semisynthetic agents that are highly active and combat Gram-positive and Gram-negative cocci and bacilli. The penicillins are a large group of antibiotics that are the most effective and least toxic of all antimicrobials. They come in many forms, to be given by different routes according to the therapeutic aim.

Natural penicillins are made from a mold that grows on bread and fruit. Penicillin G potassium and penicillin V are the most common natural penicillins. They are commonly used to treat syphilis and strep throat. Amoxicillin, a type of penicillin, may be given preventively to patients with heart disease and rheumatic fever. Infections considered susceptible to penicillins include gonorrhea, syphilis, pneumonia, meningitis, diphtheria, osteomyelitis, and otitis media. Penicillins are also effective against infections caused by *Staphylococci, Streptococci, Escherichia coli,* and *Salmonella* bacteria.

Unfortunately, some pathogens fight back when attacked by penicillin. They secrete a substance called **penicillinase**. The pathogens are then resistant in the ongoing battle against these penicillinase-producing bacteria. Protection can be provided, though, by adding a penicillin decoy. When the penicillinase attacks the decoy, it leaves the penicillin able to kill the bacteria. Examples of this penicillin and decoy strategy are: amoxicillin + clavulanate (*Augmentin*), ampicillin + sulbactam (*Unasyn*), and, most recently, piperacillin + tazobactam (*Zosyn*).

▲ Patient Education Penicillins

- Take the full course of medication even after feeling better and being symptom free.
- Take doses at the prescribed times to maintain therapeutic blood levels.
- Never take an antibiotic prescribed for someone else, because it may be for a different type of infection.
- Generally the medication should be taken on an empty stomach, but there are some exceptions. If stomach upset occurs, it may be taken with food.

- Penicillins decrease the effectiveness of estrogen-containing contraceptives. Women taking these contraceptives should be advised to use alternative forms of birth control.
- Patients with diabetes mellitus should use *Clinistix* or *Keto-Diastix* urine glucose tests instead of the *Clinitest,* because of the likelihood of false-positive results.
- The most common side effects are mild diarrhea, nausea, and vomiting.
- Notify the provider if rash, fever, or chills occur, because they may indicate an allergic reaction.

Although penicillins are usually safe and well tolerated, patient education is essential. There is the danger of penicillin allergy. Severe rashes can occur as a result of penicillin allergy. Other reactions can be life threatening. A person can go into **anaphylaxis**, which is manifested by difficulty in breathing, swelling of the throat causing suffocation, and shock symptoms. Persons who have penicillin allergies should wear a medical ID to alert the medical staff in case emergency treatment is needed.

Cephalosporins

Cephalosporins are broad-spectrum, semisynthetic drugs that are chemical modifications of the penicillin structure. They are classified into four generations. Each generation is used for specific pathogens. It wasn't until the third generation that cephalosporins were prescribed for serious infections. Generally, cephalosporins are used to treat respiratory tract infections, particularly *Haemophilus influenzae*. They may also be used in the treatment of gastrointestinal, genitourinary tract, skin and soft tissue, and bone and joint infections. Initially, they were considered advantageous over penicillin because of their resistance to the enzymatic activity of penicillinase. However, drug resistance has since been demonstrated in all four generations. Cephalosporins are often prescribed for patients who are allergic to penicillin. Generally, only about 6 to 18 percent of patients who are allergic to penicillin are also allergic to cephalosporins. An example is cephalexin (*Keflex*). Patient education is important for patients taking cephalosporins.

 Patient Education — Cephalosporins

- Take all doses of the medication even after being symptom free and feeling better.
- Take doses at the prescribed times to maintain therapeutic blood levels.
- Take the medicine with food or milk if gastrointestinal upset occurs.
- Patients with diabetes mellitus should use *Clinistix* or *Keto-Diastix* urine glucose tests instead of the *Clinitest,* because of the likelihood of false-positive results.
- Avoid alcohol or alcohol-containing medications because they interact with cephalosporins to produce abdominal pains, nausea, vomiting, decreased blood pressure, rapid pulse, and sweating.

- Read labels, such as on cough syrup, for alcohol-containing ingredients.
- Tell the provider of any history of bleeding tendencies.
- The provider may order liver and renal blood tests to monitor the drug in patients with liver or renal impairment.
- If difficulty swallowing, contents of capsules may be taken with applesauce.
- Immediately report rash, unexplained weight gain, or swelling.

Tetracyclines

The tetracyclines were the first broad-spectrum antibiotics. They are used to treat a variety of infections such as respiratory, rickettsial, venereal, and amebiasis. They are also used as an adjunct therapy in the treatment of acne. Tetracyclines pose a greater risk of superinfection than other microbials, so patients must be monitored for symptoms of secondary infections. As with all antibiotics, their effectiveness depends on the patient's compliance with treatment. Examples of this drug group are tetracycline hydrochloride and doxycycline (*Vibramycin*).

Patient Education — Tetracyclines

- Take all doses of the medication at the prescribed times until the medication is gone.
- Perform good oral and perineal hygiene to prevent *Candida* superinfection.
- Except for doxycycline (*Vibramycin*) and minocycline (*Minocin*), take the medication on an empty stomach (1 hour before or 2 hours after meals).
- Take the medication with a full glass of water to prevent gastrointestinal irritation. Take at least 1 hour before bedtime to avoid esophageal irritation.

- Avoid taking antacids, iron products, and laxatives containing aluminum, calcium, or magnesium, because they decrease absorption of the tetracyclines.
- Avoid milk and milk products for 1 hour before or 2 hours after tetracycline administration.
- Avoid direct ultraviolet light and sunlight (tetracyclines can cause a rash due to **photosensitivity**). Use sunscreen protection.
- Notify the provider if discoloration of teeth appears. Use alternative protection if taking oral contraceptives.

Macrolides

There are four macrolide antibiotics: azithromycin (*Zithromax*), clarithromycin (*Biaxin*), erythromycin, and fidaxomicin (*Dificid*). They are both bacteriostatic and bactericidal. *Zithromax* and *Biaxin* are the two newer macrolide antibiotics. *Zithromax* is used in chronic obstructive pulmonary disease (COPD), pneumonia, urethritis, cervicitis, and sinusitis. *Biaxin* is used in pharyngitis, tonsillitis, chronic bronchitis, and skin infections. Although both drugs cause gastrointestinal side effects, they have a lower incidence than erythromycin. Erythromycin may be used in respiratory infections, pertussis, pelvic inflammatory disease, diphtheria, and amebiasis. Patients receiving erythromycin should be monitored closely if also receiving theophylline (a bronchodilator), because there is a potential for increasing the serum levels of theophylline. *Dificid* is specifically given for *Clostridium difficile*. Like *Zithromax* and *Biaxin*, *Dificid* causes gastrointestinal side effects. Educating the patient about the medication is an important part of treatment success.

Patient Education — Macrolides

- Take all the medicine at prescribed times until the medicine is gone.
- Usual course of treatment is 5 days.
- Take the medicine on an empty stomach (1 hour before or 2 hours after meals) with a full glass of water, because food decreases absorption.

- Patients may be monitored closely if there is a diagnosis of liver impairment.
- Avoid excessive sunlight. Wear protective clothing and use sunscreen when outdoors.
- Report any changes in heart rate or rhythm. (May cause ventricular arrhythmias.)

Aminoglycosides

Aminoglycosides are potent bactericidal antibiotics that are generally used to treat only serious or life-threatening infections. These drugs must be used with extreme caution because of their high incidence of toxic effects on several body systems. Bacterial cultures are done to identify offending organisms and susceptibility to a certain aminoglycoside. They are generally reserved for Gram-negative bacteria causing bone infections, septicemia, skin and soft tissue infections, respiratory infections, and postoperative and intra-abdominal infections such as peritonitis. Patients who are receiving muscle relaxants or have myasthenia gravis or Parkinson's disease experience greater weakness. Extreme caution must be used with older adult patients because they are susceptible to hearing loss and to toxic effects on the kidney. Patient education is essential with these drugs to decrease the incidence of toxic side effects. Examples of aminoglycosides are amikacin, gentamicin, and tobramycin (*Tobrex*). Most aminoglycosides except ointments and drops are administered intramuscular.

 Patient Education | Aminoglycosides

- Take the full course of medication as prescribed.
- Take medication with a full glass of water to decrease the risk of toxic effects on the kidneys.
- Report any ringing or buzzing in the ears, which may indicate hearing loss.
- Report any change in urinary pattern or blood in the urine, which indicates a toxic effect on the kidney.
- Report any dizziness, numbness, tingling, twitching, vertigo, or ataxia, which indicates vestibular or nervous system toxicity (which is often irreversible).

Sulfonamides

Sulfonamides, or sulfa drugs, are useful for many different types of infection and conditions, such as urinary tract infections, chancroid, meningitis, rheumatic fever, nocardiosis, trachoma, and sexually transmitted diseases. They are primarily bacteriostatic rather than bactericidal. The combination of a sulfonamide, sulfamethoxazole, with trimethoprim makes a very powerful antibiotic regimen. It is so useful, in fact, that this combination has been given the name "co-trimoxazole," which is the active ingredient in the drugs *Bactrim* and *Septra*.

Side effects from sulfonamides are frequent. Common side effects are fever, rash, and gastrointestinal upset such as nausea, vomiting, and diarrhea. Low blood counts can also result from taking this medicine. Sulfonamides may cause crystals to form in the urine, which can cause urinary complications. For this reason, patient education is important.

Patient Education — Sulfonamides

- Take the full course of medication even after feeling better.
- Take the medication on an empty stomach and with a full glass of water to enhance absorption.
- If the common side effects of nausea and vomiting occur, medication may be taken with food.
- Avoid taking the medication with antacids because they decrease absorption of the sulfonamide.
- Drink at least 3 quarts of fluids per day to prevent urinary system complications.
- Avoid acidic juices, such as orange juice, and vitamin C (ascorbic acid), because they cause the urine to be acidic and may cause formation of urinary crystals.
- Report any skin reactions, such as a rash or itching. At first appearance of rash, stop taking and promptly report to prescribing provider.
- Fever and joint pain may occur after 7 days and must be reported immediately to the provider.
- Avoid direct sunlight and wear sunscreen.

Quinolones

Quinolones are broad-spectrum, synthetic antibiotics that are bactericidal. They are used in the treatment of respiratory, gastrointestinal, bone, skin, and urinary infections. Two commonly used quinolones are ciprofloxacin (*Cipro*) and ofloxacin. Because they have a wide range of gastrointestinal and central nervous system side effects, they are to be used with caution in older adult patients. Other side effects may be tendonitis, joint pain, and cardiotoxicity with prolonged Q-T interval. They are not to be used with infants or children. Patient education is important to enhance the effectiveness of these drugs.

Patient Education — Quinolones

- Take all doses of the medication at prescribed times.
- Take 4 hours before or 2 hours after antacids containing magnesium or aluminum or after mineral supplements such as iron or zinc because they decrease the absorption of quinolones.
- Report dizziness, lightheadedness, blurred vision, headache, insomnia, or depression immediately to the provider; they may indicate central nervous system toxicity.
- Avoid direct sunlight and tanning booths because of the possibility of a photosensitivity reaction.
- Avoid activities that require coordination and alertness because of the possibility of central nervous system symptoms.

Miscellaneous Antibiotics

Aztreonam.   Aztreonam (*Azactam*) is the first drug in a class of antibiotics known as *monobactams*. It is a synthetic bactericidal antibiotic that is effective in the treatment of respiratory, urinary, intra-abdominal, gynecological, and skin infections. The most frequent side effects are rash and itching.

Chloramphenicol.   Chloramphenicol is a potent inhibitor of protein synthesis that is generally bacteriostatic. However, in high doses, with certain susceptible organisms, it may be bactericidal. *Chloromycetin* is very toxic to the bone marrow and is reserved for use in infections for which other antibiotics have been ineffective. As a result of its bone marrow toxicity, patients should be monitored closely for bleeding tendencies.

 Pediatric Considerations | Antibiotics

- Penicillins and cephalosporins are considered safe for children but must be used cautiously in neonates because of their immature kidney function, which causes them to excrete these drugs more slowly than adults.

- Even when used with caution, aminoglycosides (e.g., gentamicin) may cause nephrotoxicity and ototoxicity in children, and neonates are at greater risk because of their immature renal function. Neomycin is not recommended for children.

- Fluoroquinolones are not recommended for children because of possible permanent damage in cartilage and joints.

- Tetracyclines are not recommended for use in children because they interfere with enamel development and may cause a permanent brownish tooth discoloration. They may also interfere with bone growth.

 Older Adult Considerations | Antibiotics

- Penicillins are considered safe for older adults.
- Use caution when administering cephalosporins because of decreased renal function. They have the potential to be nephrotoxic.
- Older adults are at an increased risk of nephrotoxicity and ototoxicity from aminoglycosides (e.g., gentamicin).

- Generally tetracyclines are contraindicated because of decreased renal function.
- Macrolides are considered safe.
- Observe for signs of bacterial or fungal superinfection.

ANTIFUNGAL DRUGS [LO 7-4]

Infections caused by fungi, which are plantlike parasitic microorganisms, are called **mycoses**, which are treated with antifungal drugs. Mycoses can range from superficial to severe and life threatening. The fungi can be orally ingested, implanted under the skin after an injury, or acquired by breathing spores from contaminated soil or bird droppings. Examples include aspergillosis, blastomycosis, coccidiomycosis, crytococcosis, and histoplasmosis.

Antifungal infections are more difficult to treat than infections caused by bacteria because fungal cell structure resembles the cell structure of human cells. As a result, drugs that are toxic to fungal cells may also be toxic to human cells. Also, when broad-spectrum antibacterial drugs are used for a prolonged time, patients may subsequently develop fungal infections. Fungal drugs may be applied topically or systemically. Topical products are available as ointments, creams, aerosols, lotions, or powders and are generally applied in the morning and evening. Oral treatment of superficial fungal infections of the skin consists of griseofulvin. It may be used in tinea infections such as tinea corporis (ringworm), tinea cruris ("jock itch"), tinea capitis (ringworm of the scalp), and tinea unguium (infection of the nails).

Yeast or yeastlike fungal organisms cause several types of dermatological infections, most often caused by *Candida albicans*. An example of an over-the-counter ointment is *Monistat-7*. Generally, these infections are common in warm, moist areas of the skin such as under the skin folds of the breasts, in diapered areas, or on the mucous membranes such as the mouth and vagina. *C. albicans* (candidiasis) may be caused by treatment with antibiotics, corticosteroids, or antineoplastics. Oral candidiasis, also called *thrush,* is common in newborns and in immunocompromised patients such as those with cancer or AIDS. Vaginal candidiasis frequently occurs in women who are taking oral contraceptives, are pregnant, or have diabetes mellitus. Nystatin and amphotericin B are used to treat yeast infections of the skin and mucous membranes. Miconazole nitrate (*Monistat-7*), clotrimazole (*Lotrimin AF*), econazole nitrate, ketoconazole (*Nizoral AD*), ciclopirox (*Loprox*), and fluconazole (*Diflucan*) are broad-spectrum antifungal drugs.

▲ Pediatric Considerations   Antifungals

- Antifungals have been used safely in children, although safety has not been established.
- Give the lowest possible dose.

▲ Older Adult Considerations   Antifungals

- Although topical antifungals are used, precautions have been established for oral and parenteral forms.
- Intravenous amphotericin B may cause serious side effects such as nephrotoxicity and hypokalemia.

ANTIVIRAL DRUGS [LO 7-4]

Antiviral drugs are synthetic and developed to fight specific viruses. The development of antiviral drugs has been much more difficult than the development of antibacterials. The reason is that the virus often reaches its peak before clinical symptoms actually appear. For an antiviral to be effective, the drug must be given before the disease begins.

Table 7.2 lists the various categories of infectious diseases.

Several theories of viral infections exist. First, there are acute viral infections such as the common cold, which are characterized by a quick onset and resolve with no aftereffects. Second, there are chronic infections such as herpes virus and AIDS in which recurrent periods of active disease are followed by latent periods when the patient is asymptomatic. Third, there are slow-growing viral infections that may grow for months or years before resulting in death. Some theorists believe that diseases such as multiple sclerosis and Alzheimer's disease may be slow-growing infections of the central nervous system. Fourth, there are serious infections such as rabies, tetanus, poliomyelitis, and

Table 7.2 Infectious Diseases

Bacterial Infections
- Anthrax
- Bacillary dysentery
- Bacterial endocarditis
- Blood poisoning
- Boils
- Botulism
- Brucellosis (undulant fever)
- Cholera
- *Clostridium difficile*
- Diphtheria
- Gastroenteritis (food poisoning)
- Gonorrhea
- Meningitis
- Osteomyelitis
- Plague
- Pneumonia
- Strep throat
- Tetanus
- Trench mouth
- Tularemia
- Typhoid fever

Chlamydial Infections
- Acute urethral syndrome
- Arthritis-dermatitis syndrome
- Bartholinitis
- Cervicitis
- Conjunctivitis

- Epididymitis
- Nongonococcal or post-gonococcal urethritis
- Perihepatitis
- Proctitis
- Reiter syndrome
- Salpingitis

Fungal Infections (Mycoses)
- Actinomycosis
- Candidiasis (moniliasis)
- Coccidioidomycosis
- Histoplasmosis

Parasitic Infections
- Flukes
- Hookworm
- Pinworm
- Roundworm
- Schistosomiasis
- Tapeworm
- Trichinosis

Protozoan Infections
- Amebic dysentery (amebiasis)
- Malaria
- Toxoplasmosis
- Trypanosomiasis (sleeping sickness)

Rickettsial Infections
- Rocky Mountain spotted fever
- Typhus

Spirochetal Infections
- Lyme disease
- Syphilis

Viral Infections
- AIDS
- Chickenpox
- Cold sores (herpes simplex)
- Common cold
- Encephalitis
- Genital herpes
- Influenza (flu, grippe)
- Lymphogranuloma
- Measles
- Mononucleosis
- Mumps
- Poliomyelitis
- Psittacosis (parrot fever)
- Rabies
- Shingles (herpes zoster)
- Viral hepatitis
- Yellow fever

smallpox that may be prevented by a vaccine. After a vaccine is administered, antibodies are formed. Antivirals have been developed at a slower rate than antibacterials because the viruses reproduce in the human host by utilizing host cell components rather than their own. As a result of this, drugs that are toxic to the virus may also be toxic to the host.

Substances called interferons are released from cells that have been attacked by a virus and T-type lymphocytes. The interferons appear to alter unaffected cells, making them resistant to the attacking virus. *Interferon alfa-2a* is used in the treatment of hairy cell leukemia and AIDS-related Kaposi's sarcoma. *Interferon alfa-2b* is used to treat chronic hepatitis and venereal warts.

The FDA has approved a once-a-day, three-drugs-in-one combination called *Atripla* to be used in the treatment of HIV/AIDS. The new pill combines the active ingredients of three antiretroviral drugs—efavirenz (*Sustiva*), emtricitabine (*Emtriva*), and tenofovir disoproxil fumarate (*Viread*)—that have already been used for some time as part of a "cocktail" therapy. Rilpivirine (*Edurant*) is a new antiviral drug used in the management of HIV infection. Amantadine and rimantadine (*Flumadine*) are antivirals proven to be effective against influenza type A virus, especially in high-risk patients such as those with chronic cardiovascular or pulmonary disease, and may also be used in Parkinson's disease and drug-induced extrapyramidal reactions. Ribavirin (*Virazole*) treats respiratory syncytial virus (RSV), influenza virus, and herpes simplex virus in hospitalized infants and young children.

Oseltamivir (*Tamiflu*) is a neuraminidase inhibitor or antiviral medication used to treat both types A and B influenza in children and adults. It may also be given prophylactically. An advantage of *Tamiflu* is that it reduces the time the patient has symptoms by approximately $1\frac{1}{2}$ days. The major side effects are nausea, vomiting, and diarrhea.

Clostridium difficile. *Clostridium difficile* is a deadly "superbug" that is more virulent and resistant than previous strains. *C. difficile* is a Gram-positive, anaerobic, spore-forming bacterium that is the major cause of nosocomial diarrhea. The organism is very infectious and transmitted by the fecal-oral route. It colonizes the intestinal tract after the normal flora has been disrupted by antibiotic therapy. Depending on the health of the patient, the range of symptoms may vary. The patient may be asymptomatic, have severe diarrhea, pseudomembranous colitis, toxic megacolon, intestinal perforation, or death from secondary sepsis.

Diagnosis is based on clinical symptoms, endoscopy, and stool testing. *C. difficile* infection should be suspected in a patient who presents with diarrhea and has received antibiotics in the last three months or has diarrhea that began 24 hours after hospitalization. The most common laboratory test is the enzyme-linked immunosorbent assay (ELISA) that checks for the presence of the toxin.

The primary drugs used to treat *C. difficile*–associated diarrhea (CDAD) are vancomycin (*Vancocin*) and metronidazole (*Flagyl*). Vancomyin is given at 125 mg four times a day for 10 to 14 days. *Flagyl* is given at 300 mg three times a day for 10 to 14 days. Antidiarrheal drugs such as diphenoxylate hydrochloride and atropine sulfate (*Lomotil*), loperamide (*Imodium A-D*), and narcotic analgesics should be avoided because they delay the clearance of the toxin from the colon.

 Pediatric Considerations Antivirals

- Although antiviral safety hasn't been established in children, some antiviral drugs may be given.
- Amantadine may be given to prevent influenza A in children 1 year of age.

- Rimantadine is given for children.
- Anti-HIV drugs must be used with extreme caution.

 Older Adult Considerations Antivirals

- Although antivirals are used for older adults, caution must be exercised because older adults may have impaired organ function or concomitant diseases and may take a lot of other medications.

- Older adults are at greater risk of toxicity; therefore, give the smallest possible dose.

ISOLATION PROCEDURES [LO 7-5]

There are two basic situations in which isolation procedures may be used:

- When a patient must be protected from any microorganisms that you carry.
- When you must be protected from any microorganisms the patient is carrying.

Depending on the specific disease or microorganism danger, there are special types of isolation requiring different precautions. The CDC's isolation guidelines are outlined in Table 7.3.

Table 7.3 CDC Isolation Guidelines

Type of Precaution	Criteria for Use	Barrier Protection
Standard Precautions	Any contact with all body fluids, secretions, excretions (except sweat), nonintact skin, mucous membranes	• Wash hands between patient contact • Gloves • Masks, eye protection, or face shield only if splash with body fluids or blood is possible • Gowns only if soiling with body fluids or blood is possible • Patient care items must be properly cleaned • Contaminated linen is placed in leakproof bag and labeled • All sharp instruments and needles are disposed of in puncture-resistant container (never recap needles after use) • Private room only if the patient's hygienic practices are careless and pose a risk to other patients
Airborne precautions	Droplet nuclei smaller than 5 microns; chickenpox, measles, tuberculosis	• Private room • Close patient room door to control direction of air flow • Mask or high-filtration respirator • Wash hands between patient contact • Gowns and gloves only if risk of exposure with body fluids or blood • Patient should wear mask when ambulating or being transported outside his or her room
Droplet precautions	Droplets larger than 5 microns; pharyngeal diphtheria, rubella, pneumonia, streptococcal phar-yngitis, pertussis, mumps	• Private room • Mask or filtration respirator • Wash hands between patient contact
Contact precautions	Direct patient or environmental contact, infection with drug-resistant organism; major wound infections, herpes simplex, scabies, varicella zoster, shigella, and other enteric pathogens	• Private room • Gloves • Gowns, hand-washing • Use disposable or dedicated, single-patient items such as stethoscopes and thermometers

Strict Isolation

The patient is kept in a separate room or shares a room with a patient who has the same disease, and the door is kept closed. All involved staff wear protective gowns, masks, and gloves. Hands must be washed upon entering and leaving the room. All equipment for drug administration must be discarded in special containers after use or must be disinfected and sterilized.

This type of isolation is ordered for hospital staph infections and serious infectious diseases that can be spread by touch and by air. It protects the medical staff (and other patients) from microorganisms the patient is carrying.

Respiratory Isolation

The patient is kept in a separate room with the door closed. Staff members wear protective masks only. The mask should be a fit-tested NIOSH-approved

N95 or higher respirator. Healthcare providers who have not been fit-tested should not perform care for a patient in respiratory isolation. Hands must be washed upon entering and leaving the room. Gloves are not necessary, but any object that is contaminated with fluids from the patient's nose and lungs must be disinfected so that the patient's microorganisms are not spread to others. Meningitis, measles, mumps, and tuberculosis are diseases requiring respiratory isolation.

Reverse Isolation (Protective Isolation)

The patient is kept in a separate room with the door closed. Gown, mask, and gloves must be worn by the staff. Hands must be washed upon entering and leaving the room. This type of isolation protects patients who have no immunity or who have weakened immunity because of leukemia or cancer chemotherapy; the patient is being protected from microorganisms you are carrying.

Special Considerations When Caring for Infectious Patients

Special procedures are also followed when handling patients with burns and skin infections (wound and skin precautions) and open sores, blood infections, and draining wounds (discharge precautions). A separate room for the patient is not required, but aseptic procedures must be followed to avoid causing or spreading infection. When a patient has a disease that is spread by direct or indirect contact with feces, enteric precautions are implemented. Generally, a private room is used, especially if the patient's hygiene is poor.

Before administering drugs to an isolation patient, you should review isolation procedures in your health facility's procedure manual. The steps are specific and should be followed. There are usually instructions for putting on and taking off gowns, masks, and gloves and for disposing of materials and equipment. Personal protective equipment is shown in **Figure 7.3**.

The procedure you will use most often, whether working with an isolation patient or not, is hand-washing. You will wash your hands both before and after administering a medication. Practice Procedure 7.1 later in the chapter will refresh your skill in the proper hand-washing technique.

When administering medications to an isolation patient, you may wonder which items are considered contaminated. The answer is everything that has been in direct or indirect contact with the patient. An example of indirect contact would be your touching a glass that has remained near a coughing patient, even if the patient had never actually touched the glass. Your gown and mask protect you (or the patient) from indirect contact. Your gloves protect you from direct contact. For additional protection, you may ask patients to take their own medications and dispose of supplies while you watch, as long as they are able to do this.

When working with a patient who has an infectious disease, it is helpful to know the main places where infection can be picked up. Infection may leave the body of a diseased person in the secretions of the nose and mouth; in material coughed up from the lungs; in the feces or anything touched by feces (bedclothes, toilet, etc.); in the urine; in the vaginal area; in drainage from infected wounds; and in the blood (as in the case of hepatitis).

You may take advantage of disposable materials to avoid carrying infection from one place to another. Where disposable materials are not available or not practical (as with permanent pieces of equipment), contaminated items must be washed and sterilized by using a special machine. Machines can kill infectious organisms by subjecting them to extreme heat, by searing them with steam, or by means of sound waves or ultraviolet rays. A common sterilizing machine is the **autoclave**, which uses steam. A variety of chemicals called *disinfectants* kill infectious organisms and are also available for sterilizing surgical tools and other pieces of equipment.

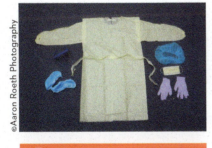

Figure 7.3

Healthcare workers may need to use various types of personal protective equipment, including gloves, masks, protective eyewear such as face shields or goggles, gowns, and caps.

Disposal procedures are also important when you work with infected patients. Equipment and disposable materials must be specially wrapped and often labeled before being discarded or sent to the facility's sterilization unit. Health facilities usually have their own disposal procedures described in a procedure manual.

UNIVERSAL BLOOD AND BODY FLUID PRECAUTIONS [LO 7-6]

Universal Precautions mean that all patients are considered potentially infectious with blood-borne pathogens. Examples are hepatitis B virus (HBV) and human immunodeficiency virus (HIV), the virus that causes AIDS. Healthcare workers are exposed to these pathogens primarily through mucous membranes, nonintact skin, and needlesticks.

Blood is the most important vehicle for transmission of these pathogens. Other body fluids that can be involved are cerebrospinal (CSF), synovial (joint), pleural (lung), peritoneal (abdominal), and amniotic fluids; semen; vaginal secretions; and human breast milk. Gloves and other protective clothing should be used routinely in handling contaminated needles and other sharp instruments. The Universal Blood and Body Fluid Precautions are frequently revised, so be sure your facility has the current, up-to-date guidelines in use (see Table 7.4).

Table 7.4 Universal Blood and Body Fluid Precautions

Employer: Protect Healthcare Worker
- Explain activities that expose workers to blood-borne pathogens.
- Develop standard operating procedures to prevent worker exposure.
- Provide initial and ongoing education on Universal Precautions.
- Follow up worker compliance with guidelines.
- Redesign the workplace and modify the workplace environment.

Healthcare Worker: Use Appropriate Barrier Precautions
- Wear gloves to reduce blood contamination to skin surface.
- Wash hands/skin immediately when exposed.
- Change and discard punctured or torn gloves.
- Change gloves between patients.
- Wear mask, gowns, and eye/face shields during procedures that are likely to generate splashes of blood or body fluids.
- Do not work if you have exudative lesions.
- If pregnant, do not risk exposing the fetus to blood-borne pathogens by lack of precautions.

Healthcare Worker: Prevent Needlestick Injuries
- Do not break, bend, or remove needles by hand from syringes.
- Do not recap needles.
- Place disposable needles in puncture-resistant containers.
- Place these containers as close to the work area as possible.
- Use safety syringes with automatic retractable needles when possible.
- Place nondisposable needles and equipment in puncture-resistant containers, and transport them to the processing area.
- Transport contaminated equipment to the appropriate area.

Healthcare for Today and Tomorrow | Antibiotic Overuse

As a result of the inappropriate use of antibiotics, organisms that were once susceptible to *all* antibiotics are increasingly becoming a serious health problem. Drug-resistant organisms have developed not only to the classic antibiotics but also to the newer line of antibiotics.

As a healthcare member, you should stress to patients the importance of taking all the prescribed antibiotic and not stopping the medication early because they feel better. Those bacteria not yet killed will multiply and become resistant to future antibiotics. You should also discourage patients from pressuring providers to order unnecessary antibiotics for colds, coughs, and other viral infections, which are not helped by antibiotics.

Legal and Ethical Issues | Monitoring Antibiotics

It is essential that patients taking antibiotics and antifungals for impaired liver and renal function be monitored to avoid toxicity. Failure to monitor a patient with compromised kidneys or liver who is receiving an antibiotic or antifungal may result in devastating and potentially life-threatening consequences.

Representative Antimicrobials

Category, Name,[a] and Route	Uses and Diseases	Actions	Usual Dose[b] and Special Instructions	Side Effects and Adverse Reactions
Antibiotics				
azithromycin (*Zithromax*) Oral, IV	Acute bacterial exacerbations of COPD due to *Haemophilus influenzae, Moraxella catarrhalis, Streptococcus pneumoniae,* pneumonia, genital ulcers, skin infections, urethritis, cervicitis	Binds to the bacterial 50S ribosomal subunit inhibiting protein synthesis (macrolide)	500 mg PO on day 1 followed by 250 mg daily on days 2–5 for a total of 1.5 g	Nausea, vomiting, diarrhea, abdominal pain, dyspepsia, anorexia, dizziness, headache
cephalexin (*Keflex*) Oral	Respiratory, genitourinary, bone, and skin infections; otitis media	Interferes with the final step in the formation of the bacterial cell wall, resulting in unstable cell membranes undergoing lysis, bactericidal (*Cephalosporin*)	250 mg q 6 hrs up to 4 g per day	Nausea, vomiting, abdominal cramps or pain, dyspepsia, glossitis, heartburn, urticaria, headache, malaise

Category, Name,[a] and Route	Uses and Diseases	Actions	Usual Dose[b] and Special Instructions	Side Effects and Adverse Reactions
amoxicillin Oral	Ear, nose, throat, genitourinary, skin, lower respiratory, and uncomplicated gonococcal infections	Inhibits cell wall synthesis, cell growth and division, bactericidal (penicillin)	500 mg q 8 hrs or 500 mg q 12 hrs	Skin rashes, diarrhea, nausea, vomiting, abdominal cramps or pain, dizziness
amoxicillin and clavulanate (Augmentin) Oral	Lower respiratory infection, otitis media, urinary tract infection, skin infections	Inhibits bacterial cell wall synthesis	250 mg PO q 8 hrs; 500 mg q 12 hrs (severe infection); watch patient closely for allergic reaction	Nausea, vomiting, diarrhea, hypersensitivity reactions such as rash, chills, shortness of breath
erythromycin Oral, IV	Acute pelvic inflammatory disease, endocarditis prophylaxis for dental work, respiratory infection	Inhibits protein synthesis	250–550 mg PO q 6 hrs	Nausea, vomiting, diarrhea, abdominal pain
gentamicin IV, IM	Bloodstream infections, serious infections, meningitis, endocarditis prophylaxis for gastrointestinal or genitourinary surgery	Inhibits protein synthesis	3 mg/kg daily in divided doses; IM or IV infusion q 8 hrs	Kidney damage, hearing loss, upset of balance; drug levels must be closely monitored
sulfamethoxazole/ trimethoprim (Septra, Bactrim) Oral, IV	Bronchitis, urinary tract infections, otitis media	Blocks folate metabolism pathway	One double-strength tablet PO q 12 hrs; encourage fluids	Nausea, vomiting, diarrhea, rash, allergic reaction to sulfa
ciprofloxacin (Cipro) Oral	Pneumonia, bone infection, urinary tract infection, skin infection	Inhibits DNA gyrase	500 mg PO q 12 hrs; do not take with antacids	Headache, nausea, diarrhea, rash
Antivirals				
amphotericin B Oral, IV	Systemic fungal infections	Damages fungal cell wall	100 mg PO QID for 7–10 days	Fever, chills, nausea, weight loss, anorexia, kidney damage, vein irritation
acyclovir (Zovirax) Oral, IV, topical	Herpes simplex, chickenpox, genital herpes	Stops viral replication	200 mg PO q 4 hrs	Kidney damage, headache, confusion, irritability, nausea, vomiting

Note: Bolded trade names are among the 50 most commonly prescribed drugs.

[a]Trade names given in parentheses are examples only. Check current drug references for a complete listing of available products.

[b]Average adult doses are given. However, dosages are determined by a provider and vary with the purpose of the therapy and the particular patient. The doses presented here are for general information only.

ADMINISTERING MEDICATION TO AN ISOLATION PATIENT

Demonstrate how to administer a medication to an isolation patient.

You may wish to practice the procedure several times using a different type of isolation each time.

Equipment

Medication order for an oral medication to be taken with water

Medication administration record

Oral medication

Disposable medication cup

Gown, mask, and gloves

Instructions for basic isolation procedures in your facility's procedure manual

Water pitcher and glass (next to patient's bed)

Procedure

1. Assemble equipment. Use disposable equipment, if possible.

2. Read the medication order and set up medication. Check to see that you have the *right dose* of the *right medication* for the *right patient* by the *right route* at the *right time* that you will administer by the *right technique* and *document right.*

3. Check to see what kind of isolation the patient is under—respiratory, strict, reverse, or special precautions (enteric, skin wounds, discharge, etc.). A sign on the door of the patient's room should tell the type of isolation.

4. Review isolation procedures for the specific type of isolation, and decide what clothing you must wear—gown, mask, and/or gloves. Here is a brief reminder:

   For reverse isolation. Wear gown, mask, and gloves. This provides protection for the patient.

   For respiratory isolation. Wear a mask only. This protects you from airborne bacteria that may be inhaled into the lungs.

   For strict isolation. Wear gown, mask, and gloves. This provides protection for you, because you must not touch anything contaminated. Remember to wash your hands before you put on the protective clothing.

5. Wash your hands using antiseptic liquid soap and warm water to make a lather, and then scrub each finger and the front and back of each hand, and the wrists, with a circular motion for a minimum of 20 seconds. Then clean fingernails by rubbing against the palm of the opposite hand. Rinse, keeping hands lower than elbows so that water flows from the cleaner area toward the dirtier area. Use a clean dry paper towel to dry each hand from the fingers (cleanest area) to the wrists (least clean area) and immediately discard the paper towel into the waste container. After drying hands, use a new, dry paper towel to turn off the water faucet and discard into the waste container. The entire washing process should last for at least 1 to 2 minutes.

6. Now put on your gown, mask, and/or gloves, following the proper procedure.

7. Carry the medication into the patient's room in a disposable medication cup.

8. Identify the patient, following health facility procedure. Explain what you are going to do (e.g., give the patient an antibiotic to help heal or fight an infection). If necessary, assist the patient into a comfortable position for taking the medication.

9. Administer the medication. Have the patient pour a glass of water from the bedside pitcher, and then watch the patient take the medication from the medication cup and swallow it with water.

10. Give any special instructions regarding the medication; for example, describe mild side effects that may be expected. Make the patient comfortable before leaving the room.

11. Remove gown, mask, and/or gloves and discard them according to the rules of your health facility. Wash your hands, following standard practice. Use a paper towel to turn off the water faucet, unless there is a foot or knee pedal.

12. Chart the medication, noting the time, dose, and anything unusual that you may have noticed or that the patient may have mentioned.

Summary

Learning Outcome	Summary Points
7-1 Distinguish between the external and internal immune systems.	• The *external immune system* protects against infection because of normally functioning defenses. • The *internal immune system* is made up of microscopic substances whose specialized function is to fight infection.
7-2 Explain why drug resistance, hypersensitivity, and superinfection are important concerns in antibiotic drug therapy.	• *Drug resistance* is the ability of a particular pathogen to resist the effects of a specific antibiotic as a result of exposure to the antibiotic for a period of time. • *Hypersensitivity* is an exaggerated response to a drug. • *Superinfection* is a secondary infection that can occur while an antibiotic is destroying the first infection.
7-3 Identify the most common types and uses of antibiotics.	• *Penicillins* are used to treat syphilis, strep throat, pneumonia, meningitis, diphtheria, osteomyelitis, and otitis media. • *Cephalosporins* are used for specific pathogens, particularly *Haemophilus influenzae.* • *Tetracyclines* are used to treat infections such as respiratory, rickettsial, venereal, and amebiasis. • *Macrolides* are used for COPD, pneumonia, urethritis, cervicitis, and sinusitis. • *Aminoglycosides* are used for only serious or life-threatening infections. • *Sulfonamides* are used for different types of infections, such as urinary tract infections, chancroid, meningitis, rheumatic fever, nocardiosis, trachoma, and sexually transmitted diseases. • *Quinolones* are used for respiratory, gastrointestinal, bone, skin, and urinary infections. • *Miscellaneous antibiotics,* such as *Azactam,* are used for respiratory, urinary, intra-abdominal, gynecological, and skin infections. *Chloromycetin* is used for a variety of infections.
7-4 Describe the antifungal and antiviral drugs and infectious diseases.	• *Antifungal drugs* are used to treat fungal infections such as dermatological infections or vaginal candidiasis. • *Antiviral drugs* are used to treat chickenpox, influenza, and viral hepatitis.

Learning Outcome	Summary Points
7-5 Describe the correct procedure for administering a medication to a patient in isolation.	• Set up the medications according to procedure, being sure to include the medication rights. • Check to see what kind of isolation the client is in. • Review the isolation procedures and decide what type of clothing to wear. • After washing hands, carry the medication to the patient's room in a disposable cup. • Give appropriate education, such as side effects. Watch the patient take the medication. • After settling the patient, remove all isolation clothing, wash your hands, and chart the medication.
7-6 Explain the primary ways a healthcare worker can be exposed to hepatitis B virus and human immunodeficiency virus.	• Mucous membranes • Nonintact skin • Needlesticks

Chapter 7 Review

Define each term.

1. (LO 7-1) Antibody _____

2. (LO 7-1) Immunization _____

3. (LO 7-1) Pathogen _____

4. (LO 7-2) Bacteriostatic _____

5. (LO 7-2) Bactericidal _____

6. (LO 7-2) Hypersensitivity _____

7. (LO 7-2) Penicillinase _____

Answer the questions in the space provided.

8. (LO 7-2) List two ways in which antibiotic drugs fight infection. _____

_____

_____

9. (LO 7-2) Which parts of the body may be damaged by aminoglycosides? _____

_____

_____

10. (LO 7-2) What classification does erythromycin belong to? _____

_____

11. (LO 7-2) Why might a provider order a Gram stain? _____

_____

12. (LO 7-5) Why are isolation procedures used? _____

_____

13. (LO 7-5) List the three main types of isolation (in which patients are kept in separate rooms).

_____

_____

_____

Match the antibiotic to the example.

_____ 14. (LO 7-3) Cephalosporins   a. *Bactrim*

_____ 15. (LO 7-3) Tetracyclines   b. *Zithromax*

_____ 16. (LO 7-3) Macrolides   c. *Tobrex*

_____ 17. (LO 7-2) Aminoglycosides   d. *Keflex*

_____ 18. (LO 7-3) Sulfonamides   e. *Vibramycin*

Match the terms to their descriptions.

_____ 19. (LO 7-2) Laboratory test to identify pathogens   a. narrow spectrum

_____ 20. (LO 7-2) Laboratory test to determine which drug   b. resistance
                 will kill a specific pathogen
                                                     c. Gram stain

_____ 21. (LO 7-2) Drugs that affect many pathogens   d. broad spectrum

_____ 22. (LO 7-2) Drugs that affect only a few pathogens   e. hypersensitivity

_____ 23. (LO 7-2) A germ's immunity to the effects of   f. culture and
                  pathogen-killing drugs   sensitivity test

_____ 24. (LO 7-2) Allergic-like reaction to a drug after taking
                  several doses

Drug Calculations—Fill in the blank with the answer.

25. (LO 7-2) The provider orders cefaclor 200 mg orally bid. Available is 125 mg/5 mL. Prepare to administer _____ mL to your patient.

26. (LO 7-2) The provider orders cephalexin (*Keflex*) 0.5 g orally bid. Available are 500-mg tablets. You will administer _____ tablets to your patient.

27. (LO 7-2) The provider orders penicillin V 500 mg orally qid. Available are 250-mg tablets. You will give _____ tablets to your patient in each dose.

28. (LO 7-2) The provider orders cefadroxil 1 g orally bid. Available are 500-mg tablets. You will administer _____ tablets to your patient.

29. (LO 7-2) The provider orders ciprofloxacin (*Cipro*) 750 mg orally bid. Available are 500-mg tablets. You will administer _____ tablets to your patient.

Multiple Choice—Circle the correct letter.

30. (LO 7-3) What are three adverse reactions to azithromycin (*Zithromax*)?
    a. Muscle weakness, hypotension, urinary frequency
    b. Dry mouth, taste alterations, constipation
    c. Weight gain, bone pain, fever
    d. Nausea, vomiting, diarrhea

31. (LO 7-3) A patient with chickenpox asks you what antiviral will most likely be prescribed. What is your most appropriate response?
    a. Acyclovir (*Zovirax*)   c. Amoxicillin
    b. Cephalexin   d. Ciprofloxacin (*Cipro*)

32. (LO 7-5) What type of protective clothing should you wear when a patient is admitted to strict isolation?
    a. Mask only   c. Gown, mask, and gloves
    b. Gown and gloves   d. Gloves only

33. (LO 7-3) A patient asks you how long the clarithromycin (*Biaxin*) will need to be taken for tonsillitis. What should be your most appropriate response?
    a. 14 days   c. 30 days
    b. 5 days   d. Until the patient feels better

34. (LO 7-4) You should monitor a patient taking amphotericin B for which of the following adverse reactions?
    a. Weight loss, fever, chills
    b. Urinary hesitancy, constipation, abdominal cramps
    c. Muscle weakness, irregular heartbeat, shortness of breath
    d. Joint pain, thirst, increased appetite

Chapter 7 Case Studies

35. (LO 7-3) You are caring for a patient taking erythromycin for a respiratory infection. What is the classification of antibiotic for erythromycin? The patient asks you what he should know to safely take the medication. What should you tell the patient? _____

_____

_____

_____

36. (LO 7-3) A patient is taking *Bactrim* and complains of nausea, vomiting, diarrhea, and urinary problems. What is the conclusion you reach from these side effects? What is the education you should give the patient? What is the classification of antibiotic? _____

_____

_____

_____

Critical Thinking

Answer the questions in the space provided.

37. (LO 7-1) Why are staph and other infections a special problem in hospitals and long-term care units? Give at least three reasons. _____

_____

_____

_____

38. (LO 7-6) List three ways in which a healthcare worker can be exposed to HBV and HIV. _____

_____

_____

_____

39. (LO 7-3) List at least three possible problems associated with the use of penicillin. _____

_____

_____

_____

40. (LO 7-3) You have just administered penicillin to Ms. Mosley. Within minutes she goes into shock, has difficulty breathing, and shows signs of swelling in the throat. What is probably the matter, and what should you do?

_____

_____

_____

41. (LO 7-3) Why should oral tetracyclines not be given to a patient who is using antacids or dairy products?

_____

_____

_____

42. (LO 7-5) How should you administer a medication to a patient in isolation? _____

_____

_____

_____

43. (LO 7-5) Why is washing your hands important with all patients you are caring for, and especially a patient in isolation? _____

_____

_____

_____

Applications

Obtain an electronic drug guide, and a current copy of a drug reference book or the *PDR*®. Use it to answer the following questions in a notebook or on index cards.

44. Choose one of the drugs from the Representative Antimicrobials table in this chapter and differentiate between the generic and brand names. _____

_____

_____

_____

45. For the drug chosen in question 46, outline the action, uses, adult dose, adverse reactions, and nursing considerations. _____

_____

_____

DRUGS FOR THE EYE AND EAR

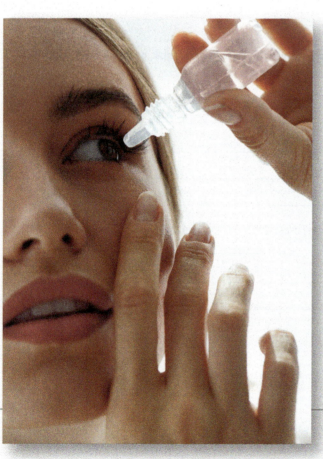

©puhhha/Shutterstock

In this chapter you will learn the functions of the various parts of the eye and ear and how sight and hearing occur. You will also learn about the disorders of the eye and ear and how drugs are used to control them. In addition, you will learn how to administer eye drops, eye ointments, and ear drops.

LEARNING OUTCOMES

8-1 Identify the external parts of the eye and ear.

8-2 Describe the major disorders of the eye and ear for which medications are given.

8-3 Describe the actions of the following drug groups: miotics, carbonic anhydrase inhibitors, beta-adrenergic blocking agents, eye antibiotics, mydriatics, and ear antibiotics.

8-4 Carry out administering eye and ear medications while performing calculations.

8-5 Carry out instilling eye drops, eye ointments, and ear drops.

acoustic

air conduction

blepharitis

canthus

cataract

central hearing loss

cerumen

conductive hearing loss

conjunctivitis

diplopia

external otitis

floaters

glaucoma

hordeolum

miotics

mydriatics

optic

otalgia

otic

photophobia

presbycusis

presbyopia

sensorineural hearing loss

tinnitus

vertigo

STRUCTURE AND FUNCTION OF THE EYE [LO 8-1]

The eye is a group of tissues that are specialized to permit vision. It is housed in a bony eye socket and is surrounded by fatty tissue and muscles that serve to protect and to move the eye. The eyelids, lashes, tears, and blinking also protect the eye. The eyelid covers the outer eye and quickly closes (blinks) to prevent a foreign body from entering the eye. Lashes on the eyelid help keep dust and dirt from entering the eye. At the edge of the eyelid is a lacrimal gland, which produces tears to keep the eye moist and to wash away dust particles. Tears are drained off through the tear ducts into the nose. The eyelids and sclera are lined with mucous membranes called the conjunctiva.

The eye itself is made up of three layers: the external protective layer (cornea and sclera); the middle layer (choroid, iris, and ciliary body); and the retina, which is sensitive to light. Within these layers are the many parts that work together to produce sight (Figure 8.1).

The cornea is the transparent anterior portion of the eye. Continuous with the cornea is the sclera, which is nontransparent and is commonly referred to as the "white" of the eye. Within the middle layer is the choroid, which is the highly vascular structure that provides nourishment to the ciliary body, the iris, and the outer part of the retina. The iris gives the eye its color. The ciliary body is the vascular section of the eye that lies between the base of the iris and the anterior portion of the choroid. The lens is transparent, lies behind the iris, and serves to ensure that a received image falls in sharp focus on the retina.

For light to reach the retina, it must pass through the cornea, aqueous humor, lens, and vitreous humor. The aqueous humor is a clear, watery fluid that fills both the anterior and posterior chambers of the anterior cavity of the eye. It bathes and nourishes the lens, the iris, and the posterior side of the cornea. The aqueous humor is the substance that usually leaks out when the eye is injured. The vitreous humor is a soft, gelatinous substance in the posterior cavity of the eye. It helps maintain sufficient intraocular pressure to prevent the eyeball from collapsing.

The **optic** nerves (one from each eye) carry information back to the brain. The brain then codes the information into visual images.

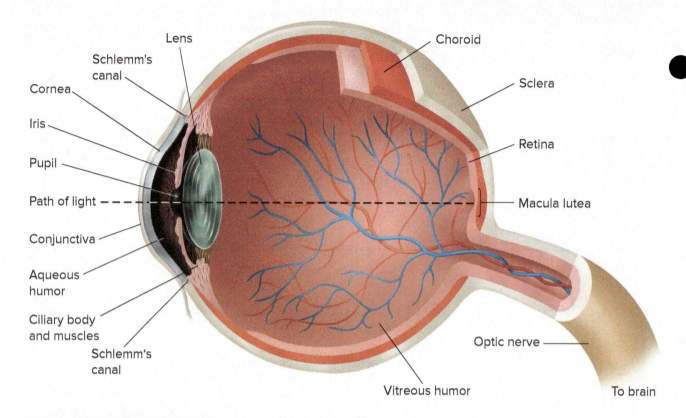

Figure 8.1

Structures of the eye.

Effects of Aging on the Visual Structures

As an individual ages, changes occur to every structure of the visual system. **Presbyopia** is farsightedness that normally occurs between the ages of 40 and 45. The eye loses its ability to accommodate, and the individual experiences eye fatigue and blurred vision. Bifocal lenses are prescribed to correct vision.

Many of the changes of aging are relatively insignificant, but some may result in a decrease in vision (Table 8.1). Someone who loses part or all of the ability to see must make a major psychological adjustment.

EYE DISORDERS [LO 8-2]

Glaucoma

Glaucoma is an eye disorder characterized by increased intraocular pressure. The increased pressure damages the optic nerve. Usually the patient has no symptoms until the loss of vision is significant. If it goes unnoticed and untreated, glaucoma can cause blindness. Glaucoma is the second leading cause of blindness in the United States. There are three types of glaucoma—primary, secondary, and congenital. All three are treatable. Primary glaucoma is either narrow-angle or wide-angle glaucoma. Drugs are needed to control narrow-angle glaucoma prior to surgery. Wide-angle glaucoma must be controlled by permanent drug therapy. Secondary glaucoma results from previous eye disease or following removal of a cataract and is also dependent on drug therapy. Congenital glaucoma is treated by surgery. The drug therapy of choice for treating glaucoma is miotics, carbonic anhydrase inhibitors, and beta-adrenergic blocking agents. The side effects of these drugs include **diplopia**, or double vision.

Cataracts

A **cataract** is an opacity that appears within the crystalline lens and may affect one or both eyes. Cataracts are the third most common cause of blindness,

Table 8.1 Effects of Aging on Visual Structures

Visual Structures	Effects of Aging
Eyebrows and eyelashes	Loss of pigmentation (brows and lashes turn gray)
Eyelids	Loss of orbital fat; weakened muscles; sensitivity to touch
Conjunctiva	Formation of small yellow spots
Sclera	Yellowing
Cornea	Yellow ring around cornea; decreased corneal sensitivity and luster; blurred vision
Lacrimal ducts	Decreased tear production; dry, irritated eyes
Iris	Decreased pupil size; slower dilation after exposure to light; decreased near vision and accommodation
Lens	Cataracts; opacity resulting in glare; yellowing
Retina	Change in color perception; decreased sharpness of vision; loss of central vision; vascular changes resulting from arteriosclerosis and hypertension
Vitreous humor	Floaters (specks)

and 50 percent of older adults over the age of 65 years have some cataract formation. In addition to a decrease in vision, abnormal color perception and glare are also common.

The treatment of choice is surgery, although preoperatively mydriatics, cycloplegic agents, nonsteroidal anti-inflammatory drugs, and topical antibiotics may be used. Postoperatively, topical antibiotics and anti-inflammatory drugs are used. Additionally, postoperatively, the provider may advise patients to avoid activities such as bending, stooping, coughing, and lifting that increase intraocular pressure. You may also instruct your patient to wear an eye shield to protect against sunlight.

Eye Infections

The treatment of eye infections is generally determined only after a laboratory test is performed to determine the infective organism. Eye infections can also cause an increase in **floaters**, which are cells in the form of nontransparent specks that float across the visual field. **Conjunctivitis** is an infection or inflammation of the conjunctiva. Conjunctival infections may be caused by bacterial, viral, or chlamydial microorganisms. Conjunctival inflammation may be caused by allergens or chemical irritants. Active bacterial conjunctivitis is an inflammation of the mucous membrane that lines the back of the eyelids and the front of the eye except the cornea. Conjunctivitis, referred to as "pink eye," is a common eye disorder and highly contagious among children. Symptoms include redness, itching, excessive tearing, and, occasionally, **photophobia**, extreme sensitivity to light. Besifloxacin (*Besivance*) is an ophthalmic solution administered by drops that is approved for use in bacterial conjunctivitis. **Blepharitis** is a bacterial infection of the eyelids that causes crusting, redness, and irritation of the eyelids. Infection of the sebaceous glands, **hordeolum**, commonly referred to as a sty, creates a hard cyst on the eyelid as a result of a blocked sebaceous duct. Tobramycin (*Tobrex*) is an ophthalmic ointment used to treat eye infections.

DRUG THERAPY FOR EYE DISORDERS [LO 8-3]

Miotics

Miotics are drugs that cause the pupil to constrict by decreasing the intraocular pressure, increasing the aqueous humor outflow, and contracting the ciliary muscles. They are used in the treatment of glaucoma. The two types of miotics are direct-acting miotics and miotics that inhibit cholinesterase activity.

Direct-acting miotics are used in narrow-angle and chronic open-angle glaucoma. The three most common types are pilocarpine HCl (*Isopto Carpine*), carbachol intraocular (*Miostat*), and acetylcholine (*Miochol_E*). The most common adverse reactions produced are local effects such as a decrease in visual acuity. They may also produce systemic effects such as flushing, sweating, gastric upset, diarrhea, and headache.

Miotics that inhibit cholinesterase activity inhibit the enzyme cholinesterase. They are longer-acting and more toxic than direct-acting miotics. Because of this property, they are reserved for patients with open-angle glaucoma who do not respond to other drugs. Like direct-acting miotics, they produce both local and systemic effects. Locally, they produce stinging, burning, ocular inflammation, lacrimation, and opacity of the lens. Systemically, they produce salivation, urinary incontinence, muscle weakness, sweating, and diarrhea.

If a toxic reaction occurs, atropine or pralidoxime chloride (PAM) are used as antidotes. An example of cholinesterase inhibitors is echothiophate iodide (*Phospholine Iodide*).

Mydriatic Drugs

Mydriatics are drugs that dilate the pupil. They are used to facilitate an eye examination, relieve inflammation associated with uveitis and keratitis, and prepare a patient for ocular surgery. The two main classes of mydriatic drugs are sympathomimetic and anticholinergic agents.

Sympathomimetic mydriatics produce pupillary dilation, increase the outflow of aqueous humor, cause vasoconstriction, relax the ciliary muscle, and decrease the formation of aqueous humor. Examples of sympathomimetic drugs include epinephrine, hydroxyamphetamine/tropicamide (*Paremyd*), naphazoline (*Albalon*), and tetrahydrozoline (*Visine Original Redness Relief*). Although serious adverse reactions to sympathomimetic drugs are rare, these drugs should be used with caution in patients with hypertension, diabetes mellitus, heart disease, and hyperthyroidism. Anticholinergic mydriatics produce pupillary dilation that interferes with the ability of the eye to properly focus, which is called paralysis of accommodation or cycloplegia, and are used in refractive examinations to determine if corrective lenses are required. Examples of anticholinergic mydriatic drugs include atropine, cyclopentolate HCl (*Cyclogyl*), homatropine HBr, scopolamine HBr, and tropicamide (*Mydriacyl*). Because of the mydriatic effects, these drugs are contraindicated in patients with glaucoma.

The adverse reactions of mydriatics include increased intraocular pressure, local irritation, blurred vision, flushing, dryness of the skin, and confusion.

 Pediatric Considerations Eye Medications

- Eye medications are rarely used in children other than to dilate the pupil and paralyze accommodation for ophthalmoscopic examination. Short-acting mydriatics and cycloplegics are used most frequently because they have fewer systemic side effects.

- Give the smallest possible dose in an effort to reduce the incidence of systemic side effects.

- Older adults need eye medications because they develop cataracts and glaucoma.
- There is an increased risk for systemic effects because many older adults have cardiovascular disorders.

- Administer the smallest possible dose to decrease the incidence of side effects (e.g., hypertension, tachycardia, and arrhythmias with adrenergic drugs and bradycardia and bronchoconstriction with beta blockers).

STRUCTURE AND FUNCTION OF THE EAR [LO 8-1]

The ear is a complex organ designed for hearing. It also plays a part in the body's sense of balance. It has three basic parts: the external ear, the middle ear, and the inner ear (**Figure 8.2**). The external ear consists of an auricle, or pinna, and the external auditory meatus, or ear canal. Ceruminous glands in the external ear produce wax, or **cerumen**. Small hairs in the canal move this wax toward the outer opening. The wax protects the ear by trapping foreign materials and dust. The function of the external ear is **acoustic**, pertaining to sound. It collects and transmits sound waves to the tympanic membrane, or eardrum.

The eustachian (auditory) tube connects the middle ear to the nasopharynx. The eustachian tube is usually collapsed, except during swallowing, chewing, yawning, or jaw movement. This tube equalizes air pressure on both sides of the eardrum, preventing it from rupturing. The external and middle ear function to conduct and amplify sound waves from the environment. This function is known as **air conduction**. Problems with either the external or middle ear cause a **conductive hearing loss**, an alteration in the patient's perception of or sensitivity

Figure 8.2

Structures of the external, middle, and inner ear.

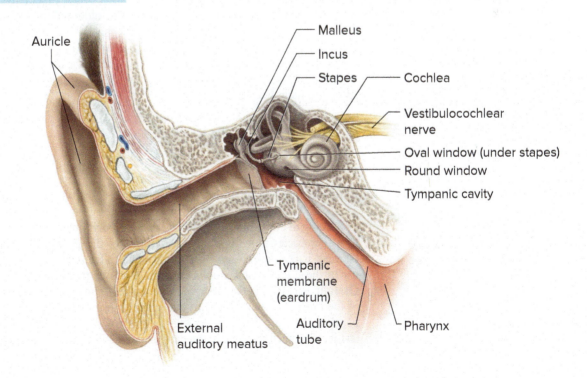

Table 8.2 Effects of Aging on Auditory Structures

Auditory Structure	Effects of Aging
External ear	Increase in cerumen; drier cerumen; increase in hair
Middle ear	Conductive hearing loss
Inner ear	Decrease in ability to hear high-pitched sounds; tinnitus; alteration in balance

to sounds. The vibrations of the eardrum are picked up by three tiny bones in the middle ear—the malleus, incus, and stapes bones. See Figure 8.2. These three bones transmit vibrations to specialized hearing cells in the inner ear.

The inner ear is also known as the labyrinth because of its complicated shape. It is made up of the bony labyrinth that contains the vestibule, cochlea, and semicircular canals and the membranous labyrinth. The vestibule is necessary to maintain equilibrium. The cochlea is the primary organ of hearing. When disease or injury occurs in the inner ear, a **sensorineural hearing loss** results, and the patient experiences an alteration in the perception of or sensitivity to high-pitched tones. Problems with the central auditory system cause a **central hearing loss**, which results in difficulty understanding the meanings of words heard or the inability to understand the meaning of incoming sounds and words. This condition results from damage to the central nervous system from the auditory nucleus to the cortex.

Effects of Aging on the Auditory Structures

Changes that occur to the structures of the auditory system as a result of aging can result in impaired hearing (Table 8.2). **Presbycusis** is a lessened ability to hear high-pitched sounds. **Tinnitus**, ringing in the ears, may accompany hearing loss. Loud noises, such as highly amplified music or noisy equipment, may cause hearing loss. When a hearing loss occurs, especially later in life, severe depression and isolation may occur. The older individual may withdraw from social contacts and neglect personal hygiene. As a result of people living longer, the incidence of hearing loss is increasing. In your role as a member of the healthcare team, helping with early identification of problems with auditory structures can contribute to patients living more active and happier lives into their 70s and 80s.

EAR DISORDERS [LO 8-2]

External Otitis

External otitis is an inflammation and infection of the epithelium of the auricle and ear canal. It is more common in the summer and is associated with swimming in contaminated water. It is called "swimmer's ear." It can be caused by either bacteria or fungi. The ear promotes the growth of microorganisms because it is a warm and dark environment. Trauma caused by picking the ear or the use of a sharp object generally causes the initial break in the skin. **Otalgia**, ear pain, is the first clinical manifestation. It is the result of swelling of the bony ear canal caused by the inflammatory process. Serosanguinous or purulent drainage from the ear may be present. After a culture and sensitivity test is performed to identify the causative organism, topical antibiotics may be administered.

Cerumen

Cerumen, or earwax, can decrease hearing when it collects in the ear canal. Cerumen becomes a greater problem with age because the earwax becomes drier, harder, and cannot be easily removed. Besides hearing loss, symptoms of cerumen impaction include otalgia, tinnitus, and vertigo. Treatment of cerumen may be irrigation of the ear canal or lubricating drops placed in the canal to soften the earwax. Instruct the patient to avoid using cotton-tipped applicators in the ear because they often impact the cerumen further. Inform the patient to clean the ear only with a washcloth and finger.

DRUG THERAPY FOR EAR DISORDERS [LO 8-3]

Topical Antibiotics

Topical antibiotics for external ear disorders include neomycin/polymyxin B/ gramicidin ophthalmic. Nystatin is used for fungal infections. Corticosteroids may be used for infections that are not fungal. After the ear canal is cleansed, a medication-soaked wick of cotton is placed in the canal to assist in the delivery of the antibiotic ear drops. Side effects of topical antibiotics such as ciprofloxacin otic are ear itching and irritation.

Otic (ear) drops should be administered at room temperature because cold drops can cause dizziness. Avoid touching the tip of the dropper to the auricle because that contaminates the remainder of the solution in the bottle. Administering antibiotics in the ear canal is an excellent opportunity to teach the patient how to prevent future ear infections or hearing problems.

 Caution Ear Wicks

Be cautious about placing a cotton wick in the ear of very young, confused, psychotic, or older adult patients because they may push the wick farther into the ear.

 Patient Education Preventing Hearing Problems

- Do not put objects in the ears. Avoid itching with something sharp like a hair pin.
- Avoid environmental noise, such as loud music, equipment, and airplanes.
- Get all childhood and adult immunizations, particularly mumps, measles, and rubella.
- Congenital deafness can occur if a pregnant woman is exposed to rubella during the first 16 weeks of gestation.
- When taking medications, report any hearing loss, **vertigo** (dizziness), nausea, or vomiting or a spinning sensation in the head while sitting.

- Instruct patients to wear hearing protection when exposed to loud noises.
- Chronic mouth breathing may result from enlarged adenoids, which may block the eustachian tubes and predispose a person to infection.
- Always take the full course of an antibiotic, even if a condition improves before the medicine is gone.
- Report any symptoms that may indicate hearing loss, such as asking others to speak up, answering questions inappropriately, or having increased sensitivity to even slight changes in noise level.
- Avoid self-medicating.

Representative Drugs for the Eye and Ear

Category, Name,[a] and Route	Uses and Diseases	Actions	Usual Dose[b] and Special Instructions	Side Effects and Adverse Reactions
Eye Medications				
bacitracin ophthalmic, neomycin/polymyxin B/gramicidin ophthalmic (*Neosporin Ophthalmic*) Topical	Superficial eye infections	Bactericidal effect against Gram-positive and Gram-negative organisms	1-cm ($\frac{1}{3}$-inch) strip every 3–4 hours	Stinging, itching, swelling, redness
pilocarpine HCl (*Isopto Carpine*) Topical	Glaucoma Induction of miosis Mydriasis caused by cycloplegic drugs	Miotic agent that causes pupil constriction; reduces intraocular pressure by increasing aqueous humor outflow	1 drop every 4–8 hrs; gently press tear duct for 1–2 minutes to prevent systemic absorption	Blurred vision, brow pain, eye irritation, myopia
pemirolast potassium (*Alamast*) Topical	Allergic conjunctivitis	Cell stabilizer that inhibits the release of inflammatory mediators from human mast cells	1–2 drops in the affected eye QID	Headache, rhinitis, cold/flu symptoms
betaxolol (Betoptic S) Topical	Glaucoma	Beta-adrenergic blocking agent that decreases production of aqueous humor	1 drop of 0.5% solution or 1–2 drops of 0.25% suspension BID	Eye stinging at time of instillation, photophobia, tearing

Representative Drugs for the Eye and Ear (continued)

Category, Name,[a] and Route	Uses and Diseases	Actions	Usual Dose[b] and Special Instructions	Side Effects and Adverse Reactions
acetazolamide PO	Glaucoma	Carbonic anhydrase inhibitor that decreases production of aqueous humor	250 mg PO q 4 hrs	Transient myopia; paresthesia, especially tingling in extremities; drowsiness; nausea; vomiting
atropine sulfate Topical	Iritis, uveitis, refraction during eye exam	Mydriatic and cycloplegic agent that dilates pupil and causes paralysis of muscles	1 drop of 1% solution or $\frac{1}{2}$ inch of ointment daily for iritis and uveitis; 1–2 drops of 1% solution before refraction examination	Blurred vision, photophobia
tobramycin (*Tobrex*) Topical	Superficial eye infections by susceptible bacteria	Bactericidal broad-spectrum antibiotic that inhibits protein synthesis	1–2 drops 2–6 times a day; 0.5 cm of ointment 2–3 times a day	Transient irritation, burning, stinging, itching, and inflammation
Ear Medications				
neomycin/polymjyxin B/ hydrocortisone otic (*Cortisporin Otic*) Topical	Bacterial infection of outer ear, postsurgical ear infection	Bactericidal effect that suppresses inflammation and itching	3–4 drops TID or QID	Superinfection, hypersensitivity
ofloxacin (*Floxin Otic*)	Infections of the ear canal	Bacteriostatic stops the spread of the organism or bactericidal kills the organism	10 drops in ears 1–2 times a day for 7–14 days	Ear itching and irritation
carbamide peroxide otic (*Murine Ear Wax Removal*) Topical	Cerumen	Softens earwax	Fill ear canal with solution and insert cotton ball	Ear redness and itching

[a]*Trade names given in parentheses are examples only. Check current drug references for a complete listing of available products.*

[b]*Average adult doses are given. However, dosages are determined by a provider and vary with the purpose of the therapy and the particular patient. The doses presented in this text are for general information only.*

Practice Procedure 8.1 (LO 8-5)

INSTILLING EYE DROPS AND EYE OINTMENT

Demonstrate how to instill eye drops and eye ointment.

Equipment

Provider's orders for eye drops and eye ointment

Medication administration record

Bottle of eye drops and sterile eyedropper

Tube of ophthalmic ointment

Sterile cotton balls or gauze

Tissues to wipe up spills

Disposable gloves

Procedure

1. Set up medications on a tray or cart. Check for the "seven rights."

2. Wash your hands.

3. Don gloves.

4. Identify the patient and explain the procedure.

5. Ask the patient about any known allergies to eye medications.

6. Gently wash the eyelid margins or inner **canthus** (angle or corner of the eye) if crusting or drainage is present. If dry, cleanse with a damp cloth. Wash from inner to outer canthus.

7. Instill eye drops:
   - Position the patient lying down or sitting back in a chair with the head slightly hyperextended, and instruct the patient to look up.
   - In your nondominant hand, gently resting on the patient's cheekbone, hold the cotton ball or tissue. With the dominant hand resting on the patient's forehead, hold the dropper $\frac{1}{2}$ to $\frac{3}{4}$ inch above the conjunctival sac (**Figure 8.3**).
   - Drop the prescribed number of drops into the conjunctival sac.
   - If the patient blinks or if a drop lands on the outer eyelid, repeat.
   - Wipe up any liquid overflow with cotton or tissue.

8. If administering a drug that causes systemic effects, cover your finger with tissue and press gently against the inner corner of the eye and the nose bone. This keeps the medication from entering the tear ducts and the nose. Do this for 30 to 60 seconds.

9. Instill eye ointment:
   - Instruct the patient to look up.
   - Holding the ointment applicator above the lower lid, apply a small layer of ointment evenly along the inner edge of the lower lid margins on the inner conjunctiva from inner canthus to outer canthus (**Figure 8.4**).
   - Instruct the patient to close the eye and rub the eyelid in a circular motion with a cotton ball to spread the ointment over the eye.
   - Wipe up excess ointment with tissue or cotton.

10. If the patient has an eye patch, replace it with a clean patch. Place the new patch over the eye in which the medication was instilled, making sure to cover the eye completely. Tape the patch securely without applying pressure.

11. Help the patient back into a comfortable position.

12. Remove gloves and wash your hands.

13. Chart the procedure, including drug name, concentration, number of drops, time, and which eye received the medication.

14. Application of eye ointment may result in temporary blurred vision.

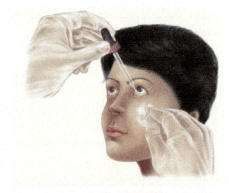

Figure 8.3

Instilling eye drops.

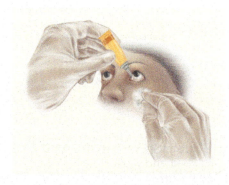

Figure 8.4

Instilling eye ointment.

INSTILLING EAR DROPS

Demonstrate how to instill ear drops in both an adult and a child.

Equipment

Medication order for ear medication

Medication administration record

Ear medication in bottle with dropper (marked with drops or milliliters)

Tissue

Cotton-tipped applicator

Cotton ball (optional)

Disposable gloves

Procedure

1. Set up medication. Make sure it is at room temperature or warmed to body temperature, according to instructions. Check for the "seven rights."

2. Wash your hands.

3. Don gloves.

4. Identify the patient, explain the procedure, and position the patient lying on the back with the head turned to the unaffected side.

5. Gently wipe out the outermost portion of the ear canal with a cotton-tipped applicator if cerumen or drainage is blocking it.

6. Instill ear drops:
   - Grasp the outer ear and pull gently to straighten the ear canal. In children, pull the auricle down and backward; in adults, pull the auricle upward and outward (**Figure 8.5**).
   - Instill prescribed drops, holding the dropper $\frac{1}{2}$ inch above the ear canal.
   - Instruct the patient to remain in the side-lying position for up to 5 minutes.
   - Gently apply pressure or massage the tragus (small cartilage projection in front of entrance) of the ear with a finger to help move medication inward.

7. Wipe up any spills with tissue.

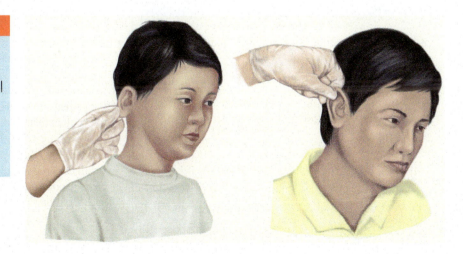

Figure 8.5

Positioning the patient's ear for instilling drops. To straighten a child's ear canal (left), pull the auricle down and back; to straighten an adult's ear canal (right), pull upward and outward.

8. If ordered, place a cotton ball in the outermost portion of the ear canal to prevent the medication from leaking out. Remove cotton in 15 minutes.

9. Remove gloves and wash your hands.

10. Chart the procedure. Be sure to record the number of drops instilled and which ear was treated.

Summary

Learning Outcome	Summary Points
8-1 Identify the external parts of the eye and ear.	• *Eye:* The external parts are the eyelid and lashes. • *Ear:* The external parts are the auricle, or pinna, and the external auditory meatus, or ear canal.
8-2 Describe the major disorders of the eye and ear for which medications are given.	• *Eye disorders* include glaucoma and eye infections. • *Ear disorders* include external otitis and cerumen.
8-3 Describe the actions of the following drug groups: miotics, carbonic anhydrase inhibitors, beta-adrenergic blocking agents, eye antibiotics, mydriatics, and ear antibiotics.	• *Miotics* cause the pupil to constrict. An example is pilocarpine HCl (*Isopto Carpine*). • *Carbonic anhydrase inhibitors* decrease production of aqueous humor. An example is acetazolamide. • *Beta-adrenergic blocking agents* decrease the production of aqueous humor. An example is betaxolol (*Betoptic S*). • *Mydriatic drugs* dilate the pupil. An example is naphazoline (*Albalon*). • *Eye antibiotics* either kill or inhibit the organism. An example is neomycin/polymyxin B/gramicidin ophthalmic. • *Ear topical antibiotics* are used for a variety of infections. An example is neomycin/polymjyxin B/hydrocortisone otic.
8-4 Carry out administering eye and ear medications while performing calculations.	• Although the processes of administering eye and ear medications are different, both share several general instructions that must be followed, such as washing hands, checking the "seven rights," identifying the patient, and explaining what will be done. • Correctly performing calculations for drugs of the eye and ear ensures patient safety.
8-5 Carry out instilling eye drops, eye ointments, and ear drops.	• *Instilling eye drops and eye ointments:* Clean the canthus from the inner corner to the outer. For eye drops, in your dominant hand, resting on the patient's cheekbone, hold a cotton ball. In the nondominant hand, gently resting on the patient's forehead, hold the dropper $\frac{1}{2}$ to $\frac{3}{4}$ inch above the conjunctival sac. • *Instilling ear drops:* In children, pull the auricle down and back. In adults, pull the auricle upward and outward. Instill ear drops holding the dropper $\frac{1}{2}$ inch above the ear canal. Upon completion, gently apply pressure or massage the tragus of the ear with a finger to help move the medication inward.

Chapter 8 Review

Match the terms to their definitions.

_____ 1. (LO 8-1) Referred to as the "white" of the eye

_____ 2. (LO 8-1) Mucous linings of the eye socket and eyelid

_____ 3. (LO 8-1) Ear canal

_____ 4. (LO 8-1) Earwax

_____ 5. (LO 8-1) Primary organ of hearing

_____ 6. (LO 8-1) Gland that produces tears

a. cochlea

b. conjunctiva

c. external auditory meatus

d. cerumen

e. sclera

f. lacrimal

Define each of the terms listed.

7. (LO 8-1) Acoustic _____

_____

_____

8. (LO 8-1) Vertigo _____

_____

_____

9. (LO 8-2) Otic _____

_____

_____

10. (LO 8-1) Optic _____

_____

_____

11. (LO 8-1) Tinnitus _____

_____

_____

12. (LO 8-2) Diplopia _____

_____

_____

13. (LO 8-1) Presbyopia _____

_____

_____

14. (LO 8-2) Glaucoma _____

_____

_____

Complete the statements by filling in the blanks.

15. (LO 8-1) The tiny bones in the middle ear that receive the vibrations of the eardrum are the

_____, _____, and

_____.

16. (LO 8-1) The covering of the outer eye that closes quickly to prevent a foreign body from entering the eye
is the _____.

17. (LO 8-1) The _____ tube connects the middle ear to the nasopharynx
and is usually collapsed except when a person is chewing, yawning, or moving the jaw.

Define the purpose of the drug categories.

18. (LO 8-3) Miotics _____

_____

_____

19. (LO 8-3) Mydriatics _____

_____

_____

Match the drug names to their use(s).

_____ 20. (LO 8-3) *Betoptic S*   a. cerumen

_____ 21. (LO 8-3) *Isopto Atropine*   b. glaucoma

_____ 22. (LO 8-3) ofloxacin (*Floxin Otic*)   c. superficial eye infections

_____ 23. (LO 8-3) *Neosporin Ophthalmic*   d. infections of the ear canal

_____ 24. (LO 8-3) *Murine Ear Wax Remover*   e. iritis, uveitis, refraction during eye exam

Complete the statements by filling in the blank.

25. (LO 8-4) Eye ointment may cause _____ for a while after application.

26. (LO 8-4) Before instilling ear medications, the ear canal must be _____.

27. (LO 8-4) For patient comfort, ear drops should be _____ in the hand
or in warm water.

28. (LO 8-4) Never administer a topical medication to the eyes unless it is labeled _____.

Answer the questions in the space provided.

29. (LO 8-2) List at least three things you can teach a patient about the prevention of hearing loss.

_____

_____

_____

30. (LO 8-1) List at least five effects of aging on the visual structures. _____

_____

_____

_____

_____

_____

Drug Calculations—Fill in the blank with the answer.

31. (LO 8-4) The provider orders acetazolamide 375 mg orally daily. Available are 250-mg tablets. You will administer _____ tablets to your patient.

32. (LO 8-4) The provider orders atropine sulfate (*Isopto Atropine*) 1 drop of 1% solution to be administered to the left eye daily. Available is 0.5% solution. You will administer _____ drops to your patient.

33. (LO 8-4) The provider orders betaxolol (*Betoptic S*) 1 drop of a 0.5% solution to both eyes daily. Available is 0.25% solution. You will administer _____ drops to your patient.

Multiple Choice—Circle the correct letter.

34. (LO 8-3) A patient taking ofloxacin (*Floxin Otic*) most likely complains of which of the following adverse reactions?
    a. Photophobia and tearing
    b. Weakness and joint pain
    c. Ear itching and irritation
    d. Urinary frequency and constipation

35. (LO 8-2) What are three symptoms that you should report immediately to prevent hearing loss?
    a. Vertigo, nausea and vomiting, spinning of the head
    b. Anorexia, taste loss, dry mouth
    c. Headache, hypotension, bradycardia
    d. Diarrhea, thirst, abdominal pain

36. (LO 8-3) You should administer which of the following drugs in the treatment of glaucoma?
    a. Atropine sulfate (*Isopto Atropine*)
    b. Tobramycin (*Tobrex*)
    c. Acetazolamide
    d. Pemirolast potassium (*Alamast*)

37. (LO 8-3) Which of the following should you include in the care of a client to prevent hearing loss?
    a. Avoid getting childhood and adult immunizations.
    b. Avoid putting objects in the ear.
    c. Discontinue the antibiotic when feeling better.
    d. Listen to loud music only once a day.

38. (LO 8-3) Which of the following medications is used for refraction during an eye exam?
    a. Atropine sulfate (*Isopto Atropine*)
    b. Betaxolol (*Betoptic S*)
    c. Tobramycin (*Tobrex*)
    d. carbamide peroxide otic (*Murine Ear Wax Removal*)

Chapter 8 Case Studies

39. (LO 8-2) You have been assigned to teach a class on the prevention of hearing loss. What should you include? _____

_____

_____

_____

40. (LO 8-3) A patient is getting carbamide peroxide otic (*Murine Ear Wax Removal*) for cerumen. The patient asks you what cerumen is. What should you tell her? What is its action? How should you administer the medication? What are the side effects you should tell the patient to watch for? _____

_____

_____

_____

Critical Thinking

Select the disorder that best matches the patient description and write it in the blank.

cerumen   external otitis   glaucoma   conjunctivitis

41. (LO 8-2) Jackie Palmer went swimming last week in a polluted stream and developed an infection in his right ear. _____

42. (LO 8-2) Mr. Brown comes to the provider's office complaining of a "hollow sensation" and decreased hearing. _____

43. (LO 8-2) Mr. Crane is having an operation to relieve increased intraocular pressure inside his eye. Without this surgery, he may become blind. _____

44. (LO 8-2) Juana, who is 5 years old, has an inflammation of the mucous membranes that line the back of the eyelids and the front of the eye except the cornea, referred to as "pink eye."

_____

Applications

Obtain an electronic drug guide, or a current copy of the *PDR*®. Use it to answer the following questions in a notebook or on file cards.

45. In Section 2 of the *PDR*®, Brand and Generic Name Index, find another brand name for each of the drugs in the Representative Drugs for the Eye and Ear table in this chapter.

46. In Section 3 of the *PDR*®, Product Category Index, identify the pages that provide detailed information about one of the drugs you listed in question 43. Read about this drug in Section 5, Product Information.

If you have trouble finding a particular drug in the *PDR*®, look in the back of the *PDR*® under Discontinued Products to see if it has been discontinued.

DRUGS FOR THE SKIN

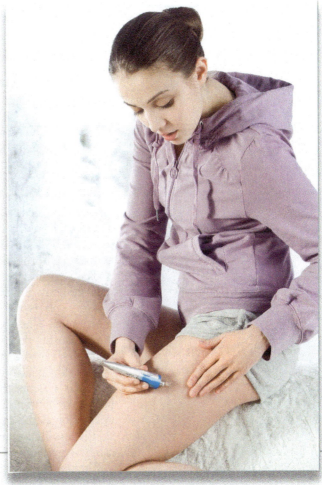

©Agencja FREE/Alamy Stock Photo

In this chapter you will learn about the structure of the skin and its functions. You will study major skin disorders, the medical terms for their symptoms, and the drugs used to treat them. You will also learn to administer topical drugs to the skin with a proper understanding of their uses and action.

antihistaminic

anti-inflammatory

antipruritic

antiseptic

astringent

comedo

contact dermatitis

corticosteroids

dermatitis

disinfectant

ecchymosis

eczema

erythema

keratolytic

keratosis

macerate

miticides

occlusive dressing

pediculicide

pediculosis

petechiae

photodermatitis

protective

pruritus

scabicide

scabies

seborrheic dermatitis

transdermal patch

vasoconstrictive/venous
insufficiency treatment drugs

INTEGUMENTARY SYSTEM [LO 9-1]

The integumentary system consists of the skin (the integument), along with the hairs, nails, and glands that are embedded in it. There are four primary functions of the skin: provide protection, sensory reception, temperature regulation, and biochemical synthesis and absorption.

The skin is the first line of defense for the immune system. It forms a waterproof, protective covering for the entire body, it protects the internal organs and acts as a barrier to microorganisms.

The skin interacts with the digestive system by absorbing and synthesizing vitamin D which facilitates the uptake of Calcium needed for healthy bones and teeth. The digestive system also needs vitamin D for the production of protective oils for the hair and skin. The skin works with the circulatory system to absorb medications applied to the skin.

The skin also senses temperature changes in the environment and helps regulate body temperature. The body's normal temperature is about 98.6°F (37°C). This is the temperature at which the cells maintain their normal functioning. When body temperature goes up, the blood vessels in the dermis dilate, causing perspiration. When body temperature goes down, blood flow decreases, causing the skin to constrict to conserve heat.

The skin is also an organ of sensation. The skin works with the neuro-muscular systems through neuron receptors that sense touch and help the body take appropriate action to protect itself. It works with the urological system for aiding in the maintenance of fluid and electrolyte balance. The skin is also important to body image. For example, conditions such as acne can have a negative impact on an adolescent's self-esteem.

The skin is the largest of all body systems in terms of its role in homeostasis, which is the internal stability and balance of all body systems and organs. Each body system depends upon the other systems to maintain balance within that specific system and within the total body as each system interacts with the others. The skin is made up of two distinct layers: the epidermis and the dermis (Figure 9.1).

Epidermis

The outermost avascular (without blood) layer, the epidermis, is made up of two types of cells, melanocytes and keratinocytes. The melanocytes contain melanin, a skin-color pigment that gives a person's skin its characteristic color. The more melanin an individual has, the darker the skin.

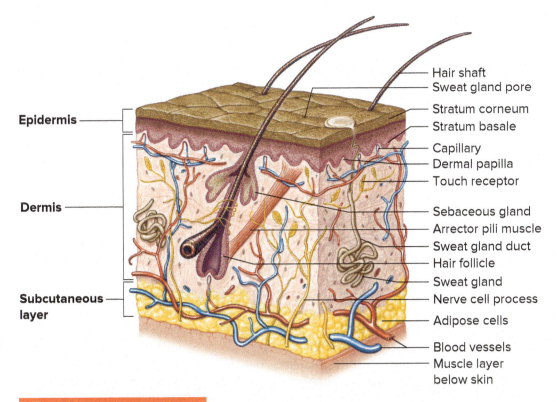

Hair shaft
Sweat gland pore
Stratum corneum
Stratum basale
Capillary
Dermal papilla
Touch receptor
Sebaceous gland
Arrector pili muscle
Sweat gland duct
Hair follicle
Sweat gland
Nerve cell process
Adipose cells
Blood vessels
Muscle layer
below skin

Epidermis

Dermis

Subcutaneous layer

Figure 9.1

Cross section of skin showing the epidermis, dermis, and subcutaneous layer that attaches skin to muscle and bone.

Keratinocytes produce a hard protein, keratin, which is waterproof and acts as a protective barrier to pathogens and chemicals.

Any break in the epidermis, such as a puncture or a cut, lets in bacteria that may attack the deeper tissues. For this reason, all skin wounds must be kept clean until they heal.

Dermis

Just beneath the epidermis lies a second layer, the dermis. The dermis is made up primarily of collagen, blood vessels, nerves, lymphatic tissue, and connective tissue. It also contains several other structures:

- Hair follicles, from which grow the tiny hairs that cover the body.
- Sebaceous glands, or oil glands, that lubricate the hairs with oil or sebum.
- Sudoriferous glands, or sweat glands, that help regulate body temperature.
- Sense receptors, which send messages to the brain when they feel pain, pressure, heat, cold, and touch.

Subcutaneous Layer

The subcutaneous layer is not actually part of the skin, but is generally discussed with the skin because it attaches the skin to muscle and bone. The nerves and blood vessels that supply the skin are also found in the subcutaneous layer. The subcutaneous layer provides support, insulation, nutrition, and cushioning or padding.

SKIN DISORDERS [LO 9-2]

The skin reflects the changes inside the body caused by infectious diseases, such as measles and chickenpox, and by irritating substances that have been touched, swallowed, or inhaled. The skin is also a mirror of human emotions, which reveal themselves through blushing, paleness, and rashes.

Disorders that are confined mainly to the skin area itself produce symptoms that are similar to those of systemic diseases. Symptoms of local irritation are the result of the body's natural response to injury: inflammation.

Inflammation is a process that occurs wherever and whenever there is cell damage. The capillaries around the damaged area expand to bring in white blood cells (leukocytes), which fight to destroy microorganisms, and cell repair is begun. Localized response to inflammation is characterized by redness, swelling, heat, and pain. An individual experiencing this reaction may be very uncomfortable, but the inflammatory process establishes an environment suitable for healing and repair.

Symptoms of Skin Disorders

The following symptoms are common to many skin disorders.

- **Pruritus** (itching), caused by the release of histamine from the skin cells during allergic reactions.

- **Erythema** (reddening), caused by an expansion of the capillaries close to the skin surface.

- Edema (swelling), caused by a buildup of fluid in the tissues.

- Scaling, which is an excess of the protein keratin in the epidermis. When a layer of dead cells builds up and becomes hard, the resulting condition is known as **keratosis**.

- Lesions, which are circumscribed areas of pathological tissue that are classified as primary or secondary. Primary lesions include macules, papules, plaques, nodules, pustules, and wheals. Secondary lesions occur as a result of primary lesions and include scales, scars, erosions, ulcers, fissures, atrophy, and crusts.

- Ulcerations, which are open lesions that are the result of tissue damage that starts below the skin and then erupts onto the skin surface.

- Hives or welts (urticaria), which are raised, irregularly shaped skin eruptions that have red margins and pale centers. Hives can appear on parts of the body or can cover the whole body. They are caused by sensitivity to some substance in the environment or by various other factors, such as fatigue and emotions.

Major Skin Diseases

Many diseases and conditions cause the symptoms of inflammation. You should be familiar with a few of the most common conditions.

Contact Dermatitis. **Contact dermatitis** is an inflammation resulting from direct contact with a substance to which the skin is sensitive (**Figure 9.2**). Most commonly, the substances are metal compounds, rubber compounds, poison oak, poison ivy, poison sumac, cosmetics, soaps, and some dyes. The main symptoms

Figure 9.2

Poison oak, poison ivy, and poison sumac are common plants that can cause contact dermatitis.

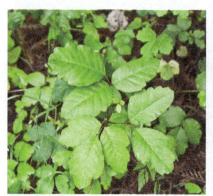

(a) Poison oak
©Steve Pridgeon/Alamy Stock Photo

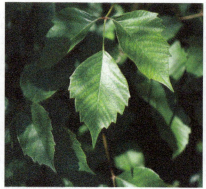

(b) Poison ivy
©Ken Samuelsen/Getty Images

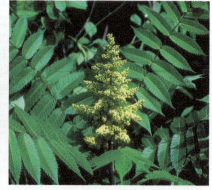

(c) Poison sumac
©Steven P. Lynch

are red, hivelike papules; itching; pain; and oozing, scaly lesions usually seen on the face, neck, hands, forearms, and genitalia. The treatment is to avoid causative agents. Other treatment includes a protective astringent lotion to prevent itching; and a topic antihistamine cream such as diphenhydramine (*Benadryl Allergy*) may be applied to the affected area to, dry up oozing and guard against infections. For serious cases, an oral antihistamine such as diphenhydramine (*Benadryl Allergy*) may be given to counteract the allergic reaction and itching.

Eczema (Dermatitis). **Eczema**, or **dermatitis**, is an inflammation with eruptions of pimplelike bumps, blisters, scales, or scabs. The lesions may be dry or "weepy" (having a watery discharge).

Eczema is a set of symptoms rather than a disease in itself. It is characterized by redness, swelling, itching, and a feeling of warmth to the touch. Eczema can be a reaction to a drug or a common substance. Creams, lotions, and ointments containing corticosteroids help suppress the inflammation of eczema. One such topical corticosteroid is clobetasol. A potential side effect is burning. Oral antihistamines may be given instead, as eczema patients often develop sensitivity to the topical preparations.

Psoriasis. Psoriasis is a chronic (long-term) dermatitis identified by its red, raised lesions covered with dry, silvery scales. The cause is unknown, but there is a family predisposition. It appears mainly on the knees, palms, soles, elbows, lower back, and scalp. The fingernails may become thick and irregular.

The aim of treatment is to retard the growth of epidermal cells. There is no cure, and psoriasis is difficult to medicate. A variety of topical medications may be prescribed, including over-the-counter and prescription treatments. Topical corticosteroids may be used. Corticosteroids may be injected into the lesions of chronically affected areas, and patients may be prescribed oral medications to treat the condition. *Tremfya* and *Taltz* (ixekizumab) treat moderate to severe plaque psoriasis in patients who are candidates who for systemic therapy or photo-therapy; given subcutaneously.

Acne. Acne lesions develop in adolescence when growth hormones speed up the secretions of the oil (sebaceous) glands. The open pores of the skin become plugged with oil (sebum) and dead cells. This produces noninflammatory lesions, such as a **comedo** (blackhead). Treatment consists of topical application of salicylic acid, benzoyl peroxide, adapalene and benzoyl peroxide (*Epiduo*), tretinoin (retinoic acid), topical or systemic long-term antibiotic therapy, and isotretinoin (*Absorica*) for long-term remission.

Seborrheic Dermatitis. **Seborrheic dermatitis** is an inflammatory skin disorder of unknown cause that begins on the scalp. It is characterized by yellow or brownish-gray greasy scales. Seborrhea is an increased amount of sebum, which is a normal secretion containing fat and epithelial cell debris. Treatment includes frequent shampooing and mild **keratolytic** agents. This can occur in infants as infantile seborrheic dermatitis and is treated with frequent shampooing.

Dandruff. Dandruff is a scaling of the scalp that produces dry, white flakes. It may sometimes be due to seborrhea. Treatment consists of regular shampooing with medicated shampoo, such as over-the-counter shampoos medicated with zinc pyrithione, selenium sulfide, and tar-based formulas; and prescription ketoconazole (*Nizoral Topical*) shampoo.

Burns. Burns are classified according to type and extent of injury. The types of burns include thermal, chemical, smoke and inhalation, and electrical burns. Thermal burns are caused by heat, such as that from a flame, scalding, or contact with a hot object. Chemical burns are the result of contact with a caustic agent such as acid. Smoke and inhalation burns occur from inhaling hot air or noxious chemicals. Electrical burns are the result of coming into contact with some kind of electrical current.

Burns are also classified as superficial, partial-thickness, and full-thickness burns (formerly known as first-, second-, third-, and fourth-degree burns).

- Never smoke in bed.
- Install smoke detectors in kitchens and near bedrooms. Detectors should be regularly checked.
- Keep a fire extinguisher in an easily accessible place.
- Avoid cooking when wearing loose-fitting clothing.

- Avoid setting the water heater too high to prevent scalding.
- Use a microwave oven appropriately.
- Identify fire exits when in public places.
- Have and practice a fire escape plan and establish a meeting point for family members.

Figure 9.3

The Rule of Nines is used to calculate the percentage of body surface affected by burns in the adult, child, and infant.

Superficial burns involve only the epidermis. The burn is painful and red, blanches (whitens) on pressure, and has mild swelling without blistering. Partial-thickness burns involve the epidermis and dermis to various depths. These burns are red, fluid-filled blisters that cause pain as a result of nerve involvement. The two most severe types of burns are the two full-thickness types. The first full-thickness burn (formerly, third-degree burn) involves the subcutaneous layer. It produces a dry, white, leathery-appearing skin without pain (because of nerve destruction). The second full-thickness burn (formerly, fourth-degree burn) involves the bone. It is characterized by variation in color, visible charring, and limited movement with loss of sensation. The Rule of Nines is used to calculate the percentage of body surface affected by burns. The body is divided into areas that are multiples of 9 percent. It is used for calculating the size of burn injury in an infant, child, or adult patient whose weight is in normal proportion to his or her height. See Figure 9.3.

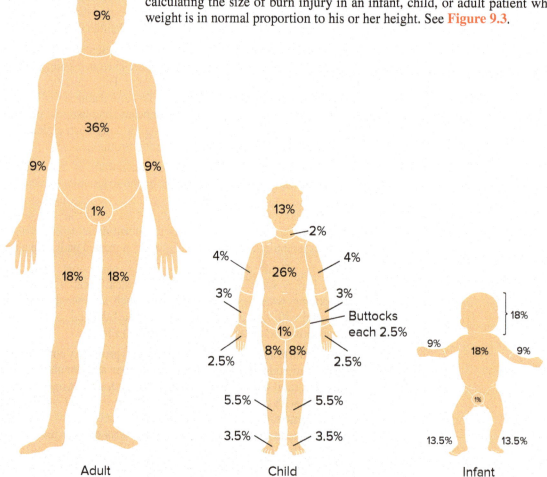

Adult   Child   Infant

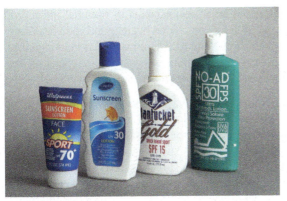

©Science Source

Figure 9.4

The general recommendation for sunblocks and sunscreens is a sun protection factor (SPF) of 15 or higher.

One of the most important elements of treating burns is prevention of infection. Silver sulfadiazine (*Silvadene*) is the preferred anti-infective agent used in most burn centers. Gentamicin sulfate has been replaced for the most part because of the development of bacterial resistance, especially to *Pseudomonas* organisms. Mafenide (*Sulfamylon*) is one of the most common agents used to treat partial- and full-thickness burns.

Extended exposure to the sun can cause sunburn, premature aging of the skin, and a predisposition to cancer. Skin preparations may be applied to absorb or reflect the sun's harmful rays. One absorbing agent is aminobenzoic acid (formerly known as para-aminobenzoic acid, or PABA). Agents that reflect rays are titanium dioxide and zinc oxide. Because they come as a thick paste and must be heavily applied, most people don't like to use them. The Food and Drug Administration has classified sun products according to their sun protection factor (SPF). The general recommendation is a minimum of SPF 15. See **Figure 9.4**.

Other sunscreens mainly block ultraviolet B (UVB) rays, which helps prevent sunburn and other types of skin damage. Ecamsule-containing *Anthelios* offers better protection from deeper-penetrating ultraviolet A (UVA) and UVB rays, which helps decrease the risk of skin cancer and sun-related wrinkling. Other sunscreen products are available containing avobenzone, oxybenzone, and others. These block UVA, UVB, or both types of rays.

Because burns are a common occurrence, especially among older adults, patient education for preventing burns is essential.

Pressure Ulcers. Pressure ulcer, *pressure sore, decubitus ulcer,* and *bedsore* are all terms used to describe impaired skin integrity caused by prolonged pressure that damages skin and underlying tissue. The most appropriate term is *pressure ulcer.* There are four stages of pressure ulcers:

- *Stage I:* Observable area of persistent redness in a pigmented area that is generally red, blue, or purple.
- *Stage II:* Partial-thickness skin loss involving epidermis, dermis, or both; superficial ulcer that appears as an abrasion, blister, or shallow crater.
- *Stage III:* Full-thickness skin loss that appears as a deep crater and damages the subcutaneous tissue to the underlying fascia.
- *Stage IV:* Full-thickness skin loss with extensive damage to the muscle, bone, and supporting structures.

This condition occurs in patients who lie in bed or sit in a chair for long periods of time without moving. Pressure ulcers develop where a bony prominence is in contact with the bed or chair (e.g., at the elbows, heels, and hips). Unrelieved pressure on the skin squeezes small blood vessels that supply the skin with oxygen and nutrients. When the skin is deprived of oxygen and nutrients for too long, the tissue dies and a pressure ulcer develops.

Prevention is the best cure for pressure ulcers. Once the tissues begin to break down, it becomes very difficult for the area to heal. Lotions may be rubbed into pressure spots to stimulate blood flow. The skin must be kept dry at all times.

Pressure ulcers that have begun to break down should be rinsed with saline. Do not use antiseptics, such as hydrogen peroxide or iodine, because they damage sensitive tissue and prevent healing.

Infections. Skin infections are caused by microbes invading the skin tissues. They may enter through a break in the skin, or they may attack when the skin's natural protective chemistry is unbalanced. The signs of infection are the same as those of inflammation: reddening, swelling, warmth to the touch, and pain. Bacterial skin infections usually exhibit pus, a thick, yellowish fluid made of dead white blood cells and debris. Impetigo and boils are examples of bacterial infections. Prevention is the best defense against infections. Good hygiene and good health are the best practices in inhibiting infections. The care administered is individualized to the specific skin infection. For example, for impetigo warm saline soaks may be used, followed by soap and water to remove crusts that develop.

Scabies and Pediculosis.   **Scabies** is a highly contagious parasitic infestation caused by the itch mite *Sarcoptes scabiei*. (Parasites are organisms that live on or in another organism.) Mites burrow under the skin, and about a month later, the patient begins to develop symptoms such as watery blisters between the fingers and severe itching. The infestation spreads quickly. Special topical insecticides called **scabicides** are used to destroy the mites. The drug of choice is the scabicide crotamiton (*Eurax*). There is no easy or fast treatment for scabies because the mites are difficult to eliminate. Bedding and clothing must be treated to help destroy the mites.

Pediculosis is caused by lice. These are insect parasites that lay eggs at the base of the hair of the head or in the pubic area. Pediculosis was once attributed to crowded housing and poor hygiene, but this theory has proven false. Lice can inhabit well-groomed and clean hair, and cleanliness and good hygiene do not prevent lice infestations. The lice are transmitted by close contact with infested individuals, clothing, combs, and bedding. Drugs called **pediculicides**, such as pediculicide lindane topical and spinosad (*Natroba*), are available to kill the lice. The FDA just passed a new lice medication called ivermectin (*Sklice*), a topical ointment used in lice infestations. Clothing, combs, and bedding must never be shared. Bedding, clothing, pillows, stuffed animals, hats, and other items must be treated for lice to prevent reinfestation on treated hair.

TOPICAL MEDICATIONS [LO 9-3]

Major Categories

Each skin disorder has its own best treatment and drugs, although many of the drugs share characteristics. They belong to certain general categories or drug groups. If you learn these categories, you will understand how many drugs operate. For instance, suppose you know that a particular drug is in the category "anti-infective." You then know that it works something like other anti-infectives, which you studied in Chapter 7. Memorizing the technical terms for these drug categories will help when you are looking up drugs in drug reference books and in electronic drug resources.

Oral drugs such as sedatives, antihistamines, and analgesics are sometimes ordered to make patients with skin diseases more comfortable. These oral drugs are described in other chapters.

Most topical drugs for the skin fall into one or more of the following drug groups.

Keratolytics.   Keratolytic drugs soften and destroy the outer layer of skin so that it is sloughed off (shed). Strong keratolytics are effective for removing warts and corns. Milder preparations are used to promote the shedding of scales and crusts in eczema, psoriasis, and acne. Very weak keratolytics irritate inflamed skin, which speeds up healing. Common keratolytics are salicylic acid and resorcinol.

Protectives and Astringents.   These drugs work by covering, cooling, drying, or soothing inflamed skin. **Protectives** do not penetrate the skin or soften it but instead form a long-lasting film. This film protects the skin from air, light, and dust. Nonabsorbable powders such as zinc stearate, zinc oxide, bismuth preparations, and talcum powder are listed as protectives, although they are not especially useful because they stick to wet surfaces. Collodion is a 5 percent solution of pyroxylin in a mixture of ether and alcohol. When applied, the ether and alcohol evaporate and leave a film on the skin. **Astringents** shrink the blood vessels locally, dry up secretions from weepy lesions, and lessen skin sensitivity. Styptic collodion contains 20 percent tannic acid, so it is both a protective and an astringent.

Antipruritics. **Antipruritics** relieve itching caused by inflammation. Calamine lotion, cornstarch, and oatmeal baths may help relieve itching. **Corticosteroid** drugs relieve itching by suppressing the inflammation itself. **Antihistaminic** drugs, such as diphenhydramine (*Benadryl Allergy*) and hydroxyzine (*Atarax*), lessen the effects of histamine, the cause of the itching.

Anti-Inflammatory Drugs (Topical Corticosteroids). The corticosteroids have three actions that relieve symptoms of skin disorders:

- **Antipruritic:** relieves itching.
- **Anti-inflammatory**: suppresses the body's natural reactions to irritation.
- **Vasoconstrictive/venous insufficiency treatment**: tightens the blood vessels in the area of the inflammation. This reduces the swelling due to edema.

Most of the top-selling prescription drugs for the skin are corticosteroids. Examples are hydrocortisone, betamethasone, triamcinolone (*Kenalog*), fluocinonide (*Lidex*), fluocinolone acetate (*Synalar*), and flurandrenolide (*Cordran*). The actions of corticosteroids are further described in Chapter 15.

Antiseptics. **Antiseptics**, such as alcohol, benzalkonium chloride, mercurochrome, and povidone-iodine (*Betadine*), inhibit the growth of microorganisms on skin surfaces. They are used only topically, never orally. Antiseptics prevent infections in cuts, scratches, and surgical wounds. **Disinfectants** are bactericidal drugs used only on nonliving objects such as surgical tools. Fungi, viruses, and spores that live on these surgical tools may, however, be resistant to destruction.

Topical Anesthetics. For pain on skin surfaces or in mucous membranes, such as wounds, hemorrhoids, and sunburns, the provider may order a topical anesthetic. It relieves pain and itching by numbing the skin layers and mucous membranes. Topical anesthetics are applied directly to the painful areas by means of sprays, creams, and suppositories. Examples are benzocaine (*Solarcaine Spray*) and dibucaine (*Nupercainal*).

Miticides. **Miticides** are drugs that kill insect parasites that infest the skin. Scabicides kill the mites that cause scabies. Pediculicides kill the lice that cause pediculosis. A miticide that is effective against both scabies and lice is lindane. One scabicide is crotamiton (*Eurax*). Malathion (*Ovide*) is a pediculicide. Permethrin (*Nix, Elimite*) is a pediculicide/scabicide considered to be an alternative to lindane.

Transdermal Delivery System. Many prescription drugs that were always taken orally are now available in **transdermal patch** form to be absorbed into the bloodstream through the skin (**Figure 9.5**). The patch is an easy and convenient way to take medicine. It may be applied on the skin near the treatment site. The mechanisms involved in the delivery of the medicine by a transdermal patch include an impermeable back that prevents the drug from leeching out, a drug reservoir, a membrane with small holes that controls the rate of the release of the drug, and an adhesive that holds the disk in place. For example, patients with high blood pressure may use a clonidine patch (*Catapres-TTS*). Other patches or transdermal (penetrating the skin) delivery system drugs include nitroglycerin (*Nitro-Dur*) and

Figure 9.5

A transdermal patch can deliver medication into the bloodstream through absorption into the skin.

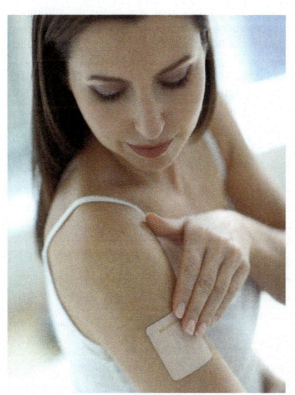

©Science Photo Library/Alamy Stock photo

Table 9.1 Selected Over-the-Counter (OTC) Drugs for the Skin

Conditions	Products	Action
Acne	*Cuticura Original Formula Medicated Antibacterial Soap, Clearasil Daily Clear Vanishing Cream, Stridex Daily Care Acne Pads*	Keratolytic
Dandruff	*Selsun Blue, Head and Shoulders*	Keratolytic/cytostatic
Diaper rash, prickly heat	*A & D Original Ointment, Desitin Rapid Relief, Vaseline, Johnson and Johnson's Medicated Diaper Rash Baby Powder*, zinc oxide	Protective/antimicrobial
Dry skin	*Keri Lotion, Corn Huskers Lotion*	Emollient
Eczema, psoriasis	*Tegrin Shampoo, Clobetasol Topical, Zetar Topical*	Keratolytic/antipruritic
Insect bites and stings	*Dermoplast Pain Relieving Spray, Nupercainal*	Anesthetic/antipruritic
Minor burns	*Solarcaine Spray, Noxzema Classic Clean*	Anesthetic/antimicrobial
Minor wounds	*Betadine, Neosporin + Pain Relief Ointment, Neo-Polycin*	Antiseptic/antibiotic
Poison ivy, poison oak	*Caladryl, Ivy Dry Cream, Ziradryl*	Antipruritic/antihistaminic

estrogen. People who are trying to stop smoking cigarettes may be prescribed nicotine patches (*Nicoderm CQ*).

An important part of applying drug patches is to mark the date and time on the patch when the patch is applied to the patient's skin. When applying a new patch, remove the old patch first and clean the skin. Leaving more than one drug patch on a patient can cause a possible overdose. Wear disposable gloves or cover the old patch with a tissue to prevent any of the remaining medication on the patch from absorbing into your skin.

Table 9.1 lists some skin preparations that are available without a prescription. You will handle these over-the-counter drugs regularly. The table of Representative Drugs at the end of this chapter lists some drugs for treating skin disorders. The table lists the drug category to which each drug belongs, its uses, actions, hints for application, and side effects. You will administer these drugs frequently. Be sure to consult drug references and package inserts when you have questions or need additional information.

 Pediatric Considerations Drugs for the Skin

- Although children develop a variety of skin disorders such as acne, atopic dermatitis, skin rashes, and skin infections, few guidelines for these drugs have been established.
- Because of the more permeable skin of infants and children, absorption is quicker than it is through adult skin.
- Absorption is also greater when the skin is broken or damaged.

- Side effects of corticosteroids are particularly common in children, so administer them with caution, in the lowest possible dose, and for the shortest period of time.
- An oral isotretinoin (*Absorica*) may be used in severe cases of acne in adolescents. If the adolescent is of childbearing age, monitor pregnancy tests very closely because *Accutane* has side effects and teratogenic effects. Pregnancy tests must be done monthly and for 6 months after the drug is discontinued.

- Older adults are more sensitive to adverse reactions of drugs for the skin. They have dry skin, limited mobility, decreased nutrition, and impaired elimination. This puts them at a greater risk of pressure ulcers.

- Teach how to apply topical drugs for the skin and report side effects.
- Use corticosteroids cautiously on thinned or atrophic skin.

Absorption of Drugs into the Skin Layers

Drugs for the skin are prepared in the form of powders, lotions, gels, creams, ointments, beads, pastes, and plasters. The form that is chosen for a topically administered drug depends on the desired therapeutic effect.

The form affects the absorption of a drug into the deeper skin layers. Few drugs used on the skin are intended to be absorbed into the bloodstream unless they are delivered via the transdermal delivery system. Some, like protectives and antiseptics, are supposed to remain only on the skin surface. Others are designed to penetrate the dermal and subcutaneous layers to provide anti-inflammatory or soothing actions. The provider must carefully choose the type of drug, its form, and the treatment that goes with it to achieve the proper effect.

When absorption into the underlying skin layers is desired, the following measures increase absorption:

- *Apply wet dressings.* Wet dressings soften or **macerate** the skin. This permits the drug to pass through the epidermis, which is normally "waterproof." These dressings are frequently used to treat wounds that require debridement, or the removal of dead tissue from the wound.

- *Use a fat- or lipid-soluble drug.* Fat- and lipid-soluble drugs are absorbed better than water-soluble drugs.

- *Rub the preparation into the skin.* Do this only when the skin is not covered with lesions that could be damaged by rubbing. Rub creams in gently; rub liniments in vigorously. Hard rubbing also stimulates the skin, which increases circulation to the area.

- *Keep medicine in contact with the skin for an extended period of time.* One way to achieve extended contact is to cover the area with a dressing that prevents the drug from being rubbed off by sheets or clothing. Another way is to reapply the medication as soon as it seems to have worn off and re-cover it.

- *Apply an occlusive dressing if ordered by the provider.* An **occlusive dressing** does not permit air to enter under the dressing. An example of an air-occlusive dressing is a plastic wrap. Petroleum jelly is an occlusive ointment. They both trap and prevent water loss (sweat) from the skin.

- *Use a stronger concentration of the drug.* A preparation that has more of the drug in it has more drug available to be absorbed.

Absorption into the skin is most complete when several techniques are used together—for example, a strong preparation held against the skin for a long period under an occlusive dressing. Absorption is also greater in young children and older adult patients because both groups have thinner layers of skin.

Drugs applied to the skin are rarely intended to be absorbed into the bloodstream. However, if the skin is cut, scratched, or scraped or if there are many open sores, the drug may readily enter the bloodstream. This is usually undesirable and can be dangerous. Safe and effective absorption of each topical drug depends on many factors. It is important that you understand and follow instructions when applying any topical medication.

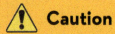
In administering medications, mucous membranes are treated differently than skin. These membranes make up the linings of body orifices such as the mouth, the eyes, the rectum, and the vagina. Unlike the skin, mucous membranes do not have a tough outer layer of dead cells to protect the underlying tissues. Instead, their surfaces are moist and easily penetrated. Therefore, drug absorption through the mucous membranes is rapid. Topical preparations for the skin are formulated differently than are those for mucous membranes. Never apply skin medications to mucous membranes, accidentally or otherwise; this invites the risk of overmedicating the patient.

GENERAL INSTRUCTIONS FOR MEDICATING THE SKIN [LO 9-4]

Psychological Support

People who have skin conditions need psychological support. Living with constant itching or pain is stressful. Patients may lose sleep because they are uncomfortable. They may become depressed about their condition, especially if it lasts for a long time. Depression may affect appetite and intake of fluids.

Because of the psychological problems associated with skin diseases, providers sometimes prescribe sedatives and tranquilizers. Patients with conditions like psoriasis, for which there is no permanent cure, may need counseling to help them live with the disease. Acne can be especially traumatic for adolescents, for whom body image is so important.

Show your support for these patients by accepting their feelings and responding to their needs with patience and understanding.

Patient Considerations

If a skin condition is painful, the provider may order an analgesic drug prior to administration of a topical medication. It is best to apply topical medications approximately 30 minutes after a dose of an analgesic, especially with burn patients.

Before giving the medication, explain to the patient what you are going to do. Inform him or her of any unusual sensations the drug may cause. For example, some gels produce warmth or a burning sensation on the skin.

Find a position that is comfortable for the patient and that lets you easily reach the skin area you need to work on. Place protective pads under the affected area to keep the bed and the patient's clothing clean. (Some skin medications cause stains.) If possible, position the affected area so that the patient cannot see it while you are applying the medication. Afterward, be sure to help the patient back into a comfortable position.

Wound Preparation

As lesions heal, the fluids that are produced dry out and crusting may appear on the skin surface. If ordered, cleanse the wound with the prescribed antiseptic solution or normal saline. Use a separate swab for each cleansing stroke. Clean from the least contaminated to the most contaminated area.

Apply medications only on the affected area. In the case of irritating substances, such as corn and wart removers, healthy skin surrounding the lesions needs to be protected. A film of petroleum jelly provides good protection against absorption and irritation.

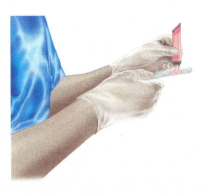

Figure 9.6

Apply ointments with a wooden tongue blade or a cotton swab.

Some drugs must be diluted (mixed with water or some other liquid) before being applied. Follow instructions carefully to prepare the drug. Check with the pharmacy if you do not understand the directions. A drug that is improperly diluted could cause irritation or poisoning or be ineffective.

Applying the Medication

Apply drugs as directed. In general, rub in creams and liniments by hand. Pat lotions onto the skin with pieces of cotton. Apply ointments with a wooden tongue blade or cotton swab (Figure 9.6). Use a glove to protect your skin. Depending on the type of wound and dressing, sterile gloves may be indicated.

When opening the medication container, place the cap upside down, with the lip of the lid up, so that the inside of the cap is not contaminated from being placed on an unsterile surface such as a medicine tray or cart. Use a sterile tongue blade or cotton swab to dip out a quantity of medication from the container. Do not dip in and out with the same applicator you are using on the patient! Then apply the medication according to instructions (the provider's or those in the package insert). Administer medication from the center outward, never going back over skin. (See Practice Procedure 9.1 later in this chapter.)

A few skin drugs are administered by means of a medicated bath (e.g., coal tar for a psoriasis patient), a special soap or shampoo (e.g., acne soaps, pediculicides), or an injection directly into a lesion.

The instruction "Apply as needed" is given only for drugs that carry no danger of overdose. Reapply the medication when symptoms flare up or when the thin film of drug has worn off or has been absorbed into the skin. A nurse or provider is frequently responsible for deciding when to reapply medication. Others may do so if they have the permission of the provider or nurse.

Dressings

Because they hold in body heat and increase absorption, dressings should be used only when ordered by the provider. Some lesions must be covered to protect them from clothing and scratching. Others must be covered to keep the medication in constant contact with the affected skin. A dressing can, however, be irritating rather than helpful. Many lesions heal more quickly when left exposed to air.

Infected lesions that are actively producing pus are usually covered with a dressing to soak up the drainage. The dressing must be changed frequently. Usually the provider orders the frequency for changing a dressing.

Be careful when removing the dressing from a wound to avoid pulling away the scab. A dressing that is sticking to a lesion may be softened by moistening it with normal saline. To avoid removing and reapplying tape each time you change a dressing, you may use butterfly tape strips.

Follow-up

Charting Observations. Each time you prepare to apply a topical medication, note the appearance of the skin. Has there been a change for better or for worse since you last saw it? If there is no change, perhaps the medication is not working. Are there signs of irritation? Chart your observations to help in evaluating the patient's progress and pinpointing problems.

Side Effects. Observe for signs of irritation that do not seem to come from the disease itself. Many people are sensitive to certain drugs. They may develop rashes, dryness, redness, tiny purplish-red spots, and ruptures of surface blood vessels (**petechiae, ecchymosis**), sensitivity to light (**photodermatitis**), and/or itching in the area where you applied the medication. Chart these signs and report them to the nurse in charge. The strength of the drug may be changed, or another drug or treatment may be ordered.

Patient Education. Instruct patients in how to apply skin medications properly. If theirs is a long-lasting condition, they will be responsible for their own skin care. A drug reference book, electronic drug guide, the *PDR®*, or the package insert are good places to look for information that will be useful to the patient.

 Healthcare for Today and Tomorrow | Safe Sun Practices

Healthcare members should be strong advocates of safe sun practices. Repeated and prolonged sun exposure is a precursor to the formation of skin cancer. Ultraviolet B (UVB) rays are a major factor in the development of skin cancer. You should advise patients to avoid the sun, but if they insist on being in the sun, advise them to use sunscreens with an SPF of at least 15 and to avoid being in the sun between 10 a.m. and 2 p.m. standard time and 11 a.m. and 3 p.m. daylight saving time.

 Legal and Ethical Issues | Acne and *Accutane*

Acne is a common condition affecting teenagers, and it often carries severe psychological consequences. Isotretinoin (*Absorica*) is used to treat acne that does not respond to other forms of therapy. However, this treatment is not without risks. It is your legal responsibility to tell your patients who are receiving *Absorica* to avoid the sun because of photosensitivity and to avoid drinking alcohol because the alcohol potentiates the serum triglyceride level. Female patients must be counseled on the risks of *Absorica* and pregnancy. Protocols for *Absorica* in female patients involve routine pregnancy monitoring due to the risk to the fetus.

Representative Drugs for the Skin

Category, Name,[a] and Route	Uses and Diseases	Actions	Usual Dose[b] and Special Instructions	Side Effects and Adverse Reactions
Keratolytics				
salicylic acid Topical	Seborrheic dermatitis, psoriasis, warts, corns, calluses	Swells and softens excess keratin for easy removal or shedding	Dosage depends on form and strength of preparation; soaking skin before use assists drug action; apply dressing as ordered; do not put drug in contact with eyes, mucous membranes, or normal skin	Irritation, burning
Astringents				
pramoxine/calamine lotion (*Caladryl*) Topical	Itching from poison ivy or poison oak, insect bites, or other skin irritations; mild sunburn	Relieves itching; soothes mild sunburns; has drying effect	Apply topically 3–4 times daily; clean and dry area before applying	Burning or itching

Representative Drugs for the Skin (continued)

Category, Name,[a] and Route	Uses and Diseases	Actions	Usual Dose[b] and Special Instructions	Side Effects and Adverse Reactions
Anti-Inflammatory Drugs (Topical Corticosteroids)				
betamethasone valerate Topical	Contact dermatitis, psoriasis	Suppresses inflammation; relieves itching and swelling	Dosage depends on form and strength of preparation; apply sparingly; massage gently into affected area; do not apply in or near eyes; available as aerosol; do not inhale spray; check skin regularly for signs of irritation; use occlusive dressing as ordered	Irritation, burning, itching, dryness, redness
triamcinolone Topical	Contact dermatitis, oral lesions	Suppresses inflammation; relieves itching and swelling	Apply TID and at bedtime	Irritation, burning, itching, dryness, redness
hydrocortisone *OTC: Hytone* 0.5% ointment, *Cortef Rectal Itch* 0.5% ointment Topical	*OTC:* Temporary relief of minor skin, genital, and anal itching and rashes; anorectal products for severe inflammation and swelling have other ingredients such as belladonna, benzocaine	Provides anti-inflammatory, antipruritic, and vasoconstrictive actions	Use sparingly and rub in lightly; cover *only as directed* with occlusive dressing; protect patient's face from aerosols; avoid inhalation	Burning and itching sensations, irritation, dryness, skin maceration, especially with occlusive dressings; systemic effects may occur with excessive or prolonged use
hydrocortisone *Prescription: Proctofoam HC* Topical	*Prescription:* Relief of inflammatory and pruritic manifestations of corticosteroid-responsive dermatosis	Provides anti-inflammatory action	Apply sparingly to affected area; apply suppository as directed	Burning, itching, irritation
Anti-Infectives, Antibacterials, Antifungals				
mafenide acetate (*Sulfamylon*) Topical	Partial-thickness and full-thickness burns	Provides broad-spectrum sulfonamide, action, bactericidal for many organisms	Cleanse area of debris before application; apply with sterile tongue blade or gloved hand to a thickness of $\frac{1}{16}$ inch; keep area covered with medication at all times; apply dressing as ordered	Pain, burning, stinging, allergic reactions, fungal superinfection

Representative Drugs for the Skin (continued)

Category, Name,[a] and Route	Uses and Diseases	Actions	Usual Dose[b] and Special Instructions	Side Effects and Adverse Reactions
Anti-Infectives, Antibacterials, Antifungals				
1% silver sulfa-diazine (*Silvadene*) cream Topical	Adjunct for prevention and treatment of wound sepsis (poisoning) in partial-thickness and full-thickness burns	Provides bactericidal and antimicrobial activity	Cleanse and debride; cover with drug at all times; reapply 1–2 times daily using sterile technique to a thickness of $\frac{1}{16}$ inch	Itching, burning, or rash; pain
Antiseptics				
povidone-iodine (*Betadine*) Topical	Surface infections, burns, minor wounds, vaginitis	Kills germs	Apply as ordered; avoid contact with eyes	Irritation, redness, swelling
Anesthetics				
benzocaine (*Solarcaine Spray*) Topical	Pruritus, minor burns; oral, nasal, and gingival mucous membranes	Inhibits conduction of nerve impulses from sensory nerves	Give smallest effective dose according to age	Sensitization

[a]*Trade names given in parentheses are examples only. Check current drug references for a complete listing of available products.*

[b]*Average adult doses are given. However, dosages are determined by a provider and vary with the purpose of the therapy and the particular patient. The doses presented in this text are for general information only.*

Practice Procedure 9.1 (LO 9-4)

APPLYING TOPICAL MEDICATION TO THE SKIN

Demonstrate applying topical medication to the skin.

Equipment

Disposable gloves; sterile gloves when changing sterile dressing

Sterile dressings and coverings

Sterile applicators: tongue blades, gauze, cotton balls, or swabs

Medication (lotion, ointment, cream, liniment, or aerosol spray)

Bag for disposal

Medication administration record

Adhesive tape or butterfly strips

Procedure

1. Assemble equipment, medication, and patient's records.

2. Read the medication administration record. Check this information against the medication label. Be sure you have the *right drug* and the *right dose* for the *right patient* at the *right time* by the *right route* by the *right technique* that you will *document right.*

3. Read the application instructions on the package insert.

4. Identify the patient and explain the procedure. Check the patient's wrist ID or follow health facility policy for identifying patients.

5. Administer a systemic analgesic (if ordered) approximately 30 minutes prior to administering topical medication.

6. Position the patient and the affected area comfortably. Protect clothing and bed linen with pads, if necessary.

7. Wash your hands and don gloves.

8. Remove old, soiled dressings. Discard them in a disposal bag. Be careful not to pull the scab from a newly healed area. If the dressing sticks to the wound, apply normal saline. Let it soak for 5 to 10 minutes.

9. Change gloves (use disposable or sterile gloves as appropriate). Open the dressings, applicators, and medication. Place the lid of the medication container upside down on the table or tray to avoid contaminating the medication.

10. Cleanse and remove dead tissue or crusts from lesions if ordered. Use a cleansing liquid ordered by the provider. Remove crusts with cotton swabs.

11. Reread the label to make sure you have the right drug.

12. Take the medication from its container using a sterile applicator (tongue blade or swab). Try to dip out the entire amount you will need for one application.

13. Apply the medication using the correct procedure:
    - *Creams:* Rub in gently.
    - *Lotions:* Pat or dab on skin.
    - *Liniments:* Rub in vigorously.
    - *Ointments:* Apply with wooden blade or cotton swab.
    - *Aerosol sprays:* Hold the can upright and spray the area from a distance of 3 to 6 inches; spray a second and a third time.
    - *Foam medication:* Hold the can inverted next to the skin and spray.
    - *Beads:* Mix with a suitable substance (e.g., glycerin), and apply directly to the wound with a sterile wooden spatula.
    - *Paste:* Puncture the tube by inverting the cap back into the tube; squeeze the paste onto the wound.

14. Apply a thin or thick amount (one-fourth the thickness for paste or beads) as ordered by the provider or as stated on the package directions. Systematically cover the affected area.

15. Cover the area with wet or dry dressings, if ordered. (See the provider's orders, package insert, or procedure manual for instructions.) Secure dressings with adhesive tape or butterfly tape strips.

16. Instruct the patient in further care of the skin. See the package directions or provider's orders. Remove your gloves.

17. Make the patient comfortable before leaving. Fluff pillows, return the patient to a comfortable position, secure the call button, and so forth.

18. Remove, clean, and/or discard equipment and supplies. Put away the medication, rereading the label as you do so. Dispose of used supplies in the appropriate area. Wash your hands.

19. Record the application of medication. Note:
    - Condition of the skin or skin lesions (on nurses' notes).
    - Reactions of the patient (on nurses' notes).
    - Date, time, medication, and dosage (on medication administration record).

Summary

Learning Outcome	Summary Points

9-1 List the layers of skin tissue and main functions of the integumentary system.	• The *epidermis,* the outer layer of the skin, is avascular (without blood) and is made up of melanocytes, which give a person's skin its color, and keratinocytes, which act as a protective barrier.
	• The *dermis* lies below the epidermis and is made up of collagen, blood vessels, lymphatic tissue, and connective tissue.
	• The main functions of the integumentary system are:
	  • Forms a protective covering for the body.
	  • Senses temperature changes in the environment and regulates body temperature.
	  • Perceives sensations such as heat, cold, pressure, and pain.

9-2 Describe the major skin disorders and symptoms.	• *Contact dermatitis* is an inflammation resulting from direct contact with a substance to which the skin is sensitive. • *Eczema* (dermatitis) is an inflammation with eruptions of pimplelike bumps, blisters, scales, or scabs. • *Psoriasis* is a chronic dermatitis identified by its red, raised lesions covered with dry, silvery scales. • *Acne* lesions develop in adolescence when growth hormones speed up the secretions of the oil (sebaceous) glands. • *Seborrheic dermatitis* is an inflammatory skin disorder of unknown cause that begins on the scalp. • *Dandruff* is a scaling of the scalp that produces dry, white flakes. • *Burns* may be thermal, chemical, smoke, and electrical. Burns are also classified according to severity. • A *pressure ulcer* is an impaired skin integrity caused by prolonged pressure that damages skin and underlying tissue. • *Infections* are caused by microbes. • *Scabies* is a parasitic infection caused by the itch mite. • *Pediculosis* is caused by lice. • Common symptoms of skin disorders are pruritus (itching), erythema (reddening), edema (swelling), scaling, lesions, ulcerations, and hives.
9-3 Articulate the actions of the following topical medication categories: keratolytics, protectives, astringents, antipruritics, topical corticosteroids, vasoconstrictor/venous insufficiency treatments, antiseptics, topical anesthetics, miticides, and transdermal patches.	• *Keratolytics* soften and destroy the outer layer of skin so that it is sloughed off. An example is salicylic acid. • *Protectives* work by covering, cooling, drying, or soothing inflamed skin. An example is zinc oxide. • *Astringents* shrink the blood vessels locally, dry up secretions from weepy lesions, and lessen skin sensitivity. An example is styptic collodion. • *Antipruritics* relieve itching caused by inflammation. An example is calamine lotion. • *Topical corticosteroids* relieve itching, suppress the body's natural reactions to irritation, and tighten blood vessels in the area of inflammation. An example is hydrocortisone. • *Vasoconstrictor/venous insufficiency treatments* tighten the blood vessels in the area of the inflammation. This reduces the swelling due to edema. • *Antiseptics* inhibit the growth of microorganisms. • *Topical anesthetics* relieve pain and itching by numbing the skin layers and mucous membranes. An example is *Nupercainal.* • *Miticides* kill insect parasites that infest the skin. An example is *Eurax.* • *Transdermal patches* enable drugs to be absorbed through the skin. An example is *Catapres-TTS.*

Learning Outcome	Summary Points
9-4 Understand the instructions for medicating the skin.	• Give patients psychological support. Accept their feelings and respond to their needs. • Prepare the patient by administering analgesic medication before administration of a topical medication and by assisting the patient to a comfortable position. • Cleanse the wound with prescribed antiseptic solution or normal saline. • Apply medication as directed by the healthcare provider. • Use a dressing only when ordered. • *Creams:* Rub in gently. • *Lotions:* Pat or dab on skin. • *Liniments:* Rub in vigorously. • *Ointments:* Apply with a wooden blade or cotton swab. • *Aerosol sprays:* Hold can upright and spray area from a distance of 3 to 6 inches; spray a second and a third time.

Chapter 9 Review

Match the functions performed to the skin structures.

_____ 1. (LO 9-1) Hair follicles

_____ 2. (LO 9-1) Epidermis

_____ 3. (LO 9-1) Subcutaneous tissue

_____ 4. (LO 9-1) Sebaceous gland

_____ 5. (LO 9-1) Sense receptor

_____ 6. (LO 9-1) Sudoriferous gland

a. grow tiny hairs covering the body

b. secretes oil

c. secretes sweat

d. feels pressure or pain

e. provides padding

f. acts as waterproof covering

Define these medical terms.

7. (LO 9-2) Pruritus _____

8. (LO 9-2) Erythema _____

9. (LO 9-2) Edema _____

10. (LO 9-1) Keratin _____

11. (LO 9-2) Inflammation _____

12. (LO 9-2) Acne _____

13. (LO 9-1) Body temperature _____

14. (LO 9-1) Sebum _____

Describe the purpose of these types of drugs.

15. (LO 9-3) Antipruritics _____

16. (LO 9-3) Keratolytics _____

17. (LO 9-3) Protectives _____

Match the drug categories to the drug names.

_____ 18. (LO 9-3) betamethasone valerate, Cordran   a. topical corticosteroids

_____ 19. (LO 9-3) *Eurax*   b. miticides

_____ 20. (LO 9-3) *Neosporin + Pain Relief Ointment,*   c. topical anesthetics
              Sulfamylon

_____ 21. (LO 9-3) Zinc oxide, calamine   d. oral antipruritics

_____ 22. (LO 9-3) *Atarax*   e. topical antibacterials

_____ 23. (LO 9-3) *Betadine,* alcohol   f. antiseptics

_____ 24. (LO 9-3) *Benzocaine*   g. protectives and astringents

Drug Calculations—Fill in the blank with the answer.

25. (LO 9-3) The provider orders diphenhydramine (*Benadryl Allergy*) 25 mg tid. Available are 50-mg tablets. You will give ____ tablets to your patient.

26. (LO 9-3) The provider orders hydroxyzine (*Atarax*) 100 mg qid. Available are 50-mg tablets. You will give your patient ____ tablets.

Multiple Choice—Circle the correct letter.

27. (LO 9-2) A patient asks if psoriasis is curable. You know that the most appropriate answer is which of the following?
   a. "It is sometimes curable."   c. "There is no cure."
   b. "A cure may be possible if appropriate treatment is followed."   d. "It may take a long time to cure."

28. (LO 9-3) Which of the following over-the-counter drugs for the skin should you use to treat dry skin?
   a. *Tegrin Shampoo* and *Zetar Topicalr*   c. Calamine and *Ziradryl*
   b. *Keri Lotion* and *Corn Huskers Lotion*   d. *Desitin* and *A & D Original Ointment*

29. (LO 9-3) After administering hydrocortisone to a patient for urticaria, you should instruct the patient to watch for what adverse reactions?
   a. Irritation, burning, itching   c. Pain, bleeding, rash
   b. Fever, swelling, stinging   d. Skin pigmentation, redness, fungal infection

30. (LO 9-3) Which of the following drugs should you administer to a patient who has poison ivy?
   a. pramoxine/calamine lotion (*Caladryl*)   c. Mafenide acetate (*Sulfamylon*)
   b. Salicylic acid   d. *Betadine*

31. (LO 9-4) As a member of the healthcare team, you should be a strong advocate of safe sun practices. You should instruct the patient to follow which of the following?
   a. Avoid being out in the sun between 10 a.m. and 2 p.m. standard time.   c. Avoid wearing a hat.
        d. Limit fluids to caffeine-containing beverages.
   b. Use a sunscreen with an SPF of 10.

Chapter 9 Case Studies

32. (LO 9-2) You have been asked to teach a class on the prevention of burns. What should you include?

_____

_____

_____

33. (LO 9-3) A patient presents with poison ivy and asks you what over-the-counter drugs may be purchased for the skin and how they work. What should you tell the patient? _____

_____

_____

_____

Critical Thinking

Select the skin disorder that best matches the patient description and write it in the blank.

decubitus   pediculosis   seborrheic dermatitis   eczema (dermatitis)   psoriasis

34. (LO 9-2) Mr. Yee has applied *Eurax* cream on his body to combat scabies. After a few hours his skin becomes dry and scaly. It is red, swollen, itchy, and warm to the touch.

_____

35. (LO 9-2) Ms. Barnett has suffered from dry scales on the backs of her hands for many years. The symptoms are kept under control with topical salicylic acid.

_____

36. (LO 9-2) Fred Entler is annoyed to find dry, white, greasy scales on his scalp.

_____

37. (LO 9-2) Fran Graham is bedridden with a muscle disease. A sore is developing where her tailbone touches the sheets.

_____

38. (LO 9-2) While washing her children's hair, Mrs. Johnson discovers tiny eggs in their scalps at the base of the hairs.

_____

Describe the procedures for applying topical medications to the skin.

39. (LO 9-4) Creams _____

40. (LO 9-4) Lotions _____

41. (LO 9-4) Liniments _____

42. (LO 9-4) Aerosol sprays _____

43. (LO 9-4) Pastes _____

Applications

Obtain an electronic drug guide, a current copy of a drug reference book, or the *PDR*®. Use it to answer the following questions in a notebook or on file cards.

44. In Section 2 of the *PDR*®, Brand and Generic Name Index, find another product name for each of the categories of drugs listed in the Representative Drugs for the Skin table in this chapter.

45. In Section 3 of the *PDR*®, Product Category Index, find Psoriasis Agents (under Dermatologicals). List all the agents found there.

If you have difficulty finding a drug in the *PDR*®, turn to the back and look under Discontinued Products to see if it has been discontinued.

DRUGS FOR THE CARDIOVASCULAR SYSTEM

LEARNING OUTCOMES

10-1 Identify the parts and functions of the cardiovascular system.

10-2 List the names of instruments used to measure blood pressure and to record the heartbeat.

10-3 List the main components of blood and the functions of the lymphatic system.

10-4 Identify the major disorders and common symptoms of the cardiovascular system.

10-5 Describe the actions and special procedures for administration of these drug groups: adrenergics, vasodilators, diuretics, antihypertensives, calcium channel blockers, antilipemics, cardiac glycosides, antiarrhythmics (antidysrhythmics), anticoagulants, thrombolytics, hemostatics, hematinics, and antiplatelets.

10-6 Know the difference between an initial and a maintenance dose.

10-7 Demonstrate administering oral and sublingual medications to patients with cardiovascular disorders.

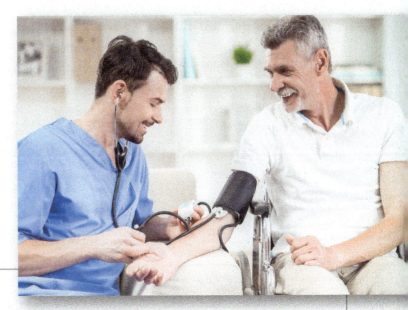

In this chapter you will learn about the organs and functions of the cardiovascular system and what goes wrong with them during common cardiovascular disorders. You will study the types of drugs used to treat each disorder and learn to classify common generic and trade-name drugs according to their drug categories. You will also practice step-by-step procedures for administering oral, buccal, and sublingual medications.

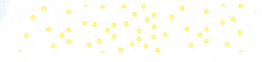

adrenergic

angina pectoris

angiotensin-converting enzyme (ACE)

anticoagulant

antihypertensive

antilipemic

antiplatelet

apical pulse

arteriosclerosis

atherosclerosis

automated external defibrillation (AED)

automatic sphygmomanometer

bradycardia

cardiac arrest

cardiac catheterization

cardiac glycoside

cardiopulmonary resuscitation (CPR)

diastolic pressure

diuretic

dyspnea

dysrhythmia

edema

electrocardiogram (ECG)

embolus

fibrillate

hematinic

hemostatic

hypercholesterolemia

hypertension

hypotension

leukemia

myocardial infarction (MI)

orthostatic hypotension

palpitations

phlebitis

point of maximum impulse (PMI)

pulmonary

pulse rate

sudden cardiac death (SCD)

systolic pressure

tachycardia

thrombolytic

thrombophlebitis

thrombosis

vasodilator

ventricular fibrillation

CARDIOVASCULAR SYSTEM [LO 10-1]

The cardiovascular system consists of the heart, the blood vessels, and the blood. It transports vital substances throughout the body. These substances include nutrients, waste products, oxygen, carbon dioxide, minerals, hormones, drugs, and body heat. The blood plays an important role in the body's defense against disease (see Chapter 7).

Blood Vessels

The three main types of vessels are the arteries, veins, and capillaries. Arteries carry blood away from the heart. Except for the pulmonary artery, the arteries carry oxygenated blood. As arteries get farther away from the heart, they branch into increasingly smaller arteries called arterioles. Veins travel toward the heart and, except for the pulmonary vein, carry deoxygenated blood. The smallest veins are called venules.

The arterioles and venules are connected by thin-walled vessels called capillaries. The capillaries serve the important function of carrying oxygen and other nutrients to the tissues and taking away the waste products.

The Heart

The heart is a hollow, muscular, four-chambered organ approximately the size of the fist that lies within the thorax and between the lungs. The heart can be felt beating at the fifth intercostal space, about 2 inches left of the midline. This area is called the **point of maximum impulse (PMI)** and is an important landmark when taking the **apical pulse** before administering certain cardiac drugs.

The wall of the heart is made up of three layers. The endocardium is the innermost layer. The myocardium is the middle layer and the most important structure of the heart. The pericardium, or pericardial sac, encases the heart. The four chambers of the heart are divided into two chambers on the right side

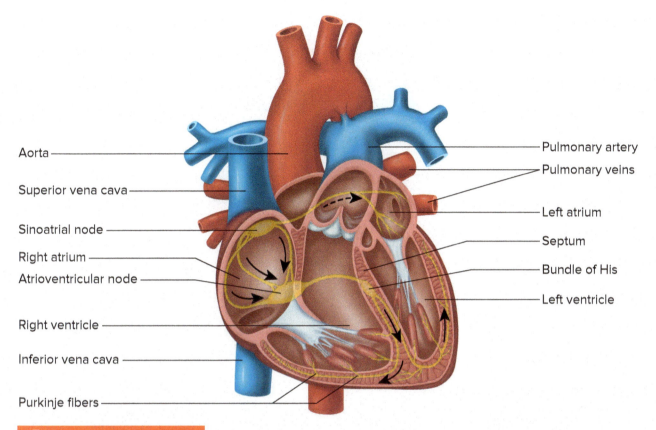

Aorta

Superior vena cava

Sinoatrial node

Right atrium

Atrioventricular node

Right ventricle

Inferior vena cava

Purkinje fibers

Pulmonary artery

Pulmonary veins

Left atrium

Septum

Bundle of His

Left ventricle

Figure 10.1

Blood flow through the cardiac chambers and valves.

and two chambers on the left side. The contractions of the chambers increase the pressure within the ventricles, which forces the blood through a system of valves and out into the general circulation (**Figure 10.1**).

Cardiac drugs are designed to affect specific parts of the heart.

- *Myocardium* (cardiac muscle). Certain cardiac drugs affect the force of myocardial contractions. Cardiac glycosides such as digoxin (*Lanoxin*) increase cardiac output.

- *Coronary arteries.* The coronary arteries supply the myocardium and heart with blood. If these arteries are narrowed, chest pain or angina pectoris occurs. If the blood flow in one or more of the coronary arteries is interrupted, that part of the heart muscle supplied may not get sufficient oxygen. Antianginal drugs such as nitroglycerin, or calcium channel blockers such as nifedipine (*Procardia*), produce coronary dilation and increase the oxygen to the heart, thereby reducing the workload on the heart.

- *Electrical conduction system.* The heartbeat is controlled by "pacemaker" cells that stimulate the heart muscle when it is supposed to contract. The heart's conduction system begins with the sinoatrial (SA) node and continues through the atrioventricular (AV) node into the bundle of His, through the left and right bundle branches and Purkinje fibers. Each heartbeat is caused by a wave of electricity that passes from the pacemaker cells to the heart muscle. The electrical signals can be picked up by a machine called an electrocardiograph. The electrocardiograph records these signals on a chart called an **electrocardiogram (ECG)**, and the signals are then used in diagnosing heart problems (**Figure 10.2**). The heart alternately contracts and then relaxes about 72 times a minute (the normal range at rest is approximately 60 to 80 beats per minute). The heartbeat you hear is the sound of the heart valves opening and closing during these contractions.

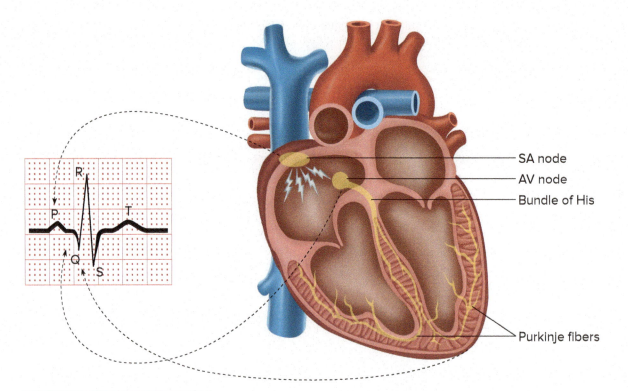

SA node
AV node
Bundle of His
Purkinje fibers

Antidysrhythmic drugs such as propranolol hydrochloride are given in the treatment of cardiac arrhythmias to decrease cardiac excitability.

After the blood has transported oxygen through the arteries, capillaries, and veins and has picked up waste products, it must go through the lungs. There it picks up new oxygen and gets rid of carbon dioxide wastes. In this way, the cardiovascular system is linked to the respiratory system, which is described in Chapter 11. The cardiovascular system is closely linked to all the other body systems, because blood is essential in all body functions.

BLOOD PRESSURE AND PULSE [LO 10-2]

One way to tell if the heart and vessels are working properly is by measuring a patient's blood pressure. This is the force of the blood against the walls of the blood vessels. Blood pressure results from a combination of two factors: the force of the heartbeat and the condition of the vessels.

The walls of normal blood vessels are elastic and able to expand. If vessels lose elasticity because of disease, such as arteriosclerosis, the heart must pump against stiff, narrow vessel walls. The heart must also pump harder if vessels are partially blocked by deposits of fat, as in atherosclerosis. Either situation results in a higher blood pressure reading.

To measure blood pressure, you will use a sphygmomanometer that consists of a pressure manometer, an occlusive (closing) cuff enclosing an inflatable rubber bladder, and a pressure bulb with a release valve to inflate the cuff (Figure 10.3). When the cuff is inflated, it tightens around the patient's arm, and you will listen for two types of sounds:

- **Systolic:** the peak pressure exerted against the arteries when the heart contracts.

- **Diastolic:** the minimal pressure when the heart is at rest between contractions.

Proper fit is essential to an adequate blood pressure reading. If the cuff is too small, the blood pressure reading will be artificially high. If the blood

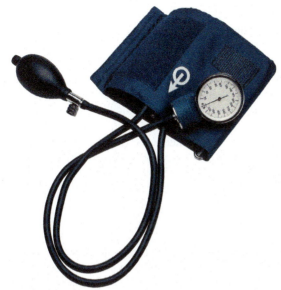

©Stockbyte/Getty Images

Figure 10.3

Blood pressure is measured by means of a sphygmomanometer.

Diastolic mm Hg
Systolic mm Hg
On/Off
Memory
Start

©Spike Mafford/Getty Images

Figure 10.4

Automatic sphygmomanometer.

pressure cuff is too large, the blood pressure reading will be artificially low.

Another method of taking a patient's blood pressure is with an **automatic sphygmomanometer**. This is a device that has all the components for taking blood pressure in one device instead of having a separate stethoscope and blood pressure cuff (**Figure 10.4**). Although the automatic sphygmomanometer is used by many hospitals and clinics, it is also very portable, easy to use, and clinically accurate and can be used independently by the patient at home. This monitor is ideal for patients with impaired vision or hearing because all the patient has to do is push a button and wait a few seconds for his or her blood pressure to display in big numbers on the screen. This also allows the patient with hypertension to monitor blood pressure at home without having to go to the provider's office. Instruct your patients to call their provider if they get an elevated reading. WiFi- and Bluetooth-enabled blood pressure monitors may be a good choice for patients who need routine home monitoring of their blood pressure as the data can be automatically uploaded to their primary care provider's office.

Blood pressure is recorded as two numbers: systolic pressure over diastolic pressure. The numbers represent the amount of mercury (Hg) that is displaced on the sphygmomanometer, measured in millimeters. The average blood pressure measures about 120/80 mm Hg (we say this as "120 over 80"). Generally, readings of 90/60 to 140/90 are parameters used when giving medications. A person is considered prehypertensive with systolic readings of 120 to 140 and diastolic readings between 80 and 90. Persons with prehypertension should follow medical treatment plans recommended by their provider that may include any combination of diet, exercise, and medications. (This is in recent literature on Medscape and adopted by the American Heart Association and the American Cardiology Association.) High blood pressure, **hypertension**, is not determined with one reading. A diagnosis of hypertension is made after two readings greater than 140/90 on two separate occasions. Hypertension is never considered normal and must be taken seriously. Report an elevated blood pressure reading immediately to your supervisor. Low blood pressure, **hypotension**, is a systolic blood pressure reading of less than 90 mm Hg. Unlike hypertension, it does not always indicate illness. There are some individuals who normally have low blood pressure. When it does indicate disease, the individual may be pale, have clammy skin, be confused, have an increased pulse rate, and have decreased urine output. This is the case with shock, such as after a blood loss.

The **pulse rate** is another way to tell how well the cardiovascular system is working. Pulse rate is most commonly measured by taking the radial pulse. Place the tips of your first two fingers along the thumb side of the patient's wrist and lightly compress so that you can feel the pulse (**Figure 10.5**). If the pulse is regular, count for 30 seconds and multiply by 2. If the pulse is irregular, take the apical pulse and count for 1 full minute. A normal pulse is strong and full. The average adult pulse is between 60 and 100 beats per minute. When administering certain medications, such as digoxin (*Lanoxin*), the apical pulse must be counted for one full minute.

If the heart or blood vessels are diseased, or if there is too little blood in the system, the pulse may be weak and irregular. A weak pulse taken at the wrist

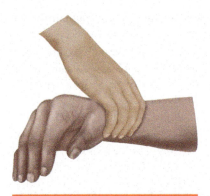

Figure 10.5

You will usually take a patient's pulse at the wrist, along the radial artery.

but a strong one taken elsewhere (foot or neck) may mean that vessels in the wrist are narrowed or blocked. These findings should be reported to the lead healthcare team member or provider.

You will often be required to take your patient's pulse and/or blood pressure before administering a cardiac drug. Review the procedures in your health facility's procedure manual to be sure you know how to do these tasks. You must chart the results each time. Charting may occur electronically in the electronic medical record (EMR) or it may occur in a paper form. Unless there is a special form for this, pulse and blood pressure (abbreviated P and B/P) are usually charted on a vital sign flow sheet or the medication administration record (MAR).

BLOOD AND THE LYMPHATIC SYSTEM [LO 10-3]

Blood

Blood has two component parts: fluid called plasma and solid elements called cells. Plasma is about 90 percent water and 10 percent solutes. Approximately 80 percent of the solutes are proteins. The remaining 20 percent is made up of glucose, amino acids, lipids, urea, creatinine, oxygen, carbon dioxide, hormones, and certain enzymes.

There are three main kinds of blood cells:

- *Red blood cells (erythrocytes)* carry oxygen. The major component of erythrocytes is hemoglobin. It is made up of iron and protein and gives blood its red appearance. The function of hemoglobin is to carry oxygen.

- *White blood cells (leukocytes)* are made up of granulocytes, monocytes, and lymphocytes. The granulocytes and monocytes consume bacteria and other foreign matter that enters the body. The lymphocytes play an important role in the development of immunity.

- *Platelets (thrombocytes)* are critical in clotting. When a blood vessel is cut or punctured, the platelets release a substance that causes fibers to form over the wound. These fibers eventually harden into a scab.

Table 10.1 summarizes the primary characteristics of blood carried by arteries and veins.

Lymphatic System

The lymphatic system is actually part of the circulatory system, because it consists of moving fluid that goes throughout the body. The lymphatic system consists of lymphatic capillaries, ducts, and lymph nodes and carries fluid from the interstitial spaces to the blood. This interstitial fluid that fills most of the cells of the body is called lymph. The system carries away waste products that the blood cannot carry, such as dead cells and debris. These wastes are removed at the lymph nodes, which act like small filtration stations. They are located mainly in the groin, the armpits, and the neck. After being filtered, the lymph is returned into the veins near where they enter the heart.

Table 10.1 Characteristics of Blood

	Color	Oxygen Level	Route
Arterial blood	Bright red	Highly oxygenated	Travels from heart to capillaries
Venous blood	Dark red	Mostly carbon dioxide and wastes; low oxygen	Travels from capillaries to heart

Unlike the blood, lymph is not pumped but merely collected from the various body parts through open-ended lymph vessels. As the body moves, the lymph is pushed through its vessels.

Another part of the circulatory system is the spleen. The spleen, a soft, purplish organ in the upper left side of the abdomen, has four functions. It plays a vital part in the body's resistance against microorganisms. It serves as a filter, removing old and defective red blood cells from the bloodstream. The spleen also has an immune function, and it stores approximately 30 percent of the body's platelets.

Effects of Aging

Heart disease is a major problem that increases with age. Most deaths from cardiovascular disease occur in the older adult population. High blood pressure, coronary artery disease, heart attacks, and congestive heart failure occur much more frequently in the over-60 age group. Certain changes in the heart are associated with aging. The heart usually becomes larger because it loses its elasticity, and it has a deeper color because there is less oxygen in the heart tissue. The endocardium becomes thicker and sclerotic (hardened), and the aorta and the arteries are less elastic. The valves thicken and are more rigid. These changes lead to problems in filling and emptying the heart, which result in decreased oxygen intake and output. Even with these changes, the heart is able to meet most demands. Under stress, however, declining heart function is apparent.

CARDIOVASCULAR DISORDERS [LO 10-4]

Anything that interferes with the functioning of the heart and vessels deprives the body of the vital nutrients that circulate in the blood. Any change in the rate, rhythm, and force of the heartbeat or in the force and quantity of blood flowing through the vessels thus endangers the entire body.

Symptoms

The presence of cardiovascular disorders is indicated by a number of symptoms.

Dyspnea is labored or difficult breathing that occurs because of fluid accumulation in the interstitial tissues and lungs. The patient becomes short of breath, with rapid and shallow respirations. Dyspnea can occur at rest or while exercising. Knowing when the dyspnea began (e.g., when the patient was lying down, sitting, or performing a strenuous physical activity) gives clues to the type of heart problem.

Angina pectoris, chest pain, is a symptom of some types of heart disease. It can be caused by a lack of blood in the heart muscle, by inflammation of the heart, or by anxiety.

Edema is an abnormal accumulation of fluid in the interstitial tissues. It occurs in cardiovascular disorders when the blood is not being pumped quickly or strongly enough. Some of the blood fluid "backs up" in the tissues, and swelling results. Edema is a common sign of congestive heart failure. It can occur in the legs, liver, abdominal cavity, or lungs.

Dysrhythmias, also known as arrhythmias, are irregular heartbeats or palpitations that may indicate a heart problem. Patients may complain that their heart is pounding or jumping or missing a beat. Disturbances of the heartbeat are **tachycardia** (very rapid heartbeat—pulse above 100 beats per minute) and **bradycardia** (very slow heartbeat—pulse below 60 beats per minute).

Hemoptysis (the coughing up of blood) may indicate serious cardiovascular disease in which blood is leaking into the lungs. A patient in congestive heart failure may cough up frothy, blood-tinged sputum.

Fainting and fatigue can be symptoms that the heart or vessels are not functioning at their best. When the brain does not receive all the oxygen it needs, syncope (fainting) may occur. When tissues do not receive all the oxygen they need, the patient may experience pain. When oxygen content in the blood is low, the skin may turn bluish, a condition called *cyanosis*.

Cardiac arrest is a sudden and unexpected stopping of the heart and circulation. It can be brought on by myocardial infarction, electric shock, severe allergic reactions, drug overdose, or surgery. Unless immediate steps are taken to restore the heartbeat, cardiac arrest is fatal. Circulation and respiration must be restored immediately. Irreversible damage occurs when the brain is deprived of oxygen for 10 minutes.

Congestive Heart Failure

Congestive heart failure (CHF) results from the inability of the heart to pump adequately enough to meet the body's metabolic needs. Congestive heart failure is not a disease but a syndrome caused by some other disease. Regardless of the cause, the ventricles of the heart are not able to contract and pump properly. The patient exhibits signs of fatigue, dyspnea, tachycardia, chest pain, and edema.

CHF is treated by giving digoxin (*Lanoxin*), a cardiac glycoside. It increases the force of and strengthens the heartbeat. Diuretic drugs are also given to help the kidneys eliminate excess fluids.

Angiotensin-converting enzyme (ACE) inhibitors are the vasodilators of choice for CHF. Amrinone (*Cordarone*) is another drug given for its vasodilating effect. It is used in patients who do not respond to the usual therapy of *Lanoxin*, diuretics, and vasodilators. Common causes of congestive heart failure are:

- Coronary artery disease.
- Myocardial infarction (heart attack).
- Cardiomyopathy (enlarged heart).
- Dysrhythmias (abnormal cardiac rhythms).
- Hypertensive heart disease.
- Anemia.

Dysrhythmias

Dysrhythmia is any deviation from the normal rhythm of the heartbeat. Such disturbances in cardiac rhythm result from an abnormality in the electrical conduction of the heart muscle. Dysrhythmias frequently occur within minutes to 72 hours after a heart attack. They can also occur in coronary artery disease or after cardiac surgery. Dysrhythmias may appear if parts of the heart vibrate (**fibrillate**), skip contractions, or beat very rapidly (tachycardia). These irregularities endanger the body because they affect the heart's ability to pump blood efficiently. Antidysrhythmic drugs are given to stabilize the heart's electrical impulses. Quinidine, procainamide, *Norpace*, and propranolol are examples of antidysrhythmic drugs.

Hypercholesterolemia

Hypercholesterolemia is a cholesterol level that is higher than the desirable level. When levels of cholesterol and triglycerides, a blood fat, become elevated, **atherosclerosis** develops, causing the arteries to narrow and the blood flow to decrease. Further narrowing of the arteries results in coronary artery disease depriving the heart from getting the oxygen-rich blood it needs. This increases the risk of heart attack. Although there are no symptoms of a high cholesterol level, there are several contributing causes. Fat circulating in the blood, which is mainly water, cholesterol, and triglycerides, must be carried by proteins called lipoproteins. There are three types of lipoproteins. The first type is called low-density lipoprotein (LDL), or bad cholesterol, because it transports cholesterol throughout the body. The second type is high-density lipoprotein (HDL), or good cholesterol, because it helps the body eliminate excess cholesterol. The third type is the very-low-density lipoprotein (VLDL), which is made up mostly of triglycerides and a small amount of protein and cholesterol. The goal is to have low levels of LDL cholesterol and high levels of HDL cholesterol.

High cholesterol levels are the result of several modifiable and nonmodifiable risk factors. The modifiable risk factors are those the patient can change such as inactivity, obesity, diet, and smoking. Nonmodifiable risk factors are medical conditions the patient cannot change; they include hypertension, type 2 diabetes, and atherosclerosis. A lipid profile that includes HDL, LDL, total cholesterol, and triglycerides is used to diagnose high cholesterol (Table 10.2). In addition to controlling total fat, limiting dietary cholesterol, eating foods high in soluble fiber (such as oatmeal) or fish and soy products, drinking alcohol in moderation, and reducing sugar intake, there are several cholesterol-lowering drugs that may be ordered. Patients are also encouraged to lose weight, exercise, and stop smoking.

Coronary Artery Disease

Coronary artery disease (CAD) is a disorder of blood vessels that falls under the category of atherosclerosis. CAD takes many years to develop. Three types of CAD are angina pectoris, myocardial infarction, and sudden cardiac death.

Table 10.2 Blood Cholesterol Tests

Total Cholesterol	Results
Below 200 mg/dL	Recommended
200–239 mg/dL	Borderline high
240 mg/dL and greater	High
Low-Density Lipoprotein (LDL)	
Below 100 mg/dL	Recommended
100–129 mg/dL	Near normal
130–159 mg/dL	Borderline high
160–189 mg/dL	High
190 mg/dL and greater	Very high
High-Density Lipoprotein (HDL)	
Below 40 mg/dL	Undesirable
40–59 mg/dL	Acceptable
Triglycerides	
Below 150	Normal
150–199	Borderline high
200–499	High

Angina Pectoris. Angina pectoris is a pressure or tightness in the chest. It results from fatty deposits that build up in the arteries that carry blood to the heart, narrowing them and temporarily restricting blood flow to the heart. It is generally brought on by physical or emotional stress. The pain, which may last up to 20 minutes, generally goes away within minutes after stopping the stressful event. The provider may prescribe aspirin, nitroglycerin, ACE inhibitors, and calcium channel blockers to treat angina. A nitroglycerin tablet placed under the tongue (sublingually) may be given every 5 minutes until three have been taken in an attempt to relieve the pain. It generally relieves pain in approximately 3 minutes and has a duration of 30 to 45 minutes. If three tablets have been taken over 15 minutes and there is no relief of the angina, the patient should seek immediate medical attention.

Myocardial Infarction. **Myocardial infarction (MI)**, or heart attack, is an injury to the heart muscle caused by a decreased blood supply generally from a blood clot blocking the flow of blood through a coronary artery. The interruption of blood flow damages or destroys a part of the muscle. The heart cells may die and scar tissue forms, replacing part of the working heart. Symptoms of an MI include a pressure, fullness, or squeezing pain in the heart. The pain may extend to the shoulder, arm, back, or even the teeth and jaw. Other associated symptoms include increased episodes of chest pain, shortness of breath, sweating, impending sense of doom, lightheadedness, fainting, nausea, and vomiting. A heart attack can occur at any time during the day or evening and may be precipitated by hours, days, or weeks of unrelieved angina. The earliest indication of an MI is recurrent angina triggered by exertion and relieved by rest. Cardiac ischemia or insufficient blood flow to the heart occurs. Tobacco and alcohol use, hypertension, hypercholesterolemia, lack of physical activity, obesity, diabetes, stress, family history, and high blood levels of homocysteine, C-reactive protein, and fibrinogen are all risk factors associated with myocardial infarction.

An electrocardiogram, cardiac enzymes, echocardiogram, or **cardiac catheterization** (angiogram) may be performed to determine the extent of the heart damage. During an angiogram, a dye is injected into the arteries of the heart with a long catheter that is generally fed through an artery in the leg to the heart. As the dye fills up the arteries visible on x-ray and videotape, a blockage of the heart may be revealed. Complications of myocardial infarction include dysrhythmias, heart failure, or valve problems. Often when a heart attack occurs, a dysrhythmia known as a **ventricular fibrillation** occurs, in which the heart quivers and death results if treatment does not ensue. Emergency treatment includes **cardiopulmonary resuscitation (CPR)** (chest compressions and breaths to reestablish circulation and breathing) or **automated external defibrillation (AED)**, which shocks the heart back into a normal rhythm (**Figure 10.6**).

Medications used during a myocardial infarction may include aspirin, thrombolytics or clot busters, anticoagulants, analgesics, nitroglycerin, beta blockers, and antilipemics. In addition to medications, coronary artery bypass surgery may be necessary.

Sudden Cardiac Death. **Sudden cardiac death (SCD)** is an unexpected death from cardiac causes in which there is a disruption in the cardiac function or malfunction of the electrical system of the heart that produces an abrupt loss of cerebral blood flow. Death usually occurs within an hour. The majority of sudden cardiac deaths are caused by ventricular dysrhythmias from ischemia that occurs during a myocardial infarction. Seventy-five percent of SCD cases are linked to a history of previous heart attack, and 80 percent of all SCD cases are linked to CAD and responsible for half of all heart disease deaths (WebMD).

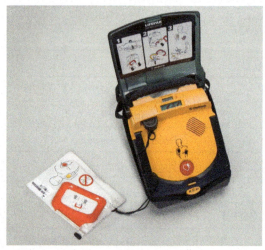

©McGraw-Hill Education/Rick Brady, photographer

Figure 10.6

An automated external defibrillator delivers an electric current to the heart to stop a chaotic rhythm such as ventricular fibrillation.

Blood Vessel Diseases

Thrombophlebitis. **Thrombophlebitis** involves the formation of a blood clot (thrombus) in a blood vessel associated with inflammation (**phlebitis**). Thrombophlebitis may be caused by pooling of blood in the veins. Pooling is associated with immobility, obesity, pregnancy, CHF, and steroid therapy. Other causes include long-term IV therapy and the administration of high-dose antibiotics, cancer drugs, potassium, and other drugs that are irritating to the veins. **Thrombosis** (thrombus formation) also occurs in certain blood disorders and in patients taking oral contraceptives. The thrombus blocks the flow of blood to the part of the body served by the particular vessel. The body part becomes pale and cold and sometimes bluish (cyanotic). If a vein is partially blocked by a blood clot, the thrombus may break off into the blood vessel and circulate back to the heart and into the **pulmonary** (pertaining to the lungs) circulation. It is then called an **embolus** (the blocking of a blood vessel is called an embolism). An embolus can also be an air bubble or any kind of particle that can block a vessel. It may travel to another part of the body and cut off blood circulation to a vital area. For example, an embolus to the brain can cause a stroke, whereas an embolus to the coronary arteries can cause a heart attack.

A patient with thrombophlebitis may exhibit warm, red skin; edema; elevated temperature; and pain upon dorsiflexing, or flexing the foot back toward the body, when the leg is raised. Treatment consists of anticoagulant therapy, large warm compresses, and bed rest for 5 to 7 days with the affected leg elevated. A deep venous thrombosis (DVT) differs from thrombophlebitis in that the clot is deeper and may be asymptomatic. Anticoagulant therapy should be administered for several months.

Arteriosclerosis. **Arteriosclerosis** is the most common arterial disorder, characterized by thickening, loss of elasticity, and calcification of arterial walls. Atherosclerosis is a form of arteriosclerosis in which fat and fibrin (white, tough, elastic, fibrous protein formed when blood clots) are deposited in the arteries. Together, these disorders are called *peripheral vascular disease*. Most of the symptoms occur in the lower extremities, such as pain on walking. Many patients with arteriosclerosis and atherosclerosis also have coronary artery disease and take vasodilators and beta blockers (drugs that decrease the heart rate and force of contraction by blocking adrenergic stimulation). Analgesics are also given for pain control.

Hypertension. High blood pressure is a chronic (long-term) disease with no single cause but many risk factors. Over time, hypertension can weaken the heart and affect vital organs such as the kidneys and eyes. Hypertension is also the leading cause of strokes. Because hypertension is called the "silent killer" and may go without symptoms for a long time, it is important to teach patients about the risk factors, which include the following:

- Men in young adulthood and early middle age
- Women after the age of 55
- African Americans
- Family history of hypertension
- Obesity
- Cigarette smoking
- Sedentary lifestyle
- Elevated blood cholesterol levels
- High-sodium diet
- Excessive alcohol consumption
- Continued stress
- Diabetes mellitus

Hypertension can be controlled by weight reduction, decreased sodium and alcohol intake, increased physical activity, stress management, and antihypertensive drugs.

Shock

Shock occurs as a result of decreased blood flow to the body's tissues that causes organs to fail. Shock has many causes. It is important not to define shock solely in terms of hypotension, because shock can occur without hypotension.

Shock may be caused by severe blood loss, surgery, trauma, heatstroke, severe infections, allergic reactions, or heart failure. Signs of shock may be low blood pressure; high pulse rate; pale, clammy skin; and mental confusion. Shock requires emergency treatment. Because patients can die rapidly from shock, the goal of treatment is to improve circulation so enough oxygen is available to the tissues and organs. Drugs called vasopressors cause vasoconstriction, which elevates blood pressure. Epinephrine and norepinephrine are two adrenergics frequently used to treat shock. Blood transfusions or intravenous fluids are also given to restore the volume of blood in the system.

Diseases of the Blood and Lymph

Blood and lymph diseases involve abnormal blood clotting processes, excessive bleeding, or disturbances in the production of blood cells.

Anemia. Anemia is a decrease in the number of erythrocytes, the quality of hemoglobin, and the volume of hematocrit, which reflects the ratio of red blood cells to plasma. The body needs a good supply of hemoglobin because this is the substance that transports oxygen to all tissues of the body. The entire body is affected by fatigue and other symptoms when too little oxygen is delivered to body tissues. Anemia can be caused by lack of iron or cyanocobalamin (vitamin B_{12}) in the diet, severe bleeding, malabsorption disorders in the gastrointestinal tract, weight-loss surgery, Crohn's disease, heavy drinking, diseases in which red blood cells are destroyed (hemolytic diseases), or failure to produce red blood cells. Treatment varies with the cause, but usually iron supplements, an iron-rich diet, treatment of underlying diseases, vitamin B_{12}, and folic acid are given. Patients on iron supplementation should be counseled that constipation and dark-colored stools are expected side effects. Transfusions may be administered.

Leukemia. **Leukemia** is a general term referring to a group of malignant disorders that affect the blood-forming tissues in the bone marrow, spleen, and lymph system. There is an elevated number of white blood cells, because they do not go through the normal cell life cycle. The symptoms of leukemia vary depending on the type, but may include fatigue, pallor, weakness, weight loss, anemia, and increased bleeding tendencies. The drugs used to treat leukemia interfere with the abnormal production of white blood cells (see Chapter 19).

Hodgkin's Disease. Hodgkin's disease is a malignant disorder characterized by the growth of abnormal giant, multinucleated cells called Reed-Sternberg cells, which are located in the lymph nodes. Hodgkin's disease makes up 15 percent of all lymphomas (malignant tumors of the lymphatic tissue). The cause is unknown. Symptoms include enlargement of lymph nodes, fever, weight loss, and night sweats. Treatment is with chemotherapeutic drugs.

Non-Hodgkin's Lymphoma. Non-Hodgkin's lymphoma is a malignant disorder of the immune system. It involves the lymphocytes and can originate outside the lymph nodes. Its method of spread is unpredictable and generally advanced at the time of diagnosis. The most common symptom is painless lymph node enlargement. Other symptoms may include fever, night sweats, and weight loss. Treatment consists of chemotherapy drugs and radiation.

DRUGS FOR CARDIOVASCULAR AND BLOOD DISORDERS [LO 10-5]

Adrenergics

Adrenergics (also known as vasoconstrictors) act by mimicking the action of norepinephrine and epinephrine by combining with alpha and beta receptors or as a result of, or regulation of, the release of neurohormones from their storage sites at the nerves' terminals. They raise blood pressure by causing the blood vessels to contract. They are used in the treatment of shock, heart block (failure of electrical impulses to stimulate the heartbeat), and adverse reactions to medications. Vasoconstrictors are powerful drugs. Many are used in the intensive care unit, where the patient must have close monitoring of heart rate, blood pressure, and kidney and pulmonary function. Patients must be assessed carefully to ensure that they are not receiving too much medication and developing hypertension. The blood pressure must be checked regularly and often. Side effects include tachycardia, palpitations, alteration in blood pressure (particularly hypertension), nausea, vomiting, heartburn, restlessness, and anxiety.

Norepinephrine (*Levophed*) is a vasoconstrictor that is given parenterally and used in hospital emergency treatment, such as for acute hypotension and shock. An IV line with two large-gauge catheters must be established as soon as possible. Other vasoconstrictors are phenylephrine (*Neo-Synephrine*), dopamine and dobutamine.

 Pediatric Considerations Adrenergics

- Adrenergics are used in pediatric patients to treat hypotension, asthma, shock, cardiac arrest, and anaphylaxis.
- Use caution when administering adrenergics to a pediatric patient. Avoid giving more than the recommended dose.
- Epinephrine is a popular drug used to treat asthma or allergic reactions in pediatric patients.

- Pediatric dosing of adrenergics is typically weight based, so an accurate weight must be obtained prior to administration. In emergency situations, dosing is typically calculated with a Broselow tape, which is based on the principle that the child's length is proportional to the child's lean body mass for drug administration.

 Older Adult Considerations Adrenergics

- Carefully monitor older adults taking adrenergics because they may have chronic cardiovascular disorders that may be aggravated by these drugs.
- In addition to being used for hypotension, cardiac arrest, and anaphylaxis, adrenergics are frequently given as bronchodilators and decongestants, which may increase the workload on the heart and cause symptoms of impaired cardiovascular function.

- Side effects such as anxiety, restlessness, nervousness, and insomnia may occur with a therapeutic dose.
- Avoid giving adrenergics to patients who are taking over-the-counter cold medicines, nasal decongestants, or appetite suppressants, because of the risk of overdose or toxicity.

Vasodilators (Nitrates)

Vasodilators relax or dilate the walls of the arteries, so less force is needed to push the blood through them. The classic vasodilators are nitrates. They are used especially in the control of angina pectoris. Nitrates dilate the arteries so that the heart receives more blood and more oxygen. Sublingual nitroglycerin (*Nitrostat*) is the most common vasodilator. Taken at the beginning of an angina attack, it takes effect within about 2 minutes. Isosorbide is another vasodilator used to treat angina.

Sublingual nitroglycerin may be left at the patient's bedside. One tablet is placed under the tongue at the first sign of an attack and may be repeated every 5 minutes until three tablets are taken in 15 minutes. You must keep track of how many tablets are taken and check on the patient—and chart the number of tablets taken. If there is no improvement or relief of chest pain (angina) after a total of three tablets in 15 minutes, the lead healthcare team member should be notified.

Time-release tablets, capsules, and topical preparations of nitroglycerin are available for longer-lasting effects. If applying nitroglycerin ointment, you will usually squeeze out 1 to 2 inches and apply it every 8 hours and at bedtime. Avoid touching the ointment with your fingers, because you will experience the vasodilating effects, such as headache. Wash off the last application. Rotate sites, which include the chest, abdomen, anterior aspect of the thigh, and the forearm. Cover the new application with a transparent wrap and tape it. Sites must also be rotated for transdermal patches. Side effects of nitroglycerin include dizziness, headaches, nausea, vomiting, facial flushing, and increased pulse rate. Patient education is important to effective nitrate therapy.

Diuretics

Diuretics are drugs that help the body eliminate excess fluids through urinary excretion (see Chapter 13). In so doing, they reduce the amount of blood that the heart has to pump. This effect is helpful for people with CHF. Certain diuretics, because they also help dilate the blood vessels, are often given along with antihypertensive drugs in the treatment of high blood pressure. Commonly used diuretics are the thiazides, potassium-sparing diuretics, and "loop" diuretics.

The thiazides are chlorothiazide (*Diuril*) and hydrochlorothiazide. Diuril is not used as much anymore. Not only is hydrochlorothiazide a diuretic, but it is also an antihypertensive. The potassium-sparing diuretics are spironolactone (*Aldactone*), triamterene (*Dyrenium*), and amiloride. Loop diuretics are furosemide (*Lasix*), metolazone, ethacrynic acid (*Edecrin*), and bumetanide.

 Patient Education Nitrates

- Avoid alcoholic beverages.
- Identify situations that precipitate attacks requiring use.
- Take a dose 5 or 10 minutes before an activity known to cause an attack.
- Side effects include dizziness, lightheadedness, and mild headache.
- Report severe headache, dry mouth, and blurred vision to the provider; they are symptoms of overdose.

- Air, heat, and moisture inactivate nitrates.
- Discard unused tablets after 6 months.
- Prevent tolerance by removing paste or patch for 8 to 12 hours—a "no nitrate" time.
- If pain occurs during the day, use the nitrate during the day and remove it at night.
- If pain occurs during the night, use the nitrate during the night.

Pediatric Considerations — Diuretics

- Diuretics are used for heart failure resulting from congenital heart disease, hypertension, and edema.
- Guidelines for thiazide diuretics have not been established, so give these drugs in small doses.

- *Lasix* is used in children, but monitor carefully.
- Spironolactone is the most commonly used potassium-sparing diuretic.

Older Adult Considerations — Diuretics

- Thiazides are frequently used with heart failure and hypertension.
- Monitor carefully for hypotension and electrolyte imbalance.
- Always give the smallest possible dose.

- Administer loop diuretics cautiously because there is an increased sensitivity for renal impairment.
- Caution older adults that they may be at increased risk for falls with diuretics.

Loop, or high-dose thiazide, diuretics can cause severe potassium loss in the urine. There are three ways of preventing this:

- Instruct the patient to eat potassium-rich foods, such as bananas and potatoes.
- Administer potassium supplements (*Micro-K*).
- Combine a potassium-losing diuretic with one that is potassium-sparing, such as hydrochlorothiazide/triamterene (*Maxzide, Dyazide*) and spironolactone (*Aldactone*).

Antihypertensives

There are several drugs that are used to lower blood pressure; they are called **antihypertensives**. The first of these are angiotensin-converting enzyme (ACE) inhibitors that suppress the renin-angiotensin-aldosterone system. They prevent the formation of angiotensin II, which normally causes the blood vessels to narrow. As a result of this, ACE inhibitors cause the vessels to become wider and the blood pressure decreases. Examples of ACE inhibitors include captopril, enalapril (*Vasotec*), and lisinopril (*Zestril*). *Entresto* is a combination of sacubitril and valsartan.

Another category of antihypertensives are the beta blockers, which have a beta-1 and beta-2 adrenergic blocking activity. They decrease the nerve impulses to the heart and blood vessels, causing the heart to beat slower and with less force. The result is a decreased workload on the heart and a decrease in blood pressure. Examples include atenolol (*Tenormin*), metoprolol tartrate (*Lopressor*), propranolol and metoprolol succinate (*Toprol XL*).

The alpha blockers inhibit alpha-adrenergic receptors by decreasing the nerve impulses to the blood vessels, resulting in easier blood flow and causing the blood pressure to lower. An example is methyldopa.

Vasodilators are a category of drugs that relax the smooth muscle and act directly on the arteries and veins to decrease the blood pressure. An example is hydralazine.

Generally, treatment of hypertension begins with a less potent antihypertensive drug, followed by changing the drug to a more potent drug or adding additional drugs to achieve a desired response. An example of a hypertensive regimen is hydrochlorothiazide and atenolol (*Tenormin*). Because these drugs work on the nervous system, which controls muscle tension, they have some general side effects that you should monitor the patient for, such as dizziness, fainting, weakness, mental depression, and **orthostatic hypotension** (a sudden lowered blood pressure when the patient stands up quickly). Caution your patient to rise slowly from a sitting or lying position to avoid dizziness or fainting. Other activities that result in orthostatic hypotension because of their vasodilating effect include hot baths and hot showers.

Like all drugs, each antihypertensive has its own list of side effects, so you should consult a drug reference book or electronic drug guide. Because there is no cure for hypertension, patients should be instructed on the need for long-term treatment and management of the adverse reactions as well as the consequences of sustained hypertension. It is important to instruct your patients to get their blood pressure checked on a regular basis.

 Pediatric Considerations Antihypertensives

- Take a child's blood pressure frequently if the child is overweight or if the parent has hypertension because there is an increased risk the child will develop hypertension.

- The incidence of secondary hypertension is greater in children than in adults, particularly the younger the child and higher the blood pressure.

- Hypertension is defined as blood pressure above the 95th percentile, so the goal of therapy is to reduce the blood pressure below the 95th percentile.

- Use antihypertensives cautiously in children, and always give the smallest possible dose.

- Beta blockers are generally the preferred drugs in cases of pediatric hypertension.

- Beta blockers should be used cautiously in pediatrics with asthma and breathing difficulties.

 Older Adult Considerations Antihypertensives

- There are two types of hypertension in older adults:
  1. Systolic hypertension, in which the systolic blood pressure is above 140 mm Hg but the diastolic pressure is below 90 mm Hg.
  2. Systolic-diastolic hypertension, in which both the systolic and diastolic pressures are elevated.

- Before initiating drug therapy, try weight reduction, decreased alcohol and sodium intake, and cessation of smoking.

- Educate patients that sodium is present in many food sources such as potato chips, pickles, soups, cheese, deli meats, canned foods, and frozen meals.

- The first drug of choice is a diuretic. ACE inhibitors and calcium channel blockers may also be used.

- Give the lowest possible dose to decrease the incidence of side effects.

- If blood pressure is decreased for 6 to 12 months, gradually decrease the dose.

Calcium Channel Blockers

Calcium channel blockers are cardiac drugs that inhibit the transport of calcium into the myocardial and vascular smooth muscle cells, which decreases myocardial contractibility and the demand for oxygen. They also dilate the coronary arteries. They are generally used to treat hypertension and angina. The calcium channel blockers include amlodipine (*Norvasc*), diltiazem (*Cardizem*), felodipine (*Plendil*), isradipine, nicardipine (*Cardene*), nifedipine (*Procardia*), and verapamil (*Calan*).

The most frequent side effects of calcium channel blockers are headaches, dizziness, fatigue, edema of the extremities, and shortness of breath. *Procardia* has the greatest effect on lowering blood pressure. Before administering calcium channel blocker drugs, it is important to take the patient's blood pressure and pulse. Caution patients to move slowly from a lying to a sitting position because of the hypotensive effect.

Antilipemics

Although the link between hypercholesterolemia, high blood cholesterol level, and heart disease is not completely understood, lowering blood cholesterol is considered part of the treatment. Many times all that is needed to lower the cholesterol level are a low-fat diet and exercise. When the cholesterol level does not decrease, an **antilipemic** drug, or drug that decreases the lipid blood level, may be prescribed.

HMG-CoA reductase inhibitors (statins) increase the HDL (good) cholesterol and decrease the LDL (bad) cholesterol, total cholesterol, apolipoprotein B, VLDL cholesterol, and plasma triglycerides. HMG-CoA reductase is normally an enzyme that catalyzes the early rate-limiting step in the synthesis of cholesterol. Examples of HMG-CoA reductase inhibitors include atorvastatin (*Lipitor*), fluvastatin (*Lescol*), lovastatin, pravastatin (*Pravachol*), rosuvastatin (*Crestor*), simvastatin (*Zocor*), and pitavastatin (*Livalo*). Pitavastatin (*Livalo*) is approved for treatment of hyperlipidemia and, along with a heart-healthy diet and regular exercise, improves overall cholesterol levels of both LDL and HDL. It is less likely to cause drug interactions. The most common side effects are back pain, constipation, diarrhea, muscle pain, and leg/arm pain.

Combination medications are sometimes prescribed for patients. Combination drugs limit the number of prescriptions and can increase adherence to drug therapy. Combination medications are sometimes prescribed for patients. Combination drugs limit the number of prescriptions and can increase adherence to drug therapy. Amlodipine and atorvastatin (*Caduet*) combine to form a calcium channel blocker and HMG-CoA reductase inhibitor. The amlodipine treats the chest pain and hypertension. Atorvastatin is used to lower cholesterol and triglyceride levels. Combination drugs can promote better compliance with medication regimens, but they are often more expensive than the drugs prescribed separately. Combination drugs can promote better compliance with medication regimens, but they are often more expensive than the drugs prescribed separately.

Bile acid sequestrants are drugs that bind with sodium cholate (bile salts), which are the primary precursors of cholesterol that are not absorbed as a result of the formation of an insoluble complex and are excreted in the feces. They decrease the cholesterol and LDL and have either no effect or increase the VLDL, HDL, and triglycerides. Examples of bile acid sequestrants include cholestyramine resin (*Questran*), colestipol (*Colestid*), and colesevelam (*Welchol*).

Other antihyperlipidemics include fenofibrate (*Tricor*) and gemfibrozil (*Lopid*). Nicotinic acid (niacin) is a vitamin B complex used as an adjunct drug in patients with a very high blood triglyceride level who are at risk for pancreatitis and do not respond to changes in diet.

Fenofibric acid (*Trilipix*) is a new drug used along with diet to lower LDL and triglycerides and raise HDL cholesterol. It is the first fibrate to be used in combination with a statin. The combination of ezetimibe and simvastatin (*Vytorin*) is also a lipid-lowering drug.

 Pediatric Considerations · Cholesterol Drugs

- Atherosclerosis develops in childhood.
- Increasing dyslipidemia is the cause of an increased incidence of obesity.

- Try nonpharmacological measures before drug therapy.
- Guidelines for cholesterol-lowering drugs have not been established.

 Older Adult Considerations · Cholesterol Drugs

- Try nonpharmacological measures first.
- Statins are given because they are well tolerated.
- Older adults frequently have chronic health issues such as diabetes, impaired liver function, and other conditions that may raise cholesterol levels.

- Monitor for side effects such as headache, nausea, vomiting, gastrointestinal disturbances, skin rashes, weakness, and muscle cramps.

Cardiac Glycosides

Cardiac glycosides strengthen the myocardium, increase the force of contraction, slow the heart, and improve the muscle tone of the myocardium. They also stimulate the pacemaker cells that control the rate (not the force) of the heartbeat. They are products of the digitalis plant. Digitalis is given to relieve some arrhythmias. Digoxin (*Lanoxin*) is by far the most commonly used digitalis product.

Digitalis therapy is begun with large doses to bring the blood level up to a certain point. This is called the period of digitalization. Thereafter, smaller doses are given—just enough to maintain the proper level of digoxin in the blood. Doses are adjusted carefully according to the needs of the individual patient. The normal therapeutic digoxin level is 0.5 to 2.0 nanograms per milliliter (ng/mL). If a patient's level is under or over this range, it is important to call the provider to get the dose adjusted. Digoxin toxicity is characterized by a wide variety of symptoms that are hard to differentiate from those of cardiac disease.

Before giving digoxin, the patient's apical pulse must be checked for 1 minute, as digoxin doses are cumulative. If the pulse is below about 60 (see the provider's order), or if it has noticeably changed in any way, do not give the drug; instead, notify the lead healthcare team member.

Patients on digitalis are weighed every day (**Figure 10.7**). A careful record is also kept of their fluid intake and output (see Chapter 13). These measures tell the medical team whether digoxin is taking effect and whether the kidneys are working properly. People who have low potassium levels are more prone to the toxicities of digoxin. This fact, along with the fact that CHF patients are commonly also taking the potassium-losing diuretic furosemide (*Lasix*), makes potassium supplements important for these patients.

Figure 10.7

Patients on digitalis must be weighed daily.

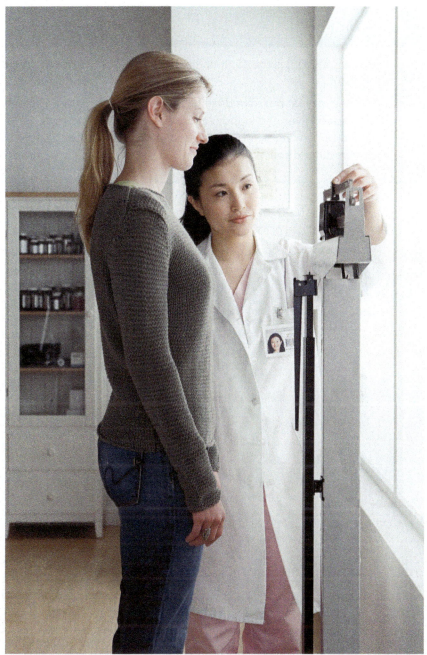

©Image Source/age fotostock

Digoxin (*Lanoxin*)—specific antibody fragments, also known by the product name digoxin immune Fab—is an antidote for life-threatening digoxin intoxication.

▲ Pediatric Considerations | Cardiac Glycosides

- The most common drug is digoxin (*Lanoxin*).

- Give the smallest possible dose because of the narrow range between the therapeutic dose and the toxic dose.

- Give according to age, weight, and renal and hepatic function.

- Newborns and infants are especially prone to toxicity.

- Monitor cautiously for side effects.

- Digoxin (*Lanoxin*) is the most common drug used.
- Give the smallest possible dose because of decreased liver and kidney function, reduced body weight, and the presence of cardiovascular disease.

- Monitor the patient's blood tests to prevent toxicity.
- Avoid giving digoxin with antacids because they decrease the absorption of digoxin. Digoxin should be taken at least 2 hours before antacids and antidiarrheals.

Antiarrhythmics

Antiarrhythmic medications also act on the heart's pacemaker cells. They are used mainly to treat atrial and ventricular dysrhythmias. They stabilize the heart muscle so that it does not flutter or beat too rapidly. Examples are quinidine, propranolol, procainamide, mexiletine, and disopyramide (*Norpace*). Propranolol is also used in the control of both hypertension and angina pectoris. There are six classes of antiarrhythmics: Class 1A, 1B, 1C, II (beta blockers), III, and IV (calcium channel blockers). Each class acts on a different phase of the cardiac-neuronal conduction rate, repolarization rate, transport of sodium ions in and out of cardiac membranes, dilatation of coronary arteries/arterioles, and oxygen demands.

Used improperly, antiarrhythmics can have serious side effects. The dosages must be adjusted individually to each patient. When an order for an antiarrhythmic says "give three times a day," check with the provider or pharmacist for the correct timing. These drugs should be given every 8 hours to ensure a constant blood level. Before administering antiarrhythmics, pulse and blood pressure usually must be taken. The response to the drug may be checked on the ECG.

Anticoagulants

Anticoagulants work quickly to prevent blood from clotting. This helps prevent or reduce the formation of a thrombus. There are two main groups of anticoagulants: those that are administered orally and those that are administered parenterally. Warfarin (*Coumadin*) is an example of an oral anticoagulant. Another anticoagulant, heparin, is given only parenterally. Enoxaparin (*Lovenox*) and dalteparin (*Fragmin*) are low-molecular-weight heparin used to prevent deep vein thrombosis after surgery. They are given subcutaneously for 7 to 20 days following surgery and may be given hours to days prior to surgery. Dabigatran (*Pradaxa*) is indicated to prevent deep vein thrombosis and in the management of atrial fibrillation. Another anticoagulant is rivaroxaban (*Xarelto*) that may be given orally to prevent deep vein thrombosis and reduce the risk of stroke and systemic embolism in patients with atrial fibrillation. Apixaban (*Eliquis*) is a newer drug and is administered orally.

If the provider wants continuous IV infusion of heparin to control the rate and volume of administration, the prescribed amount of heparin is added to 1000 mL of normal saline and an infusion pump is used. Caution should be used in administering heparin. The concentration of the heparin should be carefully reviewed, and some health facilities have protocols in place about the administration of heparin.

For subcutaneous administration, use a 25G to 26G, 1/2- or 5/8-inch needle to withdraw heparin from the container. Preferably, inject into the fatty layer of the abdomen just above the iliac crest. Pinch up a skinfold and insert the needle at a 45-degree angle; do not aspirate the syringe but inject the drug slowly. If you do not use a 45-degree angle, there will be a greater possibility of hematoma formation (collection of blood caused by a break in a blood vessel). After injection, apply pressure (do not rub) for 1 minute. Be sure to rotate administration sites.

Anticoagulants are strong drugs. Dosages must be adjusted carefully because they can lead to internal hemorrhage. Patients taking anticoagulants must routinely be monitored. Depending on the anticoagulant therapy prescribed, blood-clotting tests including prothrombin time (PT), or international normalized ratio (INR), sometimes referred to as PT-INR, are monitored. Other tests for patients on heparin-based therapies include thromboplastin time (PTT) and an activated clotting time (aPTT). They must also be observed for signs of blood in the urine and feces (red or dark brown urine and tarry stools) and bleeding from the skin or mucous membranes, which indicate overdosage. Many other drugs (including OTC drugs such as aspirin, oral contraceptives, and antacids) affect the action of warfarin. Foods high in vitamin K, including leafy green vegetables, may reduce the effect of *Coumadin*. Careful records must be kept of the various drugs a patient is taking. When using prefilled syringes, do not expel air bubbles because that could lead to loss of drug or incorrect dose.

 Pediatric Considerations Anticoagulants

- Extreme caution must be used with anticoagulants because of the risk of overdosing an infant or child with heparin.
- Warfarin is given to children after cardiac surgery to prevent thromboembolism.
- Carefully monitor the child taking warfarin; include blood tests and notify other healthcare members and parents in the child's environment to decrease the risk of trauma.

- The activity level of a child on anticoagulant therapy should be carefully monitored. Sports activities and rough play can cause serious internal bleeding.

 Older Adult Considerations Anticoagulants

- Anticoagulants are used in atherosclerosis and thrombotic disorders.
- Use these drugs, such as heparin, cautiously because of impaired renal function.
- Side effects such as hepatitis or jaundice indicate impaired liver function and decreased plasma proteins.

- Caution the patient against taking aspirin or nonsteroidal anti-inflammatory drugs unless specifically ordered.
- Older adults on anticoagulants should be carefully evaluated if a fall occurs as serious internal bleeding may occur.

Thrombolytics

Whereas anticoagulants prevent blood from clotting, **thrombolytics** are drugs that are used to dissolve clots. They are used only in a hospital setting by healthcare providers experienced in caring for patients with thrombosis. Thrombolytics are effective for the treatment of myocardial infarction if given within 6 hours of the onset of chest pain. Thrombolytics can also be used in patients with ischemic stroke to restore blood flow and tissue perfusion. An available thrombolytic agent is alteplase (*Activase*).

Hemostatics

Hemostatics help the formation of blood clots. This is useful when much blood is being lost due to injury or disease or when a patient has had an overdose of an anticoagulant. Vitamin K, a necessary ingredient in blood clotting, helps stop internal bleeding. It is sometimes given before surgery or childbirth, and is given to newborns. Vitamin K is also given to reverse the effects of warfarin toxicity. One form of vitamin K is phytonadione (*Mephyton*), but vitamin K also occurs naturally in foods such as leafy green vegetables. For this reason, patients on warfarin therapy should receive nutrition counseling. Protamine sulfate may be administered in cases of heparin overdosing to negate heparin's effects. Aminocaproic acid (*Amicar*) is useful in some cases of acute, life-threatening bleeding.

Hematinics (Antianemics)

Hematinics are used when there is a lowered red blood cell count or a lack of hemoglobin in conditions such as anemia. Hematinic medications provide the necessary ingredients for the production of red blood cells, such as iron and cyanocobalamin (vitamin B_{12}). Meanwhile, the provider must look for the underlying cause of the iron deficiency, such as a gastrointestinal bleed, a poor diet, or the effects of other drugs. Cyanocobalamin is used to treat pernicious anemia. It can be administered orally, by intranasal spray, or by subcutaneous or intramuscular injection. Popular iron preparations are ferrous sulfate, given orally, and iron, given parenterally.

Iron taken orally can irritate the mucous membranes. Tablets must be given with plenty of liquid. Patients who have trouble swallowing may need a liquid preparation. Iron supplements can stain skin, teeth, and clothing, so they must be handled carefully. Liquid preparations should be well diluted with the liquid indicated in the package insert. They should be taken with a straw and the mouth rinsed afterward to avoid staining the teeth. Patients should be warned to expect their stools to look dark and tarry. This is a harmless side effect of taking iron. However, patients should report any trouble with diarrhea or constipation.

Antiplatelets

Thromboxane A_2 is a potent platelet aggregator and vasoconstrictor. When platelets release thromboxane A_2, it constricts blood vessels and slows the blood flow, resulting in the platelets sticking to each other and to the walls of the blood vessels. **Antiplatelets** suppress platelet aggregation and prevent thrombosis in arteries. Prostacyclin is released from the membrane of a blood vessel and counteracts the action of thromboxane by dilating the vessels and inhibiting platelet aggregation. This creates a balance between thromboxane A_2 and prostacyclin that prevents platelet plugs from blocking flow and oxygenation to the tissues. Antiplatelets are used in conditions such as arterial thrombosis, deep vein thrombosis, stroke, or myocardial infarction. Examples of antiplatelets include clopidogrel (*Plavix*), dipyridamole (*Persantine*), and ticagrelor (*Brilinta*).

Aspirin is a cheap and effective drug that may be used for its antiplatelet properties. Doses not greater than 325 mg daily are used to prevent thrombi, stroke, and heart attack. *Plavix* is used to decrease the incidence of myocardial infarction and stroke in patients who are prone to gastrointestinal bleeding from aspirin. *Persantine* is commonly used for prevention of thromboembolism after heart valve replacement surgery. Common adverse reactions include headache, vomiting, rash, diarrhea, and dizziness. Thrombocytopenia may also be caused by *Plavix*. Ticagrelor (*Brilinta*) is a drug used in the management of acute coronary syndrome (ACS), history of MI, stroke, or after coronary artery stent placement.

GIVING CARDIOVASCULAR MEDICATIONS [LO 10-6]

Many of the patients to whom you will give medications suffer from some form of cardiovascular disorder. Therefore, you need to learn as much as you can about how the medications work and about how the cardiovascular system works. Read package inserts and drug references to become familiar with all the common drugs for this system.

Note that more than one dose is sometimes shown in the dosage column of the product information table. The dosage depends on whether a person is just beginning to take the drug or has been taking it for several days. When a disorder has just been diagnosed, the provider may order a fairly large dose to start the drug therapy. This quickly builds up the level of medication in the patient's bloodstream. It is called the initial or loading dose. After one or more initial doses, the dosage is lowered to a maintenance dose. This is the amount that maintains the level of drug in the blood without overdosing the patient. The maintenance dose will continue to be given for as long as the provider orders. Anticoagulants and digitalis products are both given in this way, but a loading dose of an anticoagulant is used less frequently now.

Occasionally an initial dose is lower than a maintenance dose. This is true, for example, of some antihypertensives. They must be given in small doses at first to let the body adjust to them gradually. Once the body has adjusted, the normal larger dose can be given.

Healthcare workers must give special concern to side effects and adverse reactions when administering cardiovascular drugs. The medications are strong and can be dangerous. The dosages must be absolutely correct. Most side effects of these drugs come from a sensitivity to the medication or too strong a dose.

Observe your patients, and question any who are taking a cardiovascular drug for any unusual sensations such as headache, lightheadedness, and **palpitations** (rapid, throbbing heartbeats). Chart any unusual signs and report them to your supervisor. Remember also to take and chart the pulse and/or blood pressure as ordered.

Patients who have trouble with the cardiovascular system may be very anxious. They need all the emotional support you can give. Explain procedures carefully, and answer their questions as best you can. Do not rush them. Try to gain their confidence so that they will cooperate with any special procedures you need to do.

Many patients with cardiovascular diseases must change their lifestyles if they wish to survive. The provider will have instructed them to give up lifelong habits like smoking or eating rich and salty foods. They may have to start exercise programs to lose weight and strengthen the heart. These new ways of doing things are sometimes hard to accept. Patients may be depressed or fearful. You can help by teaching them, by reassuring them, and by focusing on the benefits of their lifestyle changes.

 Healthcare for Today and Tomorrow Crushing or Not Crushing Medications

Some patients want to crush their pills and put them in liquid so that they are easier to take. However, certain common cardiovascular medications, when crushed, either will degrade and become less effective or will be absorbed too quickly. You should instruct your patients never to crush extended-release drugs (usually marked as XL, ER, or SR) such as *Procardia XL*, enteric-coated pills (usually marked as EC) such as aspirin, and sublingual drugs such as nitroglycerin.

Representative Drugs for the Cardiovascular System

Category, Name,[a] and Route	Uses and Diseases	Actions	Usual Dose[b] and Special Instructions	Side Effects and Adverse Reactions
Vasodilators				
nitroglycerin (*Nitro-Bid, Nitrostat*) Sublingual, buccal, oral, topical, ointment, patches	Angina pectoris	Reduces myocardial oxygen demand by causing peripheral vasodilation	*Sublingual:* 0.15–0.6 mg repeated at 5-minute intervals; if no relief after 15 minutes or 3 tablets, notify provider *Ointment:* 1–2 inches every 8 hours and at bedtime *Patch:* apply 1 patch every 24 hours, 12 hours on and 12 hours off or remove at bedtime.	Headache, dizziness, flushing, orthostatic hypotension, nausea, rapid pulse
clonidine hydrochloride (*Catapres*) Oral, topical, patch	Hypertension	Suppresses sympathetic outflow from the brain and decreases cardiac output	0.2–0.8 mg in divided doses daily, PO; one patch effective for 7 days	Rebound hypertension if discontinued abruptly, dry mouth, drowsiness, dizziness, constipation, pruritis
prazosin (*Minipress*) Oral	Hypertension	Decreases peripheral vascular resistance	1 mg bid or tid	Weakness, nausea, headache, palpitations, dizziness, orthostatic hypotension
hydralazine Oral, IV, IM	Hypertension	Vasodilates vascular smooth muscle	10–50 mg PO every 6 hours; take with meals	Lupuslike syndrome, headache, diarrhea, increased pulse, coma, angina, hypersensitivity, impotence; avoid abrupt discontinuance of drug; blood dyscrasia (disease)

Representative Drugs for the Cardiovascular System (*continued*)

Category, Name,[a] and Route	Uses and Diseases	Actions	Usual Dose[b] and Special Instructions	Side Effects and Adverse Reactions
Calcium Channel Blockers				
amlodipine (***Norvasc***) Oral	Hypertension, chronic stable angina	Inhibits the influx of calcium through the cell membrane, resulting in a decrease in automaticity and conduction velocity of both the smooth and cardiac muscles	5–10 mg daily	Headache, fatigue, lethargy, dizziness, nausea, abdominal distress, peripheral edema, palpitations, hypotension, muscle cramps
verapamil (*Calan*) Oral, IV	Angina, supraventricular tachycardia, hypertension, atrial flutter or fibrillation	Slows AV conduction and prolongs effective refractory period; decreases myocardial contractility and peripheral vascular resistance	80–120 mg PO tid initially, then 240–480 mg in divided doses daily	Congestive heart failure, bradycardia, hypotension, nausea, constipation, dizziness, headache, paresthesia
Antiarrhythmics/Antidysrhythmics				
quinidine Oral, IV, IM	Dysrhythmias (atrial fibrillation, flutter)	Lessens excitability of the myocardium; slows heart rate; lowers blood pressure	200–300 mg PO tid or qid; take pulse and blood pressure before administering; give with meals to avoid gastrointestinal irritation	Gastrointestinal distress, hypersensitivity (especially fever or rash), hypotension, severe headache, blurred vision, dizziness, tinnitus
propranolol Oral, IV	Arrhythmias (especially tachycardia), hypertension, migraine prophylaxis, angina	Both procainamide and its active metabolite (NAPA) lessen excitability of the myocardium; slows heart rate; lowers blood pressure	Arrhythmias, 10–30 mg PO tid or qid; give before meals and at bedtime; take pulse and blood pressure before administering	Diarrhea, nausea, dry mouth, dyspnea, hypotension, confusion, slow pulse
procainamide Oral, IM, IV	Premature ventricular contractions, ventricular tachycardia; atrial fibrillation and paroxysmal atrial tachycardia	Lessens excitability of the myocardium; slows heart rate; lowers blood pressure	PO, SR 0.5–1 g/6 hrs; IV, 25–50 mg/min; method depends on patient's condition; blood tests needed when on maintenance dose; adjust dosage to appropriate level	Hypotension, anorexia, nausea, urticaria, chills, fever, agranulocytosis, lupus syndrome after prolonged use

Category, Name,[a] and Route	Uses and Diseases	Actions	Usual Dose[b] and Special Instructions	Side Effects and Adverse Reactions
Cardiac Glycosides				
digoxin (*Lanoxin*) Oral, IV (avoid intramuscular injections because they are painful; also bioavailability of IM injection is low and has unpredictable absorption)	CHF, arrhythmias	Slows and strengthens heartbeat; increases cardiac output	Daily maintenance dose: 0.125–0.5 mg PO; usually 0.25 mg; take apical pulse for 1 minute prior to administering	Nausea, vomiting, slow or irregular pulse, loss of appetite, extreme fatigue; increased risk of side effects when blood levels are greater than 2 mg/dL, hypokalemia, and worsening renal functioning; yellow-green halos around images, blurred vision
Antihypertensives				
atenolol (***Tenormin***) Oral, IV	Angina pectoris Hypertension	(Beta-adrenergic blocking agent) Decreases cardiac output, peripheral resistance, and cardiac oxygen consumption Beta-1 and beta-2 adrenergic blocking activity	50 mg/day in single or divided doses; maintenance dose: 50–100 mg/day	Respiratory distress, bradycardia, dizziness, fatigue, pruritus, diarrhea, nausea, vomiting, hypotension
metoprolol tartrate (***Lopressor***) Oral	Management of hypertension; most effective when used with a thiazide diuretic or another antihypertensive	(Beta blocker) Decreases cardiac output, peripheral resistance, and cardiac oxygen consumption	100 mg/day in single or divided doses; maintenance dose: 100–450 mg/day	Respiratory distress, bradycardia, dizziness, fatigue, diarrhea, nausea
lisinopril (***Prinivil, Zestril***) Oral	Hypertension	(ACE inhibitor) Suppresses the renin-angiotensin-aldosterone system	20–40 mg daily	Hypotension, dizziness, headache, fatigue, vertigo, cough, asthenia, rash
losartan (*Cozaar*) Oral	HTN, CHF, and reduce risk of stroke in patients with HTN and left ventricular hypertrophy. Also used to reduce pro-gression of type II diabetic neuropathy	Angiotensin II receptor antagonist by blocking angiotensin II receptor on the surface of vascular smooth muscle, thus helping to keep blood vessels from narrowing	50 mg daily and maximum daily dose is 100 mg. May give once daily or divided dose BID. Available in 25-mg, 50-mg, and 100-mg tablets. Pediatric dose for children age 6 and older: 0.7 mg/kg up to maximum of 50 mg qd	Dry cough, cold or flulike symptoms, muscle cramps, pain in back and legs, orthostatic hypotension. May increase risk for renal impairment

Representative Drugs for the Cardiovascular System (*continued*)

Category, Name,[a] and Route	Uses and Diseases	Actions	Usual Dose[b] and Special Instructions	Side Effects and Adverse Reactions
Antihypertensives (*continued*)				
losartan/ hydrochlorothiazide (*Hyzaar*) Oral	HTN, CHF; used for severe HTN or when monotherapy with either of the component drugs is ineffective	Angiotensin II receptor antagonist, may be used in combination with other antihypertensives	Starting dose 50/12.5 mg and increased after 3 weeks to 100/25 mg/day	Dizziness and lightheadedness, dry mouth, thirst, itching, muscle cramps, abnormal high or low potassium, and increased risk of glaucoma. Should not take with *Cialis, Viagra,* or *Levitra*
metoprolol succinate (*Toprol XL*) Oral	Hypertension; chronic angina pectoris; symptomatic heart failure	(Beta-adrenergic blocking agent) Beta-1 and beta-2 adrenergic blocking activity	50–100 mg daily in a single dose for hypertension; 100 mg daily in a single dose for angina pectoris; 25 mg for CHF and up to maximum of 200 mg daily	Bradycardia, hypotension, nausea, vomiting, diarrhea, dizziness, fatigue, pruritus
nifedipine (*Procardia, Adalat CC, Procardia XL*) Oral, sublingual	Vasospastic angina; coronary artery spasm; hypertension	(Calcium channel blocker) Inhibits calcium ion influx across the cell membrane of cardiac and vascular smooth muscle, causing modest hypotension	30–90 mg/day; obtain blood pressure and pulse immediately before administration (use same arm and place patient in same position each time)	Dizziness, lightheadedness, flushing, peripheral edema, nausea, weakness, myocardial infarction
diltiazem hydrochloride (*Cardizem, Cardizem CD, Cardizem LA*) Oral	Angina and hypertension	(Calcium channel blocker) Inhibits calcium ion influx across the cell membrane during depolarization of cardiac and vascular smooth muscle	30–120 mg (up to 240 mg/day) SR	Edema, arrhythmias, drowsiness, nausea, lightheadedness
verapamil hydrochloride (*Calan*) Oral, IM, IV	Angina and hypertension; paroxysmal atrial tachycardia; atrial fibrillation or flutter	(Calcium channel blocker) Inhibits calcium ion influx and slows atrioventricular conduction; reduces supraventricular tachycardia due to atrial flutter or fibrillation	120–480 mg/day PO; 5–10 mg slow IV push. *Titrate doses:* 80 mg 3–4 times a day; up to 240–480 mg Obtain blood pressure, pulse, and respirations immediately before giving drug	Peripheral edema, bradycardia, dizziness, headache, constipation

Category, Name,[a] and Route	Uses and Diseases	Actions	Usual Dose[b] and Special Instructions	Side Effects and Adverse Reactions
Antihypertensives (continued)				
captopril Oral	Hypertension	(ACE inhibitor) Suppresses the renin-angiotensin-aldosterone system	25 mg bid; may increase to 50 mg bid	Rash, nausea, vomiting, hypotension, orthostatic hypotension
propranolol Oral	Hypertension; angina	(Beta-adrenergic blocking agent) Beta-1 and beta-2 adrenergic blocking activity	40 mg bid or 80 mg sustained release	Bradycardia, hypotension, nausea, vomiting, dizziness, fatigue, joint pain
enalapril (*Vasotec*) Oral	Hypertension	(ACE inhibitor) Suppresses the renin-angiotensin-aldosterone system	5 mg/day initially, then 10–40 mg/day either daily or bid	Abdominal pain, nausea, vomiting, hypotension, orthostatic hypotension, diaphoresis, sleep disturbances
Diuretics				
hydrochlorothiazide (*Microzide*) Oral	Edema associated with congestive heart failure; hypertension	(Thiazide diuretic) Increases water and sodium excretion	Initially, 25 mg/day; potassium supplement may be needed	Hypokalemia, hyponatremia, weakness, dizziness, fatigue, dry mouth, confusion, epigastric distress, orthostatic hypotension
furosemide (*Lasix*) Oral	Edema associated with congestive heart failure; hypertension	(Loop diuretic) Inhibits reabsorption of sodium and chloride in the proximal and distal tubules and loop of Henle	20–80 mg/day in a single dose; may be increased to 20–40 mg q 6–8 hrs; maximum daily dose should not exceed 600 mg	Dehydration, hypovolemia, hypokalemia, hypochloremia, hyponatremia, nausea, vertigo, orthostatic hypotension
triamterene and **hydrochlorothiazide** (*Dyazide, Maxzide*) Oral	Edema or hypertension associated with hypokalemia	(Combination diuretic) Acts directly on the distal tubule to promote the excretion of sodium in exchange for potassium or hydrogen ions	37.5 mg/25 mg daily; may increase to 50-mg/25 mg bid	Hyperkalemia, renal stones, nausea, vomiting

Category, Name,[a] and Route	Uses and Diseases	Actions	Usual Dose[b] and Special Instructions	Side Effects and Adverse Reactions
Diuretics (*continued*)				
spironolactone (*Aldactone*) Oral	Edema when other approaches to treatment are ineffective or inadequate	(Potassium-sparing diuretic) Acts on distal tubule to inhibit sodium exchange for potassium, resulting in increased secretion of sodium and water and conservation of potassium	100 mg/day; maintenance dose: 75–400 mg/day in 2–4 divided doses	Hyperkalemia, hyponatremia, diarrhea, cramps, drowsiness May cause gynecomastia (enlargement of male breasts)
triamterene (*Dyrenium*) Oral	Edema associated with congestive heart failure	(Potassium-sparing diuretic) Acts directly on distal tubule to promote excretion of sodium, which is exchanged for potassium or hydrogen ions	50–100 mg/day; do not give potassium supplement Dosage 50–100 mg qd-bid daily	Hyperkalemia, renal stones, nausea, vomiting
Antilipemics				
atorvastatin (*Lipitor*) Oral	Hypercholester-olemia	Decreases elevated total and LDL cholesterol and triglyceride levels while increasing HDL cholesterol	10–20 mg/day initially; then range may be 10–80 mg daily	Flatulence, dyspepsia, headache, myalgia, rash
simvastatin (*Zocor*) Oral	Hypercholester-olemia	Decreases elevated total and LDL cholesterol and triglycerides	40 mg daily in the evening or 80 mg tid	Rhabdomyolysis with renal dysfunction secondary to myoglobinuria, nausea, vomiting, diarrhea, dysfunction of certain cranial nerves, headache
rosuvastatin (*Crestor*) Oral	Hypercholester-olemia	Inhibits HMG-CoA reductase	10 mg/day	Myalgia, constipation, asthenia, muscle weakness, abdominal pain, nausea

Representative Drugs for the Cardiovascular System (*continued*)

Category, Name,[a] and Route	Uses and Diseases	Actions	Usual Dose[b] and Special Instructions	Side Effects and Adverse Reactions
Antilipemics (*continued*)				
cholestyramine (*Questran*) Oral	Hypercholester-olemia	Binds with bile salts in the intestines	4 g in a powder for suspension once or twice a day; mix with 60–180 mL of water or carbonated beverages	Constipation, nausea, vomiting, headaches, urticaria, muscle or joint pain
gemfibrozil (*Lopid*) Oral	Hypercholester-olemia	Decreases triglycerides, cholesterol, and VLDL while increasing HDL; LDL either decreases or does not change	600 mg bid; take 30 minutes before morning and evening meals	Cholelithiasis (gallstones), abdominal pain, nausea, dizziness, painful extremities
evolocumab (*Repatha*)	Subcutaneously	Decreases LDL cholesterol 140 mg	Subcutaneously every 2 weeks or 420 mg once a month	Dizziness, diarrhea, nausea, musculoskeletal pain
Anticoagulants				
warfarin sodium (***Coumadin***) Oral	Thrombus, pulmonary embolism, phlebitis, coronary occlusion	Prevents or slows formation of blood clots; prevents enlargement of existing thrombus	Dosage must be adjusted individually; 2–10 mg PO daily for maintenance (initial dose may be given IV or PO); adjust doses weekly until blood coagulation (prothrombin time) tests are 1.5–2 times normal; not to be used when there is a risk of hemorrhage (e.g., with surgery, ulcers, pregnancy); watch for signs of bleeding	Hemorrhage (blood in urine, feces, and tissues, bruising, nosebleed, bleeding gums)
rivaroxaban (*Xarelto*)	Prophylaxis of DVT and pulmonary embolism	Treatment or prevention of recurrent DVT or PE, stroke and systemic embolism risk reduction in patients with nonvalvular atrial fibrillation; patients undergoing hip and knee replacement surgery	10 mg po qd, 6–10 hrs after surgery. Treat for 35 days after hip replacement and 12 days after knee surgery	Bruise easily, and may take longer to stop bleeding. Stopping the medication increases the risk of stroke, especially if being treated for atrial fibrillation. Do not stop taking without consulting your provider

Representative Drugs for the Cardiovascular System (*continued*)

Category, Name,[a] and Route	Uses and Diseases	Actions	Usual Dose[b] and Special Instructions	Side Effects and Adverse Reactions
Anticoagulants (continued)				
heparin IV, subcut, IV bolus	Thrombosis, embolism, prophylaxis for deep vein thrombosis	Inhibits reactions that lead to clotting	5,000–40,000 units; do not give IM due to pain or risk of hematoma formation; doses adjusted to individual patient	Hemorrhage, chills, fever, hypersensitivity reactions, alopecia
Antiplatelets				
clopidogrel (***Plavix***) Oral	Reduces myocardial infarction and vascular death when atherosclerosis is present; peripheral vascular disease; acute coronary syndrome	Inhibits platelet aggregation	75 mg daily	Edema, hypertension, syncope, palpitation, abdominal pain, dyspepsia, diarrhea, nausea, vomiting, headache, dizziness

Note: Bolded trade names are among the 50 most commonly prescribed drugs.

[a]*Trade names given in parentheses are examples only. Check current drug references for a complete listing of available products.*

[b]*Average adult doses are given. However, dosages are determined by a provider and vary with the purpose of the therapy and the particular patient. The doses presented in this text are for general information only.*

Practice Procedure 10.1 (LO 10-7)

ADMINISTERING ORAL, SUBLINGUAL, AND BUCCAL MEDICATIONS

Demonstrate how to safely administer oral, sublingual, and buccal medications to a patient.

Equipment

Medication orders for three patients:

- Patient 1: digoxin, 0.25 mg p.o. q.d.
- Patient 2: ferrous sulfate, 220 mg p.o. qid with juice
- Patient 3: nitroglycerin, 0.4 mg subl p.m.

Medications

- *Lanoxin* (0.125- or 0.25-mg tablets)
- *Feosol* elixir (220 mg ferrous sulfate per teaspoonful)
- *Nitrostat* (0.4-mg sublingual tablets)

Apple juice, water, cups

Medication records

Procedure

1. Set up medications one at a time. Read drug labels as you reach for bottles, then again as you pour, and again as you put drugs away. Check and double-check the medication orders for the "seven rights."

2. Wash your hands.

3. Go to Patient 1. Identify the patient. Explain what you are going to do. Assist the patient into a position for oral administration.

4. Administer digoxin (*Lanoxin*):
   - Check the apical pulse first to make sure that it is over 60.
   - Administer one 0.25-mg tablet or two 0.125-mg tablets.
   - Give the patient water to drink. Assist the patient if necessary.
   - Chart drug, dose, time, and apical pulse.
   - Make the patient comfortable before leaving.
   - Wash your hands.

5. Go to Patient 2. Identify, explain, and assist (as in Step 3).

6. Administer ferrous sulfate:
   - Mix 1 teaspoonful of ferrous sulfate elixir with orange juice if the patient is unable to take elixir without juice.
   - Administer it to the patient (helping the patient use a straw).
   - Chart drug, dose, and time.
   - Make the patient comfortable before leaving.
   - Wash your hands.

7. Go to Patient 3. Identify the patient. Explain that you are leaving a packet of nitroglycerin tablets by the bedside. As you leave, the patient complains of angina pain.

8. Administer nitroglycerin (*Nitrostat*):
   - Put on nonsterile gloves.
   - Place one tablet (0.4 mg) of *Nitrostat* under the patient's tongue or in the buccal pouch (**Figure 10.8**). Instruct the patient not to swallow until the tablet is completely dissolved.
   - Do not give liquids.
   - Chart drug, dose, time, and reason for administration.
   - Make the patient comfortable before leaving.
   - Wash your hands.

9. Return equipment and charts to the proper location.

Figure 10.8

Sublingual (left) and buccal (right) administration.

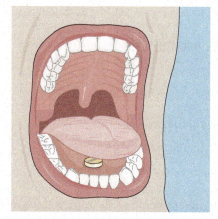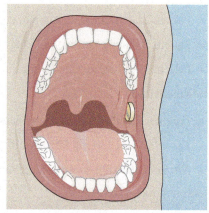

Learning Outcome	Summary Points
10-1 Identify the parts and functions of the cardiovascular system.	• *Parts:* Heart, blood vessels, and blood. • *Functions:* Transports vital substances such as nutrients, waste products, oxygen, carbon dioxide, minerals, hormones, drugs, and body heat throughout the body.
10-2 List the names of instruments used to measure blood pressure and to record the heartbeat.	• *Blood pressure* is measured with a sphygmomanometer or an automatic sphygmomanometer. • The *heart rate* is measured by placing the stethoscope over the apical pulse and counting the pulse. • The average *blood pressure* is 120/80 mm Hg. • The normal blood pressure is systolic less than 120 and diastolic less than 80. • The average *adult pulse* is between 60 and 100 beats per minute.

10-3 List the main components of blood and the functions of the lymphatic system.	• Plasma
	• Erythrocytes (red blood cells)
	• Leukocytes (white blood cells)
	• Platelets (thrombocytes)
	• The functions of the lymphatic system are:
	  • The lymphatic system carries waste products that the blood cannot carry, such as dead cells and debris.
	  • These wastes are removed at the lymph nodes.
	  • Lymph is not pumped but is collected from the various body parts through open-ended lymph vessels. As the body moves, the lymph is pushed through its vessels.

10-4 Identify the major disorders and common symptoms of the cardiovascular system.	• *Dyspnea:* labored or difficult breathing. • *Angina pectoris:* chest pain. • *Edema:* an abnormal accumulation of fluid in the interstitial tissues. • *Dysrhythmias:* any deviation from the normal rhythm of the heartbeat resulting from an abnormality in the electrical conduction of the heart muscle; irregular heartbeats are also known as arrhythmias. • *Tachycardia:* very rapid heartbeat. • *Bradycardia:* very slow heartbeat. • *Hemoptysis:* the coughing up of blood. • *Cyanosis:* bluish color of the skin when oxygen content in the blood is low. • *Cardiac arrest:* sudden and unexpected stopping of the heart and circulation. • *Congestive heart failure:* results from the inability of the heart to pump adequately enough to meet the body's metabolic needs. • *Hypercholesterolemia:* a cholesterol level that is higher than the desirable level. • *Coronary artery disease:* a disorder of blood vessels that falls under the category of atherosclerosis. • *Thrombophlebitis:* involves the formation of a blood clot (thrombus) in a blood vessel associated with inflammation (phlebitis). • *Arteriosclerosis:* the most common arterial disorder, characterized by thickening, loss of elasticity, and calcification of the arterial walls. • *Hypertension:* high blood pressure. • *Shock:* occurs as a result of decreased blood flow to the body's tissues that causes organs to fail. • *Anemia:* a decrease in the number of erythrocytes, the quality of hemoglobin, and the volume of hematocrit, which reflects the ratio of red blood cells to plasma. • *Leukemia:* a general term used to describe a group of malignant disorders that affect the blood-forming tissues in the bone marrow, spleen, and lymph system. • *Hodgkin's disease:* a malignant disorder characterized by the growth of abnormal giant, multinucleated cells called Reed-Sternberg cells, which are located in the lymph nodes. • *Non-Hodgkin's lymphoma:* a malignant disorder of the immune system.

10-5 Describe the actions and special procedures for administration of these drug groups: adrenergics, vasodilators, diuretics, antihypertensives, calcium channel blockers, antilipemics, cardiac glycosides, antiarrhythmics (antidysrhythmics), anticoagulants, thrombolytics, hemostatics, hematinics, and antiplatelets.	• *Adrenergics* raise blood pressure by causing the blood vessels to contract. Patients must be monitored for heart rate, blood pressure, and kidney and pulmonary function. Assess to make sure they are not receiving too much medication and developing hypertension. An example is *Levophed*. • *Vasodilators,* also known as nitrates, relax or dilate the walls of the arteries and are used to control angina pectoris. Place one tablet under the tongue at the first sign of an angina attack and repeat, if needed, every 5 minutes until three tablets are taken in 15 minutes. Keep track of how many tablets are taken, and notify the lead healthcare team member if more than three tablets are taken in 15 minutes. An example is *Nitrostat*. • *Diuretics* eliminate excess fluids through urinary excretion. There are loop and thiazide diuretics. An example of a thiazide diuretic is *Diuril*. An example of a potassium-sparing is hydrochlorothiazide/triamterene (*Maxzide, Dyazide*). • *Antihypertensives* lower the blood pressure. Monitor the patient for side effects such as dizziness, fainting, weakness, mental depression, and orthostatic hypotension. Caution the patient to rise slowly from a sitting or lying position. An example is captopril. • *Calcium channel blockers* inhibit the transport of calcium into the myocardial and vascular smooth muscles, and this decreases myocardial contractibility and the demand for oxygen. They also dilate the coronary arteries. An example is *Norvasc*. • *Antilipemics* lower blood cholesterol. An example is lovastatin. • *Cardiac glycosides* strengthen the myocardium, increase the force of contraction, slow the heart, and improve the muscle tone of the myocardium. An example is digoxin. • *Antiarrhythmics* stabilize the heart muscle so that it does not fluctuate or beat too rapidly. Adjust the dose individually for each patient. Administer every 8 hours to ensure a constant blood level. Take pulse and blood pressure before administering. An example is propranolol. • *Anticoagulants* prevent blood from clotting, and this helps prevent or reduce the formation of a thrombus. Carefully monitor dosages because anticoagulants can lead to internal hemorrhage. Monitor prothrombin time to determine the proper dose. An example is *Coumadin*. • *Thrombolytics* dissolve blood clots. An example is *Activase*. • *Hemostatics* help the formation of blood clots. They are used when much blood is being lost due to injury or disease or when a patient has had an overdose of an anticoagulant. A hemostatic such as vitamin K may be given before surgery or childbirth. It may also be given to reverse the effects of warfarin toxicity. An example is *Mephyton*. • *Hematinics,* also known as antianemics, are used when there is a lowered red blood cell count or lack of hemoglobin, as in anemia. An example is ferrous sulfate. Ferrous sulfate can irritate the mucous membranes. Give it with plenty of liquid. Tell patients they will have dark, tarry stools. • *Antiplatelets* suppress platelet aggregation and prevent thrombosis in arteries. An example is *Plavix*.
10-6 Know the difference between an initial and a maintenance dose.	• An *initial dose,* or loading dose, is a large dose that may be given when starting therapy to build up the level of medication in the patient's bloodstream. • A *maintenance dose* is a dosage amount that maintains the level of drug in the blood without overdosing the patient.
10-7 Demonstrate administering oral and sublingual medications to patients with cardiovascular disorders.	• *Lanoxin* is given orally after taking the apical pulse to make sure it is over 60. • Ferrous sulfate is administered as a liquid to patients who have trouble swallowing. Mix 1 teaspoon of Ferrous sulfate elixir with orange juice. • *Nitroglycerin* or *Nitrostat* is administered sublingually or buccally by placing one tablet under the patient's tongue or in the buccal pouch. The patient should not swallow until the tablet is completely dissolved.

Chapter 10 Review

Define each of the terms listed.

1. (LO 10-3) Spleen _____

2. (LO 10-4) Tachycardia _____

3. (LO 10-4) Bradycardia _____

4. (LO 10-3) Hypertension _____

5. (LO 10-3) Hypotension _____

Match the terms to their definitions.

_____   6. (LO 10-3) Blood pressure instrument   a. electrocardiogram

_____   7. (LO 10-3) Graphic record that shows the spread of   b. sphygmomanometer
electrical excitation to different parts of the heart

     c. plasma

_____   8. (LO 10-3) Important in clotting process

     d. white blood cells

_____   9. (LO 10-3) What surrounds and destroys microorganisms
and foreign matter   e. platelets

_____   10. (LO 10-3) Liquid portion of blood and lymph

Complete the statements by filling in the blank.

11. (LO 10-3) An important landmark when taking the apical pulse before administering cardiac drugs is
the _____.

12. (LO 10-3) The average blood pressure and pulse readings are _____.

13. (LO 10-3) Veins carry _____ blood.

14. (LO 10-3) Arteries carry _____ blood.

Select the cardiovascular disorder that best matches each description and write it in the blank.

angina pectoris   arteriosclerosis   myocardial infarction   atherosclerosis

thrombophlebitis   shock   embolism

15. (LO 10-4) Collapse of the circulatory system, signaled by severe hypotension; high pulse rate; pale,
clammy skin; and mental confusion.

_____

16. (LO 10-4) Fat deposited along vessel walls reducing circulation.

_____

17. (LO 10-4) Most common arterial disorder, characterized by thickening, loss of elasticity, and calcification of arterial walls.

_____

18. (LO 10-4) Formation of a blood clot in a blood vessel, associated with inflammation.

_____

19. (LO 10-4) A blood clot or air bubble that travels through the bloodstream and cuts off circulation to a vital organ.

_____

20. (LO 10-4) Chest pain that may be relieved by giving nitroglycerin.

_____

21. (LO 10-4) Death of a part of the heart muscle resulting from lack of blood circulation to that area.

_____

Describe the purpose of the drug; for example, diuretics help the body eliminate excess fluids through the urine.

22. (LO 10-5) Adrenergics _____

23. (LO 10-5) Vasodilators _____

24. (LO 10-5) Cardiac glycosides _____

25. (LO 10-5) Antidysrhythmics _____

26. (LO 10-5) Anticoagulants _____

27. (LO 10-5) Hemostatics _____

28. (LO 10-5) Hematinics _____

Match the drug categories to the drug names.

_____ 29. (LO 10-5) Verapamil, *Procardia*   a. calcium channel blockers

_____ 30. (LO 10-5) *Lopressor,* hydralazine   b. antihypertensives

Drug Calculations—Fill in the blank with the answer.

31. (LO 10-5) The provider orders clonidine (*Catapres*) 0.6 mg orally tid. Available are 0.3-mg tablets. Prepare to administer _____ tablets to your patient.

32. (LO 10-5) The provider orders metoprolol (*Lopressor*) 100 mg orally tid. Available are 50-mg tablets. You will give your patient _____ tablets.

33. (LO 10-5) The provider orders furosemide (*Lasix*) 10 mg orally bid. Available are 20-mg tablets. You will give your patient _____ tablets.

34. (LO 10-5) The provider orders digoxin (*Lanoxin*) 0.125 mg orally daily. Available are 0.25-mg tablets. Prepare to give your patient _____ tablets.

35. (LO 10-5) The provider orders heparin 6000 units subcutaneously daily. Available is 7500 units/mL. You will give your patient _____ mL.

36. (LO 10-5) The provider orders propranolol 15 mg orally tid. Available are 10-mg tablets. You will give your patient _____ tablets.

Multiple Choice—Circle the correct letter.

37. (LO 10-3) A patient asks what the white blood cells (leukocytes) do. You know that the most appropriate answer the healthcare team member should provide is which of the following?
   a. Carry oxygen
   b. Play a critical role in clotting
   c. Eliminate waste from the body
   d. Play a role in immunity

38. (LO 10-5) Which of the following instructions should be provided to a patient taking nitrates?
   a. Take a dose 30 minutes before an activity known to cause an attack.
   b. Avoid high-fiber foods.
   c. Report headache, dry mouth, and blurred vision to the provider.
   d. Use alcoholic beverages in moderation.

39. (LO 10-5) Monitor a patient taking procainamide (*Procanbid*) for which of the following adverse reactions?
   a. Hypotension, anorexia, nausea
   b. Headache, dizziness, flushing
   c. Weakness, rapid pulse, constipation
   d. Fatigue, lethargy, abdominal pain

40. (LO 10-5) A client taking furosemide (*Lasix*) is at risk for which of the following electrolyte abnormalities?
   a. Hypernatremia
   b. Hyperchloremia
   c. Hypokalemia
   d. Hypercholesterolemia

41. (LO 10-5) Administer which of the following prescribed antilipemics to a patient with hypercholesterolemia?
   a. Triamterene (*Dyrenium*)
   b. Simvastatin (*Zocor*)
   c. Warfarin sodium (*Coumadin*)
   d. Clopidogrel (*Plavix*)

Chapter 10 Case Studies

42. (LO 10-5) A patient is taking isosorbide to treat angina pectoris. What is the patient education you should give this patient? _____

_____

_____

_____

43. (LO 10-5) A patient is taking captopril (*Capoten*) and complains of dizziness, lightheadedness, and weakness. What kind of drug is *Capoten,* and what explains this effect? What is your priority action? What should you tell your patient? _____

_____

_____

_____

Critical Thinking

Complete the statements by filling in the blank.

44. (LO 10-5) Patients taking heparin or warfarin (*Coumadin*) must be watched for signs of _____ in the urine, feces, and mucous membranes.

45. (LO 10-4) _____ may be left at a patient's bedside for angina pain.

46. (LO 10-5) Because digitalis slows as well as strengthens the heartbeat, an adult patient's pulse rate must be at least _____ in order to give the drug.

47. (LO 10-5) Patients on antihypertensives may feel _____ when they get up from bed because of orthostatic hypotension.

48. (LO 10-5) Some hematinics can _____ clothing and skin, so they must be handled with care.

49. (LO 10-5) When a disorder has just been diagnosed, the provider may start the drug therapy by ordering a fairly large dose known as the _____ dose.

Applications

Obtain an electronic drug guide, a current copy of a drug reference book, or the *PDR*®. Use it to answer the questions that follow in a notebook or on file cards.

50. Use Section 2 of the *PDR*®, Brand and Generic Name Index, to find another product name for each of the drugs in the Representative Drugs for the Cardiovascular System table in this chapter.

51. Use Section 3 of the *PDR*®, Product Category Index, to locate Cardiovascular Preparations; then find the subheading Anginal Preparations. List all the drugs named.

If you have a problem finding some drugs in the *PDR*®, look in the back under Discontinued Products.

DRUGS FOR THE RESPIRATORY SYSTEM

LEARNING OUTCOMES

11-1 Describe the parts and normal functions of the respiratory system.

11-2 Describe the major respiratory disorders and related symptoms, using the correct medical terms.

11-3 Describe nicotine dependency and methods for smoking cessation.

11-4 Describe the actions of the following drug groups: antitussives, expectorants, decongestants, antihistamines, and bronchodilators.

11-5 Understand the procedures of chest physiotherapy; operating a pulse oximeter; and administering nose drops, inhalants, and oxygen.

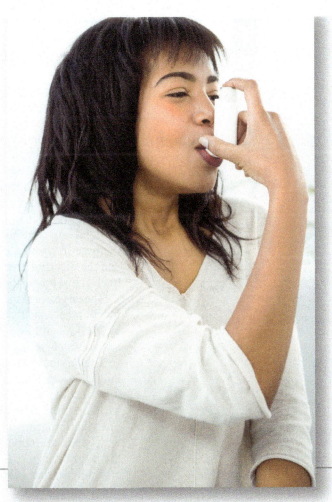

©wavebreakmedia/Shutterstock

In this chapter you will review the parts and functions of the respiratory system. You will learn how breathing takes place and how common respiratory disorders affect this process. You will study the types of drugs used to treat respiratory disorders and their actions. You will also learn to administer drugs in the form of nose drops and sprays to the mucous membranes of the nose and throat.

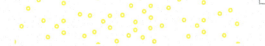

acute

antihistamine

antitussive

apnea

bronchodilator

chronic

decongestant

dyspnea

emphysema

expectorant

Fowler's position

hemoptysis

hyperpnea

hypoxia

inhaler

mucolytic

nebulizer

nicotine dependence

orthopnea

peak flow meter

percussion

pneumococcal disease

postural drainage

pulse oximeter

rebound effect

semi-Fowler's position

tachypnea

vibration

RESPIRATORY SYSTEM [LO 11-1]

The respiratory system consists of the organs that make it possible for blood to exchange gases with air. They are the nose, pharynx, larynx, trachea, bronchi, and lungs (Figure 11.1). These structures constitute the lifeline of the body, supplying a continuous, uninterrupted source of oxygen. The exchange of gases between blood and air is called respiration. If anything jeopardizes the functioning of this vital system, death is certain within a short time.

Air enters the body through the mouth or the nose. Like all of the respiratory system, the nose is lined with mucous membranes. As air enters the nose, very small hairs called cilia warm and moisten the air and trap dust particles and bacteria. The pharynx is a tubelike structure that extends from the base of the skull to the esophagus and serves both the respiratory tract and the digestive tract. The larynx, or voice box, lies at the upper end of the trachea just below the pharynx.

The larynx is responsible for making sounds. The larynx serves a protective function because the epiglottis, a leaf-shaped structure on top of the larynx, closes the airway when a person swallows. The epiglottis thus keeps food and saliva from entering the lungs.

The larynx joins a tube called the trachea, or windpipe, that leads into the lungs. C-shaped pieces of cartilage line the trachea to keep it firm and prevent it from collapsing and shutting off the airway. The trachea branches off into two tubes: the right and left bronchi, which lead to the right and left lungs. The right bronchus is slightly larger and more vertical than the left. This is why, when an individual aspirates, the aspirated object generally lodges in the right bronchus. The bronchi branch into increasingly smaller tubes, the bronchioles, that subdivide into smaller tubes. The smaller branches further divide into alveolar ducts. These terminate in several alveolar sacs whose walls consist of alveoli, small sacs that are the functional units of the lungs.

The alveolar sacs are tiny air sacs with thin walls. They are in close contact with many capillaries. This is where inhaled oxygen is picked up from the air by the red blood cells. At the same time, carbon dioxide is released from the blood into the air sacs and travels back up the air passages. During exhalation, the carbon dioxide and other waste gases pass out of the body.

The lungs are cone-shaped organs that fill the pleural portion of the thoracic cavity. They provide a place where the exchange of gases can take place between blood and air.

The average person breathes in and out about 16 to 18 times per minute. The normal respiration rate varies between 12 and 25 times per minute.

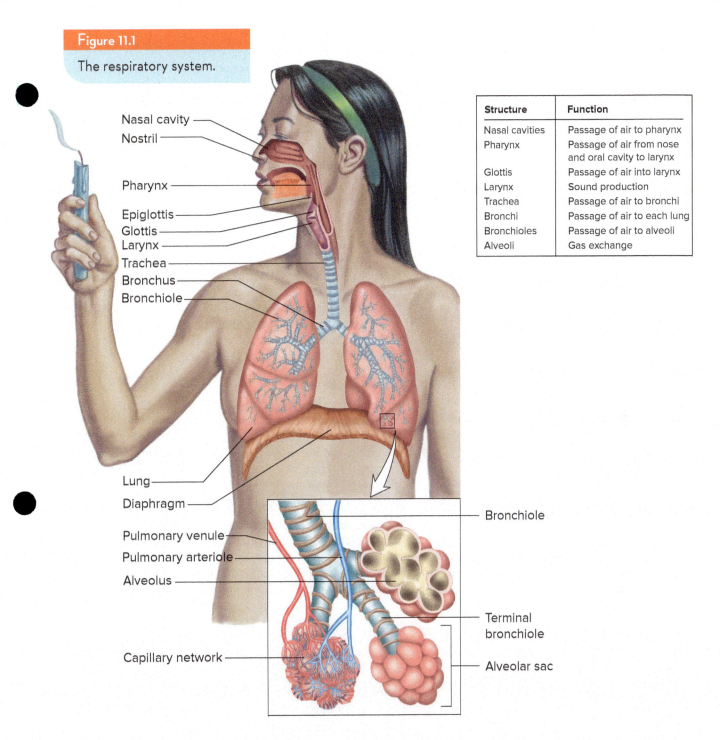

Figure 11.1

The respiratory system.

Nasal cavity
Nostril
Pharynx
Epiglottis
Glottis
Larynx
Trachea
Bronchus
Bronchiole

Structure	Function
Nasal cavities	Passage of air to pharynx
Pharynx	Passage of air from nose and oral cavity to larynx
Glottis	Passage of air into larynx
Larynx	Sound production
Trachea	Passage of air to bronchi
Bronchi	Passage of air to each lung
Bronchioles	Passage of air to alveoli
Alveoli	Gas exchange

Lung
Diaphragm

Pulmonary venule
Pulmonary arteriole
Alveolus

Capillary network

Bronchiole

Terminal bronchiole

Alveolar sac

Children tend to breathe more quickly, and older adult patients more slowly, than the average adult. Bradypnea is slowed breathing, usually less than 12 breaths per minute in adults. Tachypnea is fast breathing, usually more than 20 breaths per minute.

Breathing is accomplished by the muscles around the ribs and by the diaphragm, a layer of muscle tissue that separates the chest cavity from the other internal organs. When a person inhales, the respiratory muscles contract to lift the rib cage, and the diaphragm flattens out. These actions create a downward and outward pull on the lungs that forces them to draw in air (inhalation). When the muscles relax, the lung cavity collapses and forces the air back out (exhalation). Inside the lungs, the elastic walls of the bronchioles and the alveoli expand and contract with each breath. When this elasticity is decreased by disease, proper breathing is no longer possible.

RESPIRATORY SYSTEM DISORDERS [LO 11-2]

Respiration is crucial to sustaining life. A person cannot live more than a few minutes without oxygen. Brain damage begins after only 6 minutes without oxygen. This is why respiration rate is one of the four vital signs. The other vital signs are body temperature, blood pressure, and pulse.

As a routine part of a physical examination, the provider examines the patient with a stethoscope, an instrument that amplifies breathing sounds (**Figure 11.2**). Auscultation is the process of listening to the lung sounds to evaluate lung function. Listening to the lung sounds with a stethoscope helps to assess the movement of air throughout the tracheobronchial tree. Normally, air flows through the airways without obstruction. To the examiner, it sounds like a swish of air. Variations in lung sounds are often characteristic of certain lung diseases. Refer to **Table 11.1** for symptoms.

Several other tests help in diagnosing respiratory diseases. A chest x-ray may be taken. A patient may cough up sputum to be sent to the laboratory for microscopic examination. Blood tests called blood gases are done to check oxygen and carbon dioxide content. **Pulse oximetry** is a technique whereby a probe is attached to the ear, finger, toe, or bridge of the nose to measure the oxygen concentration of the blood.

Major Diseases

Some respiratory problems are caused by disturbances in the control centers of the brain or in the nerves that send messages to the respiratory muscles in the ribs and the diaphragm. These problems, and the drugs used to treat them, are discussed in Chapter 17. Here we will focus on disorders that affect the air passages and the lungs, or bronchopulmonary disorders (*pulmonary*, pertaining to the lungs).

Pneumonia.   There are many types of pneumonia, each named for the agent (bacterium, virus, fungus, etc.) that causes it. All pneumonias are infections of the lower respiratory tract (bronchi, bronchioles, and alveoli). Factors that predispose an individual to pneumonia include smoking, air pollution, malnutrition, bed rest, immobility, and other diseases.

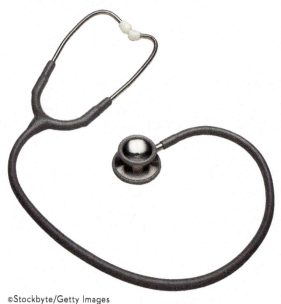

Figure 11.2

A stethoscope.

©Stockbyte/Getty Images

Table 11.1 Symptoms of Respiratory System Disorders

Symptom	Description
Coughing	Protective reflex to clear trachea, bronchi, and lungs of secretions and irritants such as mucus, pus, or fluid in the lungs. May be controlled or uncontrollled.
Sputum	Mucus that is coughed up from the lower airways. Varies in color and consistency. **Hemoptysis** refers to blood in the sputum.
Hoarseness	Difficulty making sounds when trying to speak. Causes include abnormal growth on larynx or infection in throat.
Wheezing	High-pitched, musical sound occurring through a narrow pathway. Often caused by asthma, bronchitis, or allergies.
Chest pain	Chest tightness, pain with deep breath, or stabbing pain unexpectedly.
Abnormal breathing	Types of abnormal breathing: **dyspnea**, shortness of breath or labored breathing; **tachypnea**, rapid breathing; **apnea**, cessation of breathing; **hyperpnea**, hyperventilation; **orthopnea**, difficulty breathing when lying down.

Some pneumonias are caused by bacteria that normally live in the human air passages. At times of low resistance, these bacteria may multiply and infect the lungs. Such bacterial growth may occur after surgery, anesthesia, diseases that interfere with lung drainage, and use of drugs that suppress the body's immune system. As soon as the type of bacteria is identified, antibiotics can be given to fight the infection.

Bronchitis. Bronchitis is an inflammation of the air passageways caused by irritants (e.g., smoke or chemicals), allergic reactions, flu, or viruses. It can be **acute** (short term) or **chronic** (long term). The main objective of bronchitis treatment is to keep the air passages open. They are easily plugged by sputum and pus produced by the infected bronchi. The main symptoms of bronchitis are fever, cough, tachypnea, purulent sputum (containing pus), and pleuritic chest pain. Treatment is with a broad-spectrum antibiotic, such as ampicillin, tetracycline, or erythromycin, for 7 to 10 days. The patient must drink large amounts of fluids and take drugs that keep the sputum moist and thin (**expectorants**).

Emphysema. **Emphysema** is the result of enlargement of and damage to alveolar sacs. These two problems reduce the surface of the alveoli and limit the exchange of oxygen and carbon dioxide. "Stale" air becomes backed up in the alveoli, which in turn makes it impossible to take in much air on the next breath. The alveoli are hyperinflated and overdistended. The trapped air gives the patient a "barrel chest" appearance. Although the cause of emphysema is not always understood, smoking, chronic bronchitis, and advanced age are commonly found in an emphysema patient's history. Dyspnea that continually worsens is an early symptom of emphysema.

There is no cure for emphysema, although breathing exercises are sometimes helpful. Antibiotics can be given for specific infections. Drugs that thin the sputum (expectorants) and drugs that expand the bronchioles (**bronchodilators**) are given to promote coughing up sputum that may be clogging the air passages.

Chronic obstructive pulmonary disease (COPD) is a condition that includes bronchitis and emphysema. Tiotropium bromide (*Spiriva Handihaler*) is an anticholinergic used in the maintenance treatment of bronchospasms in COPD, including chronic bronchitis and emphysema. Roflumilast (*Daliresp*) is a selective inhibitor of phosphodiesterase 4 (PDE 4) and works to decrease inflammation. A new drug *Anoro Ellipta* (umeclidinium and vilanterol) is given once a day in the treatment of airflow obstruction in patients with COPD, including chronic bronchitis and emphysema; does no relieve acute bronchospasm or asthma.

Pleurisy. Pleurisy is an inflammation of the linings (the pleura) of the lungs and lung cavities. The most common causes are pneumonia, tuberculosis, chest trauma, pulmonary infarctions, and tumors. The patient feels a knife-sharp pain in the chest that is worse on inspiration (inhalation). Pleurisy usually clears up with rest, mild sedatives, pain medication, and treatment of the primary disease. The patient is frequently taught to splint the affected side when coughing or to lie on the affected side.

Asthma. Asthma is characterized by airway obstruction, inflammation, and increased response to stimuli. Asthma attacks can be caused by substances in the environment, food additives, exercise, drug allergies, illness, or emotional upset. The attacks may occur from time to time or may last for several days (the most dangerous form). During an attack, the muscles around the bronchioles contract, narrowing the air passages. Inhaled air cannot be exhaled properly. The alveoli become plugged with unusually thick sputum that is hard to cough up. There is wheezing, shortness of breath, and coughing. The individual often has a feeling of suffocating and sits straight up or bends forward in an attempt to get more air.

The goals of asthma treatment are to relieve the constriction of the bronchioles, reduce inflammation of the airway, and prevent and control

Figure 11.3

A peak flow meter.

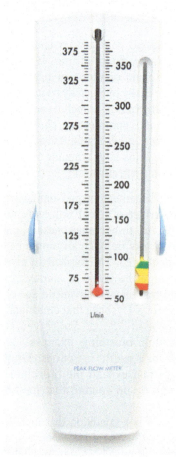

©abalcazar/Getty Images

abnormal sputum production. Bronchodilators are the drugs of choice. Theophylline was the preferred drug, but it has been replaced by other bronchodilators and anti-inflammatory drugs except in rare cases of refractory asthma in hospitalized patients. Salmeterol (*Serevent*) is an inhaled agent used in place of theophylline for reducing inflammation and maintenance bronchodilation. Currently, β_2-adrenergic agonists such as metaproterenol and albuterol (*Proventil HFA*) are used. Budesonide and formoterol (*Symbicort*) are a combination of two drugs used to help control the clinical manifestations of asthma and improve lung function. A combination of mometasone and formoterol *(Dulera)* is used for patients not controlled by other medicines or who require more than one medicine every day. This combination may also be used to treat COPD. Prevention is important in the treatment of asthma. Patients are taught to avoid the triggers of an attack. An inhaled corticosteroid such as prednisone may be given for its anti-inflammatory effect.

A **peak flow meter** is a device that measures the air flowing out of the lungs, called the peak expiratory flow rate (PEFR), as a patient blows forcefully into the device (**Figure 11.3**). It measures how well a patient's asthma is under control. It may reveal narrowing of the airways well in advance of an asthma attack. It is particularly helpful when used in moderate to severe asthma. Because a peak flow meter provides information on how well the airways are open, it aids in the determination of how effective the treatment plan is, when to stop or add a medication, when to seek emergency medical care, and what may trigger an asthma attack, such as exercise-induced asthma. You should teach your patients to use their peak flow meter daily, whenever they are experiencing early warning signs of an impending attack, and before taking any medication. The reading on the scale after the fast blow into the device helps determine the plan of care. A reading of 80 to 100 percent indicates your patient's asthma is under control. A reading of 60 to 80 percent is considered low, and medications such as albuterol (*Proventil HFA*) are started and the peak flow rate should be reassessed in 20 minutes. When the peak flow rate is less than 60 percent, it indicates the patient's asthma is out of control. The patient should begin albuterol by nebulizer or inhaler and go to the hospital emergency room.

Cancers of the Respiratory Tract. Cancers of the upper respiratory tract include cancers of the head and neck. Although cancers of the oral cavity and larynx account for only 5 percent of all cancers, their effects are devastating. Disability is great because of the loss of voice and disfigurement. The cause of head and neck cancers is unknown, but smoking and alcohol are high on the list of contributing factors. Human papillomavirus (HPV) is a risk factor becoming frequently linked to head and neck cancer. Symptoms range from pain that is aggravated by food to hoarseness. Persistent hoarseness is one of the first signs of upper respiratory cancer. It is treated by removing the growth surgically.

Cancer of the lung is the most common cancer of the lower respiratory tract. It is the leading cause of all cancer deaths. A well-known risk for lung cancer is the inhalation of cigarette smoke. Lung cancer may also spread from another cancer elsewhere in the body. It is difficult to detect because the symptoms are vague. Generally, the first symptom is a persistent, productive cough. Hemoptysis, spitting up of blood, may occur late in the disease process because of bleeding caused by the malignancy. Dyspnea and wheezing occur if the bronchioles become obstructed. Surgery to remove the cancerous tissue is the major form of treatment. Radiation and chemotherapy may also be used.

Pulmonary Embolism. Pulmonary embolism is the most common complication found in hospitalized patients. It generally begins as a thrombus deep in the vein of a leg. This is why maintaining mobility in patients is essential to prevent pulmonary embolisms, which can be fatal. Symptoms include sudden, unexplained dyspnea, tachypnea, or tachycardia. Oxygen and anticoagulant therapy are often effective in treatment.

Tuberculosis. Tuberculosis (TB) is an infectious disease caused by *Mycobacterium tuberculosis.* The body becomes sensitive to this bacterium when it is first exposed. Coughing spreads airborne droplets that contain rod-shaped bacteria known as tubercle bacilli; when droplets are inhaled, the bacteria multiply in the lungs. After initial infection, tuberculosis germs can remain dormant for long periods and then reactivate when the immune system weakens. The patient weakens, coughs up blood, and eventually dies without early treatment. Treatment consists of drugs that attack the tubercle bacillus— such as rifapentine (*Priftin*), isoniazid, rifampin (*Rifadin*), ethambutol and pyrazinamide—rest, and proper disposal of sputum in a designated waste receptacle. *Priftin* is a longer-acting form of rifampin, which has been a standard part of the treatment of TB.

The occurrence of tuberculosis in the United States fell steadily from 1953 until 1985. After that, the number of new cases began rising. The main reasons are the prevalence of the human immunodeficiency virus (HIV) infection, which impairs immunity, and new strains of tuberculosis that are resistant to drug therapy. Risk factors for tuberculosis are immigration from countries where tuberculosis is prevalent, poverty, overcrowding, poor nutrition, and homelessness. Because many cases of tuberculosis are left untreated, the disease can spread at an alarming rate. In the early stages, the patient may be free of symptoms. TB may be found accidentally on a routine chest x-ray. Later, fatigue, weight loss, anorexia, low-grade fever, and night sweats may develop. If it is thought that a patient might have tuberculosis, the patient should have a tuberculin skin test and chest x-ray.

Treatment of tuberculosis consists of a combination of at least three drugs. In high-risk areas or areas known to have a high incidence of drug resistance, three or more drugs are used. The four most commonly used drugs are isoniazid, rifampin, streptomycin, and ethambutol. The current protocol for treatment is to use isoniazid, rifampin, and ethambutol for 2 months, followed by 4 months of isoniazid and rifampin. Therapy is continued for 3 months even after a negative culture. Hospitalization is generally not necessary. If it is required, it is very brief. The patient is placed in respiratory isolation and on drug therapy for 2 weeks. Patients must show a positive response to treatment before discharge. If the tubercle bacillus develops a resistance to two of the drugs used to treat tuberculosis, the cause may be multidrug-resistant tuberculosis (MDR-TB). If MDR-TB is suspected, measures must be taken to prevent its spread. Some patients with tuberculosis may be on a directly observed therapy (DOT) protocol. This protocol requires supervision of each dose of medication by an individual trained in DOT supervision.

H1N1 Virus (Swine Flu). The H1N1 virus, more commonly known as swine flu, is a respiratory disorder caused by viruses that normally produce illness in pigs. The outbreak in 2009 involving a new H1N1 virus type-A influenza strain was a genetic combination of swine, avian, and human influenza viruses. It can spread from human to human.

The symptoms develop 3 to 5 days after exposure and include fever, cough, sore throat, body aches, headache, chills, fatigue, diarrhea, and vomiting. Swine flu may need only symptomatic treatment. If medication is needed, oseltamivir (*Tamiflu*) and zanamivir (*Relenza*), both of which are neuraminidase inhibitors, are used. These medications are most effective if treatment begins within 48 hours of symptoms beginning.

Inflammations of the Nose, Sinuses, and Throat. Rhinitis, sinusitis, and strep throat are some of the most common inflammations of the upper respiratory tract. They are caused by bacterial infections, allergies, or irritating substances. "Seasonal rhinitis," for example, is an allergic reaction to the pollen in the air during the late summer and fall. Signs of rhinitis and sinusitis include runny nose, sneezing, headache, sore throat, watery eyes, fever, and redness and swelling of mucous membranes. The symptoms can be controlled with decongestants and antihistamines. Then a systemic antibiotic is prescribed to kill that specific bacterium. Strep throat is diagnosed by a throat culture to confirm the presence of the bacteria, *Streptococcal pharyngitis*, and treated with systemic antibiotics. Ciclesonide (*Omnaris*) is a nasal spray used to treat perennial and seasonal allergic rhinitis. The common cold is the most frequent infection in all age groups. It is caused by rhinoviruses. There is no cure.

NICOTINE DEPENDENCE AND SMOKING CESSATION [LO 11-4]

Nicotine dependence is a physical vulnerability of the body to the chemical nicotine, which is brought on by tobacco products. Nicotine produces physical, mood-altering effects that are considered pleasing and reinforce the continued use of tobacco, resulting in addiction. A person with a nicotine dependence feels he or she can't quit smoking; experiences withdrawal symptoms such as anxiety, irritability, restlessness, difficulty concentrating, headache, and gastrointestinal upset when attempting to quit smoking; may give up social or recreational activities to smoke; but, most importantly, keeps smoking despite diagnosed heart and lung conditions. Tobacco smoke delivers over 60 cancer-causing chemicals including arsenic, cyanide, and nicotine, which release a brain chemical called dopamine that produces a feeling of "feeling good" that keeps the addictive process going.

The greatest at-risk population for nicotine dependence is adolescents. Over 90 percent of smokers begin smoking between the ages of 18 and 21 years. Smoking is responsible for over 85 percent of lung cancers, emphysema, and bronchitis. It is responsible for cardiovascular disease, mouth and throat cancers, infertility issues, as well as newborn complications (preterm delivery and low birth weight), wrinkles, and a deadened sense of smell and taste.

Smoking cessation generally occurs with nicotine replacement therapy and nonnicotine replacement medications. The nicotine patch, such as *Nicoderm CQ* and *Nicotrol NS,* nicotine gum (*Nicorette*), and nicotine lozenges are available without a prescription. The patch delivers nicotine through the skin into the bloodstream. A patch is applied to the upper body and is generally worn for up to 8 weeks. Nicotine gum delivers nicotine to the bloodstream through the lining of the mouth. It comes in 2-mg and 4-mg pieces, and 10 to 15 pieces are chewed daily. It is generally used for 1 to 3 months for a maximum of 6 months.

Available by prescription are nicotine sprays such as *Nicotrol NS* and a nicotine inhaler called *Nicotrol Inhaler. Nicotrol NS* delivers nicotine through the nostril into the veins, which is then transported to the heart and sent to the brain. It is a quicker delivery system generally prescribed for 3 months. The nicotine inhaler is a device like a cigarette holder that generates vapors into the mouth and is effective in relieving withdrawal symptoms.

Varenicline (*Chantix*) is available as a substitute for nicotine replacement therapy. It acts by decreasing both the cravings for nicotine and the pleasurable effect of cigarettes. The treatment period is generally 12 weeks, with another 12 weeks after successfully quitting smoking. The most common adverse reactions include abnormal dreams, nausea, vomiting, headache, and flatulence.

The antidepressant medication bupropion (*Zyban*) does not contain nicotine but it does increase the level of dopamine, which is the chemical that is also boosted by nicotine. It should not be used when a history of seizures or head injury is present, and it may cause sleep disturbances (insomnia), depression, headaches, and dry mouth.

The best way to prevent tobacco dependence is not to smoke in the first place. Since the majority of smoking begins in adolescence, the best prevention is talking to teenagers about it. Exercise, relaxation techniques, sensible nutrition, and avoiding caffeine or other stimulants may also be helpful.

Antitussives

Antitussive drugs are cough suppressants. They act on the control center in the brain that stimulates coughing. Remember that not all coughing is harmful or undesirable. Coughing clears the respiratory tract of foreign objects and sputum that interfere with breathing. A cough that brings up sputum is called a productive cough. A cough that brings up nothing is called a "dry" cough, or unproductive cough. Unproductive coughing occurs when mucus is clogged in the lower respiratory tract or when irritation in the throat stimulates repeated coughing. Despite the fact that no mucus is being brought up, a person may have a repeated urge to cough. Frequent and prolonged coughing can be exhausting, painful, and stressful to the circulatory system. Antitussives may be given to suppress the cough reflex somewhat, but never completely. There are narcotic antitussives, such as codeine, and nonnarcotic antitussives, such as dextromethorphan (*Children's Dimetapp Cold and Cough*). Increasing fluids and inhalation of steam are also utilized to thin and increase the production of secretions. Patients should be monitored for drowsiness. Patients taking narcotic antitussives should be cautioned not to drive or operate heavy machinery while experiencing the effects of the medication.

 Pediatric Considerations — Antitussives, Mucolytics/Expectorants, and Decongestants

- Upper respiratory infections, including those with increased secretions, nasal congestion, and cough, are common in children.
- Several over-the-counter cough and cold medications are available for pediatric use, although a number of others have been taken off the market because of an increased potential for overdose.
- Nasal decongestants, especially those containing pseudoephedrine, are considered safe in children older than 5 years of age. Their use in children under 2 years of age has not been established.

- The dose of pseudoephedrine in nasal decongestants for children is low, so healthcare providers can't agree on their effectiveness.
- Phenylephrine oral tablets may be given to infants to decrease their problem with nasal congestion and their ability to nurse.
- Caution parents against using acetaminophen or ibuprofen to treat any fever in a child. Some healthcare providers recommend administering them only for a fever above 101° F.

 Older Adult Considerations — Antitussives, Mucolytics/Expectorants, and Decongestants

- The effectiveness of antitussives and mucolytic/expectorants in older adults has not been proved.
- Older adults taking nasal decongestants are at risk for side effects such as hypertension, cardiac dysrhythmias, nervousness, and insomnia. Older adults with cardiovascular disease should avoid their use.

- Although there are fewer side effects from inhaled decongestants, rebound nasal congestion may occur.

Mucolytics/Expectorants

Mucolytic drugs, also called expectorants, have a disintegrating effect on mucus. They increase the amount of fluid in the respiratory tract to help liquefy and reduce the viscosity (thickness) of secretions. One of the most commonly used mucolytics is prescription inhaled acetylcysteine and another over-the-counter mucolytic is guaifenesin (*Mucinex*).

Decongestants

Decongestants are vasoconstrictors used for nasal congestion because they shrink engorged mucous membranes that are frequently present in respiratory infections.

Decongestants only relieve symptoms; they do not cure the underlying cause of congestion. They are available as nasal solutions. Adverse reactions include dryness and stinging of the nasal mucosa, sneezing, lightheadedness, headaches, palpitations, anxiety, drowsiness, anorexia, nausea, and vomiting. Examples are phenylephrine hydrochloride (*Neo-Synephrine Cold and Sinus Regular Strength Spray*) and oxymetazoline (*Afrin*). Most decongestants are available over the counter, but patients should not overuse them.

A **rebound effect** can occur with decongestants after continued use; when the drug effect wears off, the mucous membranes swell even more than before. Decongestants can also irritate the nasal passages.

Federal Legislation Covering Sales of Pseudoephedrine

As a result of drug labs using pseudoephedrine and ephedrine to make methamphetamines, drug legislation was enacted to control the sale of pseudoephedrine and ephedrine. President Bush signed the USA Patriot Improvement and Reauthorization Act of 2005 into law on March 9, 2006. In the Patriot Act is the "Combat Meth Act," which restricts the sale of over-the-counter products containing pseudoephedrine or ephedrine. Currently, products containing pseudoephedrine and ephedrine used in the treatment of cold, cough, or allergy symptoms must be purchased at the pharmacy counter because they are no longer available over the counter. So far, stastistics indicate that this process has cut down on the use of pseudoephedrine and ephedrine by methamphetamine labs.

To purchase a product containing pseudoephedrine or ephedrine, individuals must prove they are at least 18 years of age by showing a valid driver's license or some other form of identification. The pharmacist will take their name, date of birth, address, license or identification number, and the amount of pseudoephedrine or ephedrine purchased and record it in a log book. The log book contains a warning to the consumer about the use of false, forged, or altered identification.

The amount of pseudoephedrine and ephedrine that may be purchased at one time is 3.6 g daily and a total amount of 9 g may be purchased in one month. Penalties exist for violation of this federal law. There is a civil penalty of up to $25,000 for the first offense and imprisonment for up to one year in addition to a fine. Subsequent offenses may result in imprisonment for two years and a fine.

Antihistamines

Antihistamines are drugs that work against the effects of histamine, which is why they are used in allergic conditions such as hay fever and the associated symptoms such as edema, itching, redness, sneezing, and a runny nose. Recall that histamine is released by certain cells whenever there is a foreign "invader," such as an irritating substance, a microorganism, or an injury. Histamine causes the blood vessels to dilate and the smooth muscle in the bronchi to contract. Antihistamines, in contrast, shrink the blood vessels and relax the bronchial muscles.

Antihistamines are administered orally because they are easily absorbed through the intestinal lining. The major antihistamines used for respiratory problems are diphenhydramine (*Benadryl Allergy*), chlorpheniramine maleate (*Chlor-Trimeton*) and related drugs, cyproheptadine, cetirizine hydrochloride (*Zyrtec Allergy*), loratadine (*Claritin*), and fexofenadine (*Allegra Allergy 24 Hour*).

Antihistamines have the side effects of drowsiness, sedation, dizziness, dry mouth, and insomnia. Because of the sedative effect, caution patients about driving or operating hazardous equipment. Antihistamines should also be used with caution in patients with asthma, glaucoma, or urinary retention, because the side effects are potentiated (intensified). Side effects are also enhanced in older adults.

 Pediatric Considerations Antihistamines

- Use caution with first-generation antihistamines because even with a therapeutic dose, drugs such as diphenhydramine (*Benadryl Allergy*) may cause drowsiness and decreased mental alertness.
- Avoid giving antihistamines to newborns or children with chickenpox or a flulike infection.

- Give the smallest possible dose.
- Second-generation antihistamines, such as loratadine (*Claritin*), are given with caution to children of various ages.

 Older Adult Considerations Antihistamines

- Older adults are especially sensitive to side effects of first-generation antihistamines, such as diphenhydramine (*Benadryl Allergy*), which include confusion, impaired thinking, dizziness, hypotension, sedation, syncope, unsteady gait, and central nervous system (CNS) stimulation. The side effects, particularly sedation, may be confused with dementia.

- Despite the side effects of *Benadryl Allergy*, it is sometimes prescribed as a sleep aid.
- Men with prostatic hypertrophy may have difficulty voiding as a result of the anticholinergic effects of these drugs.
- Second-generation antihistamines, such as cetirizine (*Zyrtec Allergy*), may be given to older adults. They pose less risk of impaired consciousness.

Bronchodilators and Antiasthmatics

Bronchodilators improve pulmonary airflow because they cause the bronchioles to relax and expand (dilate), making it easier to breathe. This is a useful effect in conditions such as asthma, bronchitis, and emphysema. β_2-adrenergic agonists are the most effective bronchodilators. They act by relaxing the smooth muscle of the airways and increasing the cleansing of the airways by the cilia and mucus. The most common side effects are tachycardia, nervousness, palpitations, tremors, and nausea. The β_2-adrenergic agonists are most effective in the inhaled form. The main β_2-adrenergic agonist bronchodilators are metaproterenol, albuterol (*Proventil HFA, Ventolin HFA*), ephedrine and levalbuterol (*Xopenex*). A different type of bronchodilator is the anticholinergic agent ipratropium (*Atrovent HFA*). Many patients are prescribed a combination of an inhaled regimen of ipratropium and one of the β_2-adrenergic agonists.

The methylxanthine derivatives, such as theophylline and aminophylline, are another type of bronchodilator. They are considered less effective than the β_2-adrenergic agonists. These drugs are taken orally or intravenously but not by inhalation. An example of standard theophyllines for oral administration is *Elixophyllin*, which must be taken about four times a day. Sustained-release (SR) theophylline products that allow once- or twice-daily administration are available, including *Theo-24* and *Uniphyl*. Remember, the SR products should never be crushed to give the drug. Crushing would cause toxic effects because too much of the drug would be absorbed at one time.

Leukotriene receptor antagonists reduce airway edema, smooth muscle contractions, and inflammation in asthma. An example is montelukast (*Singulair*). Fluticasone/salmeterol (*Advair Diskus*) is an inhaler used to treat asthma and COPD. It should be used only when other medicines fail to control the asthma. Then they are used for long-term maintenance for asthma. Bronchodilators are given by inhalation or orally, depending on the drug (and by injection in some emergencies). Besides dilating the bronchioles, these drugs have other effects, such as stimulating the heart and respiration and stopping the release of histamine. For this reason, some of these drugs are used in emergency treatment of cardiac arrest and allergic reactions. They must be used with great care, in the proper dosages, and with close attention to side effects. Epinephrine, for example, can cause anxiety, restlessness, dizziness, weakness, pallor (pale skin), palpitations, and breathing difficulty. Patients can develop tolerance to bronchodilators, and rebound effects are also possible.

Drugs for the respiratory system are often given in combination. For example, a medicine might contain a bronchodilator to open the air passages and an expectorant to loosen the sputum so that it can be coughed up. Many cold remedies are combinations of antitussives, expectorants, and decongestants. The combination of elixir of terpin hydrate and codeine, for example, has an antitussive and expectorant action. Popular product-name remedies for allergies and colds combine antihistamines with decongestants, expectorants, and antitussives—for example, *Allegra-D 12 Hour Allergy and Congestion, Claritin-D 12 Hour, Children's Dimetapp Cold and Allergy,* and promethazine/codeine.

Other drugs often used for the treatment of respiratory diseases include cromolyn and corticosteroids. Cromolyn sodium (*Intal*) is classified as a mast cell stabilizer. These drugs act locally to inhibit the degranulation of sensitized mast cells after exposure to certain antigens. They prevent the release of histamine.

Corticosteroids are potent anti-inflammatory drugs that can help control severe asthma. When administered via inhalation, steroid activity can be provided at the needed site while minimizing systemic effects. Some examples of inhaled corticosteroids are beclomethasone, triamcinolone, flunisolide and fluticasone (*Flonase Allergy Relief*).

The Representative Drugs table at the end of this chapter lists uses, side effects, dosages, and special instructions for representative drugs used in treating respiratory disorders.

Pediatric Considerations Bronchodilators and Antiasthmatics

- Antiasthmatics are used for children much as they are for adults.
- Bronchodilators are given depending on the child's age and specific drug formulations.
- Oral drugs may be given to children as young as 2 years of age.
- Use caution with theophylline. Avoid using it for premature infants.

- Children ages 6 months to 16 years metabolize theophylline more rapidly and may need higher doses than adults.
- Long-acting theophylline is not recommended. Hyperactivity may occur because of the CNS effects.

 Older Adult Considerations Bronchodilators and Antiasthmatics

- Bronchodilators and antiasthmatics are frequently given for chronic pulmonary disorders.
- Give these drugs by inhalation because of a lower risk of side effects. Major side effects are cardiac and CNS stimulation.
- Although theophylline is given, its effects are unpredictable in older adults.

- Smoking and drugs such as phenobarbital and phenytoin (*Dilantin*) may increase metabolism and the dose requirements of theophylline.
- Drugs such as cimetidine (*Tagamet HB*) and erythromycin may decrease metabolism and, as a result, require a decrease in dose.

GIVING RESPIRATORY DRUGS [LO 11-5]

The goals of therapy in respiratory diseases are to control the rate and depth of breathing, to remove anything that may be blocking the air passages, and to clear out sputum so that it does not lead to infection. Drugs are only one part of the treatment; other important parts are to remove the source of irritation, such as having the patient stop smoking and avoid allergens, and to use physical techniques that promote normal mucous drainage and breathing.

You may be called on to assist in one of the three chest physiotherapy procedures when you administer medications to respiratory patients. Oxygen inhalation therapy may be ordered to prevent or relieve hypoxia. A ventilator may be needed to help the patient breathe regularly by mechanical means. **Postural drainage** may be ordered. The postural drainage technique consists of placing the patient in one of several positions so that gravity helps draw secretions from certain areas of the lungs and bronchi into the trachea.

Percussion is another technique for loosening clogged mucus. It involves striking the chest wall over the area being drained. Percussion is usually combined with postural drainage. Percussion is performed over a single layer of clothing but not over buttons or zippers. The single layer of clothing protects the patient's skin, but the buttons or zippers would potentially bruise the skin. Sometimes patients have to be encouraged to cough, even if it hurts, so that excess mucus does not build up in the lungs.

The third type of chest physiotherapy is **vibration**, a fine shaking pressure applied to the chest wall during exhalation. It increases the amount of air exhaled and may loosen mucus and promote a cough.

Psychological factors are important when you are administering respiratory medications. A patient who is unable to breathe properly feels threatened and frightened. But difficulty in breathing is exactly what happens with diseases of the respiratory tract, even the common cold. Patients need a calm and supportive environment.

With respiratory medications, it is especially important to watch the patient's symptoms closely. Each time you are with the patient, make a note of the rate and depth of breathing. This helps you decide which PRN drugs are needed, if any, or whether new drugs need to be ordered. Observe the following:

- Has the patient's breathing changed since you last saw him or her?
- Has the patient's respiration rate increased?
- Is it hard for the patient to take in a breath?

You can tell by looking at the patient's chest whether the soft tissues of the chest are retracting with each breath. Holding the mouth open while breathing, spreading the nostrils, and wheezing are other signs of respiratory problems. Some signs are so subtle that the patient may not be aware of them. Does the patient move more slowly, get excited easily, or have muscle twitches? Even stomach movements or changed speech patterns can be clues to the need for respiratory medications. You should always chart your observations.

Clinical Considerations

There are ways you can make respiratory medications work better and help patients breathe. Here are a few suggestions:

- Explain the effects of the drugs and the breathing exercises that are part of patients' treatment. The instructions that come with the drugs will help you.
- Assist patients into sitting or leaning positions. These positions allow the lungs to expand fully.
- Give drugs on time. Many respiratory drugs are ordered just before busy times of the day to prevent the fatigue that comes with extra activity. When getting a breath of air is an effort, any added activity can be tiring.
- Remove mucus from the nose and throat (Figure 11.4). Encourage the patient to cough. Regardless of the number of respiratory drugs a patient is taking, mucus in the respiratory tract can still prevent proper air exchange.

Figure 11.4

When a patient has a respiratory disorder, it is sometimes necessary to suction mucus from the throat and nose.

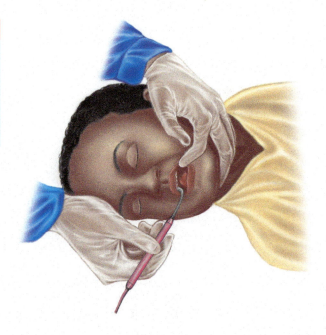

- Ask the patient to let you know whenever breathing begins to get difficult. Catching a problem early makes drug treatment more effective.

- Do not rush the patient while giving drugs. Rushing increases anxiety when the patient is already anxious because of the effort of catching a breath.

- Give the proper amounts of fluids (e.g., juice, water) with respiratory medications. Expectorants and antitussives should be given with extra fluids. Fluids help thin out respiratory secretions so that they can be coughed up and eliminated. Do not give fluids with soothing syrups (demulcents), because they are designed to coat the respiratory tract.

- If a patient has an unproductive cough, remove irritating fumes, dust, and smoke. Provide hard candy or a demulcent to get rid of tickling in the throat.

- Add moisture to the air with a humidifier. Dry mucous membranes can become irritated and are more prone to infection.

- Remember that some respiratory drugs, especially antihistamines, may cause drowsiness. Warn patients not to drive a car or operate heavy equipment while taking them. This is true of many OTC products as well as prescription drugs. Some providers avoid antihistamines because they tend to dry secretions, causing dry mouth and urinary retention.

- Instruct the family on taking measures to assist the patient's breathing. Well-informed family members can encourage a patient to cooperate in treatment.

Respiratory Therapy

Many patients with lung disorders are treated with some form of respiratory therapy. They inhale drugs such as bronchodilators, **mucolytics** (drugs that liquefy or break down tenacious mucus so that it can be coughed up more easily), corticosteroids, and antibiotics from machines that produce mist containing tiny droplets of medication.

Drugs inhaled as a mist through a **nebulizer,** a small machine used to convert a drug solution into a mist, are able to travel deep into the lungs. They are absorbed directly through the linings of the respiratory tract or through the alveoli, depending on the size of the droplets. Drugs that are absorbed by the alveoli have a rapid systemic effect because of the richness of the blood supply. Drug absorption through the linings of the respiratory tract is like that of topical applications to mucous membranes.

Breathing treatments may be delivered to patients via pocket-size, handheld **inhalers**. Because this therapy is self-administered, it is important to teach patients how to use the inhaler properly. (See Practice Procedure 11.4 later in the chapter.)

Order of Administration. Many patients are prescribed more than one drug for inhalation. When this is the case, there is a preferred order in which the drugs should be taken. Inhaled drugs should be given in this order: (1) beta-agonist [metaproterenol or albuterol (*Proventil HFA*)]; (2) anticholinergic [ipratropium (*Atrovent HFA*)]; (3) corticosteroid [beclomethasone (*Beconase AQ*), triamcinolone or flunisolide].

Use of Oxygen

Oxygen is a gas that is essential for life. It is colorless, odorless, and tasteless. Although it is not flammable, it is combustible. Without oxygen, cells die within a few minutes. Lack of oxygen is called **hypoxia**. Symptoms of hypoxia are anxiety, cyanosis, pale and cold extremities, and dyspnea. The goal of oxygen therapy is to relieve hypoxia and maximize the blood's oxygen-carrying ability.

Too much oxygen, generally 100 percent for more than 6 hours, leads to oxygen toxicity. Consistently high levels of oxygen inactivate the pulmonary surfactant and lead to acute respiratory distress syndrome. Careful assessment of the patient's needs can prevent oxygen toxicity. Symptoms of oxygen toxicity are chest pain; nausea and vomiting; malaise; fatigue; nasal stuffiness; sore throat; dry, hacking cough; and numbness and tingling of the extremities.

Oxygen should be considered a drug and should be prescribed and administered as such. There must be specific written orders for the flow rate and the method of administration. The initial dose, as well as any changes in administration and dose, including discontinuation, should be based on blood gas analysis or pulse oximetry. Pulse oximetry allows indirect measurement of the blood's oxygen content. A probe with a light and a sensor is attached to the bridge of the nose, an ear, or a fingertip. A reading occurs within 10 to 30 seconds. It emits one red and one infrared light wavelength. A light-emitting diode positioned on one side of the probe is sent to a photodetector placed on the opposite side. The probes project light differently for oxygenated versus deoxygenated blood. SpO_2 is used to indicate the oxygen saturation value determined by the pulse oximeter. The pulse oximeter is attached to a monitor that displays the SpO_2 and heart rate. A normal SpO_2 is equal to or greater than 97 percent. Oxygen therapy parameters vary, but in most cases, oxygen therapy will be administered when the SpO_2 is less than 90 percent. Pulse oximetry is particularly useful in intensive care units and perioperative areas, during exercise testing, and for monitoring or adjusting oxygen flow rates during long-term oxygen therapy (Figure 11.5).

Methods of administering oxygen include the nasal cannula, nasal catheter, oxygen mask, and possibly an oxygen tent or a face tent (Figure 11.6). In some situations, incubators or respirators may be used. An oxygen tent is used mainly with children or with patients who will not tolerate other modes of administration. To prevent dryness of the nose and throat, sterile distilled water is added to the humidifying device. Because oxygen is a dry gas, adequate humidity is crucial. You must take care to keep combustible materials away from the area where oxygen is being used. These include woolen blankets, clothing, and electrical equipment. And, of course, no one should smoke near oxygen equipment or use petroleum-based products such as certain lip balms.

Oxygen therapy is never ended abruptly. You must gradually wean the patient by alternating periods of oxygen-supplemented inspiration with periods of breathing without the oxygen.

Figure 11.5

A pulse oximeter.

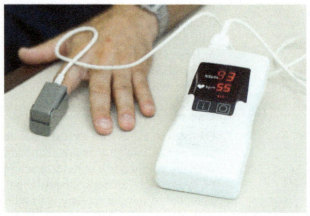

©choja/iStock/Getty Images

Figure 11.6

An oxygen mask is one method of administering oxygen.

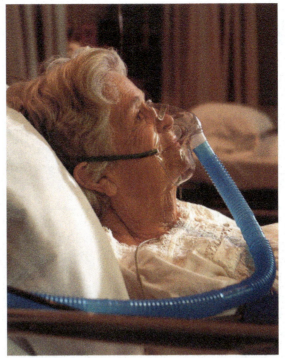

©John Foxx/Getty Images

Direct Applications, Sprays, and Nose Drops

Drugs may be painted, sprayed, or dropped onto the mucous membranes of the mouth, nose, and throat. They penetrate directly into the linings of the respiratory tract, but they treat only the sprayed area rather than traveling into the lungs. These topical applications are useful for localized inflammations and for symptoms such as sinus infections, stuffy nose, injuries of the mucous membranes, and sore throat. Decongestants, for example, may often be sprayed or dropped into the nasal cavities to reduce swelling so the patient can breathe more easily (**Figure 11.7**).

Nose drops should not be swallowed, because they are meant to give a local rather than a systemic effect. The dropper should be rinsed with hot water after use to avoid spreading germs to the medicine bottle.

Figure 11.7

Decongestants are sprayed into the nasal cavity to reduce swelling.

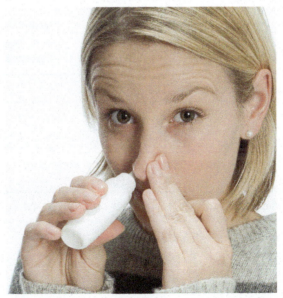

©Image Source

Healthcare for Today and Tomorrow | Pneumococcal Vaccine

Pneumococcal disease is a serious disease that leads to infections of the lungs (pneumonia), the blood (bacteremia), and the covering of the brain (meningitis). This disease kills more people in the United States every year than any other vaccine-preventable disease. Drugs such as penicillin were once effective in the treatment of pneumococcal disease, but over the years the disease has become resistant to medication therapy, making the treatment very difficult. As a result of medication-resistant strains of the disease and the high mortality rate, it is very important that you encourage your patients under 2 years and over 65 years of age, and those with certain risk factors, to get the vaccine to prevent this deadly disease.

 Legal and Ethical Issues | Influenza Vaccine

The federal Centers for Disease Control and Prevention (CDC) estimates that as many as 20,000 people may die annually from influenza, a serious respiratory virus that strikes from November through April. The CDC recommendations for flu vaccination can change annually. In some years, all individuals over the age of 6 months are recommended to take the flu vaccine. In some years when there is a shortage of the vaccine, people with priority include those between the ages of 6 months and 4 years and those over the age of 50. Also, included are those with weakened immune systems of chronic diseases of the heart, lungs, or kidneys; pregnant women; and healthcare workers.

As a healthcare team member, you should understand that a vaccine, like any medication, is capable of causing serious side effects such as an allergic reaction. Therefore, it is your responsibility to ask about any allergies and monitor the patient for an allergic reaction. In the past, the flu vaccine has been contraindicated in those with an egg allergy, but now only those with severe egg allergies should be monitored in a medical setting. Check your facility protocol regarding administration of the flu vaccine to individuals with a severe egg allergy.

Representative Drugs for the Respiratory System

Category, Name,[a] and Route	Uses and Diseases	Actions	Usual Dose[b] and Special Instructions	Side Effects and Adverse Reactions
Antitussives/Expectorants				
Narcotic codeine Oral	Antitussive	Suppresses cough; Schedule II controlled substance	10–20 mg every 4–6 hours; do not exceed 120 mg in 24 hours	Nausea, vomiting, constipation, dizziness, palpitations, drowsiness, sedation
Nonnarcotic dextromethorphan (*Delysm, Robitussin 12 Hour Cough Relief*) Oral	Suppression of unproductive cough or cough at bedtime	Inhibits cough reflex	10–20 mg every 4 hours prn	Drowsiness, dizziness, nausea, vomiting

Representative Drugs for the Respiratory System (continued)

Category, Name,[a] and Route	Uses and Diseases	Actions	Usual Dose[b] and Special Instructions	Side Effects and Adverse Reactions
Antitussives/Expectorants (continued)				
acetylcysteine Inhalant	As ancillary therapy for patients with abnormal, viscid (thick) mucous secretions	Lowers viscosity of mucus	3–5 mL of a 20% solution or 6–10 mL of a 10% solution inhaled tid or qid	Stomatitis, nausea, vomiting, drowsiness, rhinorrhea
Decongestants				
phenylephrine Oral	Nasal congestion	Shrinks engorged mucous membranes	10 mg by mouth every 4 hours as needed	Burning, stinging, sneezing, dryness of nasal mucosa
Antihistamines				
cetirizine (*Zyrtec Allergy*) Oral	Seasonal allergic rhinitis due to ragweed, grass, and tree pollens; perennial rhinitis due to dust mites, animal dander, and molds; chronic idiopathic urticaria	Potent H_1-histamine receptor antagonist; mild bronchodilator effect	5–10 mg daily	Somnolence, dry mouth, fatigue, pharyngitis, dizziness
fexofenadine (*Allegra Allergy 24 Hour*) Oral	Seasonal allergic rhinitis; skin manifestations in chronic idiopathic urticaria	Acts as potent H_1-histamine receptor antagonist	60 mg bid or 180 mg daily	Drowsiness, fatigue, headache, nausea, dyspepsia, sinusitis, throat irritation, pharyngitis
promethazine Oral	Allergic rhinitis, pruritus	Provides antihistaminic action	25 mg at bedtime or 12.5 mg before meals and at bedtime	Sedation, drowsiness, blurred vision, dryness of mouth, possible confusion, hypotension, urinary retention
chlorpheniramine Oral	Rhinitis, allergy symptoms	Provides antihistaminic action	2–4 mg every 4–6 hours	Dryness of mouth, drowsiness, dizziness, nausea, urinary retention
Bronchodilators and Antiasthmatics				
montelukast (*Singulair*) Oral	Asthma, seasonal rhinitis	Is a leukotriene receptor antagonist that relieves edema, smooth muscle contraction, and inflammation	10 mg daily	Dyspepsia, infectious gastroenteritis, abdominal pain, dental pain, headache, dizziness, asthenia, fatigue

Representative Drugs for the Respiratory System (continued)

Category, Name,[a] and Route	Uses and Diseases	Actions	Usual Dose[b] and Special Instructions	Side Effects and Adverse Reactions
Bronchodilators and Antiasthmatics (continued)				
fluticasone/ salmeterol (*Advair Diskus*) Inhaler	Asthma, COPD	Acts as potent anti-inflammatory long-acting β_2-adrenergic agonist	100/50 bid (asthma); 250/50 bid (COPD); use only if other medications fail to control the asthma	FDA issued a warning of possible increased asthma-related death; ear, nose, throat, and respiratory infections; pharyngitis; sinusitis; hoarseness/dysphonia; oral candidiasis; bronchitis; cough; headache; nausea; vomiting; abdominal discomfort; diarrhea; musculoskeletal pain
Methylxanthine Derivatives theophylline (*Elixophyllin*) Oral	Bronchial asthma, bronchitis, emphysema	Relaxes smooth muscle of bronchioles, increases mucociliary clearance	330–660 mg po every 6–8 hours; give oral form with full glass of water; should be given with food to avoid upset stomach; do not crush sustained-release tablets	Headache, dizziness, restlessness, nausea, vomiting, insomnia, tachycardia, irritability, palpitations
β_2-Adrenergic Agonists albuterol (*Proventil HFA, Ventolin HFA*) Oral, inhalation	Asthma, bronchitis	Provides bronchodilation	*Oral:* 2–4 mg tid or qid, not to exceed 32 mg daily *Inhalation:* 4–6 times daily; start with one inhalation, following with second inhalation in 3–5 minutes if no relief Rinse mouth with water between doses to prevent throat irritation and cough	Tremor, anxiety, nervousness, restlessness
epinephrine (*Primatene Mist*) Inhalation	Bronchodilation	Relaxes smooth muscles of bronchioles, increases mucociliary clearance	1 inhalation, wait at least 1 minute; if not relieved, use once more; do not repeat for at least 4 hours; if still no relief, call provider	Nervousness, headache, restlessness, palpitations, tachycardia

Category, Name,[a] and Route	Uses and Diseases	Actions	Usual Dose[b] and Special Instructions	Side Effects and Adverse Reactions
Antitubercular Drugs				
isoniazid Oral, IM	Treatment and prevention of tuberculosis	Is bactericidal; interferes with lipid and DNA synthesis	5 mg po or IM daily in active TB; 300 mg once daily; used for 1 year alone for TB prevention; used in conjunction with effective agents, rifampin and ethambutol for active TB	Peripheral neuropathy is most common adverse effect (treated with vitamin B_6); nausea, vomiting, and epigastric distress; hepatitis
rifampin (*Rifadin*) Oral	Treatment of tuberculosis and for carriers of meningitis	Is a broad-spectrum bactericidal antibiotic that inhibits RNA	600 mg once daily	Hepatotoxicity, flulike symptoms, drowsiness, epigastric distress

Note: Bolded trade names are among the 50 most commonly prescribed drugs.

[a]*Trade names given in parentheses are examples only. Check current drug references for a complete listing of available products.*

[b]*Average adult doses are given. However, dosages are determined by a provider and vary with the purpose of the therapy and the particular patient. The doses presented in this text are for general information only.*

Practice Procedure 11.1 (LO 11-5)

SPRAYING MEDICATION ONTO MUCOUS MEMBRANES OF THE MOUTH OR THROAT

Demonstrate spraying a medication onto the mucous membranes of the mouth or throat.

Equipment

Provider's medication order or medication administration record

Medication in atomizer, plastic spray bottle, or tube applicator

Flashlight, tongue blade, and cotton-tipped applicator

Medication tray or cart with appropriate chart or record

Procedure

1. Set up medications. Check for the "seven rights."

2. Wash your hands.

3. Identify the patient, explain the procedure, and assist the patient into a position for medication administration (either sitting up or lying down).

4. Apply medication as follows:
   - Tilt the head backward and open the mouth.
   - Locate the affected area visually. Use a tongue blade and small flashlight to find the area.
   - Spray the medication directly on the affected area.

5. Assist the patient back into a comfortable position.

6. Instruct the patient not to eat or drink for a certain period of time. Allow the patient to gargle with a mouthwash after a sufficient period of time for absorption (at least 15 minutes).

7. Chart the administration of medication.

8. Wash your hands.

9. Return equipment and chart to the proper location.

Practice Procedure 11.2 (LO 11-7)

INSTILLING NOSE DROPS

Demonstrate administering nose drops to a patient and instructing the patient about the process.

Equipment

Medication orders for nose drops

Medication administration record

Nose drops

Cart or tray with appropriate chart or record

Tissue wipes

Nonsterile gloves

Procedure

1. Set up medications. Check for the "seven rights."

2. Wash your hands.

3. Identify the patient. Explain the procedure. Warm the nose drops to body temperature by holding them in your hand or placing them in a bowl of warm water.

4. Instruct the patient to blow the nose to remove mucus and secretions that can block distribution of the medication.

5. Instruct the patient to assume a supine position for administration. For nose drops, the patient should lie on the back, with the head extended beyond the edge of the bed or with a pillow under the shoulders. Support the head with your hand to avoid straining the neck muscles. The head should be tilted back at a right angle to the body (**Figure 11.8**).

6. Instruct the patient on the correct administration of nose drops:
   - Measure the correct dosage on the marked dropper.
   - Hold the dropper $\frac{1}{2}$ inch above the nares.
   - Put on nonsterile gloves.
   - Instill the prescribed number of drops toward the midline of the ethmoid bone, which makes up the upper part of the nasal septum, to facilitate even distribution over the nasal mucosa. Repeat with the other nostril, if ordered.
   - Instruct the patient to stay in the supine position for at least 5 minutes to prevent loss of medication through the nares.
   - Give tissue wipes to blot any flow from the nose. Instruct the patient to avoid blowing the nose for several minutes.

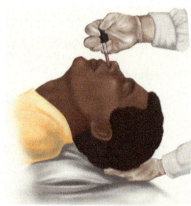

Figure 11.8

Instilling nose drops.

7. Give further instructions to the patient according to the package directions or the provider's orders.

8. Chart the medication administration, including whether you treated one or both nostrils.

9. Wash your hands.

10. Return equipment and chart to the proper location.

Practice Procedure 11.3 (LO 11-5)

USING A NASAL SPRAY

Demonstrate how to teach a patient to use a nasal spray.

Equipment

Medication orders for nasal spray

Medication administration record

Nasal spray

Cart or tray with appropriate chart or record

Tissue wipes

Procedure

1. Set up medications. Check for the "seven rights."

2. Wash your hands.

3. Identify the patient. Explain the procedure.

4. Instruct the patient on the proper position for administration. For the nasal spray, the patient should be in a sitting position.

5. Teach the patient correct administration of the nasal spray:
   - Instruct the patient to breathe through the nose with the mouth open. The patient must breathe this way as the medication is administered.
   - Instruct the patient to place the tip of the bottle at the opening of the nose, taking care not to touch the mucous membrane.
   - Tell the patient to take a deep breath and, at this time, spray the bottle two or three times quickly.
   - Wipe any excess medication from the nose.

6. Give further instructions to the patient according to the package directions or the provider's orders.

7. Chart the medication administration.

8. Wash your hands.

9. Return equipment to the proper location.

Practice Procedure 11.4 (LO 11-5)

ORAL INHALATION OF METERED-DOSE INHALANT

Demonstrate how to teach a patient to administer an oral inhalation from a metered-dose inhaler.

Equipment

Provider's medication order, medicine administration record

Medication in metered-dose inhaler

Medication tray, cart, or equipment with appropriate chart and record

Procedure

1. Set up medications. Check for the "seven rights."

2. Wash your hands.

3. Identify the patient, explain the procedure, and assist the patient into a position for medication administration (either sitting up or lying down).

4. Apply medication as follows:
   - Shake the inhaler.
   - Hold the inhaler upright.
   - Instruct the patient to tilt the head back and breathe out.
   - Instruct the patient to position the inhaler in one of two ways:
     (a) Tell the patient to open the mouth, with the inhaler 1 to 2 inches away. The patient may attach a spacer to the mouthpiece of the inhaler. (A spacer is a device that traps the medication released from the inhaler. The patient then inhales the drug from the spacer. Spacers deposit 80 percent of the medication in the lungs instead of in the oropharynx. Spacers are especially effective for patients who have trouble learning the correct way to use an inhaler and for weak or older adult patients.)
     (b) Instruct the patient to place the mouthpiece of the inhaler or spacer in the mouth.
   - Tell the patient to press down on the inhaler while inhaling.
   - Tell the patient to breathe in slowly for 2 to 3 seconds and hold the breath for 10 seconds.
   - Wait 1 minute before administering additional puffs.

5. If two inhaled medications are ordered, wait 5 to 10 minutes between inhalations.

6. If both a bronchodilator and an inhaled steroid are ordered, the bronchodilator should be administered first so that the passages will be more open for the second medication.

7. Assist the patient back into a comfortable position.

8. Instruct the patient to rinse the mouth and throat with a drink of water and spit it out and also to clean the inhaler mouthpiece.

9. Chart the administration of medications.

10. Wash your hands.

11. Return equipment and chart to the proper location.

Practice Procedure 11.5 (LO 11-5)

ADMINISTERING OXYGEN BY MASK

Demonstrate how to administer oxygen by mask to a patient and regulate the flow rate.

Equipment

Provider's order and appropriate charting record

Oxygen (tank or wall oxygen outlet system)

Humidifier equipment as ordered

Mask as ordered (Figure 11.9)

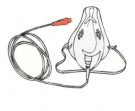 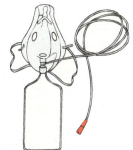 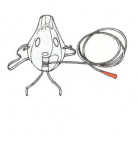 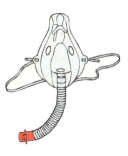

Simple face mask
(Low-flow system)

Partial rebreather mask
(Low-flow system)

Nonrebreather mask
(Low-flow system)

Venturi mask
(High-flow system)

Figure 11.9

Masks for oxygen administration.

Equipment	Percentage Oxygen	Flow Rate
Simple face mask	40–60%	Low flow: 2–3 liters/min
Partial rebreather mask	60–90%	Low flow: 6–10 liters/min
Nonrebreather mask	80–95%	Low flow: 10 liters/min
Venturi mask	24–50%	High flow: 4, 6, 8, 10 liters/min
Face tent with Venturi mask	30–55%	High flow: 4–8 liters/min

Procedure

1. Set up oxygen equipment.

2. Wash your hands.

3. Identify the patient and explain the procedure.

4. Assist the patient into an appropriate position (**semi-Fowler's position**—the patient's upper body is elevated to 30 degrees—or **Fowler's position**—45 to 60 degrees).

5. Inflate one-half of a rebreather bag with oxygen. (The rebreather bag conserves oxygen.)

6. Place the top of the mask over the nose and then over the mouth.

7. Mold the mask to the face so that oxygen does not escape from it.

8. Adjust the oxygen flow rate as ordered.

9. After 30 minutes, check the flow rate and rebreather bag.

10. Chart the procedure.

Practice Procedure 11.6 (LO 11-5)

ADMINISTERING OXYGEN BY CANNULA

Demonstrate how to administer oxygen by cannula to a patient and regulate the flow rate.

Equipment

Provider's order

Oxygen (tank or wall oxygen outlet system)

Humidifier equipment as ordered

Paper tape

Gauze pads (2 × 2)

Nonsterile gloves

Cannula (**Figure 11.10**)

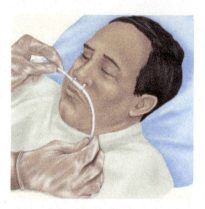

Procedure

1. Set up oxygen supply equipment.

2. Wash your hands.

3. Put on nonsterile gloves.

4. Identify the patient and explain the procedure.

5. Assist the patient into a semi-Fowler's or Fowler's position.

6. Adjust oxygen flow rate as ordered (usually 1 to 6 liters/min of a 23 to 40 percent concentration of oxygen for the cannula).

7. Check the tubing to be sure it is not twisted.

8. Place your fingertips near the opening of the cannula to check for oxygen flow.

9. Turn the nasal prongs upward and curved toward the tip of the nose.

10. Place one prong in each nostril.

11. Place tubing from the prongs over the ears.

12. Pull remainder of the tubing under the patient's chin and tighten at "Y."

13. Ask the patient if the tubing is comfortable.

14. Tape the tubing in place on the cheeks if necessary.

15. Place gauze pads under the tubing going over the ears if necessary.

16. After 30 minutes, check flow rate and humidifier water level.

17. Chart the procedure.

Correctly demonstrate administering and regulating oxygen by mask to a patient.

Practice Procedure 11.7 (LO 11-5)

ADMINISTERING OXYGEN BY NASAL CATHETER

Demonstrate how to apply oxygen by nasal catheter to a patient and regulate the flow rate.

Equipment

Provider's order and appropriate charting record

Oxygen (tank or wall oxygen outlet system)

Humidifier equipment as ordered

Paper tape

Gauze pads (2 × 2)

Lubricating (water-soluble) jelly

Flashlight

Tongue blade

Figure 11.11

Nasal catheter for oxygen administration.

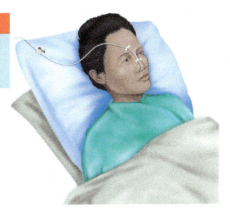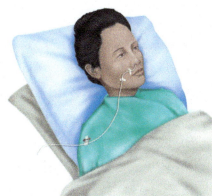

Container of sterile water

Nasal catheter as ordered for an adult or child (Figure 11.11)

Nonsterile gloves

Procedure

1. Set up oxygen equipment.

2. Wash your hands.

3. Put on nonsterile gloves.

4. Identify the patient and explain the procedure.

5. Assist the patient into a semi-Fowler's or Fowler's position.

6. Lubricate the catheter with water-soluble lubricating jelly.

7. Pass the catheter through the nose until the tip is just above the epiglottis.

8. Do not insert the catheter too far, or the patient will swallow air.

9. Tape the catheter to the forehead or nose.

10. Turn on oxygen at the ordered slow rate flow (commonly 4 to 8 liters/min of a 25 to 40 percent concentration of oxygen).

11. After 30 minutes, check the flow rate and humidifier water level.

12. Chart the procedure.

Summary

Learning Outcome	Summary Points
11-1 Describe the parts and normal functions of the respiratory system.	• The respiratory system consists of these parts: nose, pharynx, larynx, trachea, bronchi, lungs. • These organs make it possible for blood to exchange gases with air. • The normal respiration rate for an adult is 18 times per minute (may range between 12 and 25 times per minute).

Learning Outcome	Summary Points

11-2 Describe the major respiratory disorders and related symptoms, using the correct medical terms.	• Symptoms of respiratory disorders:
	  • *Coughing:* protective reflex to clear the trachea, bronchi, and lungs of secretions and irritants.
	  • *Sputum:* secretions brought up by coughing.
	  • *Hemoptysis:* spitting up of blood.
	  • *Hoarseness:* roughness in voice when talking.
	  • *Wheezing:* high-pitched, musical sound that occurs throughout a narrowed airway.
	  • *Chest pain:* pain in the chest area.
	  • *Dyspnea:* shortness of breath or labored breathing.
	  • *Tachypnea:* rapid breathing.
	  • *Apnea:* cessation of breathing.
	  • *Hyperpnea:* hyperventilation.
	  • *Orthopnea:* condition in which the patient must sit or stand to breathe deeply and comfortably.
	• Descriptions of major respiratory disorders:
	  • *Pneumonia* is an infection of the lower respiratory tract (bronchi, bronchioles, and alveoli).
	  • *Bronchitis* is an inflammation of the air passageways that is caused by irritants such as smoke or chemicals, allergic reactions, flu, or viruses.
	  • *Emphysema* is the result of enlargement of and damage to alveolar sacs. The surface of the alveoli is reduced and limits the exchange of oxygen and carbon dioxide.
	  • *Pleurisy* is an inflammation of the linings of the lungs and lung cavities.
	  • *Asthma* is characterized by airway obstruction, inflammation, and increased response to stimuli.
	  • *Cancer* of the respiratory system includes cancers of the head and neck.
	  • *Pulmonary embolism* is a sudden, unexplained dyspnea, tachypnea, or tachycardia that begins as a thrombus deep in the vein in the leg.
	  • *Tuberculosis* is an infectious disease caused by *Mycobacterium tuberculosis.*
	  • *Inflammations* of the nose, sinuses, and throat include rhinitis (inflammation of the nasal passageways), sinusitis (inflammation of the sinuses), and strep throat (strep infection of the throat).

11-3 Describe nicotine dependency and methods for smoking cessation.	• *Nicotine dependency* is a physical vulnerability of the body to the chemical nicotine from the use of tobacco products. • *Smoking cessation* occurs with nicotine replacement therapy and nonnicotine medications.
11-4 Describe the actions of the following drug groups: antitussives, expectorants, decongestants, antihistamines, and bronchodilators.	• *Antitussives* are cough suppressants. Dextromethorphan (*Children's Dimetapp Cold and Allergy*) is an example. • *Expectorants* (mucolytics) have a disintegrating effect on mucus. An example is acetylcysteine. • *Decongestants* are vasoconstrictors that reduce nasal congestion. An example is oxymetazoline (*Afrin*). • *Antihistamines* work against the effects of histamine and are used to relieve allergy symptoms. An example is diphenhydramine (*Benadryl Allergy*). • *Bronchodilators* cause the bronchioles to relax and expand (dilate). An example is albuterol (*Proventil HFA*).

Learning Outcome	Summary Points
11-5 Understand the procedures of chest physiotherapy; operating a pulse oximeter; and administering nose drops, inhalants, and oxygen.	• Chest physiotherapy procedures are: • *Postural drainage* consists of placing the patient in a position that enables gravity to help draw secretions from the lungs into the trachea. • *Percussion* involves striking the chest wall over the area to be drained. • *Vibration* is a fine shaking pressure applied to the chest wall during exhalation. • A pulse oximeter allows indirect measurement of the blood's oxygen content. • A reading occurs within 10 to 30 seconds after a probe with a light and a sensor is attached to the bridge of the nose, an ear, or a fingertip. • *Nose drops:* After the supine client blows the nose, and nose drops are measured in the dropper, hold the dropper $\frac{1}{2}$ inch above the nares and instill the number of drops toward the midline of the ethmoid bone. • *Inhalants:* Hold the inhaler upright and instruct the patient to tilt back the head and breathe out. Have the patient open the mouth, with the inhaler 1 to 2 inches away. The patient may use a spacer. Have the patient push the button to deliver the dose while inhaling. The patient should breathe in for 2 to 3 seconds and hold the breath. Wait 5 to 10 minutes between inhalations if two are ordered. • For oxygen through a nasal catheter, place the patient in a Fowler's or semi-Fowler's position, lubricate the catheter, and pass it through the nose until the tip is just above the epiglottis. Tape the catheter to the forehead or nose. • Other oxygen administration methods include via mask and cannula.

Chapter 11 Review

Define each of the terms listed.

1. (LO 11-2) Pulmonary _____

2. (LO 11-2) Dyspnea _____

3. (LO 11-2) Tachypnea _____

4. (LO 11-2) Apnea _____

5. (LO 11-2) Hyperpnea _____

6. (LO 11-2) Orthopnea _____

7. (LO 11-2) Pleura _____

8. (LO 11-6) Rebound effect _____

9. (LO 11-2) Peak flow meter _____

10. (LO 11-3) Nicotine dependence _____

Complete the statements by filling in the blank.

11. (LO 11-1) Inhaling and exhaling air so that gases can be exchanged in the lungs is called _____ _____.

12. (LO 11-1) The normal respiratory rate is _____ _____.

13. (LO 11-1) The part of the respiratory system that produces speech sounds is called the _____ _____.

14. (LO 11-1) The flap of tissue that keeps food from going down into the lungs when it is swallowed is the _____ _____.

15. (LO 11-1) The tube that leads to the lungs and is known as the windpipe is the _____ _____.

16. (LO 11-2) Coughing is important for maintaining a patient's airway because _____ _____.

17. (LO 11-1) The tiny sacs where gases are exchanged between the blood and inspired air are the _____ _____.

18. (LO 11-2) The instrument used to listen to breathing sounds is the _____ _____.

19. (LO 11-5) A handheld device that produces a drug mist for inhalation is called a(n) _____ _____.

20. (LO 11-2) A device that monitors the oxygen saturation by means of a probe on the finger, toe, ear, forehead, or bridge of the nose is called a(n) _____ _____.

21. (LO 11-4) The law that regulates the sale of pseudoephedrine and ephedrine is _____ _____.

Tell what these types of drugs do; for example, *Demulcents coat mucous membranes and soothe irritation that causes coughing.*

22. (LO 11-4) Antitussives _____

23. (LO 11-4) Mucolytics _____

24. (LO 11-4) Decongestants _____

Match the drug categories to the drug names.

_____ 25. (LO 11-4) *Afrin*

_____ 26. (LO 11-4) *Benadryl Allergy,* chlorpheniramine, cyproheptadine

_____ 27. (LO 11-4) Isoniazid, ethambutol, rifampin, rifapentine

_____ 28. (LO 11-4) theophylline

a. decongestants

b. tuberculosis drugs

c. bronchodilators

d. antihistamines

Match the treatments to their descriptions.

_____ 29. (LO 11-5) Positioning the patient so that clogged mucus is drawn out by gravity

_____ 30. (LO 11-5) Clapping the patient's chest or back to loosen mucus

_____ 31. (LO 11-5) Machine that helps a patient breathe by artificial means

_____ 32. (LO 11-5) Device that produces a mist for inhalation

_____ 33. (LO 11-4) May cause drowsiness as a side effect

a. antihistamines

b. inhaler

c. percussion

d. postural drainage

e. ventilator

Drug Calculations—Fill in the blank with the answer.

34. (LO 11-4) The provider orders amoxicillin suspension 500 mg orally bid. Available is 400 mg/5 mL. Prepare to give your patient _____ mL.

35. (LO 11-4) The provider orders cefadroxil 0.5 g orally bid. Available are 500-mg tablets. You will give your patient _____ tablets.

36. (LO 11-4) The provider orders amoxicillin/clavulanate potassium (*Augmentin*) suspension 270 mg orally tid. Available is 250 mg/5 mL. Prepare to administer _____ mL to your patient.

37. (LO 11-4) The provider orders theophylline 600 mg orally qid. Available are 300-mg tablets. You will administer _____ tablets to your patient.

38. (LO 11-4) The provider orders azithromycin (*Zithromax*) suspension 500 mg daily. Available is 200 mg/5 mL. Prepare to administer _____ mL to your patient.

Multiple Choice—Circle the correct letter.

39. (LO 11-2) You assess a patient who hyperventilates when breathing as experiencing which of the following conditions?

a. Dyspnea

b. Apnea

c. Orthopnea

d. Hyperpnea

40. (LO 11-2) Which of the following respiratory disorders do you suspect when a patient presents with fever, cough, tachypnea, purulent sputum, and pleuritic chest pain?

a. Bronchitis

b. Cancer of the lung

c. Pulmonary embolism

d. Rhinitis

41. (LO 11-3) A patient with a nicotine dependency experiences which of the following side effects after prolonged smoking?

a. Runny nose and sneezing

b. Difficulty concentrating and gastrointestinal upset

c. Constipation and abdominal pain

d. Productive cough and hemoptysis

42. (LO 11-4) For an individual to purchase a product containing pseudoephedrine or ephedrine, which of the following criteria must be met?

a. Be at least 25 years of age

b. Have a provider's order

c. Show a valid driver's license or legal document

d. Purchase at least 9 g at one time

43. (LO 11-4) Which of the following are side effects of chlorpheniramine maleate?

a. Difficulty breathing, hypotension, palpitations

b. Drowsiness, sedation, dry mouth

c. Stinging of the nasal mucosa, lightheadedness, headache

d. Diarrhea, anorexia, vomiting

Chapter 11 Case Studies

44. (LO 11-4) A patient comes to the clinic and tells you he is bothered by a dry, hacking cough. He can't bring up anything, yet the cough continues. He wants to know what is causing this. What should you tell him? The provider orders dextromethorphan (*Delsym*). What is this drug, and what is its purpose? The patient asks you what else he can do to bring up secretions. What is the side effect you should monitor the patient for? _____

_____

_____

_____

45. (LO 11-4) A patient taking theophylline for bronchial asthma is complaining of headache, dizziness, restlessness, and palpitations. What do you suspect is going on? What should your plan of action be?

_____

_____

_____

Critical Thinking

Answer the questions in the space provided.

46. (LO 11-2) Give at least three reasons why tuberculosis is becoming more common. _____

_____

_____

_____

47. (LO 11-4) Describe the difference between bronchodilators and expectorants. _____

_____

_____

_____

48. (LO 11-5) Describe the procedures for administering nose drops and inhaled steroids. _____

_____

_____

_____

49. (LO 11-5) Compare and contrast the similarities and differences in the methods of oxygen delivery. _____

_____

_____

_____

Select the disorder that best matches each description and write it in the blank.

      bronchitis   asthma   pneumonia   tuberculosis   emphysema

50. (LO 11-2) In a small town in Asia, Grandfather Kim has had a lung disease for a long time. He is very weak and is coughing up blood. The public health worker is worried that Kim's grandchildren will catch the disease from him.

_____

51. (LO 11-2) Nancy Epstein suffers from frequent attacks of wheezing, coughing, and shortness of breath. She can control these attacks by inhaling epinephrine and avoiding dust and mold.

_____

52. (LO 11-2) Mr. Smith can never take a deep breath because he cannot exhale completely. He does breathing exercises every day and takes expectorants and bronchodilators to help his condition.

_____

53. (LO 11-2) Sue Bosworth has a viral infection of the upper respiratory tract. Her provider instructs her to drink plenty of fluids so that she can cough up the sputum that is clogging her air passage.

_____

54. (LO 11-2) Frank Fernandez was recovering from the flu when he developed a bacterial infection. The infection has now blocked his alveoli with pus, making it difficult for him to breathe.

_____

Applications

Obtain an electronic drug guide, a current copy of a drug reference book, or the _PDR_®.

55. Use Section 2 of the _PDR_®, Brand and Generic Name Index, to find another product name for each of the drugs in the Representative Drugs for the Respiratory System table in the chapter.

56. In Section 3 of the _PDR_®, Product Category Index, find the Allergy Relief Products. List all the drugs named.

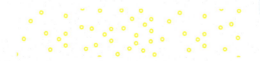

DRUGS FOR THE GASTROINTESTINAL SYSTEM

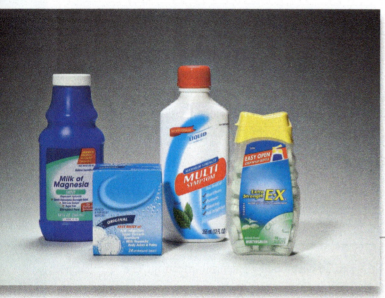

©Matt Meadows/McGraw-Hill Education

In this chapter you will learn about the organs of digestion and elimination. You will learn what they do, what happens to them when they are diseased, and how drugs are used to treat these disorders. You will also learn procedures to follow in giving gastrointestinal medications.

antacid

anticholinergic

antidiarrheal

antiemetic

antiflatulent

anthelmintic

antispasmodic

astringent

chyme

cirrhosis

Crohn's disease

demulcent

digestant

dyspepsia

emetic

endoscope

eructation

flatulence

gastroscope

gastrostomy tube

hepatitis

histamine H_2-receptor antagonist

hyperacidity

laxative

nasogastric tube

peristalsis

stoma

ulcerative colitis

villi

GASTROINTESTINAL SYSTEM [LO 12-1]

Food is vital to survival. Every cell requires nourishment to carry on its life functions. But cells cannot use the food we eat in the form it's in when it enters the body. The food must first undergo mechanical and chemical changes that break it down into particles small enough to pass through cell walls. This function is carried out by the gastrointestinal system, also known as the digestive system. There are five steps in the digestive process.

Step 1. Breaking up food into smaller pieces. This mechanical action is performed by the mouth and its accessory parts, the tongue and the teeth, with the aid of the salivary glands.

Step 2. Transporting food through the GI tract. The gastrointestinal (GI) tract (also known as the digestive tract or alimentary canal) is one long tube passing from the mouth to the rectum. Rhythmic contractions of the lining of the GI tract push food along this passageway. These muscle movements are called **peristalsis**. By moving food along, peristalsis puts the food in contact with physical and chemical processes that take place in different parts of the system.

Step 3. Secreting digestive enzymes. Glands in the mouth, in the lining of the stomach, and in the accessory organs (liver, small bowel, and pancreas) all secrete enzymes, which are chemical substances that aid digestion. Digestion is a series of chemical changes that break down food particles into basic nutrients that can be used by cells: namely, amino acids (proteins), fats, minerals, vitamins, sugars, and water.

Step 4. Absorbing nutrients into the blood. After being broken down into its smallest parts, food is absorbed from the small intestine into the bloodstream. From there it circulates to all the cells of the body to supply fuel for energy production and growth.

Step 5. Excreting solid waste products. This function takes place in the large intestine and the rectum. Undigested substances, like plant fibers, are not absorbed into the blood but pass into the large intestine. The large intestine prepares these substances for elimination from the body.

Figure 12.1 shows the major organs of the gastrointestinal tract.

Figure 12.1

The digestive system.

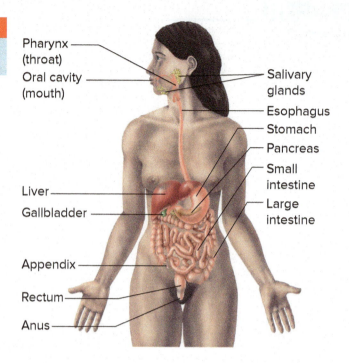

Pharynx (throat)

Oral cavity (mouth)

Liver

Gallbladder

Appendix

Rectum

Anus

Salivary glands

Esophagus

Stomach

Pancreas

Small intestine

Large intestine

Organs of Digestion

Mouth. The teeth and the tongue work together to break food into small pieces. The tongue moves food into position so that it can be chewed by the teeth. Teeth have different shapes that make them suitable for cutting, tearing, and grinding food. Even before chewing begins, the salivary glands start to produce a fluid called saliva. Saliva helps dissolve food and coats it so that it can be easily swallowed. Saliva also begins to act on carbohydrates (starchy foods) to turn them into sugars.

Esophagus. As discussed in Chapter 11, when a person swallows, the epiglottis closes to prevent food from entering the lungs. The food then passes into the esophagus, the part of the GI tract that extends from the pharynx to the stomach. Chunks of food are pushed down the esophagus by peristaltic movements of the tube lining. When the stomach is irritated, peristalsis may take place in the opposite direction, and vomiting will probably result.

Stomach. The stomach is a gourd-shaped pouch that can expand to hold up to 2 quarts of food and liquid. Valves at the entrance and exit of the stomach control the intake and outlet of food. The stomach lining is dotted with over 35 million tiny glands that secrete gastric (pertaining to the stomach) juice. Gastric juice consists of stomach acid and digestive enzymes. Stomach acid is an important factor in digestion. It dissolves food, destroys bacteria, and breaks down connective tissue in meats. After entering the stomach, food is churned around by muscles in the stomach wall and mixed with gastric juice. Food remains in the stomach for about 3 hours, with a range of 1 to 7 hours. By this time it has become an acidic, liquefied mass (**chyme**).

Small Intestine. The section of the small intestine closest to the stomach is called the duodenum. As soon as food enters the duodenum, it is mixed with strong digestive enzymes from the liver and pancreas. These juices complete the process of breaking down food into molecules of protein, sugar, fat, minerals, and so on. The small intestine is a long, coiled tube about 20 feet long. It also secretes a fluid rich in digestive enzymes that helps to break down fats, proteins, and carbohydrates. Its walls are lined with tiny, fingerlike projections called **villi**. The villi are responsible for absorbing nutrients into the bloodstream. They have thin walls and, because of their shape, provide a huge surface area for absorption to take place. Tiny capillaries and lymph ducts in the villi take in the nutrients and transport them to the liver. From there they are released into the bloodstream as needed. By the time food has passed through all 20 feet of the small intestine, most of the nutrients have been absorbed. All that is left are indigestible materials mixed with water. The other sections of the small intestine include the jejunum and ileum. The jejunum is the middle part of the small intestine and makes up two-fifths of the whole small intestine. The lowest part of the intestine is the ileum. It connects two folds of intestinal membrane, which make up an exit and entryway or valve. This is the ileocecal valve, which prevents the backflow of contents of the colon, feces, into the ileum.

Large Intestine.   The large intestine, also known as the colon, is much shorter and wider than the small intestine. It is about 5 to 6 feet long. In the large intestine, excess water is absorbed into the bloodstream, leaving undigested wastes. These are collected and compacted into semisolid masses, called feces or stools. The feces leave the body by way of the rectum and its opening, the anus.

Liver and Gallbladder.   The liver is the largest gland in the body and serves many functions. Its role in the GI system is to secrete bile, a substance that aids in digesting fats. Bile is collected in a storage pouch called the gallbladder until it is needed for digestion. The liver stores nutrients absorbed from the small intestine. The liver also removes certain waste products from the blood, and it produces important substances for blood clotting and the immune system.

The liver is important in drug action because it breaks down or inactivates many drugs. Patients with poor liver function can become overdosed with some routinely administered drugs because their livers are unable to break down the drugs quickly.

Pancreas.   The pancreas is another large glandular organ that has several functions. It produces digestive juices that complete the chemical changes that turn fats, proteins, and carbohydrates into particles that can be absorbed. The pancreas also secretes insulin, a hormone that regulates the amount of sugar used by the cells (see Chapter 15). Insulin is released directly into the bloodstream. It does not enter into digestion.

Autonomic Control

Peristalsis and the secretion of digestive enzymes are both under the control of the autonomic nervous system. This means that people cannot consciously control what goes on in their stomachs and intestines. It also means that digestion is affected by stress.

When the autonomic nervous system prepares the body to meet danger or stress, the muscular movements of the stomach and intestine slow down. Digestive enzyme production slows down, too. In other cases, peristalsis and enzyme secretion are stimulated needlessly by nervous tension. Therefore, chronically nervous or anxious people tend to have overactive digestion. Mild sedatives or tranquilizers are sometimes used to calm these reactions and restore normal digestion.

DISORDERS OF THE GASTROINTESTINAL SYSTEM [LO 12-2]

Symptoms

The symptoms of GI disorders are quite familiar. Common symptoms are occasional nausea, vomiting, constipation, diarrhea, indigestion (**dyspepsia**), heartburn (**hyperacidity**), flatulence, stomachache, and abdominal cramps. The symptoms have many causes. They can be the result of passing irritations, flu, mild food poisoning, psychological stress, or side effects of drugs. Or they can signal more serious underlying diseases. Drugs can relieve some GI symptoms, but the underlying disease must be treated to achieve permanent relief.

Nausea is a queasy feeling in the stomach arising from many causes, such as infection, radiation treatment, psychological stimulation, reaction to a drug, pregnancy, poisoning, or stomach irritation. Sometimes this feeling leads to vomiting, or emesis. Vomiting is a protective mechanism to rid the body of spoiled or irritating foods and liquids. The contents of the stomach are emptied as peristalsis switches direction and carries food back up the esophagus. Too much vomiting is dangerous because it can remove essential fluids and electrolytes, such as potassium and sodium, from the body. It is also dangerous because it keeps the body from digesting and absorbing needed nutrients.

Heartburn is a burning sensation in the stomach that may be felt in the esophagus and the throat as well. It is often felt along with sour belching. Indigestion is a gassy or bloated feeling in the stomach. Both heartburn and indigestion may be the result of poor eating habits or psychological tension. A bland diet, mild sedatives, and simple antacids help to relieve passing symptoms. Of course, if symptoms persist, an underlying cause may be indicated.

Burping, belching (**eructation**), and passing gas are common symptoms of GI irritation. The gas (flatus) comes from chemical reactions that release gases into the GI system. It also comes from swallowing air along with food and drink. Excess gas can cause pressure, pain, and a bloated feeling. Treat with over-the-counter *Gas-X extra Strength*. Cramping or griping of the digestive tract is also common with many disorders. Cramps are the result of muscle spasms in the walls of the stomach and intestines. It is commonly treated with hyoscyamine (*Levsin*).

Constipation is the failure to have regular bowel movements. It can be due to hardened feces, slow movement of the intestine, lack of fiber and fluids in the diet, psychological factors, or lack of physical activity. Constipation is of concern when it causes straining at stool or when it threatens to block the intestines. Normal bowel elimination may vary from three times a day to once every three days. Different people have different schedules, and no one should be concerned if he or she does not have a bowel movement every single day. **Laxatives** (drugs that promote bowel movement, such as bisacodyl) are much overused. Older adults who do not have a daily bowel movement may take laxatives every day and become dependent on the drug, which can cause serious problems. Laxatives can further potentiate constipation and irregularity but may cause lazy bowel syndrome, which means the colon needs a laxative to artificially cause stimulation to produce a bowel movement. Stool softeners should always be used before turning to laxatives.

Diarrhea means passing loose, watery stools or passing stools too often. It is often accompanied by abdominal cramps, which signal irritation in the large intestine. Diarrhea is the result of increased peristalsis. It has many underlying causes, including:

- Intestinal infection.
- Psychological factors (stress, anxiety).
- Food allergies.
- Food intolerance (greasy and spicy foods, alcohol, coffee).
- Certain medications (antacids containing magnesium; overuse of laxatives; antibiotics; antineoplastics).
- Certain diseases (irritable bowel syndrome, diverticulitis, cancer).

As in the case of diarrhea, many disorders either result from or cause changes in the speed at which nutrients are carried through the GI tract. The term used to refer to the speed of peristalsis is *intestinal motility*. Changes in motility lead to either diarrhea or constipation. Nervous tension, infections, drugs, and many other factors affect intestinal motility.

Abdominal or stomach pain sometimes accompanies GI disorders. The pain can be the result of gas pressure, irritation, or more serious problems. Especially in the case of abdominal pain, it is important not to give medications until a search has been made for an underlying cause. Treating abdominal pain with an analgesic may delay discovery of something serious, such as appendicitis.

Other symptoms to look for are difficulty in swallowing (dysphagia), loss of appetite (anorexia), sudden or severe weight loss, and change in the appearance of the stools (bloody, tarry, clay-colored, or containing excess mucus).

Major Disorders

GI symptoms may be similar for minor problems and serious problems. A provider may order tests (x-rays, blood tests, etc.) to find an underlying cause for the symptoms. Special flexible fiber-optic instruments (**endoscopes**) may be used to visually examine the walls of the stomach, intestine, or rectum.

Tooth and Gum Disorders. Problems with the teeth, gums, or dentures can lead to GI problems. Unless the teeth and gums are in good condition, eating and drinking may be painful or inefficient. Patients may avoid hard-to-chew foods, including foods that would help keep their bowel movements regular (e.g., fruits, vegetables, and grain products high in bulk and fiber content). Some of the main tooth and gum disorders are dental abscess (which can result from neglect or severe tooth decay), gingivitis, pyorrhea, trench mouth (Vincent's infection), and stomatitis. They are treated with antibiotics, surgical removal of diseased tissue, or special cleaning procedures. Many toothpastes have fluoride added to them and are recommended by the American Dental Association. Fluoride rinses and tablets are also available. Fluoride helps prevent tooth decay (caries). Older adults, patients in long-term care, and patients who are being fed with a tube may require your help in maintaining their oral hygiene.

Gastritis. Gastritis is an inflammation of the stomach, signaled by epigastric tenderness, nausea, vomiting, and a sense of fullness. It may be caused by accidentally swallowing caustic substances. It also results from normal use of irritants such as coffee, alcohol, and tobacco. The condition may be temporary, or it may persist for months, causing damage to the stomach lining. Treatment involves removing the cause as well as treating the symptoms.

Peptic Ulcer Disease. Peptic ulcer disease is a broad term encompassing both gastric (stomach) and duodenal (duodenum) ulcers. (*Peptic* pertains to digestion in the stomach.) An ulcer is an open sore in the stomach or duodenal lining. The mucous membranes have been broken down by digestive acids so that the underlying tissue is exposed and can be destroyed by the acids.

The causes of ulcers are excessive secretion of hydrochloric acid (HCl), insufficient stomach protection—a breakdown in the gastric mucosal barrier (which normally protects the stomach from autodigestion)—or the presence of *Helicobacter pylori* (*H. pylori*). Hypersecretion of hydrochloric acid can be caused by prolonged use of alcohol, cigarettes, coffee, or drugs such as aspirin, ibuprofen, and corticosteroids and by psychological factors. Part of the treatment is to remove the source of irritation (food sources or psychological causes). Drug therapy is aimed at reducing the stomach acid or improving stomach protection. There are three drug therapies used in the treatment of peptic ulcer disease caused by *H. pylori*. The dual therapy includes ranitidine bismuth citrate and clarithromycin (*Biaxin*) for a period of 7 days. The triple-drug therapy includes the use of a proton pump inhibitor or ranitidine bismuth citrate, amoxicillin, and clarithromycin (*Biaxin*) for 14 days. Both the dual and triple therapies have a 90 percent success rate of treatment. The quadruple therapy includes a proton pump inhibitor, bismuth, tetracycline, and metronidazole (*Flagyl*) given over a period of 14 days, with a success rate ranging between 60 and 80 percent. **Antacids** (drugs that neutralize HCl in the stomach) and **histamine H$_2$-receptor antagonists** (drugs that inhibit gastric acid secretion) are also used. Anticholinergics and tricyclic antidepressants are occasionally used. There is divided opinion as to their efficacy in preventing recurrences and in alleviating symptoms. They also have a high incidence of undesirable side effects and must be used with caution.

Liver Disorders.   A symptom of many liver disorders is jaundice, a yellowing of the skin. Jaundice is due to bilirubin (a yellow pigment) entering the bloodstream, usually because the bile duct is blocked. **Cirrhosis** is a chronic, progressive disease of the liver characterized by degeneration and destruction of the liver cells. This condition is accompanied in the early stages by nausea, weight loss, vomiting, and difficulty in digesting fats. Jaundice, anemia, spider angiomas or telangiectasia (spiderlike markings on the skin), and a loss of sensation occur in the later stages. Cirrhosis is caused by drinking too much alcohol, toxins to the liver such as large doses of drugs, obstruction of the biliary ducts, and advanced heart failure. Complications include enlarged veins, fluid in the abdomen, and renal and liver failure. It is treated with rest and a high-calorie, high-carbohydrate, low-fat diet. There is no specific drug therapy for cirrhosis.

Hepatitis is an inflammation of the liver, with acute viral hepatitis being the most common cause. Other causes of hepatitis are certain drugs such as alcohol, chemicals, and autoimmune liver disease. The types of hepatitis are A, B, C, D, E, and recently G. Hepatitis A virus (HAV) is transmitted by the fecal-oral route and occurs in instances of crowded living conditions and poor sanitation. Hepatitis B virus (HBV) is of great concern to the healthcare worker because it is blood-borne and may be transmitted through accidental needlesticks. The Centers for Disease Control and Prevention (CDC) recommends immunizing healthcare workers with the hepatitis B vaccine. HBV also occurs in IV drug users or through sexual contact. Hepatitis C virus (HCV) is primarily spread percutaneously such as through IV drug use, transfusion with infected blood products, and high-risk sexual behavior. Hepatitis D virus (HDV) is a type of hepatitis that cannot survive on its own. It requires hepatitis B to replicate. Hepatitis E virus (HEV) is also transmitted by the fecal-oral route and is most commonly caused by drinking contaminated water in developing countries. Lastly, hepatitis G virus (HGV) is a poorly characterized virus that is spread parenterally or sexually.

Although a large number of patients may be asymptomatic, there are three phases of symptoms. The first phase is the preicteric phase because it precedes jaundice and is characterized by anorexia, weight loss, malaise, headache, low-grade fever, joint pain, and skin rashes. It may last from 1 to 21 days. The icteric phase is the second phase, lasting 2 to 4 weeks, and jaundice is the classic feature. The third phase, or posticteric, is also known as the convalescent phase and lasts 2 to 4 months. Malaise and fatigue are the most common symptoms.

There is no specific drug therapy for viral hepatitis, although certain drugs such as antiemetics and sedatives may be used supportively. Dimenhydrinate (*Dramamine*) and trimethobenzamide (*Tigan*) are used for nausea. Phenothiazines should not be used because of the toxic effects on the liver. Vaccination is an effective protection against HAV. Lamivudine (*Epivir*) is a reverse transcriptase inhibitor used to treat HBV. It is taken orally for 1 year to decrease the damage to the liver. Although vaccines are available for hepatitis A and B, education and prevention are the best measures to decrease the prevalence of hepatitis.

Gallbladder Disorders. Gallstones are small granules, consisting primarily of cholesterol, in the gallbladder. They are thought to be the result of high amounts of concentrated bile. They are common in people over the age of 40, but they do not necessarily cause symptoms. Gallstones can cause trouble if they block the opening of the gallbladder or the tube that carries bile to the intestine. Inflammation of the gallbladder (cholecystitis) most commonly occurs with stones. Cholangitis (inflammation of the biliary ducts) is a complication of stones. Symptoms of gallbladder disease include fever, vomiting, jaundice, and pain in the upper right quadrant of the abdomen. Surgery is frequently indicated for cholelithiasis (gallstones) only. Treatment for cholecystitis is aimed at treating the symptoms. Analgesics and anticholinergics are the most common drugs used to control gallbladder disease. A drug used to dissolve certain types of gallstones is ursodiol (*Actigall*).

Pancreatitis. Pancreatitis is an inflammation of the pancreas that causes severe pain in the left upper quadrant of the abdomen, vomiting, fever, hypotension (low blood pressure), tachycardia (rapid pulse), and jaundice. Shock may occur as a result of hemorrhage. Pancreatitis is treated with analgesics to relieve the pain, IV fluids, bed rest, withdrawing foods, and antibiotics to prevent infections. **Digestants** are used as pancreatic enzyme replacement therapy in chronic pancreatitis. (Two other disorders of the pancreas, diabetes and hypoglycemia, are described in Chapter 15.)

Ulcerative Colitis. **Ulcerative colitis** is a disease of the colon and rectum characterized by inflammation and ulceration with alternating periods of remissions and exacerbations. The major symptoms are abdominal pain and bloody diarrhea. The stools may range from 1 or 2 semisoft stools with small amounts of blood to 10 to 20 bloody stools per day. The primary drug used to treat ulcerative colitis is sulfasalazine (*Azulfidine*), which is a sulfonamide antibiotic. It is administered orally. Corticosteroids and immunosuppressive drugs may also be used. Other treatments include rest and a high-calorie, high-protein, low-residue diet with vitamin and iron supplements. Although the majority of patients respond to medical management, a small percentage of patients may require surgery to remove the diseased portion of the colon or rectum.

Crohn's Disease. **Crohn's disease** is a chronic, nonspecific inflammatory bowel disease of unknown etiology that can affect any portion of the GI tract from the mouth to the anus, but generally it affects the terminal ileum, jejunum, and colon. It is classically characterized by periods of remissions and exacerbations. Discontinuous skip lesions with segments of normal bowel occurring between diseased portions are found. The major symptoms are abdominal pain and diarrhea. A drug used to treat Crohn's disease is infliximab (*Remicade*), which is a monoclonal antibody against tumor necrosis factor-alpha. It is administered intravenously. As with ulcerative colitis, corticosteroids and immunosuppressive drugs may also be used. A high-calorie, high-nitrogen, fat-free, no-residue diet is generally prescribed and used even during exacerbations. Surgery may be used as a last resort in patients unresponsive to therapy or in those with life-threatening complications.

Peritonitis. Peritonitis is an acute inflammation of the membranes that line the abdomen. It is caused by trauma or rupture of an organ, releasing bacteria into the abdominal cavity. Abdominal pain and tenderness are the main symptoms. The treatment is surgery to repair the damage and antibiotics to stop the infection.

Irritable Bowel Syndrome. Irritable bowel syndrome (IBS) is not a disease but a group of symptoms characterized by intermittent abdominal pain associated with changes in bowel patterns (diarrhea or constipation). It seems to be related to an intolerance to certain foods or to psychological factors. The condition is generally harmless. Anticholinergics such as dicyclomine (*Bentyl*) may be given before meals to relieve the pain associated with food intake. A mild sedative may be given, but only for a short time.

Diverticulosis. Diverticulosis is a condition in which multiple pouches (diverticula) develop in the walls of the large intestine. There are generally no symptoms until the pouches become inflamed (diverticulitis). The main symptoms are crampy, left-sided abdominal pain and alternating diarrhea and constipation. Treatment of diverticulitis consists of rest, a high-fiber diet, antibiotics, and bulk laxatives such as psyllium (*Metamucil*). Anticholinergics such as *Bentyl* and *Donnatal* are used to decrease cramping.

Hemorrhoids. Hemorrhoids are enlarged hemorrhoidal veins. They can become swollen and painful, and blood clots may form in them. Problems with hemorrhoids can be averted by not straining during bowel movements and by avoiding heavy lifting and prolonged sitting and standing. Suppositories, ointments, and warm sitz baths (immersion of thighs, buttocks, and abdomen) are used to relieve pain in severe cases. Some hemorrhoid preparations, such as *Anusol-HC,* include anti-inflammatory ingredients as well as soothing and lubricating ingredients. Stool softeners such as docusate sodium (*Colace*) may be given to promote regular bowel movements.

Tumors. Tumors, either benign or malignant, may grow in any part of the GI tract, causing obstruction, bleeding, pressure, or rupture and producing a variety of symptoms. Small outgrowths on the inside of the large intestine, most often found in the rectum or sigmoid colon, are called polyps. All polyps are abnormal and should be biopsied or removed because of their link to colon cancer.

Intestinal Parasites. Intestinal parasites are worms that live in the intestines, such as tapeworms, hookworms, trichina worms, pinworms, and roundworms. Some of these parasites are quite common, and others are found only in certain parts of the world. Most may be prevented by eating properly cooked meats (especially pork), by keeping the hands and nails clean, and by wearing shoes. Children may pick up parasites from playing in dirt or sandboxes. Teach children to avoid nail biting and to keep their hands out of their mouths.

DRUGS THAT AFFECT THE GASTROINTESTINAL SYSTEM [LO 12-3]

Antacids

Antacids relieve gastritis and ulcer pain by neutralizing hydrochloric acid in the stomach. Many people take OTC antacids to relieve indigestion as well. Remember, however, that stomach acid is necessary to digestion. Overuse of antacids may actually interfere with proper digestion.

The substances used to neutralize stomach acid are alkaline. When these substances are combined with acids, they cancel each other out chemically. Certain antacids are absorbable. If too many of these antacids are taken, excess alkali can pass into the intestine and be absorbed. This may cause an imbalance in the body's natural chemistry called alkalosis (see Chapter 13).

The major ingredients in antacids include aluminum salts, calcium carbonate, magnesium salts, and sodium bicarbonate, alone or in combination. Sodium bicarbonate is seldom prescribed because of its high sodium content and because it causes an increase in gastric acid. Common antacids are calcium salts (e.g., calcium carbonate), aluminum salts (e.g., aluminum hydroxide), and magnesium salts (e.g., magnesium hydroxide, oxide, carbonate, and trisilicate). Aluminum hydroxide is sold both generically and under the brand name *Amphojel*. Magnesium hydroxide is the familiar preparation milk of magnesia.

Aluminum salts and calcium salts tend to cause constipation as a side effect. Magnesium salts, on the other hand, tend to cause diarrhea. It is generally believed that combining these substances cancels out the side effects, so many preparations contain both. *Maalox Regular Strength, Gelusil,* and *Mylanta Maximum Strength,* for example, are combinations of magnesium salts and aluminum hydroxide. Because antacids are OTC drugs and require no medical supervision, patient education is important. Antibiotics such as tetracycline or quinolones such as ciprofloxacin (*Cipro*) and levofloxacin (*Levaquin*), antifungals such as itraconazole (*Sporanox*), as well as digoxin (*Lanoxin*), and iron supplements interact with antacids. To reduce these drug interactions, tell your patient to take the antacid 2 hours before or after other medications.

Patient Education   Antacids

- Aluminum- and calcium-based antacids cause constipation.
- Magnesium-based antacids cause diarrhea.
- When using chewable antacids, chew them thoroughly.
- Avoid milk and milk products when using calcium carbonate antacids.
- Avoid antacids containing sodium if high blood pressure, cardiac disease, or renal disease exists.

- Antacids may interact with certain antibiotics, such as tetracycline, or quinolones and reduce the absorption of the antibiotic.
- Do not take extra doses of antacids without a provider's direction.
- Antacids may interact with antifungals, digoxin, and iron supplements, decreasing the effect of these drugs.

Histamine H₂-Receptor Antagonists

These drugs block the action of histamine, which produces hydrochloric acid secretion, and promote ulcer healing. Examples of histamine H_2-receptor antagonist drugs include cimetidine (*Tagamet HB*), ranitidine (*Zantac*), famotidine (*Pepcid*), and nizatidine (*Axid*).

Proton Pump Inhibitors

Proton pump inhibitors are drugs that block the final step of acid production and are used in active ulcer disease, erosive esophagitis, and pathological

Pediatric Considerations | **Acid Suppressant Drugs**

- Although proton pump inhibitors are not approved by the FDA for use in children, omeprazole (*Prilosec*) is the only proton pump inhibitor approved for use in children 2 years of age or older.
- Use a 10-mg dose of *Prilosec* for children weighing less than 20 kg and a 20-mg dose for children weighing more than 20 kg.

- Antacids in doses of 5 to 10 mL may be used every 3 to 6 hours or after meals and at bedtime.
- The safety and effectiveness of other acid suppressant drugs have not been established.

 Older Adult Considerations | **Acid Suppressant Drugs**

- All antiulcer drugs may be safely used in older adults, although confusion is an increased side effect with cimetidine (*Tagamet HB*).
- Because older adults secrete less gastric acid, they require a decreased dose of antacids.
- Monitor closely for decreased renal function, particularly with magnesium-containing antacids.

- Calcium carbonate antacids may be used to prevent osteoporosis.
- Be aware that long-term use of proton pump inhibitors may be associated with an increased risk of hip fractures.

hypersecretory conditions. Examples include omeprazole (*Prilosec*), lansoprazole (*Prevacid*), rabeprazole (*Aciphex*), esomeprazole (*Nexium*), and pantoprazole (*Protonix*).

Digestants

The category of digestants includes a variety of drugs that promote the process of digestion in the gastrointestinal tract and serve as replacement therapy in deficiency conditions. Pancreatic enzyme replacement may be necessary for people with certain pancreatic diseases, such as pancreatic insufficiency and cystic fibrosis. Pancrelipase (*Pancreaze*) aids in the digestion and absorption of fats, carbohydrates, and triglycerides.

Antiflatulents (Carminatives)

The main function of **antiflatulents** is to reduce the gas in the stomach and intestines (**flatulence**) that accompanies indigestion. They facilitate the passing of gas by mildly stimulating intestinal motility. Simethicone (*Infant's Mylicon*), a common antiflatulent, relieves flatulence by dispersing and preventing the formation of gas pockets in the gastrointestinal tract. Other examples of simethicone are *Phazyme Ultra Strength, Gas-X Extra Strength,* and *Mylanta Maximum Strength*. These are over-the-counter antiflatulents that don't require a prescription. *Beano* is a food enzyme supplement taken right before the first bite of food to decrease flatulence. Patients can reduce the need for antiflatulents by avoiding gas-forming foods, such as cabbage, onions, and beans, and by avoiding the use of straws to drink liquids, because straws cause air to be swallowed.

Emetics

Emetics are drugs that produce vomiting in cases of poisoning. Calling Poison Control is the best thing to do. Parents are not recommended to keep activated charcoal at home. Another emetic is apomorphine hydrochloride, which is given by injection and stimulates the brain center that controls vomiting.

Antiemetics

Antiemetics suppress nausea and vomiting by acting on the brain's control center to stop the nerve impulses. These drugs have various uses, including motion sickness, "morning sickness" of pregnancy, and nausea and vomiting that occur with various diseases, after surgery, and with chemotherapy and radiation treatments.

The main antiemetics are antihistamines and phenothiazines. For example, dimenhydrinate (*Dramamine*), frequently used for motion sickness, is an antihistamine. Other antiemetics are cyclizine and meclizine (*Bonine*). The phenothiazines include prochlorperazine, chlorpromazine, and *Phenergan*. Drowsiness is their main side effect. An anticholinergic, scopolamine, is especially effective against motion sickness. Ondansetron (*Zofran*) is a powerful drug for the prevention of nausea and vomiting associated with cancer chemotherapy. Other antiemetics include trimethobenzamide (*Tigan*), the marijuana-derived agent dronabinol (*Marinol*), propantheline bromide, and metoclopramide (*Reglan*).

Anticholinergics and Antispasmodics

These drugs act on the autonomic nervous system to slow peristalsis in the GI tract. They make the smooth muscle contract less often and less forcefully.

 Pediatric Considerations Antiemetics

- Because their safety has not been identified, antiemetics should not be used long term.
- Use antiemetics cautiously, only after the etiology of the symptoms has been identified.
- Promethazine (*Phenergan*) may be used cautiously but should not be used for children under the age of 2 years.

- Avoid scopolamine-containing products in children under the age of 12 years.
- Avoid metoclopramide (*Reglan*) in children because of an increased risk of extrapyramidal side effects.
- Although dronabinol (*Marinol*) may be used to treat or prevent nausea accompanying chemotherapy, use with caution because of its psychoactive effects.

 Older Adult Considerations Antiemetics

- Use antiemetics cautiously because they cause drowsiness and older adults are especially susceptible.
- There is an increased need to prevent vomiting in older adults because they are

at greater risk for fluid loss and electrolyte imbalance than younger adults.
- Use dronabinol (*Marinol*) cautiously because older adults are prone to its psychoactive effects.

This is useful in the treatment of ulcers and irritable bowel syndrome because it allows the bowel to rest.

In addition to slowing intestinal motility, **anticholinergics** block the action of acetylcholine, a chemical substance that helps transmit nerve impulses, including those that stimulate the acid-secreting glands of the stomach. By blocking these nerve impulses, anticholinergics cause less stomach acid to be produced. This action is important in ulcer treatment.

The anticholinergics are a group of natural and synthetic alkaloids. The major natural alkaloids are atropine sulfate, belladonna, and scopolamine hydrobromide. Because these drugs affect the entire autonomic nervous system, they have many side effects. Blurred vision, dilated pupils, dry mouth, heart palpitations, constipation, and inability to urinate are some of the effects. Eluxadoline (*Viberzi*) is given for irritable syndrome with diarrhea. Main side effects are nausea and abdominal pain.

Antispasmodics have an effect on the smooth muscle and very little effect on the secretion of acid. An example is dicyclomine hydrochloride (*Bentyl*). Because of the seriousness of the side effects, special care must be taken with older adults.

Many combinations of anticholinergics or antispasmodics with sedatives are available, including *Donnatal* and *Librax*. Changes in diet and eating habits to decrease the stimulation of the colon or peristalsis are usually ordered along with these drugs.

 Caution Anticholinergics and the Older Adult

Use extreme caution when administering anticholinergic drugs to older adult patients who have hypertension or coronary artery, renal, or liver disease. Anticholinergics are also contraindicated for patients with glaucoma, urinary retention, and obstruction in the gastrointestinal tract.

Anticholinergics can aggravate these conditions by drying out both the urinary and GI tracts, which in turn causes further urinary retention and constipation, fecal impaction, and possible obstruction.

Antidiarrheals

Antidiarrheals work by:

- Absorbing the bacteria and toxins that cause the diarrhea and passing them out with the stools (absorbent action).
- Inhibiting intestinal motility, which slows the movement of fecal material through the intestine so that there is more time to absorb water and make formed stools.
- Coating the walls of the gastrointestinal tract.

Before treating diarrhea, it is important to identify the cause. Some antidiarrheals also contain ingredients that shrink swollen tissues (**astringent** action) or coat and soothe the tissues (**demulcent** action).

An example of absorbents is bismuth (*Pepto-Bismol*). It is found in many combinations, for example, bismuth subsalicylate (*Kaopectate*).

Drugs that slow intestinal motility also have a depressant effect on the central nervous system. One such drug is loperamide (*Imodium A-D*). The main group is the opiates, including opium tincture and codeine. Because of the cumulative effects, use caution when administering codeine and paregoric to patients who are receiving other central nervous system (CNS) depressants that cause sedation.

Anticholinergics such as atropine are often used as adjuncts in the treatment of diarrhea because they relieve painful intestinal spasms. They are found in combination with absorbents and opiates, for example, *Lomotil*. Other preparations suppress the growth of diarrhea-causing pathogens and reestablish the normal lining of the intestinal tract.

▲ Pediatric Considerations   Antidiarrheal Drugs

- Antidiarrheals are used to prevent fluid loss and electrolyte imbalance in small children.
- In addition to antidiarrheals, oral rehydration solutions such as *Pedialyte* should be used.

- Use caution with diphenoxylate (*Lomotil*); overdose can occur with usual doses because of the atropine it contains.
- *Lomotil* is contraindicated in children under the age of 2 years.

▲ Older Adult Considerations   Antidiarrheal Drugs

- Diarrhea occurs in older adults much less frequently than does constipation.
- Diarrhea most commonly occurs in older adults from laxative abuse or from GI preps before surgery or a special procedure such as a colonoscopy.

- Older adults are at risk for fluid loss and electrolyte imbalance.
- When diarrhea occurs due to illness, antidiarrheals may be used with caution to prevent constipation.

Anti-Inflammatory Agents

Diarrhea can also be caused by inflammation of the GI tract, such as ulcerative colitis. The use of steroids such as methylprednisolone (*Solu-Medrol*) and prednisone is one way to decrease inflammation. Sulfasalazine (*Azulfidine*) taken orally is changed into mesalamine, an aspirinlike drug, when it reaches the colon. Olsalazine sodium (*Dipentum*) is used with patients who have an intolerance for *Azulfidine*. The anti-inflammatory activity provided by these drugs makes them commonly used drugs for the treatment of colitis. Colitis closer to the anus can be treated either with mesalamine (*Rowasa*) suppositories or enemas or with a hydrocortisone retention enema (*Cortenema*) or intrarectal foam (*Cortifoam*). Vedolizumab (*Entyvio*) also reduces inflammation in the treatment of moderate to severe ulcerative colitis or Crohn's disease.

Laxatives

Laxatives (also called cathartics or purgatives) are drugs that promote defecation (bowel movement). There are different types: stimulants, saline, bulk-forming, lubricants, stool softeners, combination stool softener/stimulant, and osmotic drugs.

Stimulants. One group of laxatives stimulates peristalsis in the intestines to push fecal material through faster. When intestinal motility is increased, there is less time for water to be absorbed by the large intestine, so the stools are watery. Drugs that stimulate peristalsis include castor oil, docusate sodium/sennosides (*Senokot-S*), cascara sagrada, and several synthetics including bisacodyl (*Dulcolax*). Foods and beverages such as prunes, prune juice, and coffee also act as stimulants.

Saline.   Another group of laxatives holds liquid in the large intestine to soften feces and stimulate bowel movements. These are the saline cathartics, or salts of sodium, magnesium, and potassium. Although milk of magnesia is classified as both an antacid and a laxative, it is primarily used as a saline laxative. Epsom salts are another type of saline laxative.

Bulk-Forming (High-Fiber).   A third family of laxatives includes drugs that increase bulk. They absorb water to increase the bulk and moisture content of the stools. Bulk-forming laxatives are indigestible substances. They take from 12 hours to 3 days to be effective. Whole-grain cereals and breads that contain bran and other fibers relieve constipation in this way. So do extracts of the plantain weed (psyllium) found in such preparations as *Metamucil* and *Citrucel*. There are also several synthetic compounds. These should be taken with plenty of water to prevent constipation and possible fecal impaction.

Lubricants.   A fourth group of laxatives coats the surface of the stool and softens the stool to ease defecation. Lubricants such as mineral oil allow the feces to pass more easily through the intestine, but they are thought to interfere with the absorption of some vitamins.

Stool Softeners.   Drugs in this category incorporate the liquid in the bowel to soften stool. Examples of stool softeners are docusate calcium (*Surfak Stool Softener*) and docusate sodium (*Colace*). These drugs may cause throat irritation when administered in liquid form and should be diluted with fruit juice.

Lubiprostone (*Amitiza*) works by increasing the fluid secretion that aids in the passage of stool. It is used in chronic constipation and irritable bowel syndrome.

Combination of Stool Softener and Stimulant.   These drugs combine the action of both a stool softener and a stimulant. An example is docusate sodium and sennosides (*Peri-Colace*).

Osmotic Drugs.   Polyethylene glycol (*MirLAX*) is an osmotic drug that is used for short-term treatment of constipation; it causes water to be retained in stool. It is given as 1 heaping tablespoon of powder mixed in water or juice. The most common side effects are abdominal bloating, cramping, diarrhea, excess stool frequency, flatulence, and nausea. It may have to be taken for 2 to 4 days before a bowel movement occurs. *Movantik* (naloxegol) belongs to a class of drugs known as narcotic antagonists. It is a new one of its kind of medication to treat constipation caused by narcotic (opiate type) medications such as hydrocodone/ acetaminophen and *Vicodin* in people with ongoing pain that is caused by cancer. It blocks the effects of narcotics on the gut without blocking the effect on pain.

 Caution   Laxative Abuse

Regular laxative use leads to laxative abuse. Excessive laxative use develops over some years, and dependency goes unnoticed. This situation is especially common in older adult patients.

Laxative abuse is also seen in patients with eating disorders, such as anorexia nervosa and bulimia. Patients generally deny the overuse of laxatives. If laxative abuse is not discovered, permanent bowel and bone damage and electrolyte imbalances (particularly potassium) result. Arrhythmia (irregular heartbeat) and cardiac arrest can result from severe and prolonged potassium depletion.

Pediatric Considerations   Laxatives

- Glycerin suppositories may be used with infants and children.
- Lactulose and sorbitol are the stool softeners of choice for infants.
- Avoid mineral oil or stimulants with infants.

- Mineral oil, magnesium hydroxide, lactulose, and sorbitol may be used for older children.
- Use stimulants only for short-term therapy for children.
- Avoid giving a child a laxative more than once a week.

Older Adult Considerations   Laxatives

- Constipation is a frequent problem in older adults, and laxatives are either used or overused.
- *Metamucil* is the preferred laxative among healthcare professionals for older adults because it is not a stimulant.

- Avoid stimulant laxatives because these cause the colon to become laxative-dependent.
- Avoid the use of mineral oil in bedridden patients because of the risk of aspiration.

Anthelmintics

Anthelmintics are drugs given for helminthiasis, an intestinal infestation of worms. These parasites belong to the animal group helminths (worms). The drugs are effective against worms, but they can be toxic to the body, so they must be used with care and according to the provider's orders. Usually a provider instructs an infected person on hygienic practices to prevent future episodes. A drug used for pinworms and roundworms is pyrantel pamoate.

Anorexiants

Anorexiants, also called appetite suppressants, help the patient eat less and lose weight. (Recall that the term *anorexia* means loss of appetite.) Anorexiants are used only to treat extreme obesity. The main anorexiants are amphetamines or related drugs. They act by stimulating the central nervous system, as this has an appetite-suppressing effect. An example of these drugs is diethylpropion. These drugs are not prescribed frequently because they are potentially harmful and often abused. Appetite suppressants should be prescribed only in combination with an increase in physical activity, behavior modification, and caloric restriction. Many OTC diet products contain caffeine or phenylpropanolamine, both mild central nervous system stimulants.

Patient Education   Hygienic Practices to Prevent Helminthiasis

- Wash hands before and after eating and using the toilet.
- Avoid walking barefoot (hookworm).
- Take showers instead of baths.

- Change underclothes, bedclothes, and towels daily.
- Wash perianal area daily.
- Take medicine for the full course of therapy to prevent reinfestation.

Weight-Loss Drugs

Prescription weight-loss drugs are generally reserved for people who have been unable to achieve weight loss through diet and exercise, have a body mass index (BMI) of 27 and health problems as a result of the weight, or have a BMI of 30 or higher. The primary prescription weight-loss drug for long-term weight loss is orlistat (*Xenical*). *Xenical* prevents the absorption of fat in the intestines. The usual dose is 120 mg tid and may result in frequent oily bowel movements, diarrhea, and bloating. Phentermine (*Adipex-P*) is a weight-loss prescription drug that generally is used for less than 12 weeks to achieve short-term weight loss. Lorcaserin *(Belviq)* and phentermine/topiramate *(Qsymia)* are new weight-loss drugs. *Belviq* is to be used in conjunction with diet and exercise. *Qsymia* is prescribed for weight-loss management in adults who are also obese or overweight with at least one weight-related comobidity.

Prescription weight-loss drugs need to be taken indefinitely so that much or all of the weight is not gained back. The problem associated with long-term drug management is that the long-term effects are not known. Because *Xenical* decreases the absorption of fat-soluble vitamins, a vitamin supplement may be prescribed. It is important to tell your patient that some insurance companies may not cover these drugs and prior authorization may be necessary. It is also important to tell your patient that weight-loss drugs don't take the place of a sensible diet and exercise.

One over-the-counter weight-loss drug is orlistat (*Alli*), a weaker version of the prescription drug orlistat (*Xenical*), available to adults over the age of 18 years. It promotes weight loss by decreasing absorption of fat by the intestine. It should be given with food, up to three times a day. Although it may sound like a miracle drug, it is not. It must be taken only in combination with a reduced-calorie, low-fat diet and exercise. The most common adverse reactions are diarrhea and gas with oily spotting. Like *Xenical*, *Alli* should be taken with a daily multivitamin, including vitamins A, D, and E, to counteract the loss of fat-soluble vitamins. It should not be taken by anyone who is of normal weight, who has taken cyclosporine, had an organ transplant, or can't absorb food. It should also be used with caution in patients who take a blood-thinning medication or have diabetes mellitus or thyroid disease.

Table 12.1 lists common OTC products that affect the GI system.

 Pediatric Considerations | Weight-Loss Drugs

- Drug therapy generally is not recommended for children.

- Orlistat (*Xenical*) may be used for children 12 to 16 years of age.

 Older Adult Considerations | Weight-Loss Drugs

- Being overweight is a problem for older adults because of slower metabolism, decreased physical activity, and eating habits similar to when younger and more active.
- Diet and increased physical activity are the treatment of choice.

- Weight-loss drugs should be used only with caution, if at all. Older adults are especially prone to cardiovascular, renal, and hepatic disorders that increase the risk of side effects.

Table 12.1 Selected OTC Medications for Gastrointestinal Disorders

Conditions	Products	Actions
Toothache, cold sores, canker sores	Benzodent, Orabase	Anesthetic/astringent
Diarrhea	Kaopectate, Pepto Bismol Maximum Strength, Imodium A-D	Antidiarrheal
Acid indigestion, heartburn	Aluminum hydroxide, Maalox Regular Strength, Gelusil, Mylanta Maximum Strength, Phillips' Milk of Magnesia, Rolaids, Tums	Antacid/antiflatulent
Constipation	Metamucil, Sennokot-S, Dulcolax	Laxative
Motion sickness	Bonine, Dramamine	Antiemetic
Hemorrhoids	Anusol, Nupercainal, Preparation H	Antiseptic/astringent/anesthetic/protectant

GIVING GASTROINTESTINAL MEDICATIONS [LO 12-4]

With most GI disorders, drug therapy is only an adjunct to physical measures. Someone with constipation needs to get on a regular bowel movement schedule; eat a high-fiber diet consisting of fresh fruits and vegetables and whole-grain cereals and breads; take in 1500 to 2000 mL of fluids daily; and increase physical activity. Likewise, someone with diarrhea may get relief by eating small portions of bland foods that are low in fiber and high in calories and protein; avoiding very hot or very cold drinks; resting; and replacing lost fluids. People with ulcers or gastritis should follow a bland diet consisting of six small meals daily and eliminate irritating substances like tobacco, coffee, and alcohol. As a healthcare worker, your role is to make sure that patients understand how these practices will help them feel better and make the drugs work better.

Avoiding stress is also important for good digestion. Psychological factors such as stress and anxiety can worsen constipation, nausea, ulcers, and many other disorders. You should strive to create a pleasant, nonstressful atmosphere around the patient. Arrange the environment for comfort and privacy, with empathy for the patient's worries and fears, and be supportive and encouraging.

There are some general principles to remember when giving medications for the GI system. Table 12.2 describes the general principles to remember when giving medications for the GI system.

Table 12.2 Principles for Giving GI Medications

Time
- Digestive medications must be given before meals (a.c.), during meals, or after meals (p.c.).
- Some medications must be taken with food, others without food.

Liquids
- Give recommended amount of liquids with each medication.

Abdominal Pain
- Check with supervisor before administering p.m. analgesic medication.

PROCESSES FOR SUPPOSITORIES AND FEEDING TUBES [LO 12-5]

Suppositories

Suppositories may be ordered when a patient is unconscious or cannot take oral medication and is nauseated, has a fever, or is in pain. They may also be ordered when a laxative effect on the large intestine is desired, to promote defecation within 15 to 60 minutes.

The insertion of a suppository can be unpleasant and embarrassing for a patient. After identifying the patient, close the room curtain or door to maintain privacy and minimize embarrassment. Explain what you are doing and why it is necessary. Remove the wrapper, and lubricate the rounded end of the suppository to make it enter the rectum as smoothly and gently as possible. The suppository must be inserted gently through the anus, past the internal sphincter and against the rectal wall. Insert the suppository, with your gloved index finger, 4 inches in an adult and 2 inches in infants and children. To be effective, the suppository must be placed along the wall of the rectum, rather than into fecal matter, to increase absorption.

If the patient has pain or irritation in the rectal area after you have inserted the suppository, chart it and inform the lead healthcare team member or provider. Either reaction may be a sign of local inflammation caused by the drug. When the patient has a bowel movement, note and chart the appearance of the stools.

Feeding Tubes

When a patient is unable to ingest, chew, or swallow food but still has a functioning GI tract, a feeding tube is ordered. Many conditions may call for a feeding tube, such as facial fractures; head and neck cancers; neurological conditions, such as stroke; psychological conditions, such as anorexia nervosa; extensive burns; and chemotherapy. A **gastroscope** is used to provide direct visualization of the interior of the stomach. There are two types of tubes: (1) A **nasogastric tube** is inserted through the nose or mouth and passes through the esophagus to the stomach (**Figure 12.2**); (2) a **gastrostomy tube** is inserted directly into the stomach through a surgical opening (**stoma**) in the left upper quadrant of the abdomen.

When a feeding tube is in place, oral medications are also given through the tube. These medications must be in liquid form. For this reason, tablets and caplets must be crushed with a pill crusher or mortar and pestle (**Figure 12.3**). Capsules should be pulled apart and their contents emptied into a medication cup. Once in powder form, tablets, caplets, or capsules should be mixed with 1 ounce of water before administering through a feeding tube. Remember, in no case should you crush or dissolve a buccal, sublingual, timed-release, or enteric-coated pill. If this is the prescribed medication, consult the lead healthcare team member or provider as to what to do.

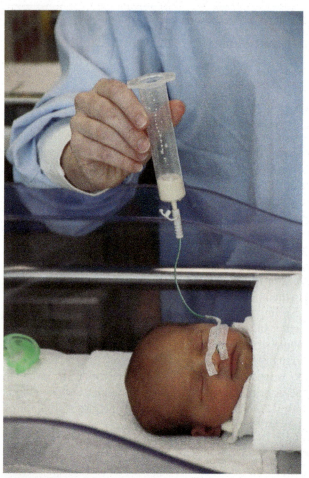

©paintings/Shutterstock

Figure 12.2

When a patient must use a feeding tube, medications are also administered through the tube.

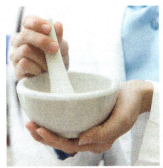

©Steve Debenport/Getty Images

Figure 12.3

Pill crusher and mortar and pestle.

Before beginning medication administration, put on disposable gloves and elevate the head of the bed 30 degrees. This is to prevent aspiration into the lungs. It is also important to check the placement of the tube. Attach the 30-mL cone-tipped syringe to the end of the tube and gently pull back on the syringe to obtain gastric contents. If you obtain 100 mL or more of gastric contents, notify your supervisor and do not proceed with the medication administration. This amount indicates the stomach has too much fluid in it and you may cause the patient to aspirate.

After determining that the tube is in the stomach, flush the tube with 30 to 60 mL of warm tap water to establish patency, meaning that the tube is open and not blocked. Administer one medication at a time. Never mix medications. Mixing medications may cause incompatability among the medications and render them useless. Administering medications together can also cause the tube to become clogged. After administering one medication, flush the tube with 5 to 10 mL of warm tap water to wash any residual medication down the tube and to maintain patency of the tube. Following the last medication, flush the tube again with 30 to 60 mL of warm tap water. It is important to keep track of how much water you use during the medication administration procedure because it is part of the patient's intake for the day. Record the intake on the patient's intake and output sheet and report it, as well as how the patient tolerated the procedure. This is particularly important in patients with certain cardiac or renal diseases, to prevent fluid overload. The same procedure is followed for the gastrostomy tube. Observe for redness, pus, or drainage around the insertion site of the tube and report them to your supervisor if found.

Keep in mind that tube-fed patients are dependent on others for eating and taking medications. This is not a pleasant experience for them. Try to make them as comfortable as possible and maintain a calm environment. Explain the procedure to patients to alleviate their fears.

Tube-fed or unconscious patients need special care with oral hygiene because they are mouth breathers and the tube is in one side of the nose. Their mouths are usually open, allowing the mucous membranes to dry out. Be alert to the need for rinsing their mouths and caring for their teeth. Cleanse the patient's mouth with a swab containing a solution of sorbitol, sodium, carboxymethylcellulose, and electrolytes. These swabs are effective in treating dry mouth. Do not use glycerin or lemon swabs. Glycerin swabs further dry the mouth and cause the gums and mucous membranes to shrink. They also promote bacterial growth. Lemon swabs change the chemical composition of the mouth and wear away tooth enamel.

 Healthcare for Today and Tomorrow   Limited Use of *Lotronex*

Alosetron (*Lotronex*) was approved by the Food and Drug Administration in February 2000 for the treatment of inflammatory bowel syndrome. However, in November 2000, *Lotronex* was taken off the market because of serious adverse side effects such as severe constipation and ischemic colitis. Although it is extremely rare for a drug to be taken off the market and then placed back on the market, *Lotronex* is now available again through a restricted marketing program. It is available only for women who meet the criteria of inflammatory bowel syndrome with chronic bowel habits, predominantly diarrhea. Patients who take *Lotronex* sign an agreement that they understand all the benefits and risks associated with the drug.

The majority of drug trial studies in America are done on Caucasians. As a result, many healthcare providers are unaware of how ethnicity affects the body's reaction to many drugs. One such drug is omeprazole (*Prilosec*).

Studies have shown that four times as much *Prilosec* accumulates in the blood of Asian Americans as it does in Caucasians. Therefore, a smaller dose of *Prilosec* should be administered to Asian Americans.

Representative Drugs for the Gastrointestinal System

Category, Name,[a] and Route	Uses and Diseases	Actions	Usual Dose[b] and Special Instructions	Side Effects and Adverse Reactions
Antiflatulents				
simethicone Oral	Flatulence in the digestive tract, diverticulitis, peptic ulcer	Has a defoaming action; prevents formation of gas pockets	40–160 mg; 1–2 tablets qid after meals and at bedtime, as needed	Excessive expulsion of gas, belching
Antiemetics				
ondansetron hydrochloride (*Zofran*) Oral	Nausea and vomiting associated with chemotherapy; postoperative nausea and vomiting	Is a serotonin antagonist	8 mg PO, 30 minutes before chemotherapy, then 8 mg every 8 hours PO	Diarrhea, headache
dimenhydrinate (*Dramamine*) Oral, IM, dermal patch	Nausea, vomiting, motion sickness	Exact mechanism of action is unknown	Give 30 minutes to 1 hour before activity; 50–100 mg PO every 4–6 hours; 50 mg IM prn; advise against driving and other activities that require mental alertness	Dizziness, drowsiness, confusion, dry mouth
prochlorperazine Oral, rectal, IM	Severe nausea, vomiting; also used for severe anxiety and psychosis	Controls vomiting reflex by depressing the CNS	5–10 mg PO 3–4 times a day; 10–20 mg IM once, then repeat in 1–4 hours if needed	Orthostatic hypotension, drowsiness, blurred vision, urine retention, constipation, dry mouth
meclizine Oral	Motion sickness, dizziness, nausea, and vomiting; management of vertigo associated with diseases affecting vestibular system	Has antihistaminic properties	5–10 mg tid or qid; 25 mg rectally bid; 5–10 mg IM every 3–4 hours	Drowsiness, dry mouth, blurred vision

Representative Drugs for the Gastrointestinal System (*continued*)

Category, Name,[a] and Route	Uses and Diseases	Actions	Usual Dose[b] and Special Instructions	Side Effects and Adverse Reactions
Antispasmodics/Anticholinergics				
propantheline bromide Oral	Adjunctive therapy in treatment of peptic ulcer disease, irritable bowel syndrome	Inhibits gastrointestinal motility, diminishes acid secretion	15 mg 30 minutes before meals and 30 mg at bedtime	Dry mouth, decreased sweating, blurred vision, mydriasis (excessive pupil dilation), urinary retention, tachycardia, headache, nervousness
dicyclomine (*Bentyl*) Oral, IM	Adjunctive therapy in treatment of peptic ulcer disease, irritable bowel syndrome	Unknown; appears to relieve smooth muscle spasm, reduce intestinal motility	20-40 mg PO qid	Constipation, drowsiness, dizziness
Antidiarrheals				
diphenoxylate HCl and atropine sulfate (*Lomotil*) Oral	Diarrhea	Reduces intestinal motility	5 mg qid; do not exceed 20 mg/day; maintenance dose lower; adjusted individually	Abdominal distention, dry mouth, sedation, urine retention, dizziness
Laxatives				
bisacodyl (*Dulcolax*) Oral, rectal	Chronic constipation, preparation of bowel for surgery or examination	Increases intestinal motility through direct effect on smooth muscle of intestine	*Tablets* (enteric-coated): 10-15 mg PO at bedtime or early morning; to be swallowed whole; do not give within 1 hr of giving an antacid or milk (these can dissolve the enteric coating) *Suppository:* 10 mg	Abdominal cramps, nausea, vomiting, burning sensation in rectum
psyllium (*Metamucil*) Oral	Chronic constipation; bowel management	Is bulk-forming; absorbs water and expands to increase bulk and moisture content of stool	1-2 rounded tsp stirred into 8-oz glass of liquid 1-3 times a day followed by another full glass of liquid	Nausea, vomiting, diarrhea after excessive use; obstruction of colon if not taken with plenty of water

Category, Name,[a] and Route	Uses and Diseases	Actions	Usual Dose[b] and Special Instructions	Side Effects and Adverse Reactions
Laxatives (continued)				
docusate sodium (*Colace*) Oral	Constipation and hard stools, in patients with painful anorectal conditions, after a heart attack, and in cardiac and other conditions where patients should not strain during defecation (Note: stool softener, not a laxative)	Softens stools; decreases surface tension by increasing liquid content of stool	50–300 mg/day; full effect may take 1–3 days	Bitter taste, throat irritation; mild abdominal cramping; diarrhea
Histamine H$_2$-Receptor Antagonists				
ranitidine (**Zantac**) Oral	Duodenal and gastric ulcers, gastroesophageal reflux disease, hypersecretory conditions	Inhibits histamine at H$_2$-receptor site in the gastric parietal cells; inhibits gastric acid secretion	150 mg bid for 6 weeks, then 150 mg at bedtime; there is an over-the-counter product	Headache, drowsiness, agitation, depression, constipation, abdominal pain
cimetidine (*Tagamet HB*) Oral	Short-term maintenance of duodenal and gastric ulcers; management of gastroesophageal reflux disease	Inhibits histamine at H$_2$-receptor site in the gastric parietal cells; inhibits gastric acid secretion	300 mg qid with meals and at bedtime for 8 weeks or 400 mg bid, 800 mg at bedtime; after 8 weeks give bedtime dose only; not the drug of choice for older adults because of the increased incidence of central nervous system alterations; give 1 hour before or after antacids because antacids decrease the absorption of *Tagamet*; there is an over-the-counter product	Confusion, headache, depression, agitation, psychosis, diarrhea
nizatidine (*Axid*) Oral	Gastric and duodenal ulcers, gastroesophageal reflux disease	Blocks H$_2$-receptors, which reduces gastric acid output	150 mg bid for 4–8 weeks or 300 mg at bedtime; there is an over-the-counter product	Headache, somnolence, pruritis, sweating

Representative Drugs for the Gastrointestinal System (continued)

Category, Name,[a] and Route	Uses and Diseases	Actions	Usual Dose[b] and Special Instructions	Side Effects and Adverse Reactions
Histamine H$_2$-Receptor Antagonists (continued)				
famotidine (*Pepcid*) Oral	Short-term treatment of active duodenal ulcers; maintenance therapy for duodenal ulcers, hypersecretory conditions, gastroesophageal reflux disease	Inhibits histamine at H$_2$-receptor site; reduces secretion of gastric acid but pepsin remains stable	40 mg every day at bedtime for 4–8 weeks; 20 mg every day for maintenance therapy; there is an over-the-counter product	Headache, dizziness, altered taste, constipation
Proton Pump Inhibitors				
lansoprazole (***Prevacid***) Oral	Gastroesophageal reflux disease, severe erosive esophagitis, pathological hypersecretory conditions	Suppresses gastric acid	30–60 mg every day before meals for up to 8 weeks	Headache, dizziness, diarrhea, abdominal pain
esomeprazole (***Nexium***) Oral	Treatment for active duodenal ulcers with anti-infectives for *Helicobacter pylori* infection; gastroesophageal reflux disease	Suppresses gastric acid	20–40 mg every day for 4–8 weeks in the treatment of gastroesophageal reflux disease; 40 mg bid for 10 days in combination with an antibiotic	Headache, dizziness, diarrhea, flatulence, cough, rash
pantoprazole (***Protonix***) Oral	Erosive esophagitis associated with gastrointestinal reflux disease, pathological hypersecretory conditions	Suppresses gastric acid	40 mg every day for up to 8 weeks	Diarrhea, flatulence, abdominal pain, headache, urinary frequency, rash
omeprazole (*Prilosec*) Oral	Gastroesophageal reflux disease, severe erosive esophagitis, pathological hypersecretory conditions	Suppresses gastric acid; classified as gastric acid pump inhibitor because it blocks the final stage in the acid production	20–40 mg every day for 4–8 weeks; there is an over-the-counter product	Headache, dizziness, diarrhea, abdominal pain, nausea

Note: Bolded trade names are among the 50 most commonly prescribed drugs.

[a]Trade names given in parentheses are examples only. Check current drug references for a complete listing of available products.

[b]Average adult doses are given. However, dosages are determined by a provider and vary with the purpose of the therapy and the particular patient. The doses presented in this text are for general information only.

INSERTING A RECTAL SUPPOSITORY

Demonstrate how to administer a rectal suppository to an adult patient and a pediatric patient.

Equipment

Provider's order for a rectal medication

Medication administration record, patient chart

Medicine tray or cart

Rectal suppository

Nonsterile gloves

Lubricating (water-soluble) jelly

Protective pad or paper towel

Procedure

1. Assemble the equipment and set up the medication. Check for the "seven rights."

2. Identify the patient according to health facility policy. Explain the procedure. Make sure that the patient understands that the suppository must be held in for at least 20 minutes. You will need the patient's cooperation.

3. Wash your hands. Unwrap the suppository and place it on the wrapper.

4. Assist the patient into a left side-lying (lateral) position with the upper leg bent. Drape the patient so as to expose only the anal area. Place a paper towel or pad under the hip to protect the sheet. Help the patient relax in preparation for the procedure.

5. Put on gloves. Lubricate the smooth or rounded tip of the suppository. Also lubricate your gloved index finger on your dominant hand.

6. Insert the suppository as shown in **Figure 12.4**:

   - With the nondominant hand, spread the buttocks apart and locate the anus.

   - Instruct the patient to breathe through the mouth. This will help relax the anal sphincter.

   - With the dominant hand, insert the suppository through the anus, past the internal sphincter and against the rectal wall. The suppository must be placed against the wall of the rectum for proper absorption and therapeutic action. Insert the suppository 4 inches in adults and 2 inches in children and infants. Withdraw the finger and wipe the anal area.

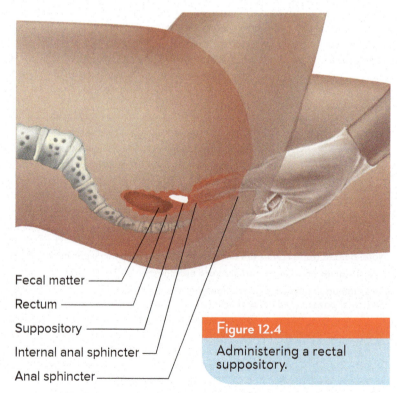

Fecal matter

Rectum

Suppository

Internal anal sphincter

Anal sphincter

Figure 12.4

Administering a rectal suppository.

7. Instruct the patient to remain flat in the left side-lying or Sims position for 5 minutes to prevent expulsion of the suppository.

8. Remove gloves by turning them inside out. Wash your hands.

9. Return in 5 minutes to determine if the suppository remained in place.

10. Chart the medication.

11. After this procedure has been completed, watch for signs of pain or irritation in the rectal area; chart and report them. Observe for the effects of the suppository, such as a bowel movement or relief of nausea or pain 30 minutes after administration.

Practice Procedure 12.2 (LO 12-5)

ADMINISTERING MEDICATION THROUGH A NASOGASTRIC OR GASTROSTOMY TUBE

Demonstrate how to administer a medication through a nasogastric or gastrostomy tube.

Equipment

Provider's order

Medication (tablet, capsule, powder, or liquid; no timed-release or enteric-coated forms)

Medication administration record, patient chart

Medicine tray or cart

Pitcher containing 2 to 4 oz of water at room temperature

30-mL cone-tipped syringe

Protective cover such as a small towel or disposable protective pad

Tube clamp on patient tubing

Nonsterile gloves

Procedure

1. Assemble the equipment and set up the medication. Check for the "seven rights."

2. Wash your hands.

3. Prepare the medication. Crush one tablet or pill with a pill crusher or mortar and pestle or between two spoons, using the top spoon to press down on the tablet. Never crush buccal, sublingual, or timed-release capsules or enteric-coated tablets. Then mix with 10 to 20 mL of lukewarm tap water in a medicine cup. If the medication is in capsule form, empty the capsule contents into water and mix.

4. Identify the patient according to health facility policy. Explain the procedure.

5. Place the patient in the proper position for administration.
   - In bed: semi-Fowler's or Fowler's position; elevate head of bed at least 30 degrees.
   - In a chair or wheelchair: sitting position.

6. Put on nonsterile gloves.

7. *Nasogastric:* Place a towel over the patient's chest, and remove the clamp from the tube.
   Gastrostomy: Remove the dressing from the abdomen, and unclamp the tube.

8. Check placement of the tube by attaching a 30-mL cone-tipped syringe to the end of the tube. Aspirate gently back on the syringe to obtain gastric contents.

9. Before administering medications, flush the tube with 30 to 60 mL of water.

10. Administer each medication separately. (Never mix medications together.) Between each medication, administer 5 to 10 mL of tap water.

11. After administering the last medication, flush the tube with 30 to 60 mL of warm tap water.

12. Clamp the tube. With a corner of a towel, wipe the end clean of any liquid.

13. *Nasogastric:* Tape the tube to the forehead or cheek.
Gastrostomy: Replace the dressing over the stoma. Check for leakage and report it to the supervisor if present. Lay the tube down over the abdomen.

14. Keep the patient in the semi-Fowler's position for 30 to 45 minutes following the procedure.

15. Wash your hands and clean the equipment.

16. Chart the medication. Chart any signs of redness, pus, or drainage around the insertion site of the tube, and report to the supervisor.

17. Chart the amount of water used during the procedure on the patient's intake sheet.

Summary

Learning Outcome	Summary Points
12-1 Describe the five main functions and the major parts of the gastrointestinal system.	<ul><li>The main functions of the gastrointestinal system:<ul><li>Breaking food into smaller pieces.</li><li>Transporting food through the GI tract.</li><li>Secreting digestive enzymes.</li><li>Absorbing nutrients into the blood.</li><li>Excreting solid wastes.</li></ul></li><li>The major parts of the gastrointestinal system:<ul><li>*Mouth:* Breaks the food into small pieces so it can be chewed by the teeth.</li><li>*Esophagus:* When a person swallows, the epiglottis closes to prevent food from entering the lungs. Allows food to the stomach.</li><li>*Stomach:* Dissolves food, destroys bacteria, and breaks down connective tissue in meats. Food remains in the stomach for about 3 hours and becomes an acidic, liquefied mass, or chyme.</li><li>*Small intestine:* Food mixes with digestive enzymes from the liver and pancreas. By the time the food has passed through the small intestine, most of the nutrients are absorbed.</li><li>*Large intestine:* Excess water is absorbed into the bloodstream, leaving undigested wastes. These are collected and compacted into feces that leave by way of the rectum and anus.</li><li>*Liver:* Secretes bile, stores nutrients absorbed from the small intestine, removes wastes from the blood, and produces substances for blood clotting and the immune system. Also important in drug action because it breaks down or inactivates many drugs.</li><li>*Gallbladder:* Collects bile.</li><li>*Pancreas:* Produces digestive juices that complete the chemical changes that turn fats, protein, and carbohydrates into particles that can be absorbed. Also secretes insulin that regulates the amount of sugar used by the cells.</li></ul></li></ul>

Learning Outcome	Summary Points

12-2 Describe the major disorders and related symptoms of the gastrointestinal system.	• The major gastrointestinal disorders:
	  • *Gastritis* is an inflammation of the stomach.
	  • *Peptic ulcer disease* is an open sore in the stomach or duodenal lining.
	  • *Liver disorders* include cirrhosis, which is a degeneration and destruction of the liver cells.
	  • *Gallbladder disorders* include gallstones, which are small granules consisting primarily of cholesterol.
	  • *Pancreatitis* is an inflammation of the pancreas.
	  • *Peritonitis* is an acute inflammation of the membranes that line the abdomen.
	  • *Crohn's disease* is a chronic, nonspecific inflammatory bowel disease of unknown etiology that usually affects the terminal ileum, jejunum, and colon.
	  • *Irritable bowel syndrome* is a group of symptoms characterized by intermittent abdominal pain associated with either diarrhea or constipation.
	  • *Diverticulosis* is a condition in which multiple pouches (diverticula) develop in the large intestine.
	  • *Hemorrhoids* are enlarged hemorrhoidal veins.
	• The symptoms of gastrointestinal disorders:
	  • Dyspepsia (indigestion)
	  • Hyperacidity (heartburn)
	  • Emesis (vomiting)
	  • Eructation (belching)
	• Correctly performing calculations ensures patient safety and decreases the incidence of adverse reactions.

12-3 Describe the actions of the following drug groups: antacids, histamine H_2-receptor antagonists, digestants, antiflatulents, emetics, antiemetics, anticholinergics and antispasmodics, antidiarrheals, laxatives, anthelmintics, anorexiants, and weight-loss drugs.	• *Antacids* neutralize hydrochloric acid in the stomach. Example: *Maalox Regular Strength*.
	  • *Histamine H_2-receptor antagonists* block histamine. Example: *Tagamet HB*.
	  • *Digestants* aid in digestion.
	  • *Antiflatulents* decrease the gas in the stomach. Example: *Mylanta Maximum Strength*.
	  • *Emetics* induce vomiting.
	  • *Antiemetics* suppress nausea and vomiting. Example: *Tigan*.
	  • *Anticholinergics* block acetylcholine.
	• *Antispasmodics* have an effect on the smooth muscle and very little effect on the secretion of acid. Example: *Donnatal*.
	  • *Antidiarrheals* decrease intestinal motility. Example: *Lomotil*.
	  • *Laxatives* promote defecation. Example: *Dulcolax*.
	  • *Anthelmintics* are used for intestinal infestation.
	  • *Anorexiants* decrease appetite. Example: *Adipex-P*
	  • *Weight-loss drugs* aid in weight loss. Example: *Xenical*.

12-4 Identify the important conditions to be aware of when giving medications for the gastrointestinal system.	• Verify the correct time to give medication. • Give liquids. • Question whether abdominal pain is present.

Learning Outcome	Summary Points

12-5 Describe and follow proper procedure for inserting rectal suppositories and for giving medications through a nasogastric or gastrostomy tube.	• Inserting rectal suppositories:
	  • With a gloved index finger, insert the rectal suppository through the anus, past the internal sphincter and against the rectal wall; insert it 4 inches in an adult and 2 inches in an infant or child.
	• Giving medications through a nasogastric or gastrostomy tube:
	  • Start by determining placement.
	  • Place the patient in a 30-degree position.
	  • Administer a gastrointestinal medicine through a feeding tube.
	  • Flush the tube with 30 to 60 mL of warm tap water before starting.
	  • Flush with 5 to 10 mL of warm tap water after each drug.
	  • Flush with 30 to 60 mL of warm tap water at the completion of medications.

Chapter 12 Review

Match the medical terms to their definitions.

_____ 1. (LO 12-2) Yellow color of the skin due to liver bile in the bloodstream

_____ 2. (LO 12-2) Instrument for looking into the stomach

_____ 3. (LO 12-2) Belching

_____ 4. (LO 12-4) Tube inserted into the stomach through a hole

_____ 5. (LO 12-4) Tube inserted into the stomach through the nose and esophagus

_____ 6. (LO 12-4) Moving the bowels

_____ 7. (LO 12-2) Vomiting

a. emesis

b. eructation

c. jaundice

d. nasogastric tube

e. gastrostomy tube

f. gastroscope

g. defecation

Complete the statements by filling in the blank.

8. (LO 12-1) Another name for the gastrointestinal system is the _____ system.

9. (LO 12-1) The tube that passes through the body from the mouth to the rectum is the _____.

10. (LO 12-1) The muscular movement that carries food through the gastrointestinal system is called _____.

11. (LO 12-1) Glands in the mouth, stomach, liver, and pancreas secrete _____ that help break down food.

12. (LO 12-1) Nutrients are absorbed into the blood mainly from the _____.

13. (LO 12-1) The fluid that coats and dissolves food in the mouth is called _____.

14. (LO 12-1) The body tube that connects the mouth to the stomach is the _____.

15. (LO 12-1) When peristalsis moves in the opposite direction, the result is _____.

16. (LO 12-1) Powerful juices from the pancreas and liver are mixed with food in the _____ _____, which is the entryway to the small intestine.

17. (LO 12-1) Because of their fingerlike shape, the _____ of the small intestine provide a huge area for absorption.

18. (LO 12-1) Undigested waste products that collect in the large intestine are called _____.

19. (LO 12-1) The opening that allows material from the rectum to pass out of the body is the _____ _____.

20. (LO 12-1) Bile, an enzyme that breaks down fat, is produced in the _____.

21. (LO 12-1) Bile is stored in the _____.

22. (LO 12-1) Powerful digestive juices that complete the digestion of carbohydrates, fat, and protein are produced in the _____.

23. (LO 12-2) The disorder that is a chronic, nonspecific bowel disease, which is characterized by discontinuous skip lesions with segments of normal bowel occurring between diseased portions is _____.

Answer the questions in the space provided.

24. (LO 12-1) What are the five functions of the gastrointestinal system?

_____

_____

_____

25. (LO 12-1) How is digestion related to psychological stress?

_____

_____

26. (LO 12-2) List all the symptoms you can think of that signal some disorder of the digestive tract.

_____

_____

27. (LO 12-2) What is intestinal motility, and what happens if it is too fast or too slow?

_____

_____

28. (LO 12-2) How can tooth and gum disorders lead to other gastrointestinal problems?

_____

_____

29. (LO 12-3) What is the primary drug used to treat ulcerative colitis?

_____

Describe the drug action; for example, *Emetics cause vomiting.*

30. (LO 12-3) Antacids _____

31. (LO 12-3) Digestants _____

32. (LO 12-3) Antiflatulents _____

33. (LO 12-3) Antiemetics _____

34. (LO 12-3) Anticholinergics _____

35. (LO 12-3) Antidiarrheals _____

36. (LO 12-3) Laxatives _____

37. (LO 12-3) Anthelmintics _____

38. (LO 12-3) Anorexiants _____

Place a T in the blank if the statement is true. Place an F in the blank if the statement is false.

39. _____ (LO 12-2) Hepatitis B is a major concern for healthcare workers because it is a blood-borne disease that may occur through needlesticks.

40. _____ (LO 12-2) The first phase of hepatitis is the icteric phase, characterized by anorexia, weight loss, malaise, headache, low-grade fever, joint pain, and skin rashes.

41. _____ (LO 12-3) The dual-drug therapy for peptic ulcer disease includes metronidazole (*Flagyl*) and tetracycline.

42. _____ (LO 12-2) The major symptoms of ulcerative colitis are abdominal pain and bloody diarrhea.

43. _____ (LO 12-3) *Xenical* is a weight-loss drug that increases the absorption of fat-soluble vitamins.

Match these drug categories to their drugs.

_____ 44. (LO 12-3) Pyrantel pamoate	a. anticholinergics and antispasmodics
_____ 45. (LO 12-3) *Metamucil,* bisacodyl	b. laxatives
_____ 46. (LO 12-3) Bismuth, *Lomotil*	c. antacids
_____ 47. (LO 12-3) Atropine, *Bentyl*	d. antiflatulents (carminatives)
_____ 48. (LO 12-3) *Zofran, Dramamine,* prochlorperazine	e. antidiarrheals
_____ 49. (LO 12-3) Simethicone, *Infant's Mylicon*	f. anthelmintics
_____ 50. (LO 12-3) Pancrelipase	g. digestants
_____ 51. (LO 12-3) *Maalox Regular Strength,* aluminum hydroxide, *Gelusil,* sodium bicarbonate	h. antiemetics
_____ 52. (LO 12-3) *Tagamet HB, Zantac,* famotidine	i. histamine H_2-receptor antagonists
_____ 53. (LO 12-3) Apomorphine	j. emetics
_____ 54. (LO 12-3) *Reglan*	k. GI stimulants
_____ 55. (LO 12-3) *Solu-Medrol,* sulfasalazine	l. anti-inflammatories
_____ 56. (LO 12-3) Orlistat, *Adipex-P*	m. weight-loss drugs

Drug Calculations—Fill in the blank with the answer.

57. (LO 12-3) The provider orders ranitidine (*Zantac*) 50 mg intramuscularly tid. Available is 25 mg/mL. Prepare to administer _____ mL to your patient.

58. (LO 12-3) The provider orders diphenoxylate HCl with atropine sulfate (*Lomotil*) 2.5 mg orally bid. Available is 5.0 mg. You will give your patient _____ tablets.

59. (LO 12-3) The provider orders cimetidine (*Tagamet HB*) 800 mg orally at bedtime. Available are 200-mg tablets. You will give _____ tablets to your patient.

60. (LO 12-3) The provider orders ondansetron (*Zofran*) 4 mg intramuscularly tid. Available is 2 mg/mL. Prepare to administer _____ mL to your patient.

61. (LO 12-3) The provider orders dicyclomine (*Bentyl*) 15 mg orally tid. Available is a 10-mg/5-mL syrup. You will administer _____ mL to your patient.

Multiple Choice—Circle the correct letter.

62. (LO 12-2) When taking a medication history, you learn that the patient is taking sulfasalazine (*Azulfidine*). On the basis of your knowledge of medications, you know that this drug is the primary drug used to treat what condition?

    a. Pancreatitis
    b. Crohn's disease
    c. Ulcerative colitis
    d. Diverticulosis

63. (LO 12-3) Which of the following instructions should you give to a patient who is taking antacids?

    a. Magnesium-based antacids cause constipation.
    b. Chew a chewable tablet thoroughly.
    c. If the antacid isn't working as prescribed, it is safe to take extra doses.
    d. Take a calcium carbonate antacid with a glass of milk.

64. (LO 12-3) Which of the following instructions must be told to a patient taking *Beano*?

    a. Avoid gas-forming foods.
    b. Use a straw to drink liquids.
    c. Take with food.
    d. Take extra doses if the diarrhea does not stop.

65. (LO 12-3) Monitor a patient taking propantheline bromide for which of the following side effects?

    a. Diarrhea, flatulence, nausea
    b. Abdominal distention, burning sensation in the rectum, vomiting
    c. Orthostatic hypotension, bradycardia, dyspnea
    d. Dry mouth, urinary retention, decreased sweating

66. (LO 12-3) Which instruction is important to tell a patient taking psyllium (*Metamucil*)?

    a. Take mixed in an 8-oz glass of water followed by another glass of liquid.
    b. Avoid antacids.
    c. Take with a small amount of food.
    d. Avoid high-fiber foods.

Chapter 12 Case Studies

67. (LO 12-3) A patient with gastroesophageal reflux disease has been prescribed omeprazole (*Prilosec*) 20 mg orally 3 times a day. The patient asks you how *Prilosec* works. What should you tell the patient? How do you administer *Prilosec*? What are the side effects you should watch for? _____

_____

_____

_____

68. (LO 12-3) *Maalox Advanced Maximum Strength Liquid* 30 mL has been ordered p.m. for a patient with heartburn. After reviewing this patient's medication record, you discover tetracycline is also ordered. How should you administer these two drugs? The patient asks you if constipation or diarrhea will be experienced. How should you respond? _____

_____

_____

_____

Critical Thinking

Answer the questions in the space provided.

69. (LO 12-3) State the four ways that laxatives (cathartics) work.

_____

_____

_____

70. (LO 12-3) What are some of the physical measures that help gastrointestinal drugs work better?

_____

_____

71. (LO 12-3) List three things to remember when giving gastrointestinal medications.

_____

_____

_____

_____

_____

72. (LO 12-5) Describe the procedure for administering a rectal suppository.

_____

_____

_____

73. (LO 12-5) What signs should you look for, chart, and report after inserting a suppository?

_____

_____

74. (LO 12-5) How should you prepare a tablet or capsule for administration through a nasogastric or gastrostomy tube?

_____

_____

75. (LO 12-5) What signs should you look for, chart, and report when administering medications through a nasogastric or gastrostomy tube?

_____

_____

76. (LO 12-3) Explain what a laxative does.

_____

_____

77. (LO 12-3) List two different antacid combinations.

_____

_____

Select the disorder that best matches the patient description and write it in the blank.

gastritis	hepatitis	duodenal ulcer	hemorrhoids
gallstones	peritonitis	cirrhosis	irritable bowel

78. (LO 12-2) Mrs. Phillips has been straining at stool. The large veins around her anal opening are swollen, itching, and beginning to bleed.

_____

79. (LO 12-2) Following a transfusion of blood, Mr. Mann develops a liver infection. The provider suspects that a blood donor also had the infection and passed it on to Mr. Mann through the transfusion.

_____

80. (LO 12-2) Mrs. Merriweather has small grains of cholesterol building up in her gallbladder. They cause mild spasms from time to time. The provider will not remove them unless they begin to block the tube that leads to the intestine. The provider prescribes a drug to reduce the intestinal spasms.

_____

81. (LO 12-2) Mr. Hale is an alcoholic. His provider has been warning him about the damage to his liver for years. Now Mr. Hale has developed a severe inflammation of the liver. The provider orders rest and a high-calorie, high-carbohydrate, low-fat diet.

_____

82. (LO 12-2) Ms. Yang has an inflammation of the stomach. The epigastric tenderness and nausea have been coming and going for several weeks. Her provider suggests that she cut out smoking and coffee to give her stomach relief.

_____

83. (LO 12-2) Mr. Hruban has developed an open sore at the entrance of the small intestine. The provider prescribes antacids to calm his nervous tension. She also orders Mr. Hruban to quit smoking.

_____

84. (LO 12-2) Because of an injury to the Nelson child's intestine, bacteria are released into the abdominal cavity. This has caused a serious inflammation of the abdominal linings. Surgery and antibiotics are ordered at once.

_____

85. (LO 12-2) Miss Perez is troubled by abdominal cramping and flatulence. She is under a great deal of stress in her job as a junior high school teacher. After a careful examination, the provider reassures her that the condition is not serious and prescribes an antispasmodic to reduce the cramping.

_____

Applications

Obtain an electronic drug guide, a current copy of a drug reference book, or the *PDR*®. Use it to answer the following questions in a notebook or on file cards.

86. Where would you look in the *PDR*® to find other product names for the antacids listed in the Representative Drugs for the Gastrointestinal System table in this chapter? Find another product name for each antacid listed.

87. In Section 3 of the *PDR*®, Product Category Index, find Antacids. Make a list of any antacid and combination drugs that are not in the Representative Drugs for the Gastrointestinal System table in this chapter.

88. In Section 5 of the *PDR*®, Product Information, look up the page number and locate the detailed information about one of the antacids you listed in question 87. What is the adult dosage? Pediatric dosage? How is the drug supplied? Who is the manufacturer of this drug?

89. Find the picture of your antacid and combinations in Section 4 of the *PDR*®, Product Identification Guide.

DRUGS FOR THE URINARY SYSTEM AND FLUID BALANCE

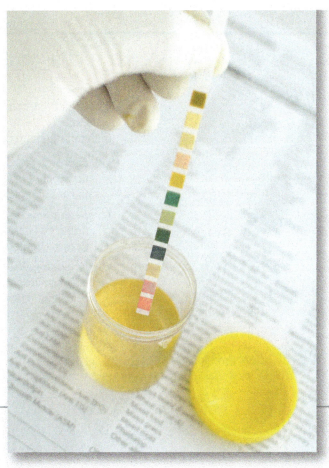

©jarun011/Getty Images

In this chapter you will learn how the urinary system excretes liquid wastes from the body. You will study how the kidneys maintain the proper balance of fluids and salts to meet the needs of the cells. You will also learn about the disorders that arise in the urinary system and how drugs are used to control them. In addition, you will learn how to administer drugs into an indwelling catheter and how to give diuretics.

acidifier	electrolytes	oliguria
acidosis	hematuria	pH
alkalizer	homeostasis	pyelonephritis
alkalosis	hypercalcemia	pyuria
anuria	hyperkalemia	residual urine
azotemia	hypernatremia	urea
cystitis	hypocalcemia	ureter
cystoscopy	hypokalemia	ureteritis
dialysis	hyponatremia	urethritis
diuretic	indwelling catheter	urinary catheter
dysuria	nephritis	urge incontinence (overactive bladder)

URINARY SYSTEM [LO 13-1]

The urinary system includes two kidneys, two ureters, a urinary bladder, and a urethra (Figure 13.1). The system has three major functions: excretion, maintaining homeostasis, and regulating pH balance.

- *Excretion of waste products.* The kidneys excrete waste products by filtering them out of the blood. The main waste products are **urea**, a by-product of the use of proteins by body cells; certain mineral salts; and water.

- *Regulating the amount of water.* By eliminating excess water, the urinary system helps maintain a proper balance of fluids in the body tissues (**homeostasis**).

- *Regulating the pH balance.* Body cells work best in a neutral or slightly basic environment. The kidneys help maintain the proper balance of acids and bases no matter what types of foods one eats.

Figure 13.1
The urinary system.

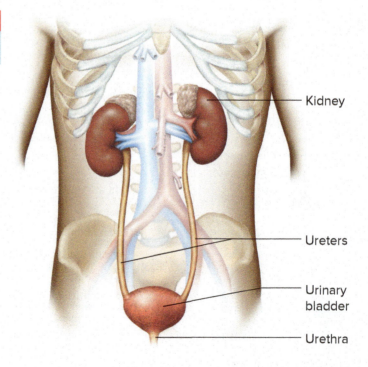

Kidney

Ureters

Urinary bladder

Urethra

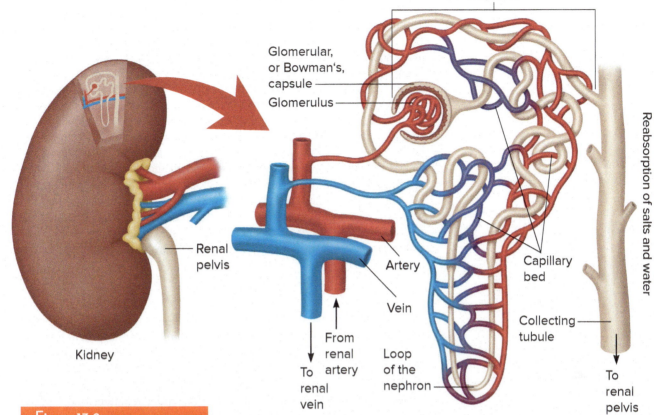

Nephron

Glomerular,
or Bowman's,
capsule

Glomerulus

Renal
pelvis

Artery

Vein

From
renal
artery

To
renal
vein

Loop
of the
nephron

Capillary
bed

Collecting
tubule

Reabsorption of salts and water

To
renal
pelvis

Kidney

All three functions of the urinary system are carried out through the same process of filtering the blood. This process takes place in the kidneys. Urine is produced and leaves the body by way of the ureter, the bladder, and the urethra, which are the organs of elimination. The two kidneys are bean-shaped organs located on either side of the vertebral column, posterior to the peritoneum and against the deep muscles of the back. They are supported by a layer of fatty connective tissue and are partially protected by the ribs. An adrenal gland lies on top of each kidney. Each kidney has two layers, the cortex (the outer layer) and the medulla (the inner layer). The functional unit of the kidney is the nephron. Each kidney contains 1 million nephrons. Each nephron has a bulb at one end, the glomerulus, which contains many capillaries (**Figure 13.2**). The glomerulus is the initial site of urine formation.

As blood circulates through the glomerulus, water and dissolved substances pass out of the blood through the capillary walls and into the nephron. This liquid then travels through the coils of the nephron tube, and some of the water, nutrients, and minerals are reabsorbed into the bloodstream through the nephron walls. This process leaves behind only waste products, certain salts, and varying amounts of water. The resulting liquid is called urine. The nephrons dip into the second layer of the kidney, the medulla. There, urine collects in a tube called the **ureter** that leads out of the kidney. The ureter is about 10 to 13 inches long.

PARTS OF THE URINARY SYSTEM [LO 13-2]

The two ureters, one from each kidney, carry the collected urine to the bladder, a collapsible storage bag for urine. Located directly behind the symphysis pubis (the junction of the pubic bones in front), the muscular walls of the bladder are able to stretch out and hold as much as 600 mL of urine. Nerve endings in the bladder signal to the nervous system when the bladder contains about 250 mL of urine. This signal creates the urge to urinate, or void.

During urination, urine passes out of the body by way of the urethra. The urethra is about $1\frac{1}{2}$ inches long in the female. It opens to the outside of the body between the labia in the female genital area, just above the vaginal opening. The urethra is about 8 inches long in the male and opens to the outside at the tip of the penis. The male urethra is shared by the urinary and reproductive systems.

Urine is a medically important substance. Examining and testing urine give clues to many types of diseases and disorders, show how well the kidneys are functioning, and indicate imbalances in the body's water and pH levels. Urine is about 90 to 95 percent water and 5 to 10 percent salts, urea, and other waste products. Normally, urine is amber or straw-colored and clear. When allowed to stand for any period of time, urine becomes cloudy. It normally has an ammonia odor. The kidneys produce about 1500 to 2000 mL of urine in a 24-hour period. The bladder voids approximately 250 mL at a time. When there is an excess of water, the kidneys allow more water to be eliminated. This shows up in urine tests because there is a smaller percentage of waste products per unit of liquid.

ABNORMAL ALTERATIONS IN URINE [LO 13-3]

There are several ways to tell if the kidneys and other parts of the urinary tract are working properly. The urine is inspected for color, clarity, and odor. Normal urine is pale yellow to amber, clear, and has an ammonia odor. Abnormalities in the appearance or smell of urine may indicate possible illness. Red urine may indicate bleeding from the kidney or bladder. Cloudy or foamy urine may alert the provider to possible renal disease or infection. A patient whose urine sample has a sweet, fruity odor may be showing a sign of diabetes mellitus or starvation. A routine urinalysis is also useful to measure other elements (Table 13.1). If any of the results of the urinalysis are abnormal, further tests may be ordered to evaluate the functioning of the urinary system.

When patients cannot empty the bladder on their own, catheterization may be necessary. Catheterization of the bladder involves passing a rubber or plastic tube, the catheter, through the urethra into the bladder. The catheter allows

Table 13.1 Routine Urinalysis Values

	Normal Value	Abnormal Results
pH	4.6–8.0	Acid-base imbalance
Protein	Negative	Renal disease (may occur temporarily after activity)
Glucose	Negative	Diabetes mellitus
Ketone	Negative	Diabetes mellitus, starvation, dehydration
RBCs	Up to 2	Trauma
Specific gravity	1.010–1.030	*High values:* dehydration, renal disease *Low values:* overhydration
WBCs	0–8	Infection
Bacteria	Negative	Infection
Casts	Negative	Infection

the bladder to empty. The amount of urine obtained from catheterization can be an indication of a medical problem. Finally, much can be discovered just by examining the urine. A visual examination of a urine sample may reveal traces of blood (**hematuria**) or pus (**pyuria**) in the urine.

X-rays may be ordered. A kidney, ureter, bladder (KUB) x-ray is used to evaluate the structures of the urinary system. It may detect trauma to a structure, such as a lacerated kidney following an auto accident, or the presence of stones, such as kidney stones. Another test, an intravenous pyelogram (IVP), uses a radiopaque dye to visualize the kidneys, renal pelvis, ureters, and bladder. X-ray films are taken over a 30-minute period to evaluate the flow of dye through the kidneys, ureters, and bladder. A defect in the passage of the dye through the various structures may indicate a tumor or a problem with the glomerular filtration. Other x-rays the provider may order are a renal scan, an ultrasound, and a CT scan. These procedures are noninvasive.

Invasive tests may also be used to evaluate the blood supply to the kidney (renal arteriogram), to conduct a microscopic examination of the renal tissue (renal biopsy), and to provide direct visualization of the interior of the bladder (**cystoscopy**).

Outward signs of urinary tract disorders are changes in the act of urinating. Inability to completely empty the bladder is called retention. Urine remaining in the bladder after voiding (volumes of 100 mL or more) is called **residual urine**. Inability to control urination is incontinence. Having to urinate very often (frequency) or feeling a great urge to urinate even when the bladder is empty (urgency) are common symptoms of disorders. Urination may be difficult or painful (**dysuria**). There may be a burning sensation during urination. Or there may be decreased urine output of 100 to 400 mL in a 24-hour period (**oliguria**) or less than 100 mL in 24 hours (**anuria**).

These symptoms may be the result of urinary tract disorders or of more serious kidney disease, as is the case with anuria. Some symptoms may appear as side effects of a drug; for example, frequency may be a side effect of taking a diuretic. When these conditions appear after giving a drug, they should be charted.

MAJOR DISORDERS OF THE URINARY SYSTEM [LO 13-4]

Obstructions

Obstructions of the urinary tract may occur at any point in the urinary system, from the urinary meatus to the kidney. They may be congenital or caused by tumors or injuries. Kidney stones are also responsible for some obstructions. These stones are formed from salts in the urine. Crystals form and precipitate the formation of a stone. Kidney stones may be large enough to block the ureters. Typically the patient experiences severe abdominal or flank pain. A procedure, lithotripsy, may be performed to crush the stone.

In men, the prostate is a donut-shaped gland that surrounds the urethra. An enlarged or inflamed prostate can squeeze the urethra, which also impairs normal urination.

Infections

Urinary tract infections (UTIs) may occur in the kidneys, ureters, bladder, and urethra. Women are more often affected by urinary tract infections than men because of the close proximity of the urethral meatus to the anus. Men are somewhat protected because prostatic secretions contain an antibacterial substance. Older adults are especially prone to urinary tract infections because of underlying conditions such as obstructions, catheterization, or nosocomial infection (hospital-acquired infection).

Personal cleanliness is important to prevent microorganisms from entering the urinary tract. Once microorganisms gain entry, they can cause infections that may travel up the urethra to the bladder and other parts of the system. Bladder infections are frequently accompanied by pain or burning on urination. These are other infections of the urinary tract:

- **Pyelonephritis**: kidney infection.
- **Nephritis**: inflammation of the kidney.
- **Cystitis**: inflammation of the bladder.
- **Ureteritis**: inflammation of the ureter.
- **Urethritis**: inflammation of the urethra.

In addition to treating urinary tract infections with antibiotics and analgesics for pain, you must educate patients about prevention.

Urge Incontinence/Overactive Bladder

Urge incontinence is a condition that is caused by uncontrolled contraction or overactivity of the detrusor muscle. It is also called an **overactive bladder** and is precipitated by a warning of only a few seconds to minutes. Leakage is both frequent and periodic. Incontinence or urinary frequency during the night (nocturnal) is common. Urge incontinence may also be accompanied by varying degrees of psychological stress. Tolterodine (*Detrol*) is the drug of choice in the treatment of an overactive bladder. It works as a muscarine receptor antagonist in the bladder to cause increased bladder control. Fesoterodine (*Toviaz*) is a antimuscarinic drug used to treat an overactive bladder. Mirabegron (*Myrbetriq*) also treats overactive bladder.

Renal Failure

Renal failure is the severe impairment or total lack of kidney function. There is an inability to excrete metabolic waste products and water. Renal failure may be acute or chronic. Acute renal failure has a rapid onset and may be reversible. Chronic renal failure is a progressive, irreversible destruction of both kidneys. Renal failure is characterized by an accumulation of nitrogenous waste products in the blood, **azotemia**. This buildup of waste products leads to uremia, in which the patient starts to exhibit signs of the disease. In acute renal failure, the urinary output decreases to less than 400 mL in 24 hours. Initially, there is an increase in urine, followed by oliguria and anuria. Unless kidney function can be restored, patients with renal failure often undergo **dialysis**. Mechanical filtering of the blood using a machine is called hemodialysis. Peritoneal dialysis involves the clearing of waste products by means of fluid exchanges across the abdominal lining, the peritoneum. Continuous ambulatory peritoneal dialysis (CAPD) frees the patient from having to sit for hours while attached to a machine. CAPD is done by the patient, who instills the dialysis solution from a collapsible bag into the peritoneal cavity through a disposable plastic tube. The patient does this four times a day. The bag is on an IV pole, so the patient can be ambulatory. In between treatments, the patient is completely free of all equipment. CAPD can be done easily at home.

Another danger in renal failure is that drugs are not excreted from the body as rapidly as with healthy kidneys. This is important to remember when giving medications. The renal system is one of the main ways drugs are removed from the body. A kidney that does not work properly fails to eliminate the drugs as expected, and the drugs build up (accumulate) in the body with each dose. Dosages must thus be carefully adjusted and the patient watched closely for drug toxicity whenever there is a suspected problem with the kidneys.

Some drugs, especially antibiotics, are damaging to the kidneys. Infections also cause damage. Either kind of damage can lead to kidney failure. But kidney function is also affected by diseases in other parts of the body. These diseases may slow the work of the kidneys, even though the kidneys themselves are not damaged. For example, if a patient is in congestive heart failure, not enough blood flows through the kidneys. As a result, the kidneys cannot do a proper job of excreting water and salts. Water is retained in the tissues, and edema occurs.

IMBALANCES OF BODY FLUIDS, ELECTROLYTES, AND PH [LO 13-5]

The body of an average adult ranges from 50 to 60 percent water (more in children and less in older adults). Most of this water is contained within the body cells, but about a quarter of it is in the spaces between cells or in the blood plasma. Maintaining enough water in the body tissues is important, because water is the medium for many chemical exchanges that are crucial to life.

To ensure adequate water, a balance is kept between fluids taken in (through food and drink) and excreted (through sweat, urine, and exhalation). The body usually does this naturally. But when there is disease, especially disease of the kidneys, the body may not be able to maintain a balance between intake and output. This is why it is sometimes necessary to keep track of fluid intake and fluid output.

An intake and output chart is used to record the quantity of fluids taken in through food, drink, IV infusion, and so on (Figure 13.3). The chart is also used to record the quantity of fluid excreted in the urine and during vomiting. To maintain balance, each day's intake should equal the day's output. If water taken in exceeds water lost, an abnormal accumulation of fluids in the interstitial spaces of the tissues, or edema, results. If too much water is excreted, the body may experience dehydration. Either condition interferes with proper functioning. By keeping track of fluid intake and output, the medical staff can decide what treatment is necessary to maintain proper balance. A vomiting patient who loses too much water this way may need IV infusions. A patient with edema may need a **diuretic** to make the kidneys excrete more urine.

For the important chemical exchanges of living cells to take place, the water must contain the proper amount and kind of **electrolytes**. Electrolytes are electrically charged particles (ions) of dissolved salts. They are a means of carrying chemicals through the body fluids. Because salt attracts water, these salt ions are also a way to hold fluids in the body tissues. The electrolytes are potassium, calcium, sodium, magnesium, chloride, bicarbonate, phosphate, and sulfate. All the electrolytes must be present in proper amounts for adequate body functioning. IV solutions with electrolytes should be given when the patient has vomiting or diarrhea.

Tranel HEALTHCARE

INTAKE AND OUTPUT RECORD

DATE	IN					OUT					IN					OUT					IN					OUT				
	ORAL	IV	IV	TF	OTHER	URINE	EMESIS	LIQ. STOOL	TUBE	OTHER	ORAL	IV	IV	TF	OTHER	URINE	EMESIS	LIQ. STOOL	TUBE	OTHER	ORAL	IV	IV	TF	OTHER	URINE	EMESIS	LIQ. STOOL	TUBE	OTHER
DAYS 7-8																														
8-9																														
9-10																														
10-11																														
11-12																														
12-1																														
1-2																														
2-3																														
8 HR TOT																														
EVENINGS 3-4																														
4-5																														
5-6																														
6-7																														
7-8																														
8-9																														
9-10																														
10-11																														
8 HR TOT																														
NIGHTS 11-12																														
12-1																														
1-2																														
2-3																														
3-4																														
4-5																														
5-6																														
6-7																														
8 HR TOT																														
24 HR TOT																														

| 24-HOUR GRAND TOTAL _____ | 24-HOUR GRAND TOTAL _____ | 24-HOUR GRAND TOTAL _____ | 24-HOUR GRAND TOTAL _____ | 24-HOUR GRAND TOTAL _____ | 24-HOUR GRAND TOTAL _____ |

FLUID EQUIVALENTS

1 oz = 30 mL

Full container ice = 1/2 container liquid

Coffee/tea = 240 mL

Custard/Ice cream/sherbet = 120 mL

Juice = 120 mL

Milk = 240 mL

Nectar = 165 mL

Popsicle (1 whole) = 75 mL

Soda = 360 mL

Soup = 180 mL

Standard milkshake/shakeup = 240 mL

Styrofoam cup = 240 mL

Small plastic cup = 150 mL

Large plastic cup = 360 mL

Water pitcher = 800 mL

Form No. 2300-00115

Figure 13.3

An intake/output record charts fluids taken in and excreted.

In addition, there must be proper balance between the amount of fluids (water) and the amounts and kinds of salts. The kidneys are sensitive to both water and salts. They compensate for an excess of salts by not allowing salts to be reabsorbed after the blood has been filtered. The unabsorbed salts, in turn, attract water. Thus, both salts and water remain in the kidney tubules, to be carried away through the urinary tract.

The kidneys, then, regulate both the amount and the makeup of body fluids. Ordinarily, the kidneys are able to keep the right proportion of salts and fluids. In disease, kidney malfunction, improper diet, or unusual physical activity, however, fluid-electrolyte imbalances occur. The types of imbalances are shown in the following table:

Hypercalcemia	High blood calcium level	Greater than 11 mg/dL
Hyperkalemia	High blood potassium level	Greater than 5.5 mEq/L
Hypernatremia	High blood sodium level	Greater than 145 mEq/L
Hypocalcemia	Low blood calcium level	Less than 9 mg/dL
Hypokalemia	Low blood potassium level	Less than 3.5 mEq/L
Hyponatremia	Low blood sodium level	Less than 135 mEq/L

Another type of necessary balance is the body's acid-base balance. This is the rate at which the body produces acids and bases equivalent to the rate at which acids and bases are excreted. This balance results in a stable concentration of hydrogen ions in body fluids. The concentration of hydrogen ions in a body fluid is called the pH value. The **pH** is a scale for measuring the acidity and alkalinity of fluid. Normal pH is 7.0. A pH below 7.0 is acid; above 7.0 is alkaline, or base. The body cannot tolerate more than very small changes in pH. The body has balancing mechanisms to ensure that strong acids and bases do not upset this balance. The kidneys are very much a part of this process. They are responsible for getting rid of excess acids or bases when required. The lungs also assist in this process. When they exhale carbon dioxide, they are eliminating acids from the bloodstream.

Disorders of the acid-base balance are called acidosis and alkalosis. **Acidosis** means too acid an environment for the cells; **alkalosis** means too alkaline an environment. Drugs may be administered to restore proper pH. **Acidifiers** (e.g., ammonium chloride and sodium biphosphate) make the pH more acid, in the case of alkalosis. **Alkalizers** (e.g., sodium bicarbonate) make the pH more alkaline, in the case of acidosis. Acidifiers and alkalizers may be given to prevent pH imbalances caused by certain drugs. They are also given to help certain drugs produce their strongest effects. For example, sodium bicarbonate is given with certain sulfonamides that work best in an alkaline pH. Acidifiers such as cranberry juice or ascorbic acid (vitamin C) may be given with methenamine (*Mandelamine*) to provide an acid urine, which enhances the action of the drug.

DRUGS FOR THE URINARY TRACT AND FLUID IMBALANCES [LO 13-6]

Antibiotics

The primary drugs used to treat urinary tract infections (UTIs) include penicillins, cephalosporins, sulfonamides, and fluoroquinolones. Ampicillin and amoxicillin are two penicillin drugs used for UTIs. Cefaclor and cefadroxil monohydrate are just two of the many cephalosporins used with UTIs.

Sulfonamides are among the most widely used antibiotics, particularly for UTIs. Sulfonamides are primarily bacteriostatic and effective against a wide variety of organisms. Sulfamethoxazole and trimethoprim (*Bactrim, Septra*) are frequently prescribed for UTIs. Newer sulfonamides such as sulfisoxazole have also proved effective. Urinary tract antiseptics such as methenamine are commonly used. Ciprofloxacin (*Cipro*) and ofloxacin are two broad-spectrum fluoroquinolones that are effective against a wide range of microorganisms.

Special analgesics are sometimes given with the antibiotic to relieve the low back pain that accompanies infection. A frequently used urinary analgesic is phenazopyridine (*Pyridium*). Pyridium may also be purchased over the counter without a prescription. You should warn the patient that phenazopyridine may cause the urine to become orange and may stain clothing. Urine discoloration is normal and not a reason for concern.

Urinary antimicrobials are sometimes administered directly into the bladder through a **urinary catheter.** (See Practice Procedure 13.1 later in the chapter.)

Diuretics

Diuretics are drugs that increase the output of water from the body. They decrease reabsorption of salts and water from the kidney tubules, with the result that more urine is produced. Increased urination removes excess water from the system. Diuretics are used to control edema in congestive heart failure. They are also used in the treatment of hypertension. In kidney disorders, diuretics are given to promote normal urine production. There are many types of diuretics with different modes of action. Examples of thiazide diuretics are chlorothiazide (*Diuril*) and hydrochlorothiazide.

The thiazides act primarily by inhibiting reabsorption of sodium in the distal tubules of the nephron. They therefore promote excretion of sodium, chloride, and water. When the increased sodium is presented to the distal tubules, there is a corresponding increase in potassium excretion. Although the thiazide diuretic achieves the goal of reducing edema, excretion of potassium can cause other problems.

The body cannot stand to lose too much potassium, because potassium is needed for chemical processes inside the cells. Too low a level of potassium (hypokalemia) results in fatigue, muscle weakness, and cardiac changes such as disturbances in the electrical impulses that stimulate the heartbeat. Hypokalemia also potentiates (increases the effect of) the action of digitalis. To avoid these problems, the patient should be instructed to eat potassium-rich foods such as bananas, an excellent source of potassium (Table 13.2).

There are also diuretics available that prevent potassium loss. In severe cases of low potassium, a medication of potassium chloride such as *Klor-Con* may be prescribed. These are called potassium-sparing diuretics. Examples are spironolactone (*Aldactone*) and triamterene (*Dyrenium*). Potassium-sparing diuretics can lead to an excess of potassium (hyperkalemia), and patients are instructed to avoid potassium-rich foods. *Aldactazide* and *Dyazide* combine a potassium-sparing diuretic with a thiazide.

Two strong loop diuretics that inhibit reabsorption of both sodium and chloride are furosemide (*Lasix*) and bumetanide. Like the thiazide diuretics, they cause a corresponding excretion of potassium. Because loss of potassium in the urine can be so extensive, potassium supplements are often prescribed in combination with these potent loop diuretics. There are also carbonic anhydrase inhibitors such as acetazolamide and osmotic diuretics such as mannitol (*Osmitrol*). Miscellaneous diuretics include chlorthalidone, metolazone, and indapamide, whose diuretic actions are similar to those of the thiazide diuretics.

Older adult patients are more susceptible to the effects of diuretics and should be monitored closely.

Table 13.2 Potassium-Rich Foods

Food	Amount	Potassium (mg)
Avocado	1	1097
Banana	1	451
Beets	1 cup	532
Cantaloupe	1 cup	494
Lima beans (frozen)	1 cup	694
Orange juice	1 cup	474
Potato	1	610
Prunes	1 cup	706
Raisins	1 cup	1089
Spinach (fresh)	1 cup	838
Squash (acorn)	1 cup	896
Tomato juice	1 cup	535

Pediatric Considerations | Diuretics for Kidney Disorders

- Diuretics are frequently given in heart failure, hypertension, and bronchopulmonary dyplasia.
- Thiazides are given to children and have the advantage of not causing hyperglycemia, hyperuricemia, or hypercalcemia as they do in adults.
- Metolazone is rarely used but does have advantages over thiazides. Although it is a stronger diuretic, it causes less hypokalemia. Generally used in combination with furosemide (*Lasix*), it works best when given 30 to 60 minutes before *Lasix*.

- *Lasix* is a loop diuretic that is frequently given to children. Monitor electrolytes closely for fluid and electrolyte imbalances as a result of frequent kidney function and fluid distribution related to growth and development.
- Bumetanide causes less ototoxicity than *Lasix*. It is a preferred diuretic when children are taking other ototoxic drugs. It also causes less hypokalemia.
- Spironolactone (*Aldactone*), the most frequently used potassium-sparing diuretic, is used primarily to decrease the incidence of hypokalemia. Avoid its use in renal failure.

 Older Adult Considerations | Diuretics for Kidney Disorders

- Thiazides are commonly given to older adults for heart failure and hypertension.
- Monitor closely for hypotension and electrolyte imbalances. Older adults are more likely to have adverse reactions.
- Give the smallest possible dose.

- Loop diuretics cause excessive diuresis in older adults, as well as hypotension and fluid volume depletion.
- Hyperkalemia is a risk with a potassium-sparing diuretic.

Replacement Electrolytes and Fluids

Normally, fluids are replaced simply by drinking water and eating foods that contain moisture. Electrolytes can be replaced by eating a diet rich in potassium, calcium, sodium, and magnesium. When a patient is unable to replace lost fluids and electrolytes through diet, they are replaced through oral supplements or IV therapy. Various parenteral and oral preparations are available. Potassium, calcium (calcium gluconate), magnesium, and other electrolytes can be given orally in the form of tablets and solutions, or they can be prepared as IV solutions for infusion. IV fluids are given routinely before and after surgery to maintain the proper amount and composition of body fluids. Dextrose 5% solution, Ringer's solution, and sodium chloride (saline) solution are fluids that are commonly administered in IV infusions.

 Caution | Older Adult Implications of Diuretics

- Begin treatment with the lowest possible dose.
- Diuretics increase the need to urinate, especially at night.
- Always consult with a provider on the appropriate fluid intake. Fluids are not necessarily increased and may be restricted if heart or kidney diseases are present.

- Monitor closely when a potassium-sparing diuretic is given, because it may cause hyperkalemia.
- Diuretics often lower blood pressure, which may cause lightheadedness, dizziness, fatigue, and muscle weakness.
- When discontinuing the diuretic, withdraw it gradually to avoid development of fluid retention.

ADMINISTERING DIURETICS [LO 13-7]

The administration of diuretics must be timed to avoid keeping the patient up all night going to the bathroom. Check the drug's onset of action so that it takes effect during the daytime. Warn the patient that he or she will be urinating more often than normal because of the diuretic. Make it easy and comfortable for the patient to urinate frequently. Keep a urinal or bedpan close by for patients who should not or are unable to get out of bed. Keep a bell or a call button handy, too, so that the patient can summon help if needed. One way to make sure that a patient gets to the bathroom often enough and in time is to set up a schedule. Tell the patient that you will come to help every 2 hours, or according to whatever schedule you work out together. Keep a commode or urinal at bedside in case the patient cannot make it to the bathroom in time.

Keep an accurate record of fluid intake and output (**Figure 13.4**). A record is necessary to make sure the diuretic is working. If it is taking effect, water leaving the body should be equivalent to the water taken in. The patient should also be weighed daily to confirm that the diuretic is removing excess water. Weigh at the same time every day.

Your observations of the patient's physical condition are important: swollen arms and legs and possibly a swollen abdomen are signs of edema. If you press your finger into the patient's skin, you will leave an indentation. This is called pitting edema. When a diuretic is working, you should notice a decrease in the edema and less pitting of the skin.

Be alert for side effects that signal an electrolyte imbalance. Diuretics can remove too much potassium from the body. Observe the patient for hypokalemia, a low potassium level. The patient may exhibit nausea, thirst, fatigue, dry mouth, muscle weakness, muscle cramps, and irregular pulse. It is important to chart these signs. Administer oral potassium as ordered. In severe cases, potassium chloride (KCl) may have to be given intravenously.

A possible side effect of some diuretics is hypotension. Patients should move slowly when sitting up or standing from a lying-down position, to avoid the dizziness of orthostatic hypotension.

PEDIATRIC CONCERNS [LO 13-8]

Small children are more susceptible than adults to sudden changes in body temperature and to diarrhea, vomiting, and dehydration. An infant's body composition is approximately 75 percent water as compared to 50 to 60 percent in adults. Infants also have less fat content than adults. Their skin is thin and permeable, and their livers and kidneys are immature or not fully developed and therefore cannot metabolize and excrete drugs as well as those organs in older children and adults. The most accurate way to determine pediatric drug dosages is to measure body surface. As a result of the larger percentage of water in children's body weight, smaller children require larger doses of some drugs such as gentamicin. Small children also have poor absorption of drugs and fluids as a result of dehydration. Drugs are most effective when administered intravenously.

Diuretics must be carefully administered to children. Obtain daily weights and vital signs to prevent fluid and electrolyte loss. Hypotension, shock, and even death can occur if children are not closely monitored. Children are more susceptible to the effects of diuretics because of their larger percentage of total body water.

Oral rehydration therapy (ORT) is a major advance in today's healthcare in the treatment of dehydration. Oral replacement solutions (ORSs) contain glucose and carefully determined amounts of sodium. ORT is very effective, safer, less painful, and less costly than IV rehydration. Nutrient-based solutions, such as *Pedialyte,* are the most frequently used solutions for oral rehydration. These solutions are rich in electrolytes and are frequently used

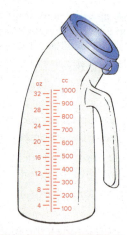

Figure 13.4

Measure fluid intake and output by means of clearly marked containers.

in children with diarrhea. After rehydration, an ORS is used for maintenance therapy, alternating with low-sodium fluids, water, breast milk, and half-strength or lactose-free formulas. An ORS may be given as a supplement with older children. One cup of ORS is used as the replacement amount to be given for each diarrhea stool resulting in dehydration.

⚠ Patient Education — Pediatric Implications in the Management of Dehydration

- Avoid a clear-liquid intake, including fluids such as fruit juices, carbonated beverages, and gelatin. These fluids have a high carbohydrate content but are very low in electrolytes.
- Avoid beverages containing caffeine because the caffeine has a diuretic effect, causing further loss of water and sodium.
- Avoid broths because they are high in sodium and have inadequate carbohydrate content.
- Oral rehydration solutions, such as *Pedialyte*, are the recommended therapy.
- Encourage small sips of fluid instead of a large amount of fluid at one time.

INSTILLING BLADDER MEDICATION [LO 13-9]

A bladder irrigation, including instillation of an antiseptic or antibiotic solution, may be ordered to wash out the bladder of a patient with a severe bladder infection.

An **indwelling catheter** (also called a retention or Foley catheter) remains inside the bladder for an extended time. It allows urine to flow into a bag hung at the side of the bed. There are several types of indwelling catheters available with outlets for drainage and irrigation. The Foley catheter (**Figure 13.5**) is held in place by inflating a small balloon inside the bladder after inserting the catheter.

Figure 13.5

Bladder medication can be instilled through an indwelling catheter.

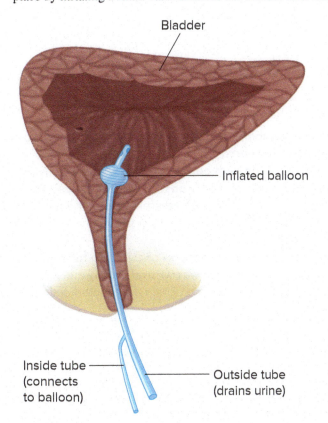

Bladder

Inflated balloon

Inside tube (connects to balloon)

Outside tube (drains urine)

Because the catheter opens a passageway between the bladder and the outside environment, sterile technique must be used to avoid letting microorganisms enter the bladder. Special sterile kits are available containing all the equipment needed for irrigating or instilling medication into the bladder.

These are points to keep in mind when instilling bladder medications into an indwelling catheter:

- Follow aseptic procedure; do not let the catheter or medication become contaminated.

- Give special consideration to the patient's privacy. Draw the curtain around the bed and drape the patient's genital area. You can ease the patient's embarrassment by being tactful and considerate.

- Make sure medication is at the proper temperature. Usually room temperature is correct, but check the medication order to be sure.

- Leave the medication in the bladder for the proper amount of time, as shown on the medication order.

- Remember to hook up the drainage tube after you finish giving medication, so that urine can be carried away into the drainage bag.

 Healthcare for Today and Tomorrow Important Drug Histories

When you care for patients in both inpatient and outpatient settings, it is essential that you assess the patient's current and past medication history for medications that can cause urinary retention. Urinary retention results in urinary stasis, leading to urinary infections. You should question your patients as to whether they take antihypertensives; *Levodopa*, an antiparkinsonian drug; anticholinergic drugs such as *Atropine* and belladonna; antihistamines; antispasmodics; or sedatives. All these drugs may cause urinary retention and may require a change in the drug prescribed.

 Legal and Ethical Issues Wrong Drugs

As a healthcare team member, you must be knowledgeable about drugs that are similar in spelling and may result in medication errors.

You are caring for a patient with benign prostatic hypertrophy, a condition that causes an enlarged prostate resulting in a urinary obstruction. Tamsulosin (*Flomax*) is a drug that is often prescribed to shrink the size of the prostate, relieve the urinary obstruction, and restore a normal urinary pattern. You discover that the pharmacy sent alendronate (*Fosamax*) for this patient to receive. What is your responsibility?

You should question the appropriateness of this drug for your patient and consult the provider's order. You find that an illegible order was written and was interpreted incorrectly. It is your responsibility to notify the provider and obtain a corrected order for *Flomax*.

Representative Drugs for the Urinary System and Fluid Imbalances

Category, Name,[a] and Route	Uses and Diseases	Actions	Usual Dose[b] and Special Instructions	Side Effects and Adverse Reactions
Urinary Antiseptics/Antibacterials/Analgesics				
ciprofloxacin (*Cipro*) Oral, IV	Urinary tract infections; respiratory, bone, and skin infections	Inhibits DNA gyrase	250–500 mg PO every 12 hours; 400 mg IV every 12 hours	Nausea, headache, diarrhea, rash
trimethoprim/ sulfamethoxazole (*Bactrim, Septra*) Oral, IV	Urinary tract infections, otitis media, bronchitis, traveler's diarrhea	Blocks two consecutive steps in the biosynthesis of nucleic acids and proteins essential for many bacteria	1–2 double-strength (DS) tablets taken in one dose; 2 regular-strength tablets, or 4 teaspoons (20 mL) of suspension, every 12 hours for 10–14 days; do not give if patient is allergic to sulfa	Nausea, vomiting, diarrhea, skin rashes, anorexia, blood disorders, headache, muscle weakness
nitrofurantoin (*Furadantin, Macrodantin*) Oral	Urinary tract infections	Interferes with bacterial enzyme systems	50–100 mg tid or qid; give with food or milk to avoid gastric irritation; rinse mouth after giving liquid form to avoid staining teeth	Anorexia, nausea, diarrhea; may turn urine brown or darker, abdominal pain
cefadroxil monohydrate (*Duricef*) Oral	Urinary tract infections	Inhibits cell wall synthesis	500 mg daily	Nausea, diarrhea, dyspepsia
ampicillin Oral, IV	Urinary tract infections (pyelonephritis)	Is bactericidal; inhibits cell wall formation	1–4 g PO daily every 4 hours	Rash, itching, shortness of breath, diarrhea, nausea, vomiting
phenazopyridine (*Pyridium*) Oral	Pain with urinary tract irritation or infection	Anesthetizes mucous membranes of urinary tract	100–200 mg tid p.c.	Headache, vertigo, orange discoloration of urine
Diuretics				
hydrochlorothiazide (***Hydrodiuril***) Oral	Edema, hypertension	Increases sodium and water excretion, lowers blood pressure	25–100 mg 1–2 times daily; give early in day because of increased urination; monitor weight and fluid intake/output	Gastric irritation, muscle weakness, hypokalemia, orthostatic hypotension, pancreatitis
furosemide (***Lasix***) Oral, IM, IV	Edema, hypertension, chronic renal failure	Is a potent loop diuretic; inhibits reabsorption of sodium and chloride	20–80 mg PO initially and then gradually increased to 600 mg/ day in patients with severely edematous states	Dizziness, headache, dehydration, anemia, leukopenia (decreased white blood cells), rash, orthostatic hypotension, hypokalemia

Representative Drugs for the Urinary System and Fluid Imbalances (continued)

Category, Name,ᵃ and Route	Uses and Diseases	Actions	Usual Doseᵇ and Special Instructions	Side Effects and Adverse Reactions
Diuretics (continued)				
triamterene (*Dyrenium*) Oral	Edema	Conserves potassium and excretes sodium	Individualized; 100 mg bid after meals; avoid excessive intake of potassium-rich foods	Nausea, vomiting, weakness, rash, dry mouth, hypotension, dizziness
Replacement Electrolytes				
potassium Oral	Potassium deficiency	Is a potassium ion replacement	20 mEq/day for prevention of hypokalemia; 40–100 mEq/day or more for treatment of potassium depletion	Nausea, vomiting, diarrhea, abdominal distress, hyperkalemia, phlebitis

Note: Bolded trade names are among the 50 most commonly prescribed drugs.

ᵃ*Trade names given in parentheses are examples only. Check current drug references for a complete listing of available products.*

ᵇ*Average adult doses are given. However, dosages are determined by a provider and vary with the purpose of the therapy and the particular patient. The doses presented in this text are for general information only.*

Practice Procedure 13.1 (LO 13-9)

INSTILLING MEDICATION INTO THE BLADDER THROUGH AN INDWELLING CATHETER

Demonstrate how to administer a medication into the bladder through an indwelling catheter.

Equipment

Provider's order for bladder medication

Medication administration record, patient chart

Medicine tray or cart

Sterile catheter irrigation/instillation set, containing tray or basin (to catch drainage), plastic sheeting, syringe, catheter tip covers, bottle for diluting medication (in some sets), alcohol wipes, sterile gloves

Medication in sterile solution, 50 or 60 mL

Procedure

1. Assemble equipment.

2. Read the provider's order and set up the medication. Check for the "seven rights."

3. Identify the patient, following health facility policy. Explain what you are going to do. Curtain off the area to provide privacy.

4. Wash your hands.

5. Assist the patient to lie down on his or her back, with bent legs spread apart to expose the genital area. Drape the patient so that only the catheter is showing.

6. Open the sterile packaging of the irrigation set and establish a sterile field. Protective plastic sheeting should be set down on the bed first, to prevent soiling the bed. Pour the desired amount of sterile solution into the sterile container. Put on sterile gloves.

7. Arrange the catheter tip so that it is hanging over the edge of the tray but not touching the bottom. (This would contaminate the catheter.) Some bladder instillation sets have a notched edge on the tray to hold the catheter in place.

8. Disconnect the catheter from the drainage tube. (The drainage tube is the one that carries the urine to a bag at the side of the bed.) Allow the urine to flow into the sterile collection container. Cover the exposed end of the drainage tube with the special sterile covering in the instillation set. This keeps microorganisms from entering the tube while it is detached. Then lay the tube down on top of the bed, anchoring it with tape so that it does not slide off and drop to the floor.

9. Lift the end of the catheter, and insert the sterile syringe into the opening used for irrigation. Hold the syringe and catheter tube together with the same hand. This keeps them from separating when you administer the medication.

10. Pour the measured amount of medication into the open end of the syringe. Let it drain through the catheter into the bladder. Do not force it in with the syringe bulb.

11. Follow with extra sterile water, if ordered.

12. Before putting down the catheter, clamp it if the medication is to stay in the bladder for a certain time. The provider's order should state how long the medication should be retained. If no special length of time is ordered, you may leave the tube unclamped.

13. Put down the catheter in the same position as before, with the end resting over the edge of the tray but not touching the bottom. If unclamped, the catheter will begin to drain right away. If the catheter is clamped, remember to unclamp it after the proper amount of time so that it can drain.

14. When the medication has drained out, reattach the drainage tube to the end of the catheter. Use a sterile alcohol wipe to clean both the end of the tube and the catheter as you reattach them.

15. Remove and clean or discard the equipment, supplies, and gloves.

16. Give the patient any special instructions, and assist him or her into a comfortable position. Make sure that the tubing is not pinched or blocked in any way so that urine can drain freely into the collection bag.

17. Wash your hands.

18. Chart the medication. If you noticed any unusual substances draining from the bladder or irritation around the catheter, be sure to chart this and notify your supervisor.

Summary

Learning Outcome	Summary Points
13-1 Identify three functions of the urinary system.	• Excreting wastes. • Regulating the amount of water. • Regulating the pH balance.
13-2 Identify the parts and functions of the urinary system.	• Two *kidneys* are bean-shaped organs containing the functional unit of the kidney called the nephron. Each nephron has a glomerulus that allows water and dissolved substances to pass out of the blood. These substances travel through the coils of the nephron tube, and some of the water, nutrients, and minerals are reabsorbed into the bloodstream. This process leaves behind only waste products, certain salts, and varying amounts of water called urine. • Two *ureters* carry the collected urine to the bladder. • The *urinary bladder* stores urine and serves as a means for urine to exit the body. • The *urethra* allows urine to exit the body.

Learning Outcome	Summary Points
13-3 Describe how abnormal alteration in the urine gives an indication of disorders in the urinary system.	• *Normal urine* is pale yellow to amber and has an ammonia odor. • *Cloudy urine* indicates renal disease. • *Sweet, fruity odor* of urine is a symptom of diabetes mellitus or starvation.

13-4 Describe the major disorders and symptoms of the urinary system, including fluid imbalances.	• Infections such as pyelonephritis (kidney infection), nephritis (kidney inflammation), cystitis (inflammation of the bladder caused by bacterial infection), ureteritis (inflammation of the ureter), and urethritis (inflammation of the urethra).
	• Obstructions.
	• Urinary incontinence.
	• Renal failure.
	• Medical terms for symptoms:
	  • Hematuria
	  • Pyuria
	  • Urinary retention
	  • Frequency
	  • Urgency
	  • Dysuria
	  • Oliguria
	  • Anuria

13-5 Identify imbalances of body fluids, electrolytes, and pH.	• Intake and output. • Fluids (water) and salt. • Body's acid-base balance.
13-6 Describe the actions of the following drug groups: urinary antibiotics, diuretics, and replacement electrolytes and fluids.	• *Urinary antiseptics* treat infections. Examples: penicillins, cephalosporins, sulfonamides, and fluoroquinolones. • *Diuretics* increase the output of water from the body. Example: hydrochlorothiazide. • *Replacement electrolytes and fluids* are supplied orally or intravenously when electrolyte and fluid status cannot be maintained. Example: potassium such as *Klor-Con.*
13-7 Carry out administering diuretics using correct procedures.	• Avoid administering diuretics at a time when they would keep the patient up all night. • Instruct the patient that voiding more often than normal is common. • Keep a bedpan or urinal close to the patient. • Maintain an accurate record of intake and output. • Monitor the patient for electrolyte imbalance and hypotension.
13-8 Describe the causes and treatment of dehydration in the pediatric patient.	• *Causes:* The primary cause of dehydration in the pediatric patient occurs because a child's body is composed of 75% water compared to 50% in an adult. • *Treatment:* Avoid a clear-liquid intake, broths, and beverages containing caffeine. Administer oral rehydration solutions.
13-9 Illustrate administering medications through an indwelling catheter.	• Maintain aseptic procedure. • Give special consideration to the patient's privacy. • Make sure the medication is at room temperature. • Leave the medication in the bladder for the proper amount of time. • Hook up the drainage tube after giving the medication.

• **Define these terms that describe symptoms of urinary tract disorders.**

1. (LO 13-3) Hematuria _____

2. (LO 13-3) Pyuria _____

3. (LO 13-3) Incontinence _____

4. (LO 13-3) Retention _____

5. (LO 13-3) Dysuria _____

6. (LO 13-3) Anuria _____

Match the medical terms to their definitions.

_____ 7. (LO 13-4) Mechanical filtering of blood.   a. cystoscope

_____ 8. (LO 13-3) Instrument for looking into the urinary tract   b. dialysis

_____ 9. (LO 13-3) Tube for bladder irrigation and medication   c. nephritis

_____ 10. (LO 13-4) Inflammation of the kidney   d. catheter

Complete the statements by filling in the blank.

• 11. (LO 13-2) The tubes that connect the kidneys to the bladder are the _____.

12. (LO 13-2) Urine passes out of the body by way of the _____.

13. (LO 13-2) A full bladder creates the urge to _____.

14. (LO 13-2) In 24 hours, the kidneys normally produce about _____ mL of urine.

15. (LO 13-2) About _____ mL of urine are passed during normal urination.

16. (LO 13-6) When a patient is on thiazide diuretics, there is a danger of excreting too much _____, which could cause hypokalemia.

17. (LO 13-6) A lack of potassium can be corrected by giving foods such as _____.

18. (LO 13-9) A catheter that is designed to stay in place over a long period of time is called a(n) _____ catheter.

Answer the questions in the space provided.

19. (LO 13-1) List the three functions of the urinary system. _____

_____

• _____

20. (LO 13-5) What are electrolytes? Name at least four electrolyte ions. _____

_____

_____

21. (LO 13-9) Discuss the procedure for administering a medication through an indwelling catheter.

_____

_____

22. (LO 13-5) List the types of fluids you would record on an input and output record.

Input: _____

Output: _____

Match the drug categories to the drug names.

_____	23. (LO 13-6) Spironolactone, *Dyrenium*	a. alkalizers
_____	24. (LO 13-6) *Lasix, Edecrin*	b. acidifiers
_____	25. (LO 13-6) *Diuril*	c. thiazide diuretics
_____	26. (LO 13-6) Potassium, calcium, sodium	d. replacement electrolytes
_____	27. (LO 13-6) *Furadantin, Septra*	e. potassium-sparing diuretics
_____	28. (LO 13-6) Sodium bicarbonate	f. replacement fluids
_____	29. (LO 13-6) Ammonium chloride, sodium biphosphate	g. loop diuretics
_____	30. (LO 13-6) Sodium chloride solution, dextrose solution	h. urinary antiseptics

Drug Calculations—Fill in the blank with the answer.

31. (LO 13-6) The provider orders ampicillin 1 g orally every 4 hours. Available are 500-mg capsules. You will administer _____ capsules to your patient.

32. (LO 13-6) The provider orders phenazopyridine (*Pyridium*) 200 mg orally tid. Available are 100-mg tablets. You will give _____ tablets to your patient.

33. (LO 13-6) The provider orders ciprofloxacin (*Cipro*) 250 mg orally bid. Available are 500-mg tablets. Prepare to administer _____ tablets to your patient.

34. (LO 13-6) The provider orders hydrochlorothiazide 150 mg orally daily. Available are 100-mg tablets. You will give _____ tablets to your patient.

35. (LO 13-6) The provider orders potassium gluconate and potassium citrate 15 mEq orally tid. Available is 20–45 mEq/15 mL oral solution. Prepare to give your patient _____ mL.

Multiple Choice—Circle the correct letter.

36. (LO 13-4) Which of the following should you include in the patient instructions for preventing urinary tract infections?

    a. Females should wipe from back to front when going to the bathroom.

    b. Wear synthetic undergarments.

    c. Drink 3 to 4 glasses of water per day.

    d. Avoid bath salts, oils, and vaginal sprays.

37. (LO 13-6) Which of the following drugs should you administer for an overactive bladder?

a. Tolterodine (*Detrol*)

c. Hydrochlorothiazide

b. Ampicillin

d. Nitrofurantoin (*Macrodantin*)

38. (LO 13-6) You should monitor a patient taking cefadroxil (*Duricef*) for which side effects?

a. Rash, itching, dyspnea

c. Headache, orange discoloration of urine

b. Weakness, dizziness, hypotension

d. Nausea, diarrhea, dyspepsia

39. (LO 13-8) Which of the following pediatric instructions should you give a child's parent for the management of dehydration?

a. Offer a clear-liquid diet including fruit juices and gelatin.

c. Encourage chicken and beef broth.

d. Avoid solutions such as *Pedialyte*.

b. Avoid beverages containing caffeine.

40. (LO 13-6) For a patient with edema, which diuretic should you administer to conserve potassium and sodium?

a. Furosemide (*Lasix*)

c. Triamterene (*Dyrenium*)

b. Hydrochlorothiazide

d. Chlorthalidone

Chapter 13 Case Studies

41. (LO 13-6) A patient is taking hydrochlorothiazide for hypertension and has a potassium level of 3 mEq/L and a sodium level of 129 mEq/L. What do these levels reflect? What is the cause of this? What type of diuretic is hydrochlorothiazide, and how does it act? What are some foods that increase the potassium level?

_____

_____

_____

42. (LO 13-6) You are caring for an older adult taking furosemide (*Lasix*). What kind of drug is *Lasix*? The patient has congestive heart failure and is edematous. What is the most likely reason that the patient is taking *Lasix*? Are there any special indications for giving this drug to an older adult?

_____

_____

_____

Critical Thinking

Select the disorder that best matches the patient description and write it in the blank.

renal failure   kidney stones   electrolyte imbalance

pyelonephritis   cystitis

43. (LO 13-4) Fred Byers must be put on dialysis to eliminate toxic waste products from his bloodstream.

_____

44. (LO 13-4) Mr. Bernardi has had painful abdominal spasms for a day due to an obstruction in the ureter. Now the obstructing material has passed into the bladder. His provider will insert an instrument into the bladder to crush and flush out the material.

_____

45. (LO 13-4) Ms. Yamamoto has a severe bladder infection with painful, frequent urination. To keep the bladder empty, a urinary catheter has been inserted. The provider has ordered regular bladder irrigation and an anti-infective to be administered into the catheter.

_____

46. (LO 13-4) Mr. Wincenz has a severe kidney infection that is damaging to the nephrons. Antibiotics are being administered with caution to avoid further damage that could lead to kidney failure.

_____

47. (LO 13-6) After several days on diuretics, a heart patient develops fatigue and muscle weakness. Dr. Bland then orders potassium chloride.

_____

Applications

Obtain an electronic drug guide, a current copy of a drug reference book, or the *PDR*®. Use it to answer the questions that follow in a notebook or on file cards.

48. Use an electronic drug guide or the *PDR*® to locate another product name for each of the urinary antibacterials listed in the Representative Drugs for the Urinary System and Fluid Imbalances table in this chapter.

49. In Section 3 of the *PDR*®, Product Category Index, find the Diuretics. Make a list of the loop diuretics listed there.

DRUGS FOR THE REPRODUCTIVE SYSTEM

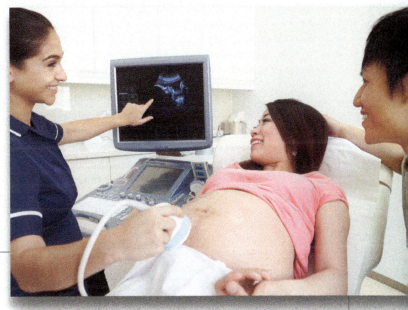

©Monkey Business Images/Shutterstock

14-1 Identify the functions of the male and female reproductive systems.

14-2 Identify the main parts and functions of the female and male internal and external genitalia using correct medical terminology.

14-3 Recall the hormones produced by the female and male gonads and describe their functions.

14-4 Describe the actions of gonadotropins, oxytocin, and prolactin.

14-5 Describe major disorders that affect the reproductive system.

14-6 Describe the main uses and major side effects of sex hormones in drug therapy.

14-7 Summarize the various types of contraceptives available, including the effects on adolescent patients.

In this chapter you will review the parts of the reproductive system and learn about the hormones produced by the male and female gonads. You will also learn what disorders affect this system and which drugs are used to treat them.

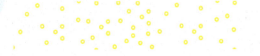

abortifacients

amenorrhea

benign prostatic hyperplasia or hypertrophy (BPH)

cervicitis

dysmenorrhea

endometriosis

engorgement

estrogen

fetus

gonadotropins

gonads

herpes simplex (genital)

libido

menopause

menorrhea

osteoporosis

ova

ovulation

oxytocic

postpartum

progesterone

prostatitis

puberty

sexually transmitted diseases (STDs)/ sexually transmitted infections (STIs)

spermatozoa

testosterone

vaginitis

REPRODUCTIVE SYSTEM [LO 14-1]

Creating the next generation of human life is the responsibility of the male and female reproductive systems. Of all the body systems, the reproductive system is the least alike in males and females. The two systems have different structures that must work together for reproduction to take place. One basic function of both the male and female systems is to produce sex cells. The other function is to engage in sexual intercourse, the act that makes it possible for those sex cells to join together. The female system has an added function: to nourish and protect the fetus thus created until it is fully developed for life outside the womb.

The external and internal reproductive organs in both males and females are called genitalia. Some of the male and female genitalia have similar functions, but their anatomy is different.

FEMALE AND MALE GENITALIA [LO 14-2]

Female Reproductive System

Internal Genitalia. The internal genitalia of the female reproductive system consists of two ovaries, two fallopian tubes, the uterus, and the vagina (Figure 14.1). The ovaries are two almond-shaped glands located in the pelvis, one on each side of the uterus. The ovaries produce **ova**, the female reproductive cells. Normally once a month, **ovulation** takes place. That is, a single ovum is expelled from the surface of one ovary and is pulled into a fallopian tube by the fingerlike projections at the end nearest the ovary that released the egg, where fertilization by the sperm may occur. It takes the fertilized ovum anywhere from 24 to 72 hours to travel down the fallopian tube until it implants in the wall of the uterus, where it begins development into a human embryo (Figure 14.2).

The uterus is designed to contain and nourish the fertilized ovum as it develops. The uterus is a pear-shaped, hollow, muscular organ that lies in the pelvis between the bladder and rectum. It opens through the cervix into the vagina. The vagina is a collapsible tubular structure capable of great distention that gives access from outside the body to the internal genitalia. The vagina serves as the lower part of the birth canal and the organ that receives the seminal fluid carrying sperm from the male.

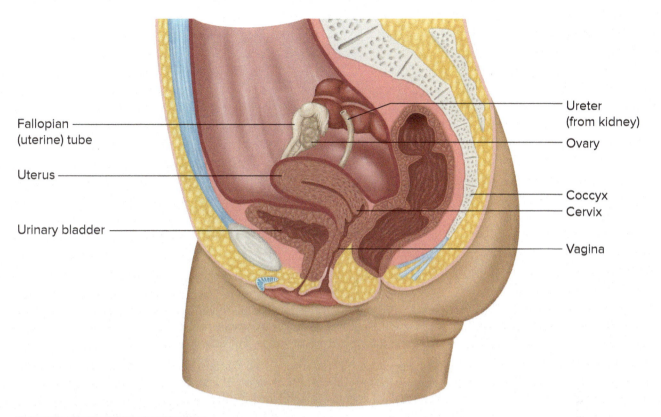

Figure 14.1

Internal genitalia of the female reproductive system.

Fallopian (uterine) tube

Uterus

Urinary bladder

Ureter (from kidney)

Ovary

Coccyx

Cervix

Vagina

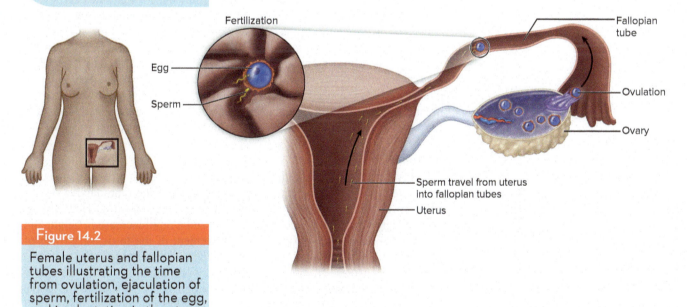

Figure 14.2

Female uterus and fallopian tubes illustrating the time from ovulation, ejaculation of sperm, fertilization of the egg, and implantation in the uterus.

Fertilization

Egg

Sperm

Fallopian tube

Ovulation

Ovary

Sperm travel from uterus into fallopian tubes

Uterus

External Genitalia. The external female genitalia, commonly called the vulva, consists of the mons pubis, the labia majora, the labia minora, the clitoris, the urethral meatus, the vaginal opening, Bartholin's glands, and the Skene's glands (**Figure 14.3**). The mons pubis is a pad of fat that lies over the pubic bone. It is covered with coarse hair. Just below it are the labia, the labia majora and labia minora, that surround the opening of the vagina. Farther toward the back is the opening to the rectum, called the anus. The entire female genital area between the vulva and the anus is the perineum.

Figure 14.3

External genitalia of the female reproductive system.

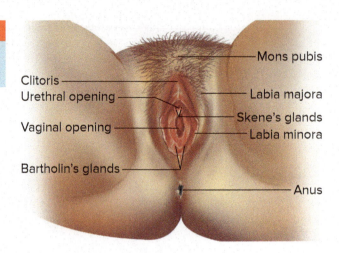

Mons pubis

Clitoris

Urethral opening

Labia majora

Skene's glands

Vaginal opening

Labia minora

Bartholin's glands

Anus

At the forward tip of the labia is a small organ composed of erectile tissue called the clitoris. It is a sensitive nerve center that becomes engorged during sexual excitation. Two glands called Bartholin's glands are located on either side of the vaginal opening. During sexual excitement, they secrete a lubricating mucus that helps the penis enter the vagina. The Skene's glands have no known function.

Pregnancy and Childbirth. If an ovum is fertilized and attaches itself to the lining of the uterus, it begins to develop into a **fetus**, and pregnancy is the result. The fetus is nourished by the mother's blood and cushioned by a surrounding sac of fluid. After approximately 266 days, or 9 months, development is complete. Several weeks before delivery, the uterus lowers into the pelvis. This descent is called "lightening," because it gives the mother a sense of decreased abdominal pressure and distention. Labor begins with rhythmic contractions of the uterus that push the baby toward the cervix. The cervix dilates to 8 to 10 cm to allow the baby to pass through the vagina (also called the birth canal) into the outside world.

While the fetus develops inside the uterus, changes also take place in the pregnant woman's breasts. The breasts are composed of fatty tissue and mammary (milk) glands. During pregnancy, they grow larger and the mammary glands prepare to secrete the milk that will nourish the baby through the first few months of life. A few days after birth, the milk glands go into full production, and the breasts swell with milk. The baby obtains the milk by sucking on the nipples.

Puberty

Puberty refers to the maturational, hormonal, and growth process that occurs when the secondary sex characteristics develop and the reproductive organs begin to function. In girls, it is marked by the first menstrual flow. Breast changes, growth of pubic and axillary hair, and a rapid increase in height and weight also occur. Boys experience enlargement of the testicles, growth of pubic and axillary hair, rapid increase in height, and a change in the voice.

One in 10 adolescent girls—approximately 1 million girls under the age of 20—become pregnant every year. Of these pregnancies, 550,000 result in live births and 450,000 are terminated. This statistic has markedly decreased with a continuous decline every year since 2005. In the 2017 Centers for Disease Control and Prevention (CDC) National Vital Statistics report this number of teenage pregnancies was 229,715 and no statistics found for live births versus births that were terminated. This decline is attributed to improved sexual education, more teens abstaining from sexual activity, and those who are sexually active using birth control measures. Teenage pregnancy is no longer considered biologically disadvantageous to the unborn child, but it continues to be socially, educationally, psychologically, and economically disadvantageous to the mother. Although the incidence of teenage pregnancy is high, the mortality rate has decreased. Teenage mothers and their babies are at greater risk for complications of both pregnancy and delivery, such as premature labor and low birth weight. When good care is available early in pregnancy, however, the risks to the pregnancy and its outcome are equal to those of a mature woman.

Contraceptive counseling is necessary as part of a comprehensive health education program for adolescents. The contraceptive method must be individually suited to each teenager. Motivation is essential, but sometimes difficult. The pill is effective, but the teenager must remember to take the pill. *Implanon* is an implantable device that is a good choice for some people because it is effective and eliminates the need for compliance. It is important, however, to stress the use of condoms in the prevention of sexually transmitted diseases. All patients using contraceptive devices other than condoms should be taught that these devices do not prevent sexually transmitted diseases.

Male Reproductive System

The male reproductive system consists of the external structures, the penis and scrotum, and the internal structures, the prostate gland and the seminal vesicles (Figure 14.4). The testes produce millions of tiny sex cells called **spermatozoa**, or sperm. The sperm collect and mature in a series of coiled tubes called the epididymis. They then pass through a larger tube, the vas deferens. The vas deferens leads from the testes to several storage areas called the seminal vesicles and to the two ejaculatory ducts. These two ducts pass through the prostate gland and terminate in the urethra, a tube that serves as the terminal portion of the reproductive tract and the passageway for eliminating the reproductive fluid, semen, from the body. The prostate gland, the seminal vesicles, and the Cowper's glands located on either side of the urethra all produce mucus and fluids that, together with the sperm, make up semen. During ejaculation, which is a muscular contraction that occurs with a peak of sexual excitement, the semen is propelled out of the body.

Figure 14.4

Internal and external genitalia of the male reproductive system.

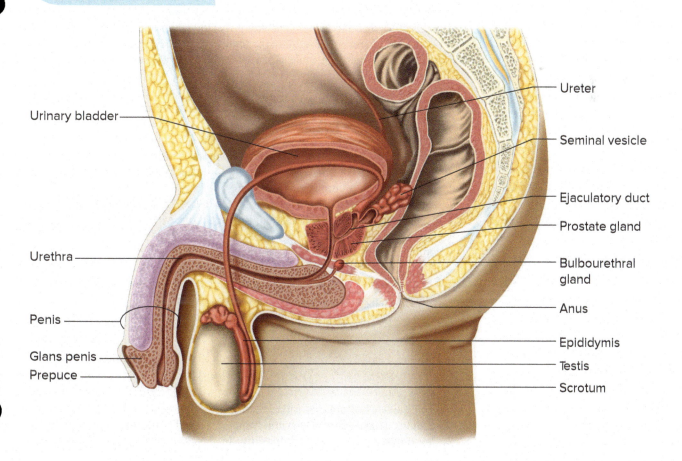

The external genitalia include the scrotum, a thin, loose, outer layer of skin in which the two testes are suspended, and the penis. During sexual excitement, the spongy tissue of the penis fills up with blood. This makes the penis lengthen and become rigid in preparation for sexual intercourse.

SEX HORMONES [LO 14-3]

Sex hormones come from the male and female sex glands, or **gonads**. These hormones—estrogen, progesterone, and testosterone—are not single hormones, but represent groups of related hormones.

The female gonads, the ovaries, secrete the hormones **estrogen** and **progesterone**. Estrogen is responsible for the higher voice, breast development, and shapeliness that are characteristic of women. It also stimulates the monthly development of an ovum. Progesterone is produced during a normal cycle even if fertilization does not occur or after the ovum is fertilized. This hormone prepares the uterus to carry and nourish the fetus as it grows. If the egg is not fertilized, the hormones cause the uterine lining to be shed, resulting in menstruation (**menorrhea**, or menses). Somewhere between the ages of 45 and 52, the ovaries stop producing estrogen and progesterone, and monthly menstruation ceases. This change in hormone production is known as **menopause**.

The male gonads, the testes, produce the male hormone **testosterone**. Testosterone gives men their deeper voices and chest and facial hair. It also stimulates production of sperm cells.

A testosterone deficiency may result in erectile dysfunction (impotence), but in younger men, erectile dysfunction is most commonly attributed to an increase in substance abuse, such as alcohol and recreational drugs. In middle-aged men, erectile dysfunction is often the result of medical technologies, such as bypass surgery, chemotherapy, organ transplants, or medical treatments for cardiovascular disease and diabetes. A man over the age of 70 may experience erectile dysfunction as a result of declining testosterone levels.

Erectile dysfunction is the inability to achieve or maintain an erect penis. Treatment is based on the cause of the dysfunction. The goal of therapy is to help the male achieve a satisfactory sexual relationship after treatment. Treatment may consist of eliminating a particular drug, such as methyldopa, used for hypertension, or propranolol, used for hypertension, angina, and arrhythmias and after a heart attack. Yohimbine is a vasodilator and aphrodisiac that is given orally. When the cause of erectile dysfunction is decreased testosterone levels, testosterone is administered intramuscularly. Research has not proven that testosterone supplementation in older men is successful. Testosterone is also contraindicated in cases of cancer of the prostate, which is common in older men.

Sildenafil citrate (*Viagra*) is a drug used to treat impotence. *Viagra* increases the ability to achieve and maintain an erection. Men who take medications containing nitrates, such as nitroglycerin, should not take *Viagra*. The combination causes excessive hypotension. *Viagra* is commonly given orally 1 hour prior to sexual activity, but it may be taken anywhere from 30 minutes to 4 hours before. The most common side effects are headache, flushing, diarrhea, indigestion, nasal congestion, and increased sensitivity to light. Two other drugs given for erectile dysfunction are tadalafil (*Cialis*) and vardenafil (*Levitra*).

PITUITARY HORMONES THAT REGULATE REPRODUCTION [LO 14-4]

The pituitary hormones—follicle-stimulating hormone (FSH) and luteinizing hormone (LH)—control several functions of the gonads. For that reason they are also called **gonadotropins**. In the female, the two gonadotropins

Figure 14.5

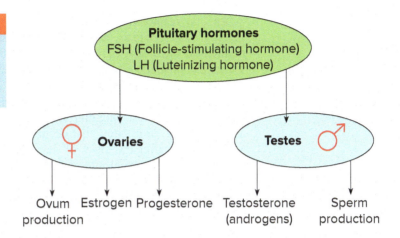

Pituitary hormones (gonadotropins) control certain functions of the gonads.

control ovulation and the production of female hormones by the ovaries; in the male, they stimulate the testes to produce sperm and secrete testosterone (Figure 14.5).

Two other pituitary hormones are involved in childbirth. Oxytocin stimulates the uterus to start contracting at the beginning of labor. A dose of oxytocin (*Pitocin*) or a similar synthetic drug (called an **oxytocic**) may be used to bring about or strengthen labor when a delay would endanger mother or child. It may also be given to slow **postpartum** (after-childbirth) uterine bleeding. When the baby is born, prolactin signals the mammary glands in the female breast to produce milk. Then oxytocin becomes involved again. It stimulates the mammary glands to "let down" the milk each time the infant begins to nurse.

After delivery, drugs such as methylergonovine (*Methergine*) may be given to minimize bleeding or postpartum hemorrhage.

Premature labor is labor that occurs before the 37th week of pregnancy and is a major problem in obstetrics. Terbutaline is used to prevent and treat premature labor by inhibiting uterine contractions.

Alternately, uterine contractions can be induced by prostaglandins for the purpose of pregnancy termination **(abortifacients).** Some prostaglandins include the vaginal suppository dinoprostone (*Cervidil*) and injectable carboprost (*Hemabate*).

DISORDERS OF THE REPRODUCTIVE SYSTEM [LO 14-5]

Vaginal Infections

Vaginal infections are common in women because microorganisms have easy access to the internal organs through the external genitalia. Yeast infection and trichomoniasis are the two most common forms of infection. Vaginal infections cause inflammation of the vagina **(vaginitis)**, and there is an unusual discharge (cheeselike, or foamy and foul-smelling). They also cause itching and burning in the vulvar area. Untreated, they may spread to other organs of the reproductive system, causing further inflammation; for example, **cervicitis**, inflammation of the cervix.

A variety of vaginal douches, creams, tablets, and suppositories are available that have antibacterial and antifungal actions. Practice Procedure 14.1 (found later in the chapter) shows how they are inserted. The specific infecting organism must be identified in the laboratory so that the proper anti-infective can be selected. Some common topical preparations are miconazole (*Monistat 7*) and clotrimazole.

An oral medication, metronidazole (*Flagyl*), is the drug of choice for treating trichomoniasis, a protozoan vaginal infection. Usually both sexual partners are infected with this organism, which can be identified in the vaginal secretions, prostatic fluid, and semen. To effect a cure, both partners must receive the drug simultaneously.

Endometriosis is a condition in which endometrial tissue grows outside the uterus. The most common symptom is low abdominal pain, described as dull, aching, or crampy, that occurs one to two days before menstruation and decreases after the onset of menstruation. Abnormal uterine bleeding, backache, painful sexual intercourse, and painful defecation can also occur. Treatment relies on surgery or hormonal medications, such as danazol, nafarelin (*Synarel*), and leuprolide (*Lupron Depot*). The patient should be informed that hormonal therapy is not a cure. It only controls symptoms.

Sexually Transmitted Diseases

Sexually transmitted diseases (STDs)/sexually transmitted infections (STIs) are infectious diseases associated with sexual contact. Diseases associated with sexual transmission may also be contracted through blood, blood products, and accidental needlesticks.

Since 1981, when public health officials identified acquired immune deficiency syndrome (AIDS) as a new disease, it has become an increasing health concern. It is transmitted from person to person by means of infected blood, semen, vaginal secretions, and breast milk. It has been identified in both heterosexual and homosexual populations and affects all races and ethnic groups. AIDS is caused by the human immunodeficiency virus (HIV). Unlike other sexually transmitted diseases, it may be latent for as many as 10 years before the onset of symptoms. Therefore, an infected person can infect another person without knowing it. Because there is currently no cure for AIDS, teaching should focus on prevention.

When symptoms do develop, they include persistent fevers, night sweats, diarrhea, headache, enlarged glands, skin rash, and fatigue. Four drugs [zidovudine (*Retrovir*), didanosine (*Videx*), stavudine (*Zerit*), and tipranavir (*Aptivus*)] have been approved to treat HIV infection. They block reverse transcriptase, an enzyme required for HIV replication. As a result, they slow the disease process.

In addition to AIDS, genital **herpes simplex** and hepatitis B are sexually transmitted viral diseases. There is currently no cure for genital herpes; however, flare-ups can be prevented and treated with acyclovir (*Zovirax*). Hepatitis B can be prevented by vaccination. Venereal warts (condylomata acuminata) are also due to a virus, human papillomavirus (HPV). One common treatment is 80 to 90 percent trichloroacetic acid applied directly to the wart surface. Podophyllin (10 to 25 percent), a cytotoxic agent, is applied to each wart and left on for 1 to 4 hours before being washed off.

The older sexually transmitted infections, such as syphilis and gonorrhea, are becoming resistant to some antibiotics and are still a problem for the healthcare community. Ceftriaxone is given for gonorrhea, and parenteral penicillin remains the treatment of choice for syphilis.

Chlamydial infections are caused by several strains of *Chlamydia trachomatis*. Infertility and pelvic inflammatory disease (PID) are two complications of chlamydial infections. Chlamydial infections may be treated with tetracycline, doxycycline (*Vibramycin*), or azithromycin (*Zithromax*).

Treatment of sexually transmitted diseases can be especially difficult for the healthcare worker. Frequently there are no symptoms, and people are reluctant to discuss existing symptoms and to involve sexual partners in the treatment plan. Prevention is preferable to trying to cure an established infection. Use of condoms (made from latex or polyurethane) by sexually active people may decrease the spread of these diseases, although recent studies by the CDC and Food and Drug Administration (FDA) state that sexually transmitted diseases may not be completely prevented because of skin-to-skin contact where there is no condom. If you are concerned about transmission of STDs, especially AIDS, you can request free, up-to-date information from the CDC.

Prostate Diseases

The prostate is the male gland that secretes mucus and other substances that help make up semen. Inflammation of the prostate, **prostatitis**, is a disease of older men and is the most common urinary tract infection. Symptoms include fever, chills, painful urination, urethral discharge, and increased urination. Prostatitis is frequently associated with infection in the urethra or lower urinary tract. Treatment consists of antibiotics, anti-inflammatory drugs, and measures to promote comfort, such as sitz baths and frequent prostatic massage.

After age 40, and especially around ages 60 to 70, the prostate tends to enlarge. An enlarged prostate may indicate cancer of the prostate, which is the second leading cause of cancer deaths in men. Treatment is generally surgery and radiation.

Benign prostatic hyperplasia or hypertrophy (BPH) is a new growth of epithelial and stromal elements within the prostate gland. *Hypertrophy* is actually an incorrect term because the condition is not an enlargement of existing cells, as this term implies. *Hyperplasia,* an increase in the number of cells, is the correct term. As the prostate grows, it creates an obstruction of the urethra, causing a decrease in the urinary stream, dribbling, and the inability to empty the bladder. Dutasteride (*Avodart*) is a drug that improves the symptoms of benign prostatic hyperplasia while decreasing the size of the enlarged prostate. It also decreases the risk of acute urinary retention, therefore decreasing the need for surgery. Finasteride (*Proscar*) is a drug that inhibits a form of testosterone responsible for the hyperplasia of cells. Tamsulosin (*Flomax*) is another drug that decreases the symptoms of benign prostatic hyperplasia. Other drugs, such as terazosin (*Hytrin*), prazosin (*Minipress*), doxazosin (*Cardura*), and alfuzosin (*Uroxatral*) cause smooth muscle relaxation and improve urinary flow. If drug therapy fails, surgery, such as transurethral resection of the prostate (TURP), is performed to remove a portion of the prostate.

Cancer

All the organs of the male and female reproductive systems can develop malignant tumors. Cancers of the breast and uterus are common in women, as is prostate cancer in men. Eighty percent of prostate cancers occur in men over the age of 65. Tumors of the testicles are rare but often malignant. The peak age for susceptibility to testicular cancer is 20 to 40 years. The treatment of choice for these cancers is surgery to remove the cancerous growth. A vaccine called *Gardasil 9* offers protection from the most dangerous types of human papillomavirus (HPV), which is the virus that causes most cervical cancers.

Infertility

Problems of infertility affect about 15 percent of couples who wish to have children. Pregnancy is ultimately achieved by about 40 percent of the couples who seek treatment.

Infertility in females can be related to cervical mucus, ovulation problems, hormonal imbalances, or endometriosis. Surgery and drugs may be used to overcome some of these problems. Infertility in the male is usually related to problems with sperm density, motility, or shape or with seminal fluid volume or viscosity. Some of the drugs used to treat infertility are clomiphene (*Clomid*), human chorionic gonadotropin (*Pregnyl*), and menotropins (*Menopur*).

- Never have sexual activity with an infected person.
- Maintain a monogamous relationship with an uninfected partner.
- Never have sexual intercourse when under the influence of alcohol or any drug that may alter the ability to make decisions.
- Use a protective barrier, such as a condom, when engaging in sexual activity with a partner of unknown HIV status.
- Abstain from all recreational or illicit drug use.

- If a drug user, never share needles or syringes.
- If a drug user who refuses to quit taking drugs, resort to smoking, snorting, or ingesting the drug instead of injecting.
- If infected, never donate blood, an organ, or semen for artificial insemination.
- Avoid sharing razors, toothbrushes, or other items that may contain blood or other body fluids.
- If infected, use birth control to avoid infecting a fetus.

USE OF SEX HORMONES IN DRUG THERAPY [LO 14-6]

Although we say that there are female hormones and male hormones, both types of hormones are secreted in both the male and female bodies. The hormones secreted by the gonads—estrogen, progesterone, and testosterone—have other uses besides regulating the organs of reproduction. They are chemically related and are involved in ongoing body processes such as growth, sexual development, bone formation, the storage of minerals, and the building of proteins. They have several uses in drug therapy as well. Hormone replacement is one use, but larger doses can be therapeutic for conditions unrelated to a lack of sex hormones. Natural sex hormones for drug therapy are gathered from the bodies of domestic animals. For example, estrogen is collected from the urine of pregnant mares. Synthetic forms are also available.

Representative drugs that affect the reproductive system are shown in the table at the end of this chapter, including their uses, actions, doses, and side effects.

Estrogen

Estrogen is administered in drug therapy for several reasons. One is to replace female hormones after menopause or following a total abdominal hysterectomy with removal of the uterus, ovaries, and fallopian tubes. At menopause, the ovaries stop producing female hormones. The pituitary produces large amounts of gonadotropins in response to the decrease in estrogen level. As a result, the most common physical changes related to menopause are hot flashes and thinning and drying of the vagina. Hormone replacement therapy (HRT) reduces these symptoms.

After menopause, estrogen may also be used to prevent bone thinning, brittleness, and spontaneous fracturing (**osteoporosis**). Estrogen is also used to treat failure to menstruate (**amenorrhea**), vaginal inflammation, and breast cancer in older women and prostate cancer in men. Women who do not wish to breast-feed their newborn babies may be given estrogen to "dry up" the milk and prevent swollen breasts (**engorgement**).

The most common side effects of hormone replacement therapy are weight gain, breast and pelvic discomfort, GI disturbances, vaginal discharge, and skin pigmentation. These symptoms usually result from an excessive dose and can be reduced by decreasing the dose. Estrogens are generally administered in cycles—for example, 3 weeks on and 1 week off. The long-term use of estrogen replacement carries an increased risk of cancer of the endometrium (the uterine lining) and some types of breast cancer. Estrogen must not be given to pregnant women because it can cause birth defects (congenital anomalies) or can later cause cancer in the female child. An important part of ensuring safe and effective therapy is patient education.

Many chemical forms of estrogen are available generically. Common forms are estradiol, estrone, and conjugated estrogens (*Premarin*). Transdermal estradiol is applied topically to intact skin. Topical forms of these drugs are available for application to the vagina to control inflammation (vaginitis) after menopause.

 Pediatric Considerations   Estrogen

- Estrogen is not recommended for use in children because little information is known about its effects.
- Because estrogen causes closure of the epiphyseal plate, it should be used with

caution before the completion of bone growth and attainment of adult height.
- The smallest possible dose of hormonal contraceptive should be given to adolescents.

 Older Adult Considerations   Estrogen

- A 1- to 2-year or short-term course of estrogen or estrogen and progestin may be used for postmenopausal symptoms.
- Long-term treatment with hormones is no longer recommended because of concerns about serious side effects.

Progesterone

Progesterone, the second female hormone, acts in partnership with estrogen to prepare the body for reproduction. While estrogen stimulates the production of egg cells in the ovary, progesterone helps prepare the uterus to receive and nourish a fertilized egg. During pregnancy, progesterone suppresses ovulation and relaxes the uterine smooth muscle.

Progesterone is given for conditions such as abnormal uterine bleeding, inflammation of the uterine lining (endometriosis), **dysmenorrhea** (painful menstruation), and amenorrhea (absence of menstruation). In postmenopausal women who are taking estrogen, the addition of progesterone for 1 week per month may provide protection from endometrial cancer. Side effects of progesterone include nausea, headache, and dizziness that usually go away with continued use. Occasionally a person may develop depression, edema, and apathy while on progesterone. Medroxyprogesterone acetate (*Provera*) and megestrol (*Megace*) are synthetic forms of progesterone.

Testosterone

Like female sex hormones, male sex hormones, also called androgens, are secreted in both males and females. The main androgen, testosterone, is used in replacement therapy for men when the testes are not producing enough hormone for proper development or sexual activity. It also helps relieve the symptoms of breast cancer. Because testosterone promotes the building of body tissues, it may be used to reverse tissue wasting and loss of protein resulting from burns, surgery, and debilitating diseases that keep patients confined to a chair or bed over long periods. As men age, aromatase, an enzyme that converts testosterone to estrogen, increases and tips the balance of testosterone and estrogen resulting in sexual dysfunction, increased abdominal fat, type 2 diabetes, loss of muscle mass, and feeling tired. Abnormal high levels of estrogen in men raise the risk for diabetes, prostate cancer, and autoimmune diseases. Abnormal low levels of estrogen in men raise the risk for cardiovascular diseases, metabolic syndrome, loss of bone strength, and fractures. When used in women, testosterone can result in masculine side effects (e.g., deepening voice, increased body hair). Its use can also lead to retention of salts and thus edema, which can usually be controlled with diuretics. Examples of testosterones are methyltestosterone and fluoxymesterone (*Androxy*).

 Patient Education | Hormone Replacement Therapy (HRT)

- Explore concerns about the risks of taking estrogen before beginning HRT.

- Inform the provider of a family history of cancer, hypertension, cardiovascular disease, or osteoporosis.

- Have regular physical exams, including a mammogram and Pap smear, every 6 months to a year during treatment.

- Perform monthly breast self-examinations.

- If pregnancy is suspected, immediately stop medication and contact the provider.

- Avoid smoking (smoking increases the side effects of HRT).

- Notify the provider if you develop severe headache, blurred vision, chest pain, shortness of breath, or leg pain.

- Weigh yourself once or twice a week, and report any sharp increase in weight or fluid retention to the provider.

- Follow a low-sodium diet.

- Maintain good oral hygiene to prevent periodontal problems.

- Avoid excessive sun exposure (sun can cause blotchy, brown skin discolorations).

- Expect uterine bleeding when stopping HRT.

- Apply transdermal forms of drugs to rotating sites on the abdomen, using the same site no more than once in 7 days.

- Learn how to take the medication (e.g., 3 weeks on, 1 week off).

- When using the vaginal form of the drug, protect clothing with a sanitary pad.

CONTRACEPTIVES [LO 14-7]

Oral Contraceptives. Oral contraceptives are a very effective method of birth control if taken as prescribed. "The Pill" contains varying combinations of estrogen and progestin. There are three combination types of pills. The first type is monophasic and provides the same amount of estrogen and progestin throughout the cycle. A few examples of monophasic pills are *Brevicon, Cryselle, Lo/Ovral, Portia, Sprintec,* and *Yasmin.* The second type of pill is biphasic, in which there is the same amount of estrogen in each tablet with less progestin in the first part of the cycle and a higher concentration in the last part of the cycle. A few examples of biphasic pills are *Necon 10/11* and *Ortho Novum 1/35.* The third type is triphasic, where both the estrogen and progestin may be the same or vary throughout the cycle of medication. A few examples of triphasic pills include *Cyclessa, Ortho-Novum 7/7/7,* and *Tri-Norinyl.* The purpose of both biphasic and triphasic pills is to provide hormonal fluctuations similar to those that normally occur physiologically. As a result, breakthrough bleeding is decreased throughout the medication cycle.

The action of oral contraceptives is to inhibit ovulation by suppressing the follicle-stimulating hormone (FSH) and luteinizing hormone (LH) that are necessary for the development of the ova. They also alter the cervical mucus so that it is not receptive to the penetration of sperm, leaving the endometrium less desirable for implantation of the blastocyst should fertilization occur. There is a wide range of controversy about the safety of oral contraceptives. Some practitioners recommend discontinuing the pill for 18 to 24 months after taking it for a certain amount of time. There is also a wide range of adverse reactions associated with the pill. The majority of adverse reactions are due to the pill's estrogen component. The major adverse reactions include hypertension, migraine headaches, depression, dizziness, nausea, vomiting, bloating, diarrhea, abdominal cramps, breakthrough bleeding, amenorrhea during and after treatment, and changes in the menstrual flow. Oral contraceptives are contraindicated in women who have experienced angina or a myocardial infarction or who have coronary artery disease, breast cancer, endometrial cancer, or thrombophlebitis. They are also not recommended for women who smoke.

Another type of oral contraceptive is the mini-pill, which is a progestin-only pill (POP) because it contains a small amount of progestin in each tablet and no estrogen. It comes in packs of 28 tablets that preferably should be taken at the same time each day. Forgetting a mini-pill and taking it late increases the chance of pregnancy more than does missing a regular birth control pill. The mini-pill's effectiveness can be increased by using a spermicide or a condom. Mini-pills prevent fertilization by affecting the mucus around the cervix, making it harder for the sperm to enter the uterus, and they also affect sperm transportation through the fallopian tubes. Mini-pills have a lower effective rate (87 to 99.7 percent) than regular birth control pills. They also do not provide any protection against sexually transmitted diseases. The most common adverse reaction is bleeding irregularities such as irregular periods, spotting between periods, or no periods at all. Interestingly, the usual adverse reactions experienced with regular birth control pills such as nausea and breast tenderness do not occur with the mini-pill. Other possible adverse reactions are mood changes, headaches, and a lowered sex drive.

Levonorgestrel/ethinyl estradiol is an oral contraceptive that eliminates menstrual periods for as long as a woman takes it. An alternative to the regular regimen of taking an active hormone pill once a day for 21 days followed by an inactive pill once a day for 7 days is to take levonmorgestrel/ethinyl estradiol for 365 days. It eliminates a woman's menstruation, which may be a welcome effect for some women but a distressing result for those concerned about pregnancy who feel reassured by the onset of menstruation. Remember: Although the failure rate for birth control measures is small, no method has a zero failure rate. Dienogest (*Natazia*) is a progestin with estradiol in a combination formulation. It is the first contraceptive that involves a four-phase dose regimen which decreases the estrogen dose and increases the progestin dose in a 28-day cycle. Its purpose is to prevent breakthrough bleeding and prevent pregnancy by suppressing ovulation.

One last type of oral contraceptive is a kit available for emergency contraception, known as *Plan B One-Step*. This product is to be used after unprotected intercourse or suspected contraceptive failure. *Plan B One-Step* contains two tablets of levonorgestrel. The recommended dose is 1 *Plan B One-Step* tablet as soon as possible, but within 72 hours of unprotected intercourse. A second dose of 1 *Plan B One-Step* tablet should be taken 12 hours later. *Plan B One-Step* may be used at any phase of the menstrual cycle. The FDA has made *Plan B One-Step* available to women age 17 years and older without a prescription.

Transdermal Birth Control System. The norelgestromin/ethinyl estradiol (*Ortho Evra*) transdermal system works similar to oral contraceptives. A new patch is applied each week for 21 days or for 3 weeks. The patch is not worn during the fourth week. The patch should be applied at the same time during the first 24 hours of menstruation. If the patch is started after the first 24 hours of menstruation, a nonhormonal contraceptive must be used for 7 days. The patch may be applied to the abdomen, upper torso (between the shoulder and neck), outer arm, or buttocks, but never on irritated or red skin. The adverse reactions of the patch are similar to those of oral contraceptives but with the addition of skin irritation.

Birth Control Ring. The birth control ring (*NuvaRing*) is an alternative to the birth control pill. It is a 2-inch-wide, transparent, flexible, one-size-fits-all ring that is inserted into the vagina once a month much like a diaphragm. Like the birth control pill, it releases both estrogen and progestin into the bloodstream at a continuous rate to prevent pregnancy. The hormones are activated and released from the ring by the moisture in the vagina and body heat. The birth control ring eliminates remembering to take a pill daily and may result in shorter, lighter, and more regular periods. Used appropriately, it has a 98 to 99 percent effective rate. The ring is still effective even if it is not placed in the exact spot. After the third week, the woman removes the ring by pinching it between the index and middle finger. This is followed by the beginning of the menstrual cycle. Even if the period is not completed in one week, the new ring should be inserted. The ring may be used with tampons.

Although the ring's slipping out of the vagina is rare, it may happen if the woman is straining for a bowel movement or has a prolapsed uterus. The ring is not recommended for women who are smokers or breast-feeding or who have a prolapsed uterus, blood clots, certain cancers, or a history of a heart attack or stroke. The ring may cause the same adverse reactions as oral contraceptives but with the addition of vaginal infections or a discharge. Like oral contraceptives and the transdermal patch, the ring does not prevent sexually transmitted diseases. A sharp pain in the chest, severe abdominal pain, coughing up blood, severe pain in the calf, swelling of the leg, severe headaches, vomiting, tingling or weakness on one side of the body, slurred speech, and double or blurred vision are all indications that there is a ring-related problem and the provider should be consulted immediately.

Implantable Device. Etonogestrel subdermal is an implantable contraceptive that has been marketed in other countries since 1998. It is now approved by the FDA for sale in the United States. It is a matchstick-sized device that is implanted in the upper arm. It works by releasing a low, steady dose of progestin to prevent pregnancy and has an effectiveness of 99 percent when used correctly. Etonogestrel subdermal may be left in place for three years and removed at any time. It may cause irregular menstrual bleeding, spotting, cessation of menstruation, acne, headaches, breast tenderness, and weight changes. As with other contraceptives, it increases the risk of blood clots, particularly in women who smoke, and it does not offer protection from sexually transmitted diseases.

 Healthcare for Today and Tomorrow   Hormone Replacement Therapy

Not only is hormone replacement therapy used to relieve menopausal symptoms and to prevent osteoporosis, but current research also indicates that estrogen protects against the development of Alzheimer's disease. Research also demonstrates some evidence that estrogen may slow the progression of Alzheimer's in individuals already diagnosed with this disease.

Although significant improvements have been made in contraceptive methods, patients must be educated regarding the various choices available so that they can make a fully informed decision on which method of birth control is right for them. Legally, failure to fully inform women about both the positive and negative effects of each method can result in long-term consequences, particularly with the longer-acting contraceptives such as injectable *Depo-Provera Cl* and implantable Etonogestrel subdermal. No counterinjection can be given to neutralize the effects of *Depo Provera Cl* and surgical removal is the only option to stop the effects of Etonogestrel subdermal. Regardless of the contraceptive method a patient selects, that patient must be given the knowledge to make an informed consent.

Representative Drugs for the Reproductive System

Category, Name,[a] and Route	Uses and Diseases	Actions	Usual Dose[b] and Special Instructions	Side Effects and Adverse Reactions
Hormones				
conjugated estrogens (*Premarin*) Oral, cream	Abnormal uterine bleeding, menopausal symptoms, breast and inoperable prostate cancer	Replaces estrogen	*Postmenopause:* 0.3–1.25 mg/day for 3 weeks, then 1 week off; repeat cycle *Cancer:* 1.25–2.5 mg tid daily as ordered by provider	Nausea, breakthrough bleeding, fluid retention, breast pain, and changes in vaginal discharge
oxytocin (*Pitocin*) IV, IM	Induction or stimulation of labor, incomplete abortion or miscarriage, and control of postpartum bleeding	Stimulates uterine and mammary glands	10–40 units in 1000 mL. Current best practice is dilute in normal saline or Ringer's lactate	Hypertension, arrhythmias, seizures, coma, effects on fetus due to decreased blood flow causing irregular heart rate, anoxia, or asphyxia
medroxyprogesterone acetate (*Provera*) Oral, IM	Dysfunctional uterine bleeding, amenorrhea, endometrial hyperplasia, endometrial cancer, contraception	Suppresses ovulation	5–10 mg PO for 5–10 days; administer with food if gastric upset occurs	Breast tenderness, weight changes, fluid retention, abdominal pain, thrombophlebitis, pulmonary embolism, dizziness, migraines, breakthrough bleeding

Category, Name,[a] and Route	Uses and Diseases	Actions	Usual Dose[b] and Special Instructions	Side Effects and Adverse Reactions
Hormones (*continued*)				
methyltestosterone Oral	*Male:* Hypogonadism, delayed male puberty, andropause (hormone decline starting at around age 35) *Female:* Cancer of the breast, postpartum breast engorgement	Stimulates spermatogenesis, development of male sex characteristics, sexual maturity	*Male:* 10–50 mg/day PO *Female:* 80 mg/day PO for 3–5 days or 40 mg/day buccal for breast engorgement; 200 mg/day PO or 100 mg/day buccal for cancer; do not swallow or chew buccal medications; do not eat, drink, or smoke until buccal medication has dissolved	*Male:* Jaundice, edema, hypercalcemia *Female:* Amenorrhea, virilization, body hair growth and male pattern baldness, acne, change in **libido** (sex drive) breast atrophy, mental status changes with moodiness
testosterone cypionate IM	*Male:* Hypogonadism, delayed male puberty, andropause (hormone decline starting at around age 35).	Stimulates spermatogenesis, development of male sex characteristics, sexual maturity	*Male:* 50–400 mg deep IM every 2–4 weeks	*Male:* jaundice, edema
Antibacterials				
miconazole (*Monistat 7*) Suppository, cream	Local vaginal yeast infections caused by *Candida* fungus	Is a fungicidal agent	1 suppository or applicator full of cream once daily at bedtime for 7 days; protect underclothing	Vaginal itching and burning
metronidazole (*Flagyl*) Oral, IV	Antibiotic for trichomoniasis, amebiasis	Is an amebicide and trichomonacidal agent	2 g as single dose or 250 mg tid for 7 consecutive days; male partner should also be treated Avoid alcohol during and for 3 days after treatment	Nausea, vomiting, anorexia, headache, diarrhea; rarely, seizures, peripheral neuropathy, tingling or prickling sensations in extremities

Category, Name,[a] and Route	Uses and Diseases	Actions	Usual Dose[b] and Special Instructions	Side Effects and Adverse Reactions
Antiretroviral				
zidovudine (azidothymidine, *Retrovir*) Oral	Human immuno-deficiency virus (HIV) infection to prevent virus from multiplying During pregnancy to prevent transfer of HIV to the fetus	Blocks reverse transcriptase	200 mg PO tid or 100 mg PO 5 times a day; drug of choice to initiate treatment	Fatigue, headache, rash, nausea, seizures, severe bone marrow depression, confusion, agitation Lowers blood cells that carry oxygen resulting in anemia and WBC needed to fight infection
Erectile Dysfunction Drugs				
sildenafil citrate (**Viagra**) Oral	Impotence	Aids in penile erection	25 mg, 50 mg, or 100 mg 1 hour before sexual activity; may interact with drugs containing nitrates such as nitroglycerin	Headache, diarrhea, flushing, dyspepsia, nasal congestion, hypertension, increased sensitivity to light, abnormal erection or ejaculation
tadalafil (**Cialis**) Oral	Impotence BPH	Aids in penile erection, reduces prostate hyperplasia	10 mg qd as needed for ED prior to sexual activity and effects last up to 36 hours or 2.5 to 5 mg qd at same time every day without regard to timing of sexual activity or meals	Prolonged erection greater than 4 hours or painful erection, dizziness, fainting, hypotension, headache, dyspepsia, blurred or double vision, sudden loss of hearing

Note: Bolded trade names are among the 50 most commonly prescribed drugs.

[a]*Trade names given in parentheses are examples only. Check current drug references for a complete listing of available products.*

[b]*Average adult doses are given. However, dosages are determined by a provider and vary with the purpose of the therapy and the particular patient. The doses presented in this text are for general information only.*

Practice Procedure 14.1 (LO 14-8)

INSERTING VAGINAL MEDICATION

Demonstrate how to insert a vaginal medication.

Equipment

Medication orders for vaginal medications

Medication administration record, patient chart

Medicine tray or cart

Vaginal medications (practice with one or all four): suppository, ointment, cream, or jelly

Applicator for inserting medication

Disposable gloves

Tissues

Perineal pad (optional)

Procedure

1. Assemble equipment.

2. Read the medication order and set up medications. Check for the "seven rights."

3. Wash your hands.

4. Identify the patient. Explain what you are going to do. Have the patient void before beginning the procedure. Curtain off the area for privacy.

5. Assist the patient into a position for insertion. She should lie on her back, with the knees bent and legs spread apart to expose the perineum. Drape the patient for privacy and warmth.

6. Put on disposable gloves, unwrap the suppository, and lubricate the rounded end with petroleum jelly (*K-Y Jelly*). Suppositories are inserted by the dominant hand. Creams, ointments, and jellies are inserted with an applicator, using the dominant hand.

7. With the nondominant hand, gently retract the labial fold to expose the vaginal opening (refer to Figure 14.3).

8. Insert medication:

   - *By hand:* Insert the rounded end of the suppository along the posterior wall of the vaginal canal, the length of an index finger (approximately 3 to 4 inches).

   - *By applicator:* Fill the applicator with cream and insert it 2 to 3 inches into the vagina. Push down on the applicator plunger to release the medication into the vagina, allowing equal distribution along the vaginal wall (**Figure 14.6**).

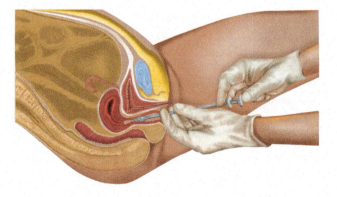

Figure 14.6

Inserting vaginal medication with an applicator.

9. Withdraw the finger or applicator, and wipe the vaginal opening with tissue, if necessary, or let the patient do this.

10. Clean or discard the applicator, and remove and discard gloves.

11. Assist the patient back into a comfortable position, and give any needed instructions. Provide perineal pads to collect excess vaginal discharge and to avoid staining underclothes.

12. Wash your hands.

13. Chart the medication.

Summary

Learning Outcome	Summary Points
14-1 Identify the functions of the male and female reproductive systems.	• One function is to produce sex cells. • Another function is to engage in sexual intercourse. • The female system has the added function of nourishing and protecting the fetus until it is fully developed for life outside the womb.

14-2 Identify the main parts and functions of the female and male internal and external genitalia using correct medical terminology.	• *Female reproductive system—internal genitalia:*
	  • Two ovaries
	  • Two fallopian tubes
	  • Uterus
	  • Vagina
	• *Female reproductive system—external genitalia:*
	  • Vulva
	  • Mons pubis
	  • Labia majora
	  • Labia minora
	  • Clitoris
	  • Urethral meatus
	  • Vaginal opening
	  • Bartholin's glands
	  • Skene's glands
	• *Male reproductive system—internal genitalia:*
	  • Prostate
	  • Seminal vesicles
	• *Male reproductive system—external genitalia:*
	  • Penis
	  • Scrotum

14-3 Recall the hormones produced by the female and male gonads and describe their functions.	• *Female hormones:*
	  • Progesterone prepares the uterus to carry and nourish the fetus as it grows.
	  • Estrogen is responsible for a higher voice. Stimulates monthly development of an ovum.
	• *Male hormone:*
	  • Testosterone gives men a deeper voice, chest hair, and facial hair and stimulates production of sperm cells.

14-4 Describe the actions of gonadotropins, oxytocin, and prolactin.	• *Gonadotropins* control ovulation and the production of female hormones by the ovaries. • *Oxytocin* stimulates the uterus to start contracting at the beginning of labor and slows postpartum bleeding. • *Prolactin* signals the mammary glands in the female breasts to produce milk.

Learning Outcome	Summary Points

14-5 Describe major disorders that affect the reproductive system.	• *Female reproductive disorders:*
	  • Vaginal infections such as vaginitis (inflammation of the vagina) and cervicitis (inflammation of the cervix).
	  • Endometriosis (endometrial tissue grows outside the uterus).
	• Sexually transmitted diseases such as acquired immune deficiency syndrome (AIDS) (transmitted from person to person by means of infected blood, semen, vaginal secretions, and breast milk); herpes simplex (enters the body through small breaks in the skin or mucous membranes); gonorrhea (affects the urethra, rectum, and throats of both men and women; it also affects the cervix in women); and chlamydial infections (caused by *Chlamydia trachomatis*).
	
	• *Male reproductive disorders:*
	  • Prostatitis (infection of the urethra or lower urinary tract).
	  • Benign prostatic hyperplasia (BPH) (new growth of epithelial and stromal elements within the prostate gland).
	• Cancer and infertility may occur in both females and males.
	  • Most common female cancers in women are breast and uterus.
	  • Most common cancer in males is prostate.
	  • Infertility in females may be related to cervical mucus, ovulation problems, hormonal imbalances, or endometriosis.
	  • Infertility in males is related to problems with sperm density, motility, or shape, or with seminal fluid volume or viscosity.

14-6 Describe the main uses and major side effects of sex hormones in drug therapy.	• *Estrogen* replaces female hormones after menopause or after a total hysterectomy. It is also used to treat osteoporosis and amenorrhea.
	  • Side effects include weight gain, breast and pelvic discomfort, vaginal discharge, and skin pigmentation.
	• *Progesterone* is used for abnormal bleeding, endometriosis, dysmenorrhea, and amenorrhea.
	  • Side effects include nausea, headaches, and dizziness.
	• *Testosterone* is used in replacement therapy for men when the testes are not producing enough hormone for sexual activity. It also relieves symptoms of breast cancer, promotes building of body tissues, and reverses tissue wasting after a variety of conditions.
	  • Side effects include deepening voice and increased body hair.

14-7 Summarize the various types of contraceptives available, including the effects on adolescent patients.	• *Pill:* consists of varying combinations of estrogen and progestin.
	• *Mini-pill:* a progestin-only pill (POP).
	• *Plan B:* an emergency contraceptive.
	• *Transdermal patch:* works similar to oral contraceptives. May be applied each week for 21 days or for 3 weeks.
	• *Birth control ring:* alternative to birth control pill. It is a 2-inch-wide, transparent, flexible, and one-size-fits-all ring inserted into the vagina once a month.
	• *Implantable device:* matchstick-sized device implanted in the upper arm.
	• *Female puberty effects:*
	  • Appearance of the menstrual flow
	  • Breast changes
	  • Growth of pubic and axillary hair
	  • Rapid increase in height and weight
	• *Male puberty effects:*
	  • Enlargement of testicles
	  • Growth of pubic and axillary hair
	  • Rapid increase in height
	  • Change in voice
	• *Contraceptive counseling* is essential as part of a comprehensive health education program.

Define each of the terms listed.

1. (LO 14-4) Oxytocic _____

2. (LO 14-6) Dysmenorrhea _____

3. (LO 14-7) Engorgement _____

4. (LO 14-7) Endometrium _____

5. (LO 14-2) Abortifacients _____

6. (LO 14-5) HIV _____

7. (LO 14-5) AIDS _____

8. (LO 14-2) Testes _____

Complete the statements by filling in the blank.

9. (LO 14-2) Female sex cells, the ova, are produced by the _____.

10. (LO 14-2) Male sex cells, the sperm, are produced by the _____.

11. (LO 14-2) The tubular structure that serves as the birth canal is called the _____.

12. (LO 14-2) The structure that holds the fertilized ovum while it develops inside the woman's body is the _____.

13. (LO 14-2) Lactation occurs when the _____ glands in the breast go into production.

14. (LO 14-2) Part of a comprehensive health education program for adolescents is _____ counseling.

15. (LO 14-2) Semen leaves the male body through a tube called the _____, which is shared with the urinary system.

16. (LO 14-7) Oral contraceptives contain varying combinations of _____ and _____.

17. (LO 14-2) The perineum consists of the entire female genital area between the _____ and the _____.

18. (LO 14-2) During sexual excitement, the _____ secrete a lubricating mucus that helps the penis enter the vagina.

Match the hormone functions in regulating human reproduction to the hormones.

_____ 19. (LO 14-2) Estrogen

_____ 20. (LO 14-2) Progesterone

_____ 21. (LO 14-2) Testosterone

_____ 22. (LO 14-2) Oxytocin

a. stimulates sperm production and development of deep voice and chest and facial hair

b. acts in partnership with estrogen to regulate ovulation and prepare the uterus for pregnancy

c. triggers the onset of labor

d. stimulates development of breasts, shapeliness, and the feminine voice

Answer the questions in the space provided.

23. (LO 14-6) List all the therapeutic uses you can think of for sex hormones (both male and female). _____

_____

_____

_____

_____

24. (LOs 14-6, 14-7) What are the possible side effects of estrogen therapy (including oral contraceptives)? ___

_____

_____

_____

_____

25. (LO 14-6) What are the possible side effects of testosterone therapy? _____

_____

_____

_____

_____

Place a T in the blank if the statement is true. Place an F in the blank if the statement is false.

_____ 26. (LO 14-5) Sexually transmitted diseases are all easily treated and cured with drugs.

_____ 27. (LO 14-5) Chlamydial infections are common but have no serious effects.

_____ 28. (LO 14-7) *NuvaRing* is an alternative to the birth control pill.

_____ 29. (LO 14-5) Endometriosis can be a factor in infertility.

_____ 30. (LO 14-7) Osteoporosis is caused by too much estrogen.

_____ 31. (LO 14-7) Oral contraceptives work by preventing ovulation.

_____ 32. (LO 14-6) Testosterone relieves the symptoms of breast cancer.

_____ 33. (LO 14-2) *Androgens* is another word for male sex hormones.

_____ 34. (LO 14-5) *Gardasil 9* is a vaccine that offers protection against human papillomavirus (HPV), which may cause cervical cancer.

_____ 35. (LO 14-5) Sexually transmitted diseases may not be completely prevented with condoms.

_____ 36. (LO 14-7) *Ortho Evra* is an implantable birth control device.

Drug Calculations—Fill in the blank with the answer.

37. (LO 14-6) The provider orders conjugated estrogen (*Premarin*) 0.625 mg orally daily. Available are 1.25-mg tablets. You will administer _____ tablets to your patient.

38. (LO 14-7) The provider orders oxytocin (*Pitocin*) 8 units intramuscularly after the delivery of the placenta. Available is 10 units/mL. Prepare to administer _____ mL to your patient.

39. (LO 14-6) The provider orders medroxyprogesterone acetate (*Depo Provera Cl*) 5 mg orally for 5–10 days. Available are 2.5-mg tablets. You will administer _____ tablets to your patient.

40. (LO 14-5) The provider orders metronidazole (*Flagyl*) 750 mg orally tid. Available are 500-mg tablets. You will give your patient _____ tablets.

41. (LO 14-6) The provider orders medroxyprogesterone acetate (*Depo-Provera Cl*) 1 g intramuscularly one time. Available is 400 mg/mL. Prepare to administer _____ mL to your patient.

Multiple Choice—Circle the correct letter.

42. (LO 14-7) The FDA has made *Plan B One-Step* available over the counter to women of what age?
    a. 18 years of age
    b. 21 years of age
    c. 17 years of age
    d. No specific age criteria

43. (LO 14-3) You should monitor a patient taking sildenafil citrate (*Viagra*) for which of the following side effects?
    a. Fluid retention, abdominal discomfort, urinary retention
    b. Bradycardia, constipation, peripheral neuropathy
    c. Hypotension, depression, confusion
    d. Headache, nasal congestion, hypertension

44. (LO 14-6) Which of the following should you include in the education given to a patient receiving hormone replacement?
    a. Have a mammogram every 5 years during therapy.
    b. Follow a low-sodium diet.
    c. Smoke in moderation.
    d. Report bleeding when stopping hormone therapy replacement.

45. (LO 14-5) Which drug is the treatment of choice for syphilis?
    a. Parenteral penicillin
    b. Ceftriaxone
    c. Stavudine (*Zerit*)
    d. Azithromycin (*Zithromax*)

46. (LO 14-7) Which of the following oral contraceptives are monophasic pills?
    a. *Necon 10/11, Ortho Novum 1/35*
    b. *Lo/Ovral*
    c. *Cyclessa, Ortho-Novum 7/7/7*
    d. *Tri-Norinyl*

Chapter 14 Case Studies

47. (LO 14-6) A patient is taking estrogen (*Premarin*) 0.3 mg orally daily for menopause. How is this patient most likely to take the estrogen? The patient tells you she has a significant history of cardiovascular disease. What should you do with this information? What should you tell this patient about how to take *Premarin*? _____

_____

_____

_____

48. (LO 14-7) You are caring for a patient who is taking an oral contraceptive and is concerned about the side effects. What are the major side effects you should tell her about? What causes the majority of the pill's side effects? The patient tells you she smokes two packs of cigarettes a day. What should you tell her? _____

_____

_____

_____

Critical Thinking

Select the disorder that best matches the patient description and write it in the blank.

cervicitis   benign prostatic hyperplasia (BPH)   genital herpes simplex
endometriosis   acquired immune deficiency syndrome (AIDS)

49. (LO 14-5) Nancy Bullock had an unusual vaginal discharge that caused itching and burning, but she ignored it. Now the provider says that the infection has spread to the opening of the uterus.

_____

50. (LO 14-5) Harry Jackson, age 62, is having more and more trouble urinating lately. The provider thinks something may be blocking the urethra. Harry says this is the same condition that several friends his age have had.

_____

51. (LO 14-5) Akiko Niki has an inflammation of the uterine lining, and her provider has placed her on progesterone therapy.

_____

52. (LO 14-5) John Sullivan, age 28, is experiencing night sweats, diarrhea, and a persistent fever. A physical examination revealed that he is an IV drug user.

_____

53. (LO 14-5) Sara Davis is diagnosed with a sexually transmitted viral disease and treated with acyclovir (*Zovirax*).

_____

Applications

Obtain an electronic drug guide, a current copy of a drug reference book, or the *PDR*®. Use it to answer the following questions in a notebook or on file cards.

54. Use the electronic drug guide or the *PDR*® to find another product name for each drug in the Representative Drugs for the Reproductive System table in the chapter.

55. In Section 3 of the *PDR*®, Product Category Index, find Endometriosis Management. Make a list of all the drugs you see listed there.

DRUGS FOR THE ENDOCRINE SYSTEM

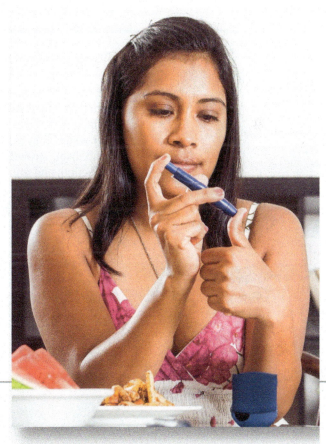

©Chris Fertnig/Getty Images

In this chapter you will learn about hormones and the glands that manufacture them. You will learn what goes wrong when the glands produce too much or too little of the hormones and how hormone therapy can help correct hormone imbalances. You will also learn about the treatment of diabetes and the uses of corticosteroid hormones and hormonelike drugs.

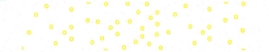

ENDOCRINE SYSTEM [LO 15-1]

The endocrine system is made up of **glands**, structures that produce and secrete chemical substances called **hormones** directly into the bloodstream. Hormones regulate many body functions. They are carried by the blood to sites where they exert their action. Hormones are the main regulators of metabolism, growth and development, reproduction, homeostasis, energy production, and immunity.

The endocrine glands include the hypothalamus, pituitary, thyroid, parathyroids, pineal, thymus, adrenal, pancreas, ovaries, and testes (**Figure 15.1**).

Figure 15.1

The major endocrine glands.

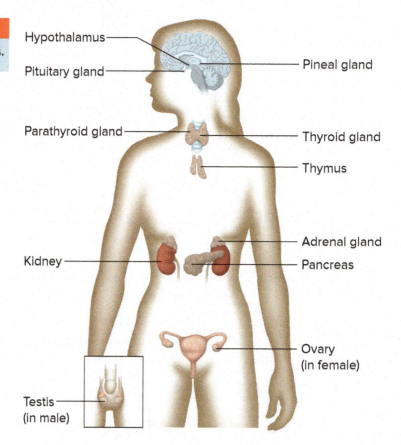

Hypothalamus

Pituitary gland

Pineal gland

Parathyroid gland

Thyroid gland

Thymus

Kidney

Adrenal gland

Pancreas

Ovary
(in female)

Testis
(in male)

Pituitary Gland

The pituitary, a small gland about the size of a pea, is located at the base of the brain. The pituitary stalk connects the pituitary to the hypothalamus. Although the pituitary is one gland, it has two lobes: the anterior and the posterior. The anterior lobe is particularly important in sustaining life. One of the hormones it secretes is the growth hormone, somatotropin, which promotes skeletal, visceral, and general growth. If too much growth hormone is produced, the body grows too fast and becomes overly large. When this occurs in a child, it is called gigantism. In adulthood, it is called acromegaly. Too little of the hormone results in stunted growth or dwarfism.

Other pituitary hormones control the secretions of the sex glands, the thyroid gland, and the adrenal glands. Because it controls the hormone production of other glands, the pituitary is known as the master gland.

Thyroid Gland

The thyroid gland is wrapped around the trachea just below the larynx, or voice box. It secretes two thyroid hormones and thyrocalcitonin. The two thyroid hormones are **thyroxine** (T_4) and triiodothyronine (T_3). These thyroid hormones control metabolism. **Metabolism** refers to the rate at which all cells produce energy (heat, muscle strength, etc.). When the thyroid produces extra thyroxine and triiodothyronine (**hyperthyroidism),** the metabolic rate is increased and there is an increase in temperature, respiration, heart rate, and nervous and muscular activity and a feeling of warmth. Too little thyroxine and triiodothyronine (**hypothyroidism**, **cretinism**, **myxedema**) causes cell metabolism to slow down. Signs of hypothyroidism include intolerance to cold, personality changes, fatigue, dry skin, brittle nails, slow speech, and weight gain.

To produce adequate thyroxine and triiodothyronine, the thyroid gland needs **iodine**, a mineral that is present in vegetables and seafood. The availability of iodized table salt helps people take in enough iodine to fulfill the needs of the thyroid. Thyrocalcitonin helps maintain a normal blood calcium level.

Parathyroid Glands

The parathyroids are four small glands located behind the thyroid gland. The hormone they produce is called parathyroid hormone (PTH). The main function of this hormone is to maintain a normal blood calcium level. A certain amount of calcium is needed in the bloodstream for muscles to work properly. Extra calcium is stored in the bones. When the level of calcium in the blood is low, the parathyroid glands produce parathyroid hormone to release stored calcium from the bones. If too much parathyroid hormone is manufactured, too much calcium may be taken out of the bones. As a result, the bones may become soft and easy to bend. If too little parathyroid hormone is produced, the muscles may go into spasms, and convulsions and gradual paralysis may occur. This condition, which affects mainly the face and the hands, is called **tetany** and can be fatal. The symptoms of tetany are relieved by administration of calcium.

Adrenal Glands (Suprarenals)

The two **adrenal** glands sit on top of (superior to) the two kidneys. Each adrenal gland has two layers: the adrenal cortex and the adrenal medulla. The adrenal cortex is the largest portion of the adrenal gland and secretes two hormones called **corticosteroids**. **Glucocorticoids** regulate the metabolism of carbohydrates and fats and have an anti-inflammatory effect. **Mineralocorticoids** maintain normal blood volume and promote sodium and water retention and urinary excretion of potassium.

The adrenal medulla secretes epinephrine and norepinephrine. These hormones help the body meet stressful situations. Epinephrine and norepinephrine prepare the body to react to emergencies by stimulating the heartbeat, increasing blood pressure, and releasing extra sugar into the bloodstream. Epinephrine and norepinephrine are produced in the body, but are also available as drugs to be administered. Epinephrine made in the body is also known as adrenaline. As a drug, it is used in the treatment of bronchial asthma, as described in Chapter 11. Norepinephrine is used in the emergency treatment of shock because of its ability to constrict blood vessels.

Pancreas

As noted in Chapter 12, the pancreas secretes enzymes as part of the digestive system. It also contains a number of secreting structures that are part of the endocrine system. These structures are called the islets of Langerhans. They secrete two hormones: insulin and glucagon.

Insulin controls the cell's use of sugar. It also stimulates the liver to store extra sugar in the form of glycogen. When the pancreas fails to produce insulin, the cells cannot burn sugar. Instead, it remains in the bloodstream and is excreted in the urine. This condition is known as **diabetes mellitus**.

The hormone glucagon stimulates the liver to release stored sugar into the bloodstream. It is administered in emergencies when diabetic patients have received too much insulin.

Ovaries and Testes

The ovaries and the testes are the sex glands, or gonads. They are responsible for the different physical characteristics of males and females and for the manufacture of sex cells for reproduction. The female gonads are the ovaries. The male gonads are the testes.

The ovaries, located in the pelvis of the female, secrete the hormones estrogen and progesterone. The testes, located in the scrotum of the male, produce testosterone, the male hormone. However, both males and females have both types of hormones in their bodies. These hormones and their uses in drug therapy are described in Chapter 14.

Hormone Control System

The level of hormones in the blood is constantly adjusted to meet the body's requirements. A large intake of carbohydrates, for example, stimulates the pancreas to release insulin to help reduce the blood sugar level. A complex chemical control system is required to ensure proper hormone levels. At the center of this control system is the pituitary gland, which stimulates other glands to produce hormones.

The pituitary, in turn, is linked to the brain's control system (the nervous system) by the hypothalamus. This portion of the brain stem lies just behind the pituitary and is connected to the pituitary by a stalk. The hypothalamus controls basic body functions such as sleep, appetite, and body temperature.

The hypothalamus and pituitary form a partnership in running the hormone chemical message system. The hypothalamus can stimulate or inhibit the pituitary according to conditions inside and outside the body. Because of this link, the endocrine system is influenced by the nervous system. Thus, emotions, fears, and moods have an impact on body processes through hormone stimulation as well as nerve stimulation.

The levels of circulating hormones provide feedback to the control system. As mentioned, hormones are distributed throughout the body via the bloodstream. When the proper hormone level is reached, the hypothalamus signals the pituitary to stop stimulating hormone production.

As an example, say the body needs extra sugar and fat for a heavy physical task. The pituitary excretes adrenocorticotropic hormone (ACTH), which is swiftly transported by the bloodstream to the adrenal cortex. The ACTH

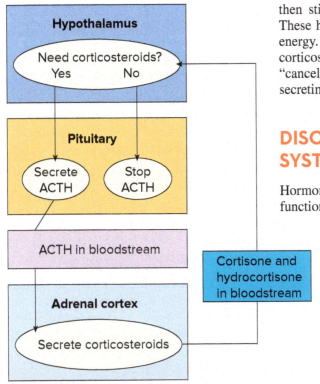

Hypothalamus

Need corticosteroids?
Yes   No

Pituitary

Secrete ACTH   Stop ACTH

ACTH in bloodstream

Cortisone and hydrocortisone in bloodstream

Adrenal cortex

Secrete corticosteroids

Figure 15.2

Hormone levels in the bloodstream determine when hormone secretion will occur.

then stimulates the adrenal cortex to produce corticosteroids. These help liberate extra sugar and fat for the body to burn for energy. When the hypothalamus senses that there are enough corticosteroids in the bloodstream, it signals the pituitary to "cancel the order" for ACTH. The adrenal cortex then stops secreting its hormones until they are needed again (**Figure 15.2**).

DISORDERS OF THE ENDOCRINE SYSTEM [LO 15-2, LO 15-3]

Hormones control body processes—growth, metabolism, kidney function, and so forth. Consequently, when there is a disturbance in the production of hormones, the body processes go out of control. If a child's pituitary produces too much growth hormone, it can result in a condition called gigantism; an adult develops diabetes mellitus because the pancreas fails to produce enough insulin to maintain sugar metabolism.

Symptoms of endocrine disorders are logically related to the specific hormones that are out of balance. That is, when a certain hormone is lacking, symptoms show that the body process it regulates is no longer working properly.

Endocrine disorders arise because a gland overproduces, underproduces, or produces its hormones too early or too late. **Table 15.1** lists examples of endocrine disorders and their symptoms. Note that the names of the various disorders usually tell you something about how hormone production has gone wrong. Recall that *hypo* means too little (less than normal) and *hyper* means too much (more than normal).

There are several reasons that a gland may secrete too much, too little, or too early. One is that the gland may be overdeveloped, a condition called **hyperplasia**. Or it may contain a tumor. Usually tumors and hyperplasia cause too much hormone production because there are far more secreting cells than normal. In these cases, surgery or radiation treatment may be needed to reduce the number of cells and thus restore normal hormone balance.

One form of radiation treatment is the radioactive "cocktail." The patient drinks a radioactive material that travels to the gland to destroy the tumor. In the case of a thyroid tumor, for example, the provider can take advantage of the fact that the thyroid traps circulating iodine to use in making thyroxine. A cocktail of radioactive isotopes of iodine can be given so that when they arrive at the thyroid, they destroy the offending cells.

Genetic factors are another reason for gland malfunctions. Some individuals are simply born with defective glands or are missing the necessary chemicals for producing certain hormones. People can inherit tendencies to develop some types of endocrine problems—for example, diabetes mellitus. Genetically caused problems can usually be treated with replacement hormones. Chances for cure are good if these conditions are discovered early enough, before growth and development are permanently affected.

Finally, there may be nothing wrong with a gland itself. The problem may be that the gland is receiving faulty messages from the pituitary. A small tumor on the pituitary, for example, can cause over- or underproduction of the hormones that direct the other glands. Underproduction is diagnosed by administering pituitary hormones to see if they successfully stimulate the other glands. If the problem lies with the pituitary, then either surgery, radiation, or appropriate hormone replacement is required.

Table 15.1 Selected Hormones and Their Disorders

Hormone	Function	Disorder	Symptoms	Treatment
Pituitary				
Somatotropin	Regulates growth	Hypersecretion in adulthood—acromegaly	Enlargement of hands, feet, face, jaws, and cheeks	Radiation, surgery
		Hypersecretion in childhood—gigantism	Growth to an extreme height	Sex hormones
		Undersecretion—dwarfism	Failure to grow to normal height, remaining small and fragile	Somatotropin (growth hormone replacement)
Follicle-stimulating hormone (FSH)	Regulates development of sex characteristics by stimulating gonads (ovaries and testes) to secrete sex hormones	Too much, too early—overdevelopment	Development of adultlike sex characteristics as early as 5 years of age	Hormone replacement
		Too little—underdevelopment	Failure to develop sex characteristics during the teens	Hormone replacement
Luteinizing hormone (LTH) (called ovulating hormone)	Stimulates ovulation	Too little—failure to ovulate	Menstrual irregularities	Hormone replacement
Antidiuretic hormone (ADH)	Regulates reabsorption of water in kidney tubules	Too little—diabetes insipidus	Polyuria, polydipsia	Hormone replacement, some diuretics
Thyroid				
Thyroxine and triiodothyronine (regulated by the thyroid-stimulating hormone [TSH] of the pituitary)	Regulates metabolism	Too much of either thyroxine or triiodothyronine—hyperthyroidism	Nervousness, weight loss, heat intolerance, tachycardia, elevated temperature, insomnia, bulging eyes, etc.	Surgery, radioactive iodine cocktail, antithyroid drugs such as propylthiouracil and methimazole (*Tapazole*)
Calcitonin	Inhibits calcium reabsorption from bone, increases calcium storage in bone, increases renal excretion of calcium and phosphorus, lowers calcium level in blood	Too little—hypothyroidism (also cretinism and myxedema, depending on when deficiency occurs)	Slowed mental and physical processes, fatigue, hair loss, constipation, intolerance to cold, weight gain, dry skin, brittle nails	Synthetic oral thyroxine (*Synthroid*)
		Enlargement of thyroid gland—goiter	Enlargement of thyroid, swelling in neck	Thyroid hormone may prevent further enlargement; surgery for large goiters

Table 15.1 (continued)

Hormone	Function	Disorder	Symptoms	Treatment
Parathyroid				
Parathyroid hormone	Regulates blood level of calcium	Too much—hyperparathyroidism	Too much calcium taken out of bones, resulting in bone weakness, loss of appetite, increased need for sleep, short attention span, calcium stones in kidneys	Antihypercalcemic agents
		Too little—hypoparathyroidism	Muscle spasms (tetany), convulsions, gradual paralysis	IV calcium salts, vitamin D
Pancreas				
Insulin	Permits body to burn sugar for energy, regulates storage of sugar in the liver	Too little—diabetes mellitus	Thirst, constant hunger, weight loss, fatigue, changes in vision, slow-healing cuts	Insulin replacement, oral hypoglycemics, management of diet, exercise
		Too much—hypoglycemia	Weakness, tachycardia, cold clammy skin, emotional changes	Sugar, food with high sugar content, glucagon
Adrenal Cortex				
Mineralocorticoids (aldosterone, desoxycorticosterone)	Regulates body's salt–water balance by stimulating kidneys to retain sodium and excrete potassium	Too much aldosterone—aldosteronism	Low serum potassium, alkalosis, high blood pressure, headache	Surgery, drugs
Glucocorticoids (cortisone, hydrocortisone)	Stimulates breakdown of protein molecules into carbohydrates	Too much—Cushing's disease	Weight gain, rounding of face, fat deposits on back of neck and on shoulders, hypertension	Surgery
		Too little of all adrenal cortex hormones—acute adrenal crisis, chronic Addison's disease	Shock symptoms in acute cases; in Addison's disease, weakness, tiredness, skin hyperpigmentation, anorexia, weight loss, gastrointestinal symptoms	Hydrocortisone
Androgenic steroids (small amounts of male and female hormones secreted in both males and females)	Is thought to contribute to development of sex characteristics (but gonads secrete most of the necessary hormones)	Too much of wrong sex hormone—feminization of males, virilization of females	Inappropriate sex characteristics (e.g., manliness, deep voice in females; loss of body hair, high voice in males)	Surgery

HORMONE THERAPY [LO 15-4]

Hormone replacement is the most common use of hormones in drug therapy. Replacement is necessary whenever hormones are missing because of either genetic defects in the glands, surgical removal of glands, or production of poor-quality hormones. Some hormones and hormonelike drugs are used because of actions that are not related to the endocrine system—for example, the anti-inflammatory action of the adrenal corticosteroids.

Most hormones used for drug therapy are taken from animals: hogs, cattle, sheep, and horses. A few hormones have been synthesized in the laboratory. Recombinant DNA technology will increase the availability of these important substances.

Drug Management of Diabetes Mellitus

Diabetes mellitus is a condition in which the beta cells of the islets of Langerhans in the pancreas do not secrete enough of the hormone insulin. Alterations in insulin production result in abnormal metabolism of carbohydrates, fats, and proteins. As a result, sugar remains in the bloodstream and is excreted in the urine. Meanwhile, body cells "starve." To compensate, they burn protein and fat. The three classic symptoms of diabetes are hunger (**polyphagia**), thirst (**polydipsia**), and frequent urination (**polyuria**). Other symptoms include weight loss and weakness. Urine tests may reveal large quantities of sugar in the urine.

Diabetes can appear in childhood as **type 1, insulin-dependent diabetes mellitus (IDDM)** or in adulthood as **type 2, non-insulin-dependent diabetes mellitus (NIDDM).** Many older adults develop some degree of diabetes along with the changes of aging. Over time, diabetes causes damage to the tissues and organs, especially the heart, kidneys, and eyes. It always carries the danger of complications, such as diseases of the blood vessels and nervous system. Gestational diabetes is the onset of glucose intolerance during pregnancy.

Many mild cases of diabetes can be managed by controlling diet, maintaining normal body weight, and exercising enough to burn off excess blood sugar. Patients with diabetes are encouraged to eat small meals throughout the day rather than a few large meals. The purpose is to avoid large fluctuations in the amount of sugar in the blood. When these measures are not enough to control the diabetes, drug therapy is indicated.

 Caution Hormone Doses

Hormones are powerful chemicals that have profound effects on the human body. They must be administered carefully, according to a provider's orders. Often the doses are very small. They may be measured in micrograms. The exception is corticosteroids, which are given in large doses to combat allergic reactions and inflammation.

INSULIN [LO 15-5]

The major drug for type 1 diabetes is insulin, which is administered by injection. Insulin must be administered by subcutaneous injection because it is destroyed by the gastric secretions. Insulin is secreted from the beta cells in the pancreas. Several oral drugs are available to control blood sugar in type 2 NIDDM. Insulin therapy replaces the missing hormone that enables the body to use sugar. More than one preparation of insulin is available, and providers prescribe different preparations according to individual cases. Dosages are highly individualized and depend on many factors. Insulin preparations are grouped into four basic categories: rapid-acting, short-acting, intermediate-acting, and long-acting. They differ according to how quickly they take effect (onset of action), how soon they reach their peak effect, and how long their effect lasts (duration of action). Table 15.2 summarizes some of these differences.

Popular drugs for diabetes control are the intermediate-acting insulins: *Lente* and *Insulin NPH*. They reach their peak effectiveness in about 7 hours and last up to 16 hours. They are thus convenient for once-a-day doses, usually administered $\frac{1}{2}$ hour before breakfast. Some providers prefer to keep closer control over insulin dosages by using the rapid-acting and regular insulins. These are given several times during the day (e.g., $\frac{1}{2}$ hour before each meal), and dosages are varied on the basis of frequent urine tests.

Biosynthetic insulin has come to be used almost exclusively. *Humulin N* and *Humulin R* are produced genetically by altering common bacteria or yeast using DNA technology. These insulins cause fewer allergic reactions, and their insulin activity is more predictable.

A diabetic person's need for insulin varies according to diet, amount of exercise, and emotions. All three factors must be kept under control for insulin-replacement therapy to be effective. Changes in these factors affect the dosage requirements for insulin and can lead to over- or underdoses. For this reason, health team members as well as patients must be thoroughly familiar with the symptoms of insulin overdose and underdose.

Table 15.2 Types of Insulin (All Administered Subcutaneously)

Type	Insulin	Onset of Action	Peak Action	Duration of Action
Rapid-acting	insulin lispro (*Humalog*)	10–15 min	1–1.5 hours	6–8 hours
	insulin aspart (*NovoLog*)	10–15 min	1–2 hours	3–5 hours
	insulin glusine (*Apidra*)	10–15 min	1–1.5 hours	5–6 hours
Short-acting	insulin regular *Humulin R* or *Novolin R*	15 min (IV) 30 min (SC)	2–3 hours	30–60 min (IV) 8–12 hours
Intermediate-acting	Neutral protamine Hagedorn (NPH)	1–3 hours	5–8 hours	Up to 18 hours
	Recombinant (*Humulin N, Novolin N*)	1–3 hours	5–8 hours	Up to 18 hours
Long-acting	insulin glargine (*Lantus*)	1.5 hours		Up to 24 hours
	insulin detemir (*Levemir*)	1.5 hours	6–8 hours	Up to 24 hours

HYPERGLYCEMICS AND HYPOGLYCEMICS [LO 15-6]

Too little insulin in the bloodstream, **hyperglycemia**, is serious and can be fatal if the situation is not caught early and corrected. The first signs are vomiting, excessive thirst, diarrhea, urine containing large amounts of sugar (**glycosuria**), and (occasionally) increased appetite and eating without weight gain. Later the patient becomes dazed (stuporous), respirations are deep, and the face is dry and flushed. There is a fruity acetone smell to the breath, signaling that the body is burning excessive amounts of fat. This is called **ketoacidosis**. If these symptoms go undiagnosed, the person becomes unconscious within a day or two, a condition referred to as **diabetic coma**. The treatment is to immediately administer insulin and replace fluid and electrolytes.

The opposite situation, too much insulin, is called **hypoglycemia**. Symptoms are increased appetite, nervousness, heart palpitations, cold sweating, shakiness, difficulty concentrating, and blurred vision. They occur as a result of strenuous physical effort, overly large doses of insulin, or eating too little food. These situations cause all the blood sugar to be burned off so that the level of sugar in the bloodstream is too low (hypoglycemia). A urine test reveals that there is no sugar in the urine either. Treatment consists of giving sugar in some easily digestible form—120 to 180 mL of orange juice, 180 to 240 mL of regular soft drink, two packets of sugar, or 5 or 6 hard candies, for example—to increase the blood sugar level quickly. In extreme cases, glucose or glucagon may be given parenterally. You should look for signs of hypoglycemia anywhere from 5 minutes to several hours after a dose of insulin. Be especially watchful for these signs during the hours of peak effect. Keep in mind that the peak effect of any insulin varies according to the individual patient's physical condition and level of activity.

The term *hypoglycemia* means low blood sugar. **Oral hypoglycemics (antidiabetic agents)** purposely lower blood sugar levels to reduce diabetic symptoms. Overdoses of hypoglycemics or of insulin result in drug-induced hypoglycemia, a dangerous adverse reaction. There is another type of hypoglycemia, however, that is unrelated to diabetes. It is called reactive hypoglycemia and is extremely rare. The symptoms are similar to those of insulin-induced hypoglycemia. A definite diagnosis can be made only after a blood glucose level of less than 50 mg/dL. Treatment consists of frequent small meals balanced in carbohydrates and protein.

Diabetic patients are largely responsible for administering their own insulin, so they and their families should be educated about all aspects of the disease and its treatment. They must learn new dietary habits and injection and testing procedures. You can help by reinforcing their attempts to moderate their diet and exercise and by encouraging them to stay on a regular schedule of medication. Caution them to read OTC medication labels, because many have high sugar content. They should also avoid alcoholic beverages.

Insulin pumps have improved the metabolic state of IDDM patients who have not achieved adequate diabetic control after a combination of dietary restrictions and insulin injections. The insulin infusion system, worn on the belt or at the side, is battery-operated and connected to a small computer programmed to release small amounts of insulin each hour (**Figure 15.3**). The amount of insulin released is based on the individual's daily needs according to diet and physical exercise. The patient pushes a button to obtain a dose of insulin after eating. Although these pumps can be effective, they present potential problems in the way of battery failure and line leakage, and they are expensive.

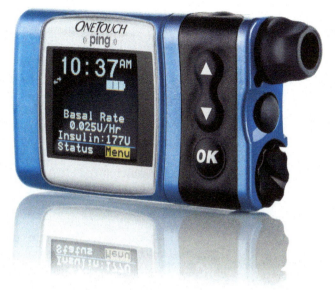
An insulin pen looks like a regular ink pen and may increase the patient's compliance with the program to take insulin. The pen has an insulin-filled cartridge and a needle, both of which are disposable (Figure 15.4). Some research has shown that insulin pens deliver a more accurate dose than the 100-unit syringe. The dose of insulin is offered by turning the dial to the number of insulin units needed. The insulin pen is more expensive than the traditional insulin syringe.

Oral Hypoglycemics

Patients with type 2 (non-insulin-dependent) diabetes mellitus are treated with oral hypoglycemics, diet, exercise, and insulin when necessary. The patient who responds best to oral hypoglycemic drugs is over the age of 40 years, has had diabetes less than 5 years, is normal weight or obese, has a consistent diet, has never received insulin, or has been controlled on 40 units or less of insulin a day. Currently there are three classifications of oral hypoglycemic agents: first- and second-generation sulfonylureas, and

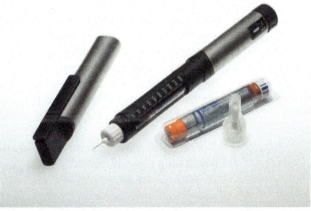

miscellaneous oral hypoglycemics. The miscellaneous oral hypoglycemics consist of the alpha-glucosidase inhibitors, biguanides, meglitinides, and thiazolidinediones. The first category of oral hypoglycemic agents introduced into the United States was the sulfonylureas. The first- and second-generation sulfonylureas are differentiated by when they were first developed and used. The second-generation sulfonylureas have the advantage over the first-generation sulfonylureas in that they have a longer action and fewer side effects. The first-generation sulfonylureas include tolbutamide, tolazamide, and chlorpropamide. The second-generation sulfonylureas include glipizide (*Glucotrol*), glipizide extended release (*Glucotrol XL*), glyburide (*DiaBeta*), and glyburide micronized (*Glynase PresTab*). The miscellaneous oral hypoglycemics include the alpha-glucosidase inhibitors acarbose (*Precose*) and miglitol (*Glyset*); a biguanide, metformin (*Glucophage*); a meglitinide, repaglinide (*Prandin*); and the thiazolidinediones, pioglitazone (*Actos*) and rosiglitazone (*Avandia*). Sitagliptin phosphate (*Januvia*) and linagliptin (*Tradjenta)* belong to a new class of oral hypoglycemics known as DPP-4 inhibitors. They are not frontline drugs for type 2 diabetes. Their use is reserved for people whose diabetes is not adequately controlled with diet, exercise, and other oral hypoglycemics. The oral hypoglycemic agents are used when the beta cells of the islets of Langerhans continue to produce some insulin. Their effect is to stimulate these cells to secrete insulin in response to rising glucose levels. There is some evidence that they may also make the body cells more receptive to the action of insulin. Table 15.3 summarizes the categories of the oral hypoglycemics.

Saxagliptin (*Onglyza*) is a new oral hypoglycemic used in the treatment of type 2 diabetes. It is used as an adjunct to diet and exercise and may be given with other oral hypoglycemics.

Urine and Blood Tests

All diabetics must monitor their condition by one of two methods (urine or blood) for testing glucose levels. Urine testing is less common since the development of home-monitoring blood glucose devices. Urine testing should be done on people with IDDM who have unexplained hyperglycemia or who are ill. Urine is tested for both glucose and ketones. Unfortunately, urine testing yields unpredictable results.

Tests for sugar in the urine include Clinitest, Diastix, and Tes-Tape. The urine must be a freshly voided specimen. Results are determined by matching the color of the test to the manufacturer's chart; the chart colors represent a range of sugar content. Precision QID is a glucose monitor marketed for home use.

Blood tests for sugar can be done with a glucose meter. This type of monitoring is more accurate than urine tests but is more expensive. Blood glucose meters include Accu-Chek, Glucometer, and OneTouch Ultra. The machines display the results digitally.

Blood glucose can also be monitored by visual examination. A drop of blood placed on special strips induces a color change. As in the urine tests, the color change is compared to the manufacturer's color scale on the side of the container. Examples of visual blood glucose tests are Chemstrip bG and Dextrostix.

Results of these tests must be charted so that the provider can properly adjust drug doses if needed.

Table 15.3 Oral Hypoglycemic Agents for NIDDM (Type 2)

	Onset of Action (hours)	Duration of Action (hours)	Daily Dose Range	Daily Doses
First-Generation Sulfonylureas				
tolbutamide[a]	1	6–12	0.25–2 g[b]	1 before meals
tolazamide	4–6	12–24	100–1000 mg	1 daily or bid
chlorpropamide	1	72	100–500 mg	1 daily
Second-Generation Sulfonylureas				
glipizide (Glucotrol)	1	10–24	Initial: 50 mg Maintenance: 5–40 mg	1 daily
glipizide extended release (Glucotrol XL)	1	24	5–20 mg	1 daily
glyburide nonmicronized (DiaBeta)	2–4	24	Initial: 2.5–5 mg Maintenance: 2.5–20 mg	1 daily
glyburide micronized (Glynase PresTab)	1	24	0.75–12 mg; over 6 mg in divided doses	1 daily
Alpha-Glucosidase Inhibitors				
acarbose (Precose)	Not absorbed	Unknown	25–100 mg	25 mg tid
miglitol (Glyset)	Unknown	Unknown	25–100 mg	25 mg tid
Biguanides				
metformin (Glucophage)	1	6–12	500–2500 mg	500–850 mg bid or tid
Meglitinides				
repaglinide (Prandin)	2–4	24	0.5–4 mg	0.5 mg before meals
Thiazolidinediones				
pioglitazone (Actos)	$\frac{1}{2}$	Unknown	15–45 mg	1 daily
rosiglitazone (Avandia)	1	24	4–8 mg	Once daily or in divided doses
linagliptin (Tradjenta) Dipeptidyl peptidase-4 inhibitor	$\frac{1}{2}$ hour	Unknown	5 mg	1 daily

[a]Trade names given in parentheses are examples only. Check current drug references for a complete listing of available products.

[b]Dosages for the older adult and the debilitated are usually smaller. Average adult doses are given here. However, dosages are determined by a provider and vary with the purpose of the therapy and the particular patient. The doses presented in this text are for general information only.

Diabetes Mellitus in the Pediatric Patient

Diabetes mellitus in childhood is type 1, or insulin-dependent, diabetes mellitus. Glycosuria, polyuria, and a history of weight loss or failure to gain weight despite a hearty appetite are indications of diabetes. The management of the child with IDDM must be a multidisciplinary approach. The child, family, provider, diabetic nurse educator, nutritionist, and exercise physiologist must be included. Often psychological support is also needed because it is generally difficult for a child of any age to accept and comply with the treatment regimen. Communication is very important among all the members of the healthcare team, the child, and the family, but it must also extend to the child's teachers, school nurse, school guidance counselor, and coach. The treatment is insulin. However, insulin needs are affected by nutritional intake, activity, stress, illness, and puberty. Therefore, successful management includes both education and support. Initially, the parents are responsible for the care of the diabetic child, but the child should assume responsibility for self-management as soon as she or he is capable. Children at age 4 or 5 years can begin to check their blood glucose levels. Children at age 9 can begin to administer their own insulin (Figure 15.5).

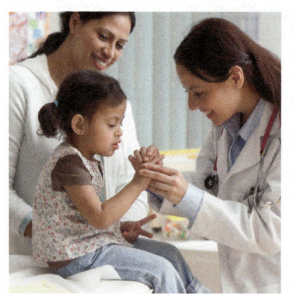

©SelectStock/Getty Images

Figure 15.5

Communication is very important among the child, the parents, and members of the healthcare team to help the child comply with the diabetes treatment regimen.

Complications of Diabetes

As the disease progresses, patients with diabetes are prone to urinary and vaginal infections and to blood vessel diseases that lead to vision problems, gangrene, foot and leg problems, and dental problems. Gangrene and amputation are extremes of diabetes that is out of control. These complications must be treated separately, keeping in mind that any added drugs may have an impact on the dosage of insulin. Many drugs may affect blood sugar and interact with insulin and oral hypoglycemics, so any drug therapy for these secondary conditions must always be carefully planned (Table 15.4). As a member of the healthcare team, you can help the patient prevent infections by teaching good habits of skin, foot, and dental care.

 Pediatric Considerations Insulin

- A child with diabetes must take insulin because the pancreas does not produce insulin. Insulin is generally given 3 to 4 times a day (this is difficult to maintain but important for growth and development).
- Children must maintain balanced meals, snacks, blood glucose, and exercise.

- Avoiding hypoglycemia is critical in infants and children because of growth and development.
- If less than 5 U is required per day, diluted insulin may be used because of more accurate administration.

 Older Adult Considerations Insulin

- Diabetes mellitus is a challenge for older adults because they may have other complicating diseases or poor dexterity for administering insulin and monitoring glucose.

- With oral sulfonylureas, hypoglycemia is an issue.
- Miglitol (*Glyset*) and metformin (*Glucophage*) are contraindicated in older adults with impaired renal function.

Table 15.4 Drugs That Commonly Affect Blood Sugar

Drugs That Increase Glucose	Drugs That Decrease Glucose
CNS stimulants	Alcohol
Corticosteroids	Salicylates
Diuretics	Sulfonamides
Estrogen	
Nicotine	

CORTICOSTEROIDS [LO 15-7, LO 15-8]

Corticosteroids are a group of hormones secreted by the adrenal cortex. Insufficient production of corticosteroids (Addison's disease) can be fatal. There are two major groups of corticosteroids, each group having different functions: (1) the glucocorticoids (cortisone, hydrocortisone, and cortisol) affect fat and carbohydrate metabolism; and (2) the mineralocorticoids (aldosterone and desoxycorticosterone) regulate the salt–water balance.

The glucocorticoids often included in drug therapy are hydrocortisone (*Cortef, Hydrocortone*), fluticasone (*Flonase Allergy Relief*), cortisone, triamcinolone, prednisone, prednisolone, dexamethasone (*Decadron*), and methylprednisolone (*Medrol, Solu-Medrol*). Fludrocortisone is used for its mineralocorticoid effects.

Corticosteroids have many uses. One important use is in hormone replacement therapy. The pituitary may not produce enough ACTH to stimulate corticosteroid production in the adrenal cortex. Or the adrenal cortex itself may not work properly (Addison's disease). In both cases, corticosteroids can be used to replace the missing hormones.

Large doses of corticosteroids are used with many conditions unrelated to adrenal functioning: allergic reactions, skin inflammations, some cancers, autoimmune reactions and suppression of immunity in organ transplants, and eye and respiratory diseases. The main reason for their use in these diseases is that corticosteroids suppress inflammation, which is the body's normal reaction to irritation or injury.

The inflammation reaction is signaled by redness, warmth to the touch, pain, and swelling. Corticosteroids change the tissue's response to irritation in such a way as to reduce these symptoms. They also reduce fever and itching. Because of their anti-inflammatory action, corticosteroids are often used in chronic inflammatory diseases such as rheumatoid arthritis; in skin, gastrointestinal, and blood disorders; or in combination with other drugs for cancer, kidney, and eye disorders and respiratory diseases.

When used in small doses for a short time, corticosteroids show beneficial effects. In long-term use and in the large doses required for suppressing inflammation, however, there are many dangers. In general, long-term systemic use of steroids is not desirable. One problem with corticosteroids is that they mask infection and may cause it to spread. Inflammation is suppressed, but the irritation or injury remains. Tissue destruction can continue even though the symptoms are not obvious. There are other dangers, too: Old infections can be reactivated and new infections can start, but the symptoms will be hidden because the drug suppresses them.

Another problem with long-term corticosteroid therapy is the side effects. Some of these are weight gain, sodium (salt) retention and edema, hypertension, facial rounding (moon face), diabetes, easy bruising, thinning of the skin, failure of wounds to heal, psychological changes, ulcers, osteoporosis, and hyperglycemia. In addition, corticosteroid therapy interferes with the feedback between the adrenal glands and the pituitary. After withdrawal of corticosteroids, the chemical signal system between the glands takes several months to return to normal. Consequently, providers taper the dose or order gradually smaller doses of a corticosteroid before the patient completely discontinues it.

If steroids can be discontinued within 7 days of when therapy is initiated, then tapering of doses is not necessary, because the drug has not yet inhibited normal feedback control. On the other hand, abrupt discontinuation of steroids after prolonged therapy can result in adrenal insufficiency. Signs of adrenal insufficiency are nausea, fatigue, shortness of breath, low blood pressure, hypoglycemia, and muscle and joint aches.

For all these reasons, providers try to prescribe the smallest dose possible for the shortest time needed to achieve the desired therapeutic effect. This principle is important, of course, in all drug therapy, but especially when giving corticosteroids. Doses must be individualized according to each patient's response to the drugs. You should monitor the patient for the side effects previously mentioned.

 Pediatric Considerations   Corticosteroids

- Corticosteroids are used for children for the same reasons they are for adults.
- Start with a moderate dose of inhaled steroid.
- Growth retardation is a problem with small doses of inhaled steroid.

- Children generally have a growth spurt when the steroid is discontinued.
- Monitor effects with weight and height measurement.

 Older Adult Considerations   Corticosteroids

- Because of other diseases older adults may have, they are at greater risk for side effects of corticosteroids.

- Lower doses are prescribed because of decreased muscle mass, plasma volume, hepatic metabolism, and renal excretion.

Other Hormones

Natural thyroid (*Armour Thyroid*), used as a thyroid replacement for many years, is not commonly used today. Synthetic thyroid preparations—levothyroxine (*Synthroid*), liothyronine (*Cytomel*), and liotrix (*Thyrolar*)—that are available today are more standardized, stable, and therefore more frequently prescribed. Thyroid supplements are used in the treatment of hypothyroidism, cretinism, myxedema, and thyroid cancer; in the prevention and treatment of goiter; and in thyroid function tests.

Somatropin (*Humatrope*) is a pituitary hormone that is used to stimulate growth in pituitary growth hormone deficiency such as hypopituitary dwarfism.

Vasopressin tannate is the antidiuretic hormone (ADH) of the pituitary that regulates reabsorption of water in the kidneys. It is given to control diabetes insipidus, a disorder in which too much water is excreted in the urine. Vasopressin causes water to be reabsorbed so that the patient urinates normally.

 Pediatric Considerations **Thyroid**

- Thyroid replacement is required with hypothyroidism for normal growth and development.
- Thyroid started at 6 weeks for congenital hypothyroidism (cretinism) and continued for life.

- Recommended dose is 10 to 15 micrograms per kilograms of body weight daily.
- Retardation occurs if replacement therapy is delayed.
- Propylthiouracil or methimazole is used for hyperthyroidism.

 Older Adult Considerations **Thyroid**

- Thyroid disease may be confusing in the older adult because it mimics other diseases such as congestive heart failure.
- Levothyroxine (*Synthroid*) is given for hypothyroidism.

- Because of an increased incidence of cardiovascular adverse reactions, an older adult needs to be given smaller doses and monitored very carefully.
- Propylthiouracil or methimazole (*Tapazole*) may be prescribed for hyperthyroidism, but radioactive iodine is preferred because it causes fewer side effects.

Diagnosis of Hormone Deficiencies

Hormones can be used to find out whether a gland is failing to produce its hormone. Suppose, for example, that the body lacks a certain adrenal hormone. Is this the fault of the pituitary or of the adrenal glands? One way to find out is to administer the pituitary hormone ACTH. If this makes the adrenals secrete the missing hormone, we know the problem lies with the pituitary; the pituitary has not been secreting enough of its own ACTH to stimulate the adrenals. On the other hand, if the dose of ACTH does not stimulate the adrenals, we know that the adrenals are not working properly. In this situation, the patient will likely be put on a regular course of hormone therapy to replace the missing adrenal hormone.

Representative hormones and hormonelike drugs used for replacement therapy and inflammation are listed at the end of this chapter. Other uses of hormones—for example, in arthritis, cancer therapy, and contraception—are discussed in Chapters 14 and 16.

ADMINISTERING INSULIN [LO 15-9]

Insulin is given parenterally, and as a healthcare worker, you should not administer it unless you are trained and permitted by law to give medications by injection. General instructions for giving injections are provided in Chapter 4. Table 15.5 identifies the instructions for giving insulin.

Insulin is most commonly given subcutaneously, although intravenous (IV) administration of regular insulin may be used when rapid onset of action is needed. Rate of absorption depends on the site of injection. Rate of absorption

Table 15.5 Instructions for Giving Insulin

- Keep insulin at room temperature for up to 4 weeks.
- Use insulin only with a good expiration date.
- Rotate insulin suspensions such as *NPH,* and *Lente,* between the palms of hands.
- Ensure that suspension insulins are cloudy, such as *NPH,* and *Lente,* check that regular insulin is clear.
- Do not shake vial. If clumps are present after rotating, discard.
- Administer insulin on time so peak action is reached when blood sugar is highest.
- Be accurate with correct prescribed dose using only insulin syringe measured in units (U).
- Do not massage site after administration.

is greatest in the abdomen, followed by the arm, thigh, and buttocks. Rotate injection sites in the same anatomical area because of the differences in absorption at the various sites (**Figure 15.6**).

Be aware of the peak action time for the type of insulin you are giving so you can be alert for signs of hypoglycemia and have juice or sugar available if necessary. With long-acting insulin, hypoglycemia may occur during the night, signaled by restless sleep and sweating.

Two different types of insulin can be drawn up into the same syringe, as long as one type is regular insulin. The regular insulin should be drawn first (Practice Procedure 15.1).

Insulin may be administered according to a sliding scale in which there are standard orders with a variety of insulin doses dependent on a patient's blood glucose. A patient's dose of insulin is determined and administered after checking the blood glucose.

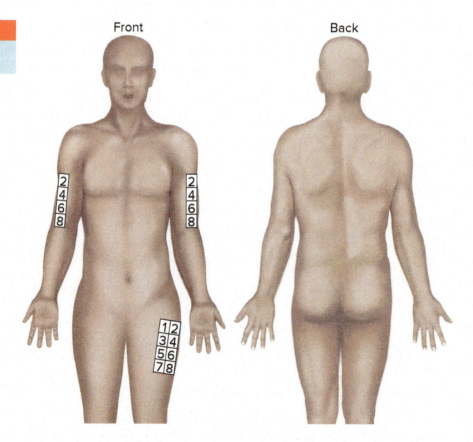

Figure 15.6

Insulin rotation sites.

Front

Back

Healthcare for Today and Tomorrow | *Lantus*

A long-acting insulin called insulin glargine (*Lantus*) is available to allow the body to maintain a steady state of insulin over 24 hours, thus eliminating the need for multiple daily injections.

Insulin glargine is a human insulin that dissolves more easily in acid than in the pH of subcutaneous tissue. Once injected, it forms a microprecipitation that releases insulin at a constant slow rate over 24 hours with no peaks. This mimics the body's natural basal rate.

Legal and Ethical Issues | Dangerous Herbal Use

As a result of the explosion of herbal therapy in the United States, it is your responsibility to assess whether your diabetic patients are taking herbal supplements. You must stress that herbs have not gone through the same rigorous research as pharmaceuticals and are not approved by the Food and Drug Administration to be sold as drugs. The use of herbs by the diabetic patient can have serious and even life-threatening results. Most herbs cause either a hypoglycemic or hyperglycemic reaction that can have devastating effects on the blood glucose level and insulin requirements. If you fail to assess whether the diabetic patient is taking herbs, the patient may receive the wrong dose of insulin, which could result in death.

Representative Hormones and Hormonelike Drugs[a]

Category, Name,[b] and Route	Uses and Diseases	Actions	Usual Dose[c] and Special Instructions	Side Effects and Adverse Reactions
Hormones				
levothyroxine sodium (**Synthroid, Cytomel, Thyrolar**) Oral	Hypothyroid conditions such as cretinism, myxedema, goiter, mild hypothyroidism, surgical removal of thyroid gland	Is a synthetic thyroid hormone replacement; stimulates metabolism	*Maintenance:* 25–100 µg PO daily in single dose; increase by 50–100 µg PO every 1–4 weeks until desired response occurs	Headache, palpitations, sleeplessness, weight loss, nervousness, tachycardia, hypertension
glucagon Subcutaneous, IM, IV	Severe insulin reaction, hypoglycemia	Raises blood sugar by stimulating liver to convert glycogen to glucose	0.5–1 mg; may be repeated 1 or 2 times as ordered	Nausea, vomiting, rash, dizziness
vasopressin tannate Subcutaneous, IM	Diabetes insipidus	Replaces ADH of pituitary, promotes reabsorption of water in kidneys	5–10 units IM or subcut, 2–3 times a day	Tremor, dizziness, headache, bradycardia, abdominal cramps, nausea, vomiting
somatropin (*Humatrope*) Subcutaneous, IM	Growth failure due to growth hormone deficiency	Stimulates growth	Up to 0.06 mg/kg subcut, or IM 3 times a week with minimum 48 hours between doses	Pain at site of injection, headache, localized muscle pain, weakness, intolerance to cold, weight gain, dry skin and hair

Category, Name,[b] and Route	Uses and Diseases	Actions	Usual Dose[c] and Special Instructions	Side Effects and Adverse Reactions
Corticosteroids				
fluticasone (*Flonase Allergy Relief*) Aerosol	Asthma	Suppresses inflammation and immune response	88–440 µg bid	Epistaxis, nasal burning, pharyngitis, irritation of nasal mucous membranes, sneezing, runny nose, nasal dryness, nasal congestion, headache, dizziness, urticaria
prednisone Oral	Hormone replacement, inflammatory diseases (e.g., arthritis, dermatitis), lymphatic cancer, allergies, ulcerative colitis, kidney disease	Suppresses inflammation and immune response; stimulates bone marrow; influences protein, fat, and carbohydrate metabolism	2.5–15 mg PO 2, 3, or 4 times a day, depending on specific disease, adjusted to lowest effective maintenance level; never abruptly discontinue drug; maintenance dose may be given daily or every other day	Euphoria, insomnia, edema, hypokalemia, GI upset (peptic ulcer), rounded (moon) face, delayed wound healing, weight gain, muscle weakness
dexamethasone Oral, IV, IM	Hormone replacement, inflammatory diseases (e.g., arthritis, dermatitis), lymphatic cancer, allergies, ulcerative colitis, kidney disease, cerebral edema	Suppresses inflammation and immune response; stimulates bone marrow; influences protein, fat, and carbohydrate metabolism	0.25–4 mg PO 2, 3, or 4 times a day depending on specific disease; never abruptly discontinue	Euphoria, insomnia, edema, hypokalemia, GI upset (peptic ulcer), rounded (moon) face, delayed wound healing, weight gain, muscle weakness
Oral Hypoglycemics				
metformin (*Glucophage*) Oral	Type 2 diabetes mellitus (NIDDM)	Stimulates release of insulin from beta cells in islets of Langerhans in pancreas	500 mg bid (one with the morning and one with the evening meal) or 850 mg q.d. with the morning meal; 500–1000 mg XR daily with the evening meal	Diarrhea, nausea, vomiting, abdominal bloating, lightheadedness, headache, asthenia, rash
glyburide (*DiaBeta, Trulicity*) Oral	Type 2 diabetes mellitus (NIDDM)	Stimulates release of insulin from beta cells in islets of Langerhans in pancreas	2.5–5 mg PO daily with breakfast	Nausea, vomiting, abdominal discomfort, flatulence, anorexia, diarrhea or constipation

Representative Hormones and Hormonelike Drugs[a] (continued)

Category, Name,[b] and Route	Uses and Diseases	Actions	Usual Dose[c] and Special Instructions	Side Effects and Adverse Reactions
Oral Hypoglycemics (continued)				
dulaglutide (*Trulicity*) Subcutaneous, IM	Type 2 diabetes, glucagon-like peptide-1 receptor antagonist	Stimulating the body's natural production of insulin Lowers blood glucose and weight loss	1.5 mg and 7.5 mg, administered subcut, only once a week in the abdomen, thigh, or upper arm Prescribed when diet and exercise have failed to lower the blood glucose May be used instead of metformin	Stomach pain, indigestion, loss of appetite, and diarrhea. Pancreatitis may occur. Serious side effects are swelling in neck, which indicates kidney problems, and includes painful urination and swelling of feet and ankles, but these are rare.

Note: Bolded trade names are among the 50 most commonly prescribed drugs.

[a]See also the hormones listed in Table 15.1.

[b]*Trade names given in parentheses are examples only. Check current drug references for a complete listing of available products.*

[c]*Average adult doses are given. However, dosages are determined by a provider and vary with the purpose of the therapy and the particular patient. The doses presented in this text are for general information only.*

Practice Procedure 15.1 (LO 15-9)

MIXING REGULAR- AND INTERMEDIATE–ACTING INSULIN IN ONE SYRINGE

Demonstrate how to mix regular- and intermediate-acting insulin in one syringe.

Equipment

Medication order (e.g., *Humulin N* 42 units and *Humulin R* 10 units subcutaneously qid)

Medication administration record

U-100 syringe

Vial of *Humulin N* insulin and vial of *Humulin R* insulin

Antiseptic wipe

Procedure

1. Read the medication order and assemble the equipment. Check for the "seven rights." Read the vials of *Humulin N* and *Humulin R* insulin by comparing them to the medication administration record or provider's order.

2. Wash your hands.

3. Select a U-100 syringe.

4. Check both vial labels against the appropriate record for the second time.

5. Remove the metal or plastic caps from the vials of insulin. If the vials have been previously opened, clean the rubber stopper by applying an antiseptic wipe in a circular motion.

6. Remove the needle cover to the U-100 syringe of *Humulin N* insulin by pulling it straight off.

7. Hold the U-100 syringe pointed upward at eye level. Pull back the plunger to take in a quantity of air equal to the ordered 42 units of *Humulin N* insulin.

   - Place the vial of *Humulin N* insulin on a flat surface. Take care not to touch the rubber stopper.
   - Insert the needle through the center of the rubber stopper of the *Humulin N* insulin vial. Inject 42 units of air into the vial's airspace by pushing in the plunger.
   - Without withdrawing any *Humulin N,* withdraw the needle from the *Humulin N* vial and replace the needle cover.

8. Hold the U-100 syringe pointed upward at eye level. Pull back the plunger to take in a quantity of air equal to the ordered 10 units of *Humulin R* insulin.

   - Place the vial of *Humulin R* insulin on a flat surface. Take care not to touch the rubber stopper.
   - Insert the needle through the center of the rubber stopper of the *Humulin R* insulin vial. Inject 10 units of air into the vial's airspace by pushing in the plunger.
   - Without withdrawing the needle from the stopper, invert the vial and draw up 10 units of *Humulin R* insulin. Be careful to withdraw only the ordered dose. Keep the tip of the needle below the surface of the insulin to prevent air from entering the syringe.
   - Check the syringe for bubbles. Remove them by tapping on the syringe.
   - Remove the needle from the *Humulin R* vial and replace the needle cover.
   - Check the vial label and the syringe of *Humulin R* against the medication administration record.

9. With the vial of *Humulin N* insulin on a flat surface, insert the needle. Be careful not to inject air into the vial. Invert the vial and withdraw the ordered 42 units of *Humulin N* insulin to achieve the combined 52-unit ordered dose. Withdraw the needle and replace the needle cover (**Figure 15.7**).

10. Check that the syringe with 10 units of *Humulin R* insulin and 42 units of *Humulin N* insulin equals the total dose of 52 units. The dose is now ready for administration.

11. Return the insulin vials back to the appropriate location.

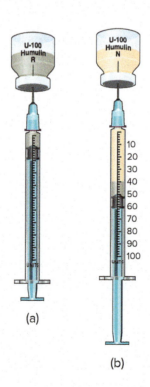

Figure 15.7

Mixing insulins. (a) Draw up the rapid-acting (clear) insulin first; (b) be careful when drawing up the second type of insulin to avoid pushing *Humulin N* into the syringe containing the regular insulin.

(a)

(b)

Summary

Learning Outcome	Summary Points
15-1 List the hormones produced by the seven major glands.	<ul><li>*Somatotropin,* secreted by the pituitary gland.</li><li>*Thyroxine (T₄)* and *triiodothyronine (T₃)*, secreted by the thyroid gland.</li><li>*Parathyroid hormone,* secreted by the parathyroid glands.</li><li>*Corticosteroids,* secreted by the adrenal glands.</li><li>*Insulin* and *glucagon,* secreted by the pancreas.</li><li>*Estrogen* and *progesterone,* secreted by the ovaries, and *testosterone,* secreted by the testes.</li></ul>
15-2 Describe the major disorders of the endocrine system, the symptoms, and the drugs used for treatment.	<ul><li>*Somatotropin* regulates growth.</li><li>*Thyroxine* regulates metabolism.</li><li>*Parathyroid hormone* regulates the blood calcium level.</li><li>*Corticosteroids* comprise two major groups: glucocorticoids (cortisone, hydrocortisone, and cortisol) and mineralocorticoids (aldosterone and desoxycorticosterone).<ul><li>*Glucocorticoids* stimulate the breakdown of protein molecules into carbohydrates.</li><li>*Mineralocorticoids* regulate the body's salt–water balance.</li></ul></li><li>*Epinephrine* is used to treat bronchial asthma.</li><li>*Norepinephrine* is used in the emergency treatment of shock.</li><li>*Insulin* controls the cells' use of sugar.</li><li>*Adrenocorticotropic hormone (ACTH)* stimulates the adrenal cortex to produce corticosteroids.</li><li>*Antidiuretic hormone (ADH)* regulates reabsorption of water in the kidney tubules.</li></ul>
15-3 Identify which hormones are lacking in the conditions of diabetes mellitus, diabetes insipidus, Addison's disease, and hypothyroidism.	<ul><li>*Diabetes mellitus:* Not enough insulin is produced, so insulin is used as a replacement therapy.</li><li>*Diabetes insipidus:* The kidneys are not able to conserve water. Characterized by intense thirst and excretion of large amounts of urine.</li><li>*Addison's disease:* Insufficient production of corticosteroids is common. A combination of a mineralocorticosteroid (fludrocortisone) and a glucocorticoid (prednisone) is used in the treatment.</li><li>*Hypothyroidism:* Disease or destruction of the thyroid gland causes an insufficient amount of thyroid hormones.</li><li>Natural thyroid preparations such as *Thyroid* or synthetic thyroid preparations such as levothyroxine (*Synthroid*), liothyronine (*Cytomel*), and liotrix (*Thyrolar*) are used in the treatment.</li></ul>
15-4 Define the parts of the endocrine system and symptoms of hormone imbalances.	<ul><li>The main parts of the endocrine system are the pituitary, thyroid, parathyroid, and adrenal glands and the pancreas, ovaries, and testes.</li><li>Symptoms of endocrine diseases such as diabetes mellitus include polyphagia, polydipsia, and polyuria.</li></ul>
15-5 List the types of insulin available for treatment of diabetes mellitus.	<ul><li>*Rapid-acting insulin: Apidra, Humalog,* and *NovoLog.*</li><li>*Short-acting insulin: Humulin* or *Novolin* and regular insulin.</li><li>*Intermediate-acting insulin: NPH* and *Lente.*</li><li>*Long-acting insulin: Lantus.*</li><li>A patient's need for insulin varies according to diet, amount of exercise, and emotions.</li></ul>

Learning Outcome	Summary Points

15-6 Identify the signs and symptoms of hyperglycemia and hypoglycemia.	• *Hyperglycemia:* The three cardinal symptoms are polyphagia, polydipsia, and polyuria. It is treated with oral hypoglycemics or insulin.
	• *Hypoglycemia:* The symptoms include increased appetite, nervousness, heart palpitations, cold sweating, shakiness, difficulty concentrating, and blurred vision. Treatment involves giving sugar in an easily digestible form.
	• The three classifications of oral hypoglycemics are first-generation and second-generation sulfonylureas and miscellaneous oral hypoglycemics.
	  • *First-generation sulfonylureas* include tolazamide and chlorpropamide.
	  • *Second-generation sulfonylureas* include *Glucotrol* and *DiaBeta.*
	  • *Miscellaneous oral hypoglycemics* include *Precose, Prandin,* and *Avandia.*
	• Oral hypoglycemics are used when the beta cells of the islets of Langerhans continue to produce some insulin. They stimulate these cells to secrete insulin in response to rising glucose levels.

15-7 List several uses of corticosteroids.	• Corticosteroids are used for hormone replacement therapy, allergic reactions, and skin inflammations. • They are also used for some cancers, autoimmune reactions, suppression of immunity in organ transplants, and eye and respiratory disorders, as well as to reduce fever, decrease itching, and suppress inflammation.
15-8 Identify five possible side effects of long-term corticosteroid therapy.	• Several side effects of long-term corticosteroid therapy are weight gain, sodium retention, edema, hypertension, and a moon face. • Other side effects include symptoms of diabetes mellitus, easy bruising, thinning of the skin, failure of wounds to heal, psychological changes, ulcers, and osteoporosis.
15-9 Describe the procedure for administering regular- and intermediate-acting insulin in one syringe, and what factors affect the insulin needs of a diabetic patient.	• When mixing regular and intermediate insulin in one syringe, draw up the regular insulin first.

Chapter 15 Review

Define each of the terms listed.

1. (LO 15-1) Tetany _____

2. (LO 15-6) Glycosuria _____

3. (LO 15-6) Hypoglycemia _____

4. (LO 15-1) Insulin _____

5. (LO 15-1) Glucagon _____

6. (LO 15-1) Glycogen _____

Match the functions to the hormones.

_____ 7. (LO 15-1) Somatotropin

_____ 8. (LO 15-1) Parathyroid hormone

_____ 9. (LO 15-1) Corticosteroids

_____ 10. (LO 15-1) Epinephrine and norepinephrine

_____ 11. (LO 15-2) ADH

a. prepare the body to cope with stress

b. regulates the reabsorption of water in the kidney

c. regulates growth

d. suppress inflammation

e. regulates the amount of calcium in the blood

Complete the statements by filling in the blank.

12. (LO 15-1) The gland that traps iodine while producing its hormone is the _____ gland.

13. (LO 15-1) The glands that sit on top of the kidneys are the _____ glands.

14. (LO 15-1) Diabetes mellitus is caused by a lack of the hormone _____.

15. (LO 15-2) Diabetes insipidus is caused by a lack of the _____ hormone.

16. (LO 15-3) Addison's disease is caused by a long-term lack of _____ hormones.

The following drugs are used in the management of diabetes mellitus. Next to each drug, place the letter that tells what drug group it belongs to, as follows:

L = long-acting insulin   R = rapid-acting insulin   S = short-acting insulin

I = intermediate-acting insulin   O = oral hypoglycemic

_____ 17. (LO 15-5) *Humalog*

_____ 18. (LO 15-5) *NPH*

_____ 19. (LO 15-5) *Glucophage*

_____ 20. (LO 15-5) Regular insulin

_____ 21. (LO 15-5) *Humulin N*

_____ 22. (LO 15-6) *Januvia*

_____ 23. (LO 15-6) Glipizide

_____ 24. (LO 15-5) *Novolog*

_____ 25. (LO 15-5) *Lantus*

Answer the questions in the space provided.

26. (LO 15-6) What is the main action of the oral hypoglycemics? _____

_____

_____

27. (LO 15-9) What are three factors that bring about changes in the diabetic patient's need for insulin?

_____

_____

_____

28. (LO 15-1) What is the difference between glucocorticoids and mineralocorticoids? _____

_____

_____

_____

29. (LO 15-7) What are the uses for corticosteroids? _____

_____

_____

_____

30. (LO 15-8) What are the possible side effects of long-term use of corticosteroids? _____

_____

_____

31. (LO 15-9) When combining *Humulin N* insulin and *Humulin R* insulin in the same syringe, which insulin should be drawn up first? _____

_____

_____

Match the drug uses to the drug names.

_____ 32. (LO 15-7) ACTH

_____ 33. (LO 15-7) Vasopressin tannate

_____ 34. (LO 15-7) *Solu-Medrol,* prednisone

_____ 35. (LO 15-6) Rosiglitazone, *Januvia*

a. replacement of pituitary hormone that stimulates production of corticosteroids

b. inflammatory diseases, allergic reaction, replacement of corticosteroids

c. diabetes insipidus

d. diabetes mellitus

Drug Calculations—Fill in the blank with the answer.

36. (LO 15-4) The provider orders *Novolin R Regular* U-100 insulin 8 U with *Novolin N* U-100 insulin 20 U subcutaneously before breakfast. Describe the setup procedure and prepare to administer _____ units to your patient.

37. (LO 15-4) The provider orders metformin (*Glucophage*) 2500 mg orally daily. Available are 1000-mg tablets. You will administer _____ tablets to your patient.

38. (LO 15-3) The provider orders levothyroxine sodium (*Synthroid*) 0.5 mg orally daily. Available are 25-μg tablets. You will give your patient _____ tablets.

39. (LO 15-3) The provider orders prednisone 15 mg orally bid. Available are 10-mg tablets. You will give your patient _____ tablets.

40. (LO 15-4) The provider orders metformin (*Glucophage*) 2 g orally daily. Available are 1000-mg tablets. You will administer _____ tablets to your patient.

41. (LO 15-9) When a patient is taking levothyroxine sodium (*Synthroid*), which of the following side effects should you monitor for?
   a. Weight gain, moon face, muscle weakness
   b. Nausea, vomiting, dizziness
   c. Palpitations, weight loss, tachycardia
   d. Tremor, abdominal cramps, drowsiness

42. (LO 15-9) Which of the following directions should you follow when administering insulin?
   a. Use an insulin syringe to draw up the insulin.
   b. Keep the insulin in the refrigerator.
   c. Shake the vial of insulin to make sure it is mixed.
   d. Massage the site after the insulin is administered.

43. (LO 15-9) A patient asks you why prednisone has been prescribed. What is the most appropriate answer to give the patient?
   a. Regulate growth
   b. Regulate the blood sugar
   c. Replace the deficient hormone
   d. Suppress inflammation

44. (LO 15-5) How long does it take for *Humalog* insulin to start working in the body?
   a. 15 minutes
   b. 30 minutes
   c. 1 hour
   d. 4 hours

45. (LO 15-9) Which of the following are side effects of glyburide (*DiaBeta*)?
   a. Euphoria, insomnia
   b. Delayed wound healing, muscle weakness
   c. GI upset, diarrhea or constipation
   d. Headache, palpitations

Chapter 15 Case Studies

46. (LO 15-6) A patient with diabetes mellitus received *Novolin R Regular* U-100 6 U subcutaneously at 0700. At 0900, he begins to experience shakiness, nervousness, heart palpitations, and blurred vision. What should you do? What is the usual treatment?

_____

_____

_____

47. (LO 15-8) Corticosteroids have been prescribed for a patient as a hormone replacement. The patient's adrenal cortex does not function properly. What condition do you suspect the patient may have? What are other conditions that may require corticosteroids? What are the side effects you should watch the patient for?

_____

_____

_____

Critical Thinking

Patients with diabetes who are on insulin must live with the risk of insulin overdose or underdose. Decide which of these two problems is signaled by each set of symptoms. Give the usual treatment for each.

Symptoms	Problem	Treatment
48. (LO 15-6) Polydipsia, polyuria, polyphagia, fruity breath, confusion	_____	_____

Symptoms	Problem	Treatment
49. (LO 15-6) Nervousness, shakiness, blurred vision, cold sweating, palpitations, increased appetite, difficulty concentrating	_____	_____

Applications

Obtain an electronic drug guide or a current copy of the *PDR*® from your school, health facility, or clinic. Use it to answer the following questions in a notebook or on file cards.

50. Use the electronic drug guide or *PDR*® to find another product name for each drug in the Representative Hormones and Hormonelike Drugs table in this chapter.

51. In Section 3 of the *PDR*®, Product Category Index, find Hypoglycemic Agents/Diabetes Agents. Make a list of all the oral hypoglycemic agents you see listed there.

DRUGS FOR THE MUSCULOSKELETAL SYSTEM

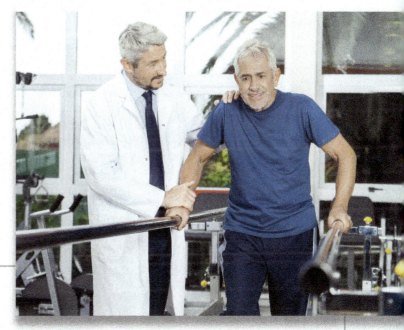

©Shutterstock/Tyler Olson

In this chapter you will review the various parts of the musculoskeletal system and the correct terms used to describe them. You will learn what disorders affect this system and what drugs are used to control them.

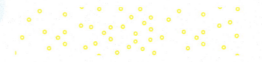

MUSCULOSKELETAL SYSTEM [LO 16-1]

The bones, muscles, joints, cartilage, ligaments, tendons, fascia, and bursae make up the musculoskeletal system. Like all body structures, the muscular and skeletal systems play a part in the body's achievement of its overall goal of survival. Its main functions are support, protection of vital organs, movement, blood cell production, and storage of minerals.

Bones form the body's supporting framework. Without this support, the body would be unable to move and would collapse. The bones and their connecting joints act like a series of levers. The muscles exert force on these levers, and the result is movement. The major bones are shown in Figure 16.1. The major muscles are shown in Figure 16.2.

Bones

Bones are made up of both organic (collagen) and inorganic (calcium, phosphate) material. Even though they appear lifeless, bones are living tissue. The reason for their hardness is that the spaces between bone cells are filled with calcium. Bones start out relatively soft and pliable in babies. During childhood, calcium is deposited in the spaces between bone cells, so the bones gradually harden. Because of their softness, young bones heal more easily than older ones. Throughout life there is constant replacement of older bone elements. This occurs because of the eating away (reabsorption) of bone in some areas along with the formation of new bone in other areas.

We think of bones mainly as a framework for the muscles, but they perform other important functions as well: They produce blood cells, act as a storage area for calcium, and protect delicate organs of the body. The skeleton is made up of 206 bones. They are classified by shape. The four classifications of bone are long, short, flat, and irregular. The femur, radius, and humerus are long bones. The carpals and tarsals are short bones. The ribs, scapula, skull, and sternum are classified as flat bones. Irregular bones include the vertebrae, sacrum, and mandible.

Inside most bones is a spongy type of tissue called bone marrow. Red bone marrow manufactures the three formed elements of the blood: all the red blood cells, certain white blood cells, and all the platelets. Yellow bone marrow, found only in the hollow parts of the long bones of the arms and legs, is a storage area for fat.

Cartilage is a rigid connective tissue that both provides support and allows joint movement. Unlike bone that has a rich blood supply, cartilage has no blood supply. Cartilage lines every joint and gives shape to the ears and nose.

Joints

A joint is the place where two or more bones come together (Figure 16.3). The primary function of a joint is to allow movement and flexibility in the body. The three types of joints are the diarthrodial, amphiarthrodial, and synarthrodial.

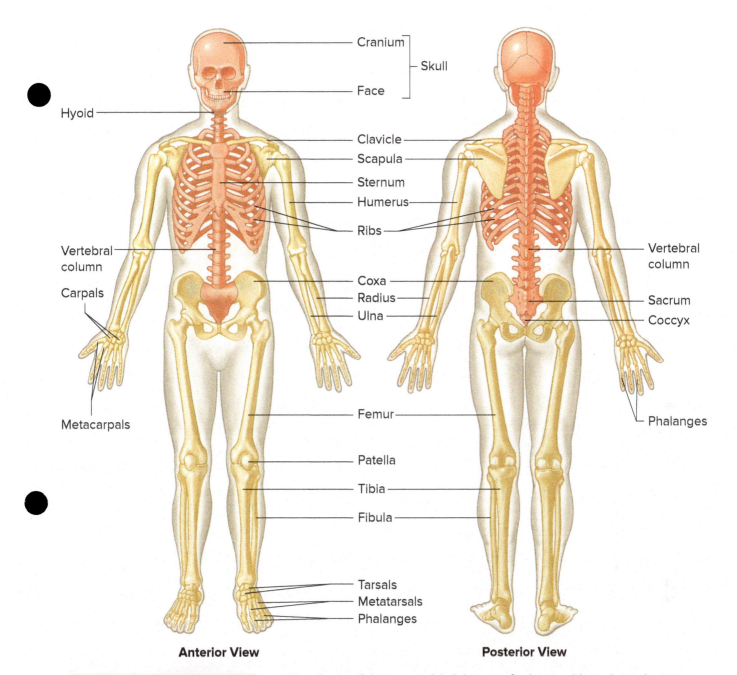

Anterior View

Cranium
Skull
Face

Hyoid

Clavicle
Scapula
Sternum
Humerus
Ribs

Vertebral
column

Carpals

Coxa
Radius
Ulna

Metacarpals

Femur

Patella

Tibia

Fibula

Tarsals
Metatarsals
Phalanges

Posterior View

Vertebral
column

Sacrum
Coccyx

Phalanges

Figure 16.1

The complete skeleton.

The diarthrodial, or synovial, joints are freely movable and are the most common joints in the body. Diarthrodial joints have a small space, the joint cavity, that lies between the articulating surfaces of the two bones that form the joint. Types of diarthrotic joints include saddle, hinge, pivot, ellipsoidal, ball and socket, and sliding joints. The shoulder, wrist, thumb, hip, knee, ankle, and proximal cervical vertebrae are all examples of diarthrodial (freely movable) joints.

The amphiarthrodial joints are only slightly movable and are found in the pelvis. Synarthrodial joints do not have a joint cavity but instead have tissue (fibrous, cartilage, or bone) growing between their articulating surfaces, preventing them from being able to move freely. Examples of synarthrotic (completely immovable) joints include those in the skull.

The ends of bones are covered with cartilage. A capsule of connective tissue joins two bones to form a cavity lined with a synovial membrane. The membrane secretes synovial fluid, which functions as a lubricant and decreases friction in the joint. **Ligaments** are dense bands of connective tissues that connect bones to bones at joints such as the elbow joint. Ligaments provide movement while maintaining stability.

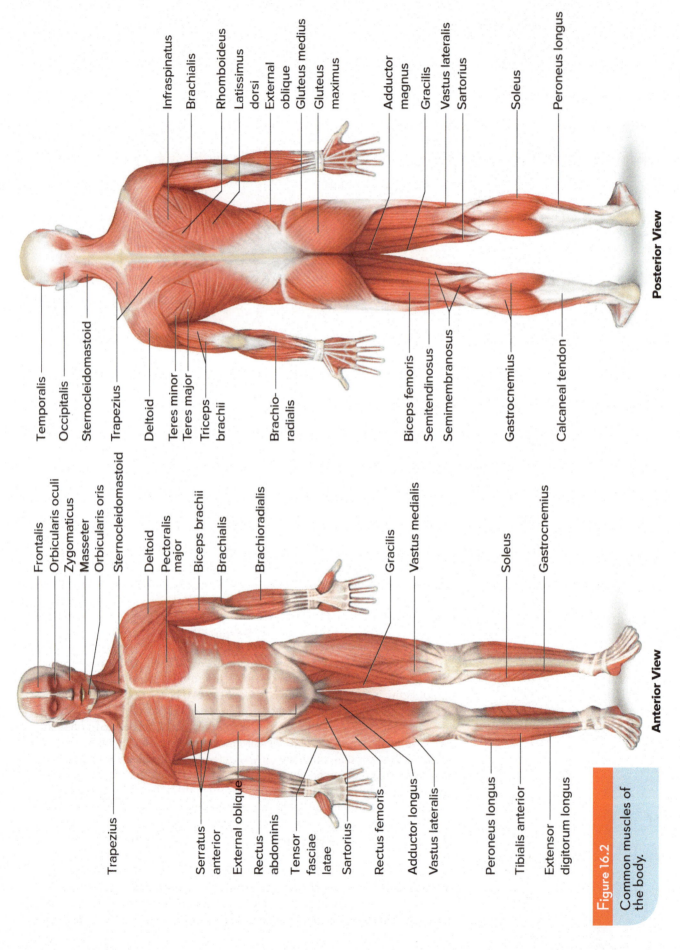

Posterior View

Infraspinatus
Brachialis
Rhomboideus
Latissimus dorsi
External oblique
Gluteus medius
Gluteus maximus
Adductor magnus
Gracilis
Vastus lateralis
Sartorius
Soleus
Peroneus longus

Temporalis
Occipitalis
Sternocleidomastoid
Trapezius
Deltoid
Teres minor
Teres major
Triceps brachii
Brachio-radialis
Biceps femoris
Semitendinosus
Semimembranosus
Gastrocnemius
Calcaneal tendon

Anterior View

Frontalis
Orbicularis oculi
Zygomaticus
Masseter
Orbicularis oris
Sternocleidomastoid
Deltoid
Pectoralis major
Biceps brachii
Brachialis
Brachioradialis
Gracilis
Vastus medialis
Soleus
Gastrocnemius

Trapezius
Serratus anterior
External oblique
Rectus abdominis
Tensor fasciae latae
Sartorius
Rectus femoris
Adductor longus
Vastus lateralis
Peroneus longus
Tibialis anterior
Extensor digitorum longus

Figure 16.2
Common muscles of the body.

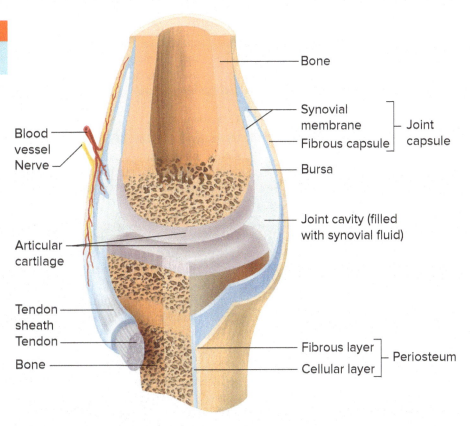

Figure 16.3

Structure of a synovial joint.

Bone

Synovial
membrane
Fibrous capsule ⎤ Joint
⎦ capsule

Bursa

Joint cavity (filled
with synovial fluid)

Blood
vessel
Nerve

Articular
cartilage

Tendon
sheath
Tendon
Bone

Fibrous layer ⎤
⎦ Periosteum
Cellular layer ⎦

Muscles

The muscles that work together with bones to allow movement are called **skeletal muscles**. There are two other types of muscle tissue: smooth and cardiac. Smooth muscle tissue lines the gastrointestinal tract, urinary tract, blood vessels, airways, and uterus. Cardiac muscle tissue is found in the heart.

Skeletal muscles are made up of long, thin muscle fibers bundled together with sheets of connective tissue called **fascia**. The muscles are richly supplied with blood, because they need great quantities of oxygen to generate the energy needed for their heavy work. The more exercise these muscles get, the more blood vessels grow into them to supply the needed nutrients and carry away wastes.

Skeletal muscles are attached to the bones by cords of connective tissue called **tendons**. The muscles exert a force on the bones by contracting, which means that the muscles become shorter and thicker. When this effort is no longer needed, the muscles relax and assume their normal size.

Muscles that are well exercised are always slightly contracted so that they will be ready for action as needed. This is referred to as **muscle tone**. Poor muscle tone is considered a sign of lack of use. If muscles are not used for a prolonged period, as in the case of bed rest, they become wasted and decrease in size **(atrophy).** Muscle atrophy is measurable within three days of disuse and contractures may develop within four to seven days of disuse. Without physical therapy, **contractures**, or a shortening of the muscle or ligament, may result and become permanent.

DISORDERS AND DRUG TREATMENT OF THE MUSCULOSKELETAL SYSTEM [LO 16-2, LO 16-3]

Physical Injuries

Muscles and bones and their accessory parts are subject to various injuries. Strains occur when a muscle is stretched. Sprains result from tearing of a ligament. The symptoms of sprains and strains are similar and generally include pain, edema, decrease in function, and bruising. Pain is worse with movement and use. A fracture is a break in the continuity of the structure of a bone. There are many different types of fractures. The type of fracture dictates the treatment. Fractures are usually accompanied by pain, decreased function, and inability to use.

Osteomyelitis

Osteomyelitis is an infection inside a bone, with symptoms usually appearing near a joint. There is pain and tenderness, and fever is present. The infection destroys bone tissue, and pus may drain through the skin. Osteomyelitis is treated with antibiotics. Surgery may be necessary to drain abscesses inside the bone.

Osteoporosis

Osteoporosis is a decrease in total bone mass. It is a major cause of fractures in women past menopause. Osteoporosis is eight times more common in women, since women have less bone mass than men because of their smaller size. Women also tend to have lower calcium intake throughout their lives. Pregnancy and breastfeeding also deplete a woman's skeletal reserve. Women, too, live longer than men, which increases the likelihood of osteoporosis.

Osteoporosis is a condition in which the bones thin out, become abnormally porous, and are easily broken or fracture spontaneously. Osteoporosis most commonly occurs in the wrists, hips, and spine. Wedging and fractures of the vertebrae cause a gradual loss of height and a humped back and are often the cause of the stooped appearance of an older adult. Osteoporosis can also result from an inadequate calcium intake (such as failure to eat calcium-rich foods or to drink milk), inactivity (as in bedridden patients), and diseases such as rheumatoid arthritis. Treatment consists of estrogen, calcium supplements, and a diet rich in calcium. Vitamin D is important to bone and calcium metabolism.

Bisphosphonates such as alendronate (*Fosamax*) and risedronate (*Actonel*) are used to prevent osteoporosis in postmenopausal women. They are nonestrogen, nonhormonal options for preventing bone loss in the early postmenopausal period. The drugs can cause hypocalcemia and significant gastrointestinal upset. *Fosamax* and *Actonel* may be taken orally. Calcitonin is also used to prevent osteoporosis in postmenopausal women. It is given by injection and also causes gastrointestinal upset. A nasal preparation of calcitonin is available and causes less GI side distress but most common side effects are runny nose, nasal sores, and headache. Raloxifene (*Evista*) is an estrogen receptor modulator designed to prevent osteoporosis and also has properties that prevent cardiovascular disease and reduce the risk of invasive breast cancer in postmenopausal women with osteoarthritis.

 Patient Education Osteoporosis

- Premenopausal women should take 1000 mg of calcium per day.
- Postmenopausal women should take 1500 mg of calcium and 5000 IU of vitamin D per day.
- Regular exercise is important to keep bones strong.

- Foods that are high in calcium include milk, yogurt, cottage cheese, ice cream, sardines, spinach, and turnip greens (**Figure 16.4**).
- Women whose diets are low in calcium should consult their provider about possible estrogen replacement therapy or calcium supplementation.

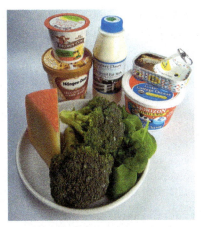

©McGraw-Hill Education/Jill Braaten, photographer

Ibandronate (*Boniva*) is the first bisphosphonate bone growth regulator for postmenopausal osteoporosis that is taken only once a month. Like *Fosamax*, it inhibits osteoblast activity, thus preventing bone resorption. Taking a pill once a month eliminates any interruptions to the patient's morning routine and the need to remember to take a pill daily. Instruct the patient to select an easy-to-remember day such as the beginning or end of the month to take the pill. It should be taken with a large glass of water 1 hour before eating or drinking anything, except plain water, and before any other drugs. Lying down should be avoided for 60 minutes after taking *Boniva*. The major adverse reactions are dyspepsia, abdominal pain, diarrhea, and pain in the extremities. The monthly dose of *Boniva* is 150 mg. Although less common, *Boniva* may also be prescribed as a daily 2.5-mg dose.

Zoledronic acid (*Zometa*, also known as *Reclast*) is a bone growth regulator and also a bisphosphonate. It is primarily used for hypercalcemia from malignancy, but it also may be used for postmenopausal osteoporosis. It is given only intravenously, generally once a year.

Teriparatide (*Forteo*) is approved for use in both men and postmenopausal women with osteoporosis who are at high risk for fractures. Unlike bisphosphonates that slow or stop bone loss, *Forteo* is the only drug that rebuilds bone. It is a unique therapy that is given subcutaneously daily for 2 years. Research has shown that *Forteo* may begin to increase bone mineral density in as little as three months. Denosumab *(Prolia)* is a human monoclonal antibody that binds to a protein that is essential for the formation, function, and osteoclasts. By doing this, bone resorption is decreased and bone mass and strength are increased. It is administered subcutaneously, once every 6 months, only for postmenopausal women with osteoporosis who are at risk for fractures or have failed on other treatments; decreases spinal fractures by 68%. Abaloparatide (*Tymlos*) is also used in the treatment of postmenopausal women with osteoporosis at risk for fracture or who have failed with other therapies.

Osteoporosis is a preventable disease; therefore, educating patients about it is essential. It often begins in a person's early 40s (postmenopause) but the obvious measurable loss of bone calcium density may not be noted for 20 to 30 years later.

Bursitis, Myositis, and Synovitis

Various inflammations arise because of repeated physical stress on joints or muscles. Bursitis involves the **bursae**, which are small, fluid-filled pouches located between bones and ligaments and between bones and muscles. The bursae are designed to keep these parts from rubbing against each other when they move. Myositis is an inflammation of the muscles. Synovitis is an inflammation of the cavity surrounding a joint (the **synovial capsule**). All these inflammations produce symptoms of pain, stiffness, redness, and swelling. Often the only needed treatment is rest. Other treatment is with oral anti-inflammatory agents, such as indomethacin (*Indocin*) and naproxen (*Naprosyn*). Sometimes hydrocortisone (a corticosteroid) is injected directly into the inflamed area. The injection reduces inflammation in the local area while avoiding the systemic effects of an oral corticosteroid.

Gouty Arthritis

Arthritis is the name for several disorders of the joints, each having different causes and treatments—gouty arthritis, osteoarthritis, and rheumatoid arthritis. Gout, or gouty arthritis, is an inflammation of the joints that starts when there is an excess of uric acid in the bloodstream. Uric acid is a normal waste product of cell metabolism. In gout, either the kidneys do not excrete uric acid efficiently or there is some reason (genetic, chemotherapy, etc.) that makes the body produce larger than normal amounts of uric acid. Because the uric acid is not completely excreted, crystals of the acid are deposited in the cartilage around the joints such as those of the big toe, ankle, knee, and elbow. The deposits cause the joints to become red, hot, swollen, and painful. The condition can flare up or become worse with heavy alcohol drinking, prolonged fasting, trauma, surgery, or infection. Uric acid crystals can also form in the urine, causing "gravel" or urate stones in the bladder and kidneys.

Chronic gout may be treated with **uricosuric** drugs. These are drugs that promote excretion of uric acid, such as probenecid. Alternately, chronic gout may be treated with **antihyperuricemic** drugs, such as allopurinol (*Zyloprim*), which decrease the amount of uric acid the body produces. These drugs are particularly beneficial for patients with uric acid stones or renal impairment.

The most common drugs for acute attacks of gout are colchicine, anti-inflammatory drugs, and corticosteroids. Colchicine produces dramatic relief of pain within 24 to 48 hours. Its exact mechanism of action is unknown. It may also reduce the frequency of gouty attacks. Caution should be used when administering colchicine to older adults because they are more likely to have cumulative toxic effects of the cardiac, renal, or gastrointestinal systems.

Patients being treated for gout must drink large amounts of fluids to help wash away the uric acid crystals. Eight glasses of water a day are recommended. Future attacks of gout are prevented by a maintenance dose of colchicine, weight reduction if necessary, avoidance of alcohol, drugs to reduce the serum uric acid, and a low-purine diet. Uric acid is the major end product of the catabolism of purines. High-purine foods include sardines, meat soups, chicken, salmon, crab, veal, bacon, pork, beef, and ham. Some vegetables that contain moderate amounts of purine include asparagus, shell beans, lentils, mushrooms, peas, and spinach.

Osteoarthritis

Osteoarthritis is also called degenerative joint disease. It is a progressive disorder that slowly destroys the mobile joints. It affects mainly the weight-bearing joints—the spine, hip, and knee. Most people over the age of 50 have some form of it, but not all show symptoms. As people grow older, the cartilage that cushions joints begins to thin out and wear away. As a result, bones rub against each other when the joints are moved. With continual rubbing and scraping, these bones thicken and become knobby or lumpy. Movement becomes painful, stiff, and limited. Symptoms are especially noticed toward evening, after a full day's wear and tear on the joints. There is pain and stiffness, but usually no inflammation. Treatment consists of relieving the pain, protecting the joints from additional injury, and restoring joint function. **Antiarthritic** drugs, which suppress inflammation in the joints, are commonly used in the treatment of arthritis. Aspirin is the drug of choice and is used for pain control and inflammation, if present. Nonsteroidal anti-inflammatory drugs are used for patients who cannot tolerate aspirin. Corticosteroids may be injected into the joint during an acute flare-up. Nonpharmacological treatment consists of application of heat or cold and range-of-motion exercises.

Rheumatoid Arthritis

Rheumatoid arthritis is a chronic inflammatory disease that affects the mobile joints. Unlike osteoarthritis, rheumatoid arthritis is systemic, involving other organs. It is characterized by periods of remissions and exacerbations. It also is a significant national health problem, particularly in women. The symptoms are pain in the joints (especially of the wrists, fingers, ankles, and other peripheral joints, such as the elbows, shoulders, knees, and hips) and stiffness. The stiffness occurs mainly in the morning and tends to improve throughout the day. There may also be fever, anorexia, weight loss, weakness, easy tiring, and aching muscles. The inflamed joints may feel warm to the touch. As the disease progresses, cartilage is slowly destroyed and the bones may even fuse together, causing loss of movement and sometimes deformity.

The cause of rheumatoid arthritis is unknown, and there is no specific cure. Some researchers think the cause may be genetic, perhaps from an infection, or a form of autoimmune response in which the body reacts to its own tissues as if they were foreign invaders like allergens and microorganisms. Treatment for rheumatoid arthritis consists of making patients as comfortable as possible, using drugs and a variety of physical measures. Nonpharmacological treatment measures include the application of ice during an acute flare-up and the application of heat for daily chronic stiffness. Alternating periods of rest and activity are scheduled both to protect the joints and to prevent further joint immobility. A procedure called arthroplasty may be a last resort. It is a surgical procedure involving reconstruction or replacement of a joint.

The drugs used to treat mild rheumatoid arthritis have changed significantly in recent years. Whereas in the past high doses of aspirin and nonsteroidal anti-inflammatory drugs were used, now drugs called disease-modifying agents are used because they decrease the permanent effects of the disease, specifically joint immobility. The most common disease-modifying drug is hydroxychloroquine (*Plaquenil*). The most common side effects are nausea, abdominal discomfort, and rash.

Corticosteroids may be given either alone or in combination with *Plaquenil*. Corticosteroids have a wide range of side effects, such as euphoria, insomnia, GI upset, muscle weakness, delayed wound healing, weakening of the bone, and hypertension, so the smallest possible dose is administered for the shortest possible time.

The drug of choice for moderate to severe rheumatoid arthritis is methotrexate (*Trexall*). It is used for its rapid anti-inflammatory action. It reduces the symptoms of rheumatoid arthritis in days. Azathioprine (*Imuran*) and penicillamine (*Cuprimine*) may be used if methotrexate fails to relieve the patient's symptoms. Both carry a high incidence of serious side effects, such as disorders of the blood. Along with these new drug regimens, aspirin and nonsteroidal anti-inflammatory drugs are still used. The nonsteroidal anti-inflammatory drugs may be used for patients who have an intolerance to aspirin.

COX-2 inhibitors are a newer class of nonsteroidal anti-inflammatory drugs that inhibit prostaglandin synthesis by decreasing the enzyme needed for biosynthesis. Celecoxib (*Celebrex*) is an example of a COX-2 inhibitor and has anti-inflammatory, analgesic, and antipyretic properties. COX-2 inhibitors should be used with extreme caution in patients with a past history of peptic ulcer disease or gastrointestinal bleeding because GI bleeding, ulceration, or GI hemorrhage may be adverse reactions. Caution should also be used in patients with a history of cardiovascular problems because COX-2 inhibitors may cause serious cardiovascular problems such as aggravation of hypertension, chest pain, coronary artery disease, palpitations, tachycardia, and possibly myocardial infarction.

Tumor necrosis factor-alpha (TNF-alpha) inhibitors or immunomodulators such as adalimumab (*Humira*), etanercept (*Enbrel*), and infliximab (*Remicade*) are given to patients with moderate to severe rheumatoid arthritis to reduce its signs and symptoms and improve physical function. They are generally given to patients who haven't adequately responded to other antirheumatoid drugs. *Enbrel* and *Humira* are administered subcutaneously. *Remicade* is administered intravenously.

 Older Adult Considerations   COX-2 Inhibitors

- Although aspirin and NSAIDs are used in the treatment of musculoskeletal disorders, a COX-2 inhibitor may be used for some people, especially those prone to bleeding, since the incidence is lower.

- Monitor the patient carefully for cardiovascular effects.

The cancer drug rituximab (*Rituxan*) is a monoclonal antibody that has been FDA-approved to treat rheumatoid arthritis. It specifically binds to CD20 antigen, which is found in both normal and malignant B lymphocytes, causing cell lysis. It is administered by IV infusion. Immune cells grow out of control in cancer patients. In rheumatoid arthritis patients, the immune cells are also overactive, and *Rituxan* has resulted in some improvement.

Another drug administered intravenously to patients with moderate to severe rheumatoid arthritis who haven't benefited from methotrexate or TNF-alpha inhibitors is abatacept (*Orencia*). *Orencia* has been proven to decrease the signs and symptoms of rheumatoid arthritis, but it can also reverse joint damage.

A new drug is tocilizumab (*Actemra*), a biological agent or interleukin-6 receptor inhibitor that is administered IV in combination with disease-modifying antirheumatic drugs such as methotrexate.

Fibromyalgia

Fibromyalgia is a musculoskeletal disorder that amplifies how the brain processes pain and sensory messages such as touch and smell. It causes widespread generalized pain in the muscles and other tissues, affecting an estimated 5.8 million people in the United States. Fibromyalgia is a specific kind of pain that's chronic, widespread, and often accompanied by tenderness. It is generally felt all over the body but there may be specific areas such as the shoulders or neck, and various pressure points, where a small amount of pressure can result in severe pain. There are no apparent causes for the pain such as trauma, injury, accident, surgery, or excessive stress, although changing weather conditions and professional or emotional stress may intensify the pain. The common symptoms are pain, sensitivity to touch, environmental sensitivity, muscle and joint stiffness that is worse in the morning, muscle spasms, exhaustion without physical or mental overexertion, trouble concentrating, chronic headaches, bowel disturbances known as irritable bowel syndrome (IBS), and depression. In general, treatments for fibromyalgia include both medications and self-care. Medications may reduce pain and promote sleep and may include pain relievers, ibuprofen, naproxen, and tramadol. Narcotics are not recommended because they can lead to dependence and may even worsen the pain over time. Antidepressants and/or muscle relaxants such as duloxetine (*Cymbalta*) or cyclobenzaprine may be used to lessen the pain and fatigue associated with fibromyalgia. Certain types of pain may be lessened by the use of antiseizure medications such as gabapentin (*Neurontin*) or pregabalin (*Lyrica*). *Lyrica* was the first drug approved by the federal Food and Drug Administration for the treatment of fibromyalgia.

Muscle Pain

There are many reasons for pain in the skeletal muscles (**myalgia**): overexercise, inflammation, sprains, degenerative osteoarthritis, multiple sclerosis, herniated vertebral disc, or other conditions causing spasms. Skeletal muscle relaxants may be prescribed for patients with these conditions. The exact action of skeletal muscle relaxants is unknown, but they do depress the central nervous system, which results in relaxation of the muscle spasm. The most common muscle relaxants used for spasticity (**antispasmodics**) are baclofen, diazepam (*Valium*), and dantrolene (*Dantrium*). Other skeletal muscle relaxants used are methocarbamol (*Robaxin*), carisoprodol (*Soma*), chlorzoxazone, and cyclobenzaprine hydrochloride. Side effects are primarily fatigue, lethargy, and sedation.

BONE MARROW DISORDERS [LO 16-4]

Because red bone marrow produces most of the important components of the blood, any disorder that affects the bone marrow can create serious problems. Failure of the bone marrow to produce enough of all three components of the blood is called aplastic anemia. Overproduction of white blood cells is called leukemia.

Bone marrow depression is a serious adverse reaction linked to many drugs, especially certain antihistamines, tranquilizers, chloramphenicol, sulfonamides, antineoplastics, thyroid medications, antidepressants, and diuretics. For this reason, you should be aware of symptoms that indicate that a drug may be affecting the bone marrow:

- Lack of red blood cells—weakness, pale skin (pallor), dyspnea.
- Lack of white blood cells—agranulocytosis, soreness of mucous membranes in the mouth and throat, fever, chills, extreme fatigue, urinary and vaginal infections.
- Lack of platelets—bleeding from the gums, nose, or gastrointestinal tract; signs of hemorrhage under the skin such as purpura, petechiae, and ecchymoses.

Like any unusual symptoms, these should be charted so that the provider can prescribe alternative drugs or treatments. Treatment of bone marrow depression involves:

- Transfusing red blood cells or platelets.
- Discontinuing the offending drug(s).
- Providing antibiotics until the white blood cell count is restored.
- Treating non-drug-induced cases, such as bone marrow infections or cancer.
- Considering erythropoietin to increase the red blood cell count and colony-stimulating factor.

CARE OF PATIENTS WITH MUSCULOSKELETAL DISORDERS [LO 16-5]

Patients with arthritis and other musculoskeletal disorders must live with pain. Sometimes every movement causes discomfort. Analgesics and anti-inflammatory drugs relieve this pain, but not completely. A person who is in pain can easily become impatient with those who are trying to help. Keep this in mind when caring for your patients. They hurt, and they may be angry that they must depend on others for routine care such as dressing and eating. There are several things you can do to make things easier for them:

- Give pain medications on time. This ensures that patients do not have to endure unnecessary pain while waiting for their next dose of medication.
- Handle patients with care. Do not bump against the bed as you prepare to administer medications. If you need to move patients for any reason, do it slowly and support their body parts. Avoid sudden, jarring movements that could cause pain.
- After moving a patient, reposition body parts in their natural alignment to reduce strain on joints and muscles.
- Attend to psychological needs. Be calm and reassuring. Explain procedures clearly beforehand. Help patients "talk out" the depression and frustration that may come with restricted movement and constant pain.
- Let your actions show that you are aware of the patient's fears and needs. You will be able to do your job better, and the patient will appreciate your help.

Healthcare for Today and Tomorrow | Anti-Inflammatory Drugs

As a result of an aging population and an increased incidence of musculoskeletal diseases and the use of anti-inflammatory drugs, members of the healthcare team must assess a patient's current and past histories of respiratory, cardiovascular, kidney, or liver diseases as well as any history of gastric ulcers or blood dyscrasias. It must be determined on an individual basis whether anti-inflammatories are appropriate for your patients.

 Legal and Ethical Issues | Older Adults and *Celebrex*

Celecoxib (*Celebrex*) has been a revolutionary drug in the treatment of osteoarthritis to reduce inflammation, pain, stiffness, and fever. However, osteoarthritis is most common in older adults, and because of the geriatric population's increased sensitivity to medications, you should closely monitor your patients for side effects. If your patient experiences side effects to *Celebrex*, you should immediately report this to the provider. The patient may need a lower dose to prevent serious or even lethal effects.

Representative Drugs for the Musculoskeletal System

Category, Name,[a] and Route	Uses and Diseases	Actions	Usual Dose[b] and Special Instructions	Side Effects and Adverse Reactions
Tumor Necrosis Factor-Alpha Drugs				
adalimumab (*Humira*) Subcutaneous	May be used alone or with methotrexate to decrease the symptoms of rheumatoid arthritis to improve physical function and inhibit the progression of structural damage	Tumor necrosis factor-alpha (TNF-alpha) or immunomodulator binds to TNF-alpha and blocks interaction with certain cell surface receptors, which results in a decrease in the inflammation, erythrocyte sedimentation rate, and serum cytokines	40 mg subcutaneously every other week	Serious infections and sepsis in patients receiving immunosuppressants, nausea, vomiting, abdominal pain, confusion, headache, hypertension, urinary tract infections

Category, Name,[a] and Route	Uses and Diseases	Actions	Usual Dose[b] and Special Instructions	Side Effects and Adverse Reactions
Tumor Necrosis Factor-Alpha Drugs *(continued)*				
etanercept *(Enbrel)* Subcutaneous	Decreases the symptoms and delays structural damage while improving physical functioning in moderate to severe rheumatoid arthritis	Binds to tumor necrosis factor and blocks its interaction with cell surface TNF receptors	50 mg subcutaneously every other week	Abdominal pain, nausea, vomiting, altered taste sensation, headache, dizziness, depression, upper respiratory infections, ocular inflammation, dry eyes, peripheral edema, anorexia, weight gain
Anti-Inflammatory Drugs (Antiarthritics)				
aspirin Oral, suppository	Mild to moderate pain, inflammatory diseases (e.g., osteoarthritis)	Reduces pain (analgesic), inflammation (anti-inflammatory), and fever (antipyretic); inhibits prostaglandin synthesis	*Mild pain:* 325–650 mg every 4 hours prn *Rheumatoid arthritis:* 3.6–5.4 g daily in divided doses; give oral forms with food, milk, or full glass of water to avoid stomach irritation unless enteric-coated	Nausea, stomach pain, indigestion, gastrointestinal bleeding; overdose: tinnitus, rapid breathing, dizziness, severe headache
Nonsteroidal Anti-Inflammatory Drugs				
ibuprofen (prescription; *Motrin IB, Advil*, OTC) Oral	Rheumatoid arthritis, osteoarthritis, mild to moderate pain	Reduces pain, inflammation, fever; inhibits prostaglandin synthesis	200–800 mg PO tid or qid, adjusted individually; give with milk or food if stomach irritation occurs; takes up to 2 weeks to show effects; if no relief in 2 weeks, consult provider	Epigastric distress, nausea, headache, dizziness, tinnitus, rash, visual disturbances, gastrointestinal bleeding, renal impairment. May inhibit platelet aggregation and prolong bleeding time; may increase bleeding time if co-administered with corticosteroids, anticoagulants, and use of alcohol
naproxen (*Naprosyn*) Oral	Rheumatoid arthritis, osteoarthritis, ankylosing spondylitis, tendonitis, bursitis, acute gout	Inhibits prostaglandin synthesis; is an anti-inflammatory agent with antipyretic and analgesic effects	250–500 mg bid in morning and evening for rheumatoid arthritis, osteoarthritis, ankylosing spondylitis; for gout: 750 mg, then 250 mg every 8 hours until attack subsides	Gastrointestinal bleeding, heartburn, nausea, headache, dizziness, itching, tinnitus, edema
celecoxib (*Celebrex*) Oral	Acute and chronic rheumatoid arthritis, osteoarthritis (COX-2 inhibitors)	Inhibits prostaglandin synthesis; has analgesic, anti-inflammatory, and antipyretic properties	100–200 mg PO qd-bid	Tachycardia, fatigue, anxiety, depression, nausea, vomiting, constipation, dry mouth, nephrotoxicity, hematuria, blood dyscrasias

Representative Drugs for the Musculoskeletal System (continued)

Category, Name,ᵃ and Route	Uses and Diseases	Actions	Usual Doseᵇ and Special Instructions	Side Effects and Adverse Reactions
Nonsteroidal Anti-Inflammatory Drugs (continued)				
indomethacin (*Indocin*) Oral	Moderate to severe rheumatoid arthritis including acute flare-ups of chronic disease, moderate to severe ankylosing spondylitis, moderate to severe osteoarthritis, bursitis, tendonitis, acute gouty arthritis	Inhibits prostaglandin synthesis; is an anti-inflammatory agent with the ability to relieve pain, swelling, fever of arthritis	25–50 mg bid–tid; may increase by 25 mg daily; do not exceed 200 mg daily	Nausea, vomiting, indigestion, dizziness, headache, fatigue, tinnitus, renal impairment, gastrointestinal bleeding
Antihyperuricemics				
allopurinol (*Zyloprim*) Oral	Gout, excess uric acid, prevention of hyperuricemia associated with cancer chemotherapy	Suppresses formation of uric acid	100 mg PO daily; take with meals and drink 10–12 glasses of fluid daily	Drowsiness, vomiting, rash, headache
colchicine (*Colcrys*) Oral, IV	Acute gout and prophylaxis treatment for gout flare-ups	Inhibits inflammatory response	Oral dose is supplied as 0.6-mg scored tablets. Usually taken as 0.6 mg qd, may be divided and taken 0.3 mg bid; in an acute flare-up, take 1.2 mg (two tablets), followed by 0.6 mg in 1 hour May be given without regard to meals Should be taken short term for 3 weeks or less	Diarrhea, nausea, vomiting, abdominal cramping, bone marrow depression, neuritis, aplastic anemia May interact with other medications, especially renal system meds, and cause high levels of colchicine; serious side effect is death when levels are too high
Muscle Relaxants				
carisoprodol (*Soma*) Oral	Acute, painful musculoskeletal conditions	Unknown; blocks interneuronal activity in descending reticular formation and spinal cord	350 mg qid with or without meals	Drowsiness, dizziness, vertigo, skin rash, fever, tachycardia, nausea, hypotension, leukopenia, gastrointestinal upset Avoid alcohol; may be addictive; observe for withdrawal symptoms if stopped suddenly
methocarbamol (*Robaxin*) Oral, IV, IM	Acute, painful musculoskeletal conditions	Unknown; depresses central nervous system	*Initial:* 1500 mg qid *Maintenance:* 1000 mg qid	Lightheadedness, dizziness, drowsiness, nausea, rash, pruritus, and other allergic manifestations; avoid alcohol

Representative Drugs for the Musculoskeletal System (*continued*)

Category, Name,[a] and Route	Uses and Diseases	Actions	Usual Dose[b] and Special Instructions	Side Effects and Adverse Reactions
Muscle Relaxants (continued)				
baclofen Oral	Muscle spasm	Reduces transmission of impulses from spinal cord to skeletal muscle	5 mg tid; increase dose slowly; do not exceed 80 mg/day; available in 10-mg and 20-mg tablets; do not discontinue abruptly; may be taken with or without meals but give with meals to decrease GI distress	Drowsiness, confusion, dizziness, nausea, constipation; avoid alcohol May cause hallucinations or seizures if stopped suddenly
Bone Growth Regulators				
alendronate (***Fosamax***) Oral	Osteoporosis	Inhibits osteoclast activity, preventing bone resorption (bisphosphonate)	5 mg daily or 35 mg once weekly, available in 5-mg, 10-mg, 35-mg, or 40-mg tablets and dosage could be 10 mg qd or 70 mg weekly. May take 1–2 months or longer to obtain full benefit Take in a.m. upon awakening with water only and at least 30 minutes before any food, beverage, or other medications	Flatulence, acid regurgitation, esophageal ulcer, dysphagia, symptomatic esophageal diseases, gastritis, duodenitis, ulcers
ibandronate (*Boniva*) Oral	Osteoporosis	Inhibits osteoclast activity, preventing bone resorption (bisphosphonate)	2.5 mg daily taken 60 minutes before any food or fluids except plain water; 150 mg taken once a month	Upper gastrointestinal disorders, dyspepsia, diarrhea, tooth disorder, vomiting, headache, myalgia, ear congestion, sore throat, urinary urgency
Antineoplastic Drug				
methotrexate Oral, IV	Severe rheumatoid arthritis	Binds with folic acid to inhibit synthesis of DNA and RNA	7.5 mg weekly, either as an initial single dose or as divided doses May take 3-6 weeks to feel any results, and 12 or more weeks to feel full benefits Dosage may be increased to 20-25 mg weekly	Blood disorders, gastrointestinal bleeding, nausea, vomiting, liver toxicity

Representative Drugs for the Musculoskeletal System (continued)

Category, Name,ᵃ and Route	Uses and Diseases	Actions	Usual Doseᵇ and Special Instructions	Side Effects and Adverse Reactions
Antiseizure Drug				
pregabalin (*Lyrica*) Oral	Fibromyalgia	Slows transmission of pain impulses in the brain and affects brain chemicals that send pain signals across the nervous system	75 mg qd to 660 mg PO qd in divided doses. *Lyrica CR* starting dose is 165 mg qd and increased to 330 mg/day within 1 week. Dose may be increased to a maximum of 660 mg/day. When stopping drug, taper for at least 1 week and only stop abruptly if having a severe hypersensitivity such as swelling of the throat and difficulty breathing	Clumsiness, unsteady gait, changes in balance, accidental injury, angioedema (swelling of face, arms, hands, lower legs, and feet), confusion, sleepiness, sensation of pins and needles. *Hypersensitivity*: hives, rash, dyspnea, wheezing

Note: Bolded trade names are among the 50 most commonly prescribed drugs.

ᵃTrade names given in parentheses are examples only. Check current drug references for a complete listing of available products.

ᵇAverage adult doses are given. However, dosages are determined by a provider and vary with the purpose of the therapy and the particular patient. The doses presented in this text are for general information only.

Summary

Learning Outcome	Summary Points
16-1 Describe major parts, functions, and disorders of the musculoskeletal system.	• *Major parts of the musculoskeletal system* are the bones, muscles, joints, cartilage, ligaments, fascia, and bursae. • *Bones* provide the framework for muscles, produce blood cells, act as a storage area for calcium, and protect organs of the body. • *Joints* allow movement and flexibility in the body. • *Skeletal muscles* work together with bones to allow movement. • *Smooth muscles* line the gastrointestinal tract, urinary tract, blood vessels, airways, and uterus. • *Disorders of the musculoskeletal system* include physical injuries, osteomyelitis, osteoporosis, bursitis, myositis, synovitis, gout, osteoarthritis, rheumatoid arthritis, and bone marrow disorders.

Learning Outcome	Summary Points
16-2 Describe major disorders that affect the musculoskeletal system.	• *Osteomyelitis* is an infection of the bone. • *Osteoporosis* is a decrease in total bone mass. It results in fractures from a decrease in total bone marrow. • *Bursitis, myositis,* and *synovitis* are inflammations. • *Gout* is an inflammation of the joints that starts when there is an excess of uric acid in the bloodstream. • In *gout,* or gouty arthritis, the kidneys do not excrete uric acid efficiently or, for some reason, the body makes large amounts of uric acid. • *Osteoarthritis* is a degenerative joint disease. This condition slowly destroys the mobile joints. • *Rheumatoid arthritis* is a chronic inflammatory disease that affects the mobile joints, but is systemic, involving other organs. • *Leukemia* is an overproduction of white blood cells. • *Fibromyalgia* is a specific kind of pain that is chronic, widespread, and often accompanied by tenderness in the muscles.
16-3 Describe the actions and side effects of drug groups commonly used in the treatment of osteoporosis, gout, osteoarthritis, and rheumatoid arthritis.	• *Bisphosphonates* are used in the treatment of osteoporosis. Examples: *Fosamax, Actonel,* and *Boniva.* The major side effects are GI upset such as dyspepsia and diarrhea. Pain in the extremities may also occur. Most of the side effects are cardiac, renal, or gastrointestinal. • *Evista* is an estrogen receptor modulator used to treat osteoporosis. • *Uricosuric drugs* are used to treat gout by promoting the excretion of uric acid. Example: *Probenecid.* • *Antiarthritis drugs* are used in the treatment of arthritis to suppress inflammation of the joints. Example: aspirin. • *Rheumatoid arthritis drugs:* The side effects are specific to the type of drug. For example, the side effects of the disease-modifying drugs such as *Plaquenil* are nausea, abdominal discomfort, and rash.
16-4 Describe malfunctions of bone marrow and their effects on blood.	• Failure of the bone marrow to produce enough of all three components of the blood is called aplastic anemia. • Overproduction of white blood cells is called leukemia. • *Bone marrow disorders* include aplastic anemia, or failure of the bone marrow to produce enough of the three components of the blood.
16-5 Describe the usual care of patients with musculoskeletal disorders.	• Care begins with giving the patient his or her medication on time. • Handle the patient with care by supporting body parts. • Avoid bumping the bed and sudden jarring movement of the patient. • Reposition the body parts in natural alignment after moving the patient. • Attend to the psychological needs of the patient.

Chapter 16 Review

Define each of the terms listed.

1. (LO 16-3) Antihyperuricemic _____

2. (LO 16-3) Antispasmodic _____

3. (LO 16-2) Atrophy _____

4. (LO 16-2) Strain _____

5. (LO 16-2) Sprain _____

6. (LO 16-2) Bursa _____

Complete the statements by filling in the blank.

7. (LO 16-1) The musculoskeletal system supports the body and gives it the ability to _____

_____.

8. (LO 16-1) Bones are connected to each other by means of _____.

9. (LO 16-1) Bones are living tissue. They get their hardness from deposits of the mineral _____.

10. (LO 16-1) Bundles of tissue that connect muscles to bones are called _____.

11. (LO 16-1) The spongy part of the bone where blood cells are produced and fat is stored is called the bone _____.

12. (LO 16-1) The skull, spinal column, sternum, ribs, and pelvis _____ the vital organs of the head, chest, and abdomen.

13. (LO 16-1) Smooth muscles allow movement in the gastrointestinal tract and blood vessels, whereas _____ muscles allow movement of the bones.

14. (LO 16-1) Healthy muscles are slightly contracted at all times. This is called muscle _____.

15. (LO 16-2) Strains are injuries to muscles and tendons, whereas _____ are injuries to ligaments.

Match the drug categories or uses to the drugs.

_____ 16. (LO 16-3) *Ecotrin*

_____ 17. (LO 16-3) *Zyloprim,* colchicine

_____ 18. (LO 16-3) Hydrocortisone

_____ 19. (LO 16-3) *Robaxin, Soma*

_____ 20. (LO 16-3) Alendronate, *Boniva, Evista*

_____ 21. (LO 16-3) *Humira,* etanercept, *Plaquenil*

a. drugs used in the treatment of osteoporosis

b. drugs that reduce the formation of uric acid crystals in the joints

c. muscle relaxants

d. corticosteroid sometimes injected into the synovial capsule to reduce joint inflammation

e. enteric-coated aspirin

f. antiarthritic drugs

Place a T in the blank if the statement is true. Place an F in the blank if the statement is false.

_____ 22. (LO 16-2) After middle age, calcium is no longer deposited in the bones, causing the development of osteoporosis.

_____ 23. (LO 16-2) Myalgia is pain in the skeletal muscles.

_____ 24. (LO 16-2) Aplastic anemia is a bone marrow disorder.

_____ 25. (LO 16-2) Gout is a condition that results from too little uric acid in the bloodstream.

_____ 26. (LO 16-2) Surgery is frequently used to treat osteoporosis.

_____ 27. (LO 16-2) Lack of estrogen is a factor in the development of osteoporosis.

_____ 28. (LO 16-1) Ligaments are strong bands of connective tissue that hold bones together.

_____ 29. (LO 16-2) An inflammation of the synovial capsule is known as synovitis.

_____ 30. (LO 16-2) Crystals of uric acid deposited in the cartilage around joints can cause the joints to become red, hot, swollen, and painful.

_____ 31. (LO 16-2) Rheumatoid arthritis is caused by wear and tear on the joints.

_____ 32. (LO 16-2) Osteomyelitis is a decrease in total bone mass.

_____ 33. (LO 16-4) Leukemia is an overproduction of white blood cells.

Answer the questions in the space provided.

34. (LO 16-3) What are three side effects of the COX-2 inhibitor celecoxib (*Celebrex*)? _____

_____

_____

_____

35. (LO 16-3) How is ibandronate (*Boniva*) taken? _____

_____

_____

_____

36. (LO 16-2) What two principles should be included in the treatment of gout? _____

_____

_____

37. (LO 16-2) What four foods are high in purine? _____

_____

_____

_____

_____

Drug Calculations—Fill in the blank with the answer.

38. (LO 16-3) The provider orders methocarbamol (*Robaxin*) 1.5 g orally qid. Available are 750-mg tablets. Prepare to administer _____ tablets to your patient.

39. (LO 16-3) The provider orders naproxen (*Naprosyn*) 500 mg orally bid. Available are 250-mg tablets. You will administer _____ tablets to your patient.

40. (LO 16-3) The provider orders indomethacin (*Indocin*) suspension 50 mg orally bid. Available is a 25-mg/5-mL suspension. You will give your patient _____ mL.

41. (LO 16-3) The provider orders alendronate (*Fosamax*) 35 mg orally weekly. Available are 70-mg tablets. You will give your patient _____ tablets.

42. (LO 16-3) The provider orders allopurinol (*Zyloprim*) 0.2 g orally daily. Available are 100-mg tablets. Prepare to administer _____ tablets to your patient.

43. (LO 16-3) A patient asks you how teriparatide (*Forteo*) works. What is the best response?
    a. It is used for hypercalcemia.
    b. It prevents osteoporosis.
    c. It rebuilds bone.
    d. It inhibits calcium uptake.

44. (LO 16-3) Patients with which two conditions should use celecoxib (*Celebrex*) with caution?
    a. Peptic ulcer disease and cardiovascular disease
    b. Rheumatoid arthritis and muscle pain
    c. Gout and osteoporosis
    d. Urinary retention and constipation

45. (LO 16-3) Monitor a patient taking aspirin for which of the following side effects?
    a. Tinnitus, visual disturbances, urinary retention
    b. Tachycardia, fatigue, constipation
    c. Pruritus, rash, stomatitis
    d. Indigestion, gastrointestinal bleeding, headache

46. (LO 16-3) Which of the following instructions should you give a patient receiving a uricosuric drug?
    a. Avoid lying down after taking a dose.
    b. Avoid high-purine foods.
    c. Restrict fluids.
    d. Increase physical activity.

47. (LO 16-3) Monitor a patient taking carisoprodol (*Soma*) for which of the following side effects?
    a. Fatigue, lethargy, sedation
    b. Heartburn, headache, tinnitus
    c. Diarrhea, nausea, vomiting
    d. Rash, dizziness, weight gain

Chapter 16 Case Studies

48. (LO 16-3) You are caring for a patient taking colchicine 0.5 mg orally daily. The patient asks you when the colchicine will make the pain go away. How should you respond? What is the teaching you should reinforce with your patient? The patient also wants to know if any foods should be avoided and why.

    _____
    _____
    _____

49. (LO 16-2) After the nurse teaches the patient what to do for osteoporosis, you reinforce the teaching by telling the patient how much calcium she should take daily. What else should you tell the patient to do? The patient asks you for a list of high-calcium foods. What should you write down on the list?

    _____
    _____
    _____

Critical Thinking

Answer the question in the space provided.

50. (LO 16-5) When administering medications to patients with painful musculoskeletal conditions, what can you do to help make them comfortable?

    _____
    _____
    _____

osteomyelitis   osteoporosis   bursitis   gout

51. (LO 16-2) An older adult patient has been instructed to eat a diet rich in calcium, and she is taking small doses of hormones. This is because her bones have become very porous and fracture easily.

_____

52. (LO 16-2) A patient has developed an infection in the leg bone near the knee joint. He is taking antibiotics, and surgery is planned to drain the infected material from the bone.

_____

53. (LO 16-2) A small, fluid-filled pouch in a patient's shoulder joint is inflamed. This is causing swelling, pain, and stiffness. The provider plans to inject hydrocortisone directly into the joint to reduce the inflammation.

_____

54. (LO 16-2) Increasing levels of uric acid in a patient are causing crystals to form in the cartilage around the joints. A dose of colchicine relieves the pain in his joints within a few hours.

_____

Applications

Obtain an electronic drug guide or a current copy of the *PDR*® from your school, health facility, or clinic. Use it to answer the following questions in a notebook or on file cards.

55. Find another product name for each of the muscle relaxants listed in the Representative Drugs for the Musculoskelatal System table in this chapter.

56. In Section 3 of the *PDR*®, Product Category Index, find the Arthritis Medications. Then find the subheading NSAIDs. Make a list of all NSAIDs (nonsteroidal anti-inflammatory drugs) you see listed there.

DRUGS FOR THE NERVOUS AND SENSORY SYSTEMS

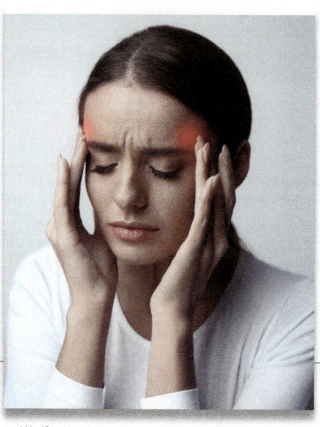

©puhhha/Getty Images

In this chapter you will learn how the nervous system coordinates all systems of the body and responds to changes inside and outside the body. You will become familiar with the disorders that affect the nervous and sensory systems, the types of drugs used to treat them, and how to administer the drugs properly.

LEARNING OUTCOMES

17-1 List the main divisions and parts of the nervous system.

17-2 Identify the basic function of the autonomic nervous system.

17-3 Know the correct medical terms for symptoms of nervous system disorders.

17-4 Recognize descriptions of the major nervous system disorders for which medications are given.

17-5 Articulate to patients how to prevent strokes.

17-6 Describe the actions of the following drug groups: central nervous system stimulants, analgesics, anticonvulsants, antiparkinsonians, Alzheimer's drugs, and anti-migraine drugs.

17-7 Know the principles for administering pain medications, long-term medications, stimulants, and emergency drugs.

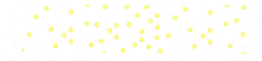

THE NERVOUS AND SENSORY SYSTEMS
[LO 17-1, LO 17-2]

The brain, the spinal cord, and the nerves make up the nervous system, which is a highly specialized system (Figure 17.1). The function of the nervous system is to control and integrate many of the body's activities. The brain interprets messages from nerves and sense organs and decides on an appropriate set of actions. The brain then sends out "action messages," which are relayed by the nerves to various parts of the body. The brain's messages can involve voluntary actions (walking, talking, etc.), feelings (fear, anger, love, etc.), or automatic actions (breathing, heartbeat, blood vessel contraction, etc.). In this way, the body is able to respond to constantly changing conditions, both within and outside the body.

The nervous system has two main parts: the **central nervous system (CNS)** and the **peripheral nervous system (PNS)**. The CNS consists of the brain and the spinal cord. The PNS consists of the cranial and spinal nerves and peripheral components of the **autonomic nervous system (ANS)**.

Figure 17.1

The nervous system: The central nervous system (CNS) consists of the brain and spinal cord. The peripheral nervous system (PNS) consists of nerves and ganglia.

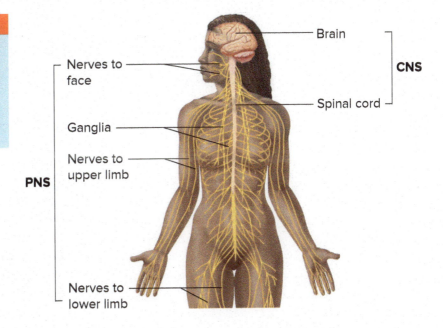

The Nerves

The nervous system is made up of two types of cells, neurons and neuroglia. Neurons are the primary functional units and have many different shapes and sizes. Neurons consist of a cell body, an axon, and several dendrites. The cell body is the metabolic center of the neuron and contains the nucleus and cytoplasm. The axon carries the nerve impulses to other neurons, and the dendrites receive the impulses from the axons and send the impulses to the cell body (**Figure 17.2**).

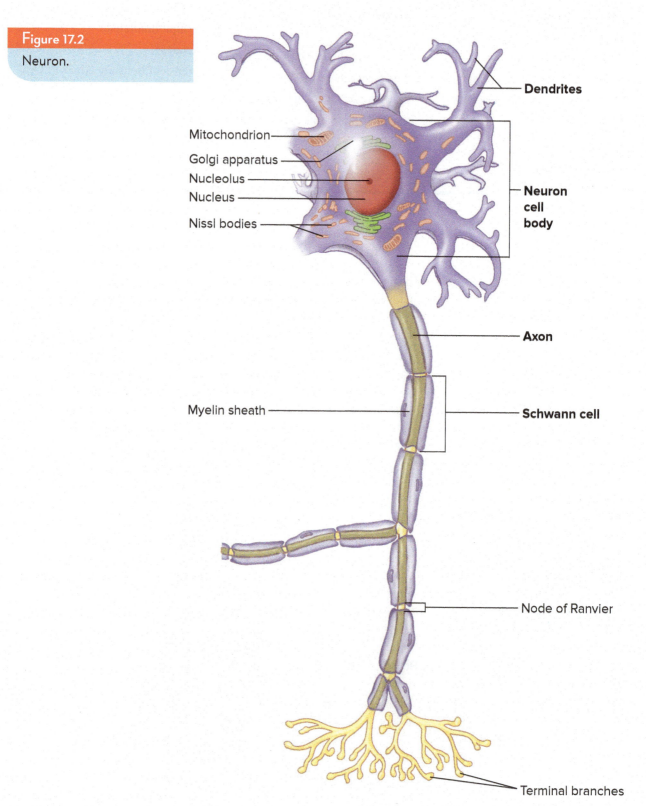

Figure 17.2
Neuron.

Dendrites

Mitochondrion

Golgi apparatus

Nucleolus

Nucleus

Nissl bodies

Neuron cell body

Axon

Myelin sheath

Schwann cell

Node of Ranvier

Terminal branches

The neuroglia are greater in number, and they serve to support, protect, and nourish the neurons.

Neurons have the ability to initiate, receive, and process messages, or **impulses**. This is done by means of special chemicals (acetylcholine, norepinephrine) in the ends of neurons and in the gaps (**synapses**) between them. Many drugs that affect the nervous system are designed to increase or decrease the concentration of these chemicals.

Nerve impulses travel along the nerve pathways at all times so that the brain and body parts are in constant communication. Some neurons are specialized for transmitting messages to the CNS; others are specialized for carrying messages away from the CNS to various tissues and organs of the body.

Brain and Spinal Cord (CNS)

The brain is the control center for all body functions. It consists of the cerebral cortex (*cerebral* means pertaining to the brain), the cerebellum, and the brain stem. As Figure 17.3 shows, different parts of the brain have special functions to carry out. Most of our conscious thought processes—plus speech, hearing, and sight—are controlled by the cerebrum. Unconscious brain activity, balance, muscle coordination, and gland stimulation are regulated in the brain stem and the cerebellum.

The spinal cord is attached to the brain stem and passes from the neck down to the lower back. It acts as a reflex center and as a pathway for impulses to and from the brain.

Peripheral and Autonomic Nervous System

The peripheral nervous system consists of somatic motor neurons and all structures that lie outside the central nervous system. These include the cranial (pertaining to the skull) and spinal nerves and portions of the autonomic nervous system. The primary function of the autonomic nervous system is to regulate the functions of the cardiac and smooth muscles.

Figure 17.3

Conscious brain activity is controlled by the cerebrum, and unconscious activity is controlled by the brain stem and cerebellum.

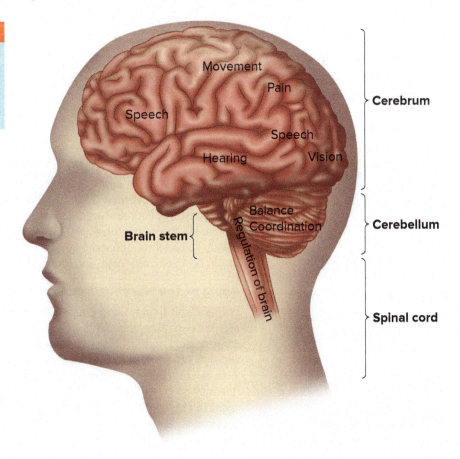

The ANS includes six visceral systems: digestive, respiratory, urinary, genital, endocrine, and vascular. It is made up of the peripheral system and the central control centers. The peripheral system is composed of the thoracolumbar (sympathetic) and craniosacral (parasympathetic) divisions.

Sympathetic or Thoracolumbar Division. The **sympathetic nervous system** is concerned with the use of energy. Under conditions of stress, it prepares the body to meet an emergency by producing epinephrine. This agent speeds up the heart rate and raises the blood pressure. The bronchial tubes dilate to allow more oxygen to enter the body, and the digestive system is slowed by the inhibition of peristalsis. With these changes, the body is ready for action. For this reason, the sympathetic portion of the ANS is called the "flight or fight" system.

Parasympathetic or Craniosacral Division. The **parasympathetic nervous system** restores and conserves body energy and brings the body back to normal conditions. It works the opposite way of the sympathetic division.

The Senses

Our ability to feel, see, hear, taste, and smell things around us is due to special nerve cells called sense receptors. They are specialized to pick up only specific sensory messages. For example, some pick up color, some react to feelings of pressure, and others respond only to odors. It is up to the brain to figure out what the messages mean according to which receptors sent the messages.

We are used to thinking of only five senses—sight, hearing, smell, taste, and touch. But there are other senses as well, including pressure, pain, temperature, body position, thirst, and hunger. Some types of sensory receptors are found in only certain parts of the body or in specialized organs such as the eyes and the ears. Other types of sensory receptors are spread throughout the body.

The Nose. The upper part of the nasal cavity is lined with olfactory cells that perform the function of smelling. These cells are connected to the olfactory nerve leading to the brain. The brain interprets messages from the olfactory cells as odors.

The Tongue. The tongue contains taste-sensitive cells inside oval-shaped taste buds. Dissolved foods and liquids stimulate the taste buds to send messages to the brain by way of the glossopharyngeal nerves and facial nerves. Taste buds on different parts of the tongue detect different tastes: sweet, sour, salty, and bitter (Figure 17.4). The olfactory cells of the nose also assist in the sense of taste because the aroma of foods is an important part of taste. A person who cannot smell properly also cannot taste properly.

Other Sense Receptors. Receptors for hunger are located in the stomach ("hunger pangs" come from these receptors). Receptors for thirst seem to be centered in the mouth, nose, and throat. A number of other sense receptors are widely spread throughout the body. These are the receptors that feel pressure, touch, heat and cold, pain, and body position.

Aging of the Nervous System

For healthful living, there must be functional nerve pathways and responsive receptors within the CNS and the peripheral nervous system. But, unfortunately, aging brings structural and functional changes to the human nervous system. Changes occur, and some nerve cells may die. Therefore, there are decreases in reception and conduction and reflex reaction. Reflexes first may become sluggish and then may disappear completely. These changes result in varying degrees of muscular incoordination, paralysis, and asthenia (weakness). Sensory receptors are less reactive unless the stimulus is much stronger.

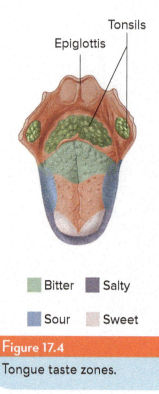

Tonsils

Epiglottis

■ Bitter ■ Salty

■ Sour ■ Sweet

Figure 17.4

Tongue taste zones.

NERVOUS SYSTEM DISORDERS [LO 17-3, LO 17-4]

Almost any disease or injury is likely to affect the nervous system in some way. There are many signs that show that the nervous system is being affected. The signs do not always mean that the nervous system itself is malfunctioning or diseased. They can signal a drug overdose or side effects, a psychological disorder, or a problem elsewhere in the body. Pain, for example, is a danger signal picked up by sensory receptors to alert the brain to a possible injury.

Some other signs that the nervous system is being affected by disease or drugs are trembling (**tremor**); **spasticity**; dizziness (**vertigo**); loss of muscle control; dry mouth; blurred vision; inability to move (**paralysis**); unusual postures and body movements; convulsions; deep sleep from which a person cannot be roused (coma); being "in a daze" (**stupor**); irritability, excitation, agitation, restlessness, and/or sleeplessness (**insomnia**); nausea; headache; speech difficulties; and changes in pulse, respiration, and pupil size.

Parkinson's Disease

Parkinson's disease is a syndrome characterized by slowing of movement (**bradykinesia**), stiffness (**rigidity**), tremor, and impaired postural reflexes. Tremor makes it hard to do simple tasks like eating and writing. Rigidity can lead to bent posture, difficulty walking, deformities of the hands and feet, and poor equilibrium.

The exact cause of Parkinson's disease is unknown. There is a degeneration of dopamine-producing neurons. Dopamine is a **neurotransmitter** necessary for normal functioning of the **extrapyramidal** motor system, which includes control of posture, physical support, and voluntary movement.

There is no cure for Parkinson's disease, so treatment is aimed at relieving symptoms. There are treatments in the form of special medicines (antiparkinsonian agents) and physical therapy. The drug of choice is often levodopa/carbidopa (*Sinemet*). The levodopa is converted to dopamine and functions as a neurotransmitter. The carbidopa prevents destruction of the levodopa. Although a levodopa/carbidopa drug regimen is the most effective treatment for Parkinson's disease, its effectiveness may diminish over time. As a result, patients fluctuate between periods of relatively good functioning and periods of poor functioning. Entacapone (*Comtan*), an antiparkinsonian drug, is used as an adjunct to levodopa/carbidopa to decrease the symptoms of Parkinson's disease. Rasagiline (*Azilect*) is an irreversible monoamine oxidase type B inhibitor. It works by blocking the breakdown of dopamine. It may be used in early Parkinson's disease as a single dose or in combination with levodopa in more advanced disease. *Azilect* may cause a hypertensive crisis, so patients should avoid a diet high in tyramine. Physical therapy is important to keep the muscles functioning despite their stiffness. Massage, stretching, and overall exercise can help keep the disease from completely crippling the patient. The only other treatment is for severe unilateral tremor. It is most effective in young patients. The role of surgical intervention is varied. Transplantation of adrenal tissue into the brain to provide dopamine-producing cells has proved unsuccessful. Experimentation with transplanting fetal tissue for the same purpose holds more promise.

Myasthenia Gravis

Myasthenia gravis is a chronic autoimmune neuromuscular disorder consisting of fluctuating weakness of the skeletal muscles in which antibodies attack the number and effectiveness of acetylcholine (ACH) at the neuromuscular junction. It is characterized by periods of remission and exacerbation. The primary symptoms are muscle weakness that increases with activity during the day but improves with rest. Other symptoms include ptosis, diplopia, dysphagia, and respiratory and speech difficulties. Anticholinesterase drugs are used in the treatment of myasthenia gravis. The most commonly used anticholinesterase drugs are neostigmine and pyridostigmine (*Mestinon*).

Multiple Sclerosis

Multiple sclerosis (MS) is a chronic, progressive, degenerative disease that attacks the outer covering (myelin sheath) of the nerves. Once the myelin sheath is gone, the nerves are unable to conduct impulses. Multiple sclerosis can attack any part of the body such as the brain and/or spinal cord. Symptoms depend on which nerves are damaged and are usually intermittent, with lengthy remissions. They include paralysis, blurring of vision, speech problems, unsteady walk, and numbness. The cause and cure of MS remain unknown. Treatment is aimed at relieving the symptoms.

Adrenocorticotropic hormone (ACTH) and prednisone are helpful during acute exacerbations of the disease. They decrease edema and inflammation at the site of myelin destruction. Immunosuppressive drugs such as azathioprine (*Imuran*) and cyclophosphamide have also been used in patients with relapsing multiple sclerosis. Interferon beta-1a (*Avonex*) and interferon beta-1b (*Betaseron*) have proved successful in controlling the disease in patients who are managed at home. Interferon beta-1b (*Extavia*) is a first-line disease-modifying drug in the treatment of the relapsing form of multiple sclerosis. Dalfampridine (*Ampyra*) is a potassium blocker that is administered orally to improve walking in patients with multiple sclerosis.

Natalizumab (*Tysabri*) was a drug used to treat multiple sclerosis that was pulled off the market in 2005 because of a possible connection between the drug and a rare but often fatal brain disorder called progressive multifocal leukoencephalopathy (PML). The FDA reconsidered its decision because natalizumab reduced the relapse rate by 70 percent. The FDA brought it back to the market under certain conditions. The patient must be enrolled in a special program called TOUCH and receive regular evaluations to receive the drug.

Mitoxantrone is an antineoplastic drug used to treat progressive, worsening, relapsing-remitting multiple sclerosis to decrease neurologic disability or the frequency of relapses.

Antispasmodics such as diazepam (*Valium*), baclofen, dantrolene (*Dantrium*), and tizanidine (*Zanaflex*) are used to decrease symptoms of spasticity. Central nervous system stimulants such as methylphenidate (*Ritalin*) and modafinil (*Provigil*) are used to control symptoms of fatigue. Tricyclic antidepressants and antiseizure drugs may be used to treat chronic pain.

Epilepsy

Epilepsy is a set of disorders that cause periodic **seizures**. Seizures are temporary losses of consciousness caused by overactivity of the nerve signals in part of the brain. Epilepsy commonly appears in the first six months of life as a result of birth defects or infections. Causes of epilepsy in childhood and young adulthood include trauma, brain tumors, and infections. Epilepsy after the age of 50 is usually the result of a cerebrovascular accident (CVA) or malignant brain tumor. Seizures occurring in childhood and young adulthood are called petit mal seizures. In this type of seizure, the patient stares into space for a few seconds and the seizure often goes unnoticed.

During tonic-clonic seizures, formerly called grand mal seizures (the most common generalized seizure), the epileptic patient suffers **convulsions** with loss of consciousness. Tonic-clonic seizures may occur in either children or adults. With convulsions, the large muscles tighten and twitch uncontrollably. Most epilepsy is controllable with medications that prevent seizures (**anticonvulsants**) such as phenytoin (*Dilantin*), carbamazepine (*Tegretol*), phenobarbital, primidone (*Mysoline*), gabapentin (*Neurontin*), and divalproex (*Depakote*). Side effects include ataxia, diplopia, nausea, vomiting, constipation, and hyperglycemia.

Epileptic patients must take their medications regularly and on time. A missed or late dose may result in a seizure. Teaching the patient the importance of regularity is part of your responsibility when administering medications.

Pediatric Concerns on Epilepsy. Typical absence seizures or petit mal seizures generally occur in children and rarely continue past adolescence. As the child grows, they may cease altogether or evolve into another type of seizure. During a petit mal seizure, the child has a brief staring spell that may go unnoticed. A brief loss of consciousness can occur. If left untreated, there can be up to 100 seizures per day. Seizures that begin before age 4 tend to result in some degree of mental retardation and behavior and learning problems. The treatment consists of antiepileptic drugs and helping the child live as normal a life as possible. When the child has been seizure-free for two years and has a normal EEG (electroencephalogram), the antiepileptic treatment may be discontinued.

Alzheimer's Disease

Alzheimer's disease (AD) is a chronic, progressive, degenerative disease of the brain. It accounts for the majority of all cases of dementia. Estimates suggest that 10 percent of all persons over the age of 65 years and 50 percent of all those over the age of 85 years are affected by AD. Women are affected more because they live longer. The exact course of AD is unknown, but age is the significant risk factor. However, it is important to understand that AD is not a normal process of aging. Physiologically, the brain cells are destroyed, which is not a normal manifestation of AD. Characteristically, there are abnormal clumps of neuritic or senile plaques and tangled bundles of fibers known as neurofibrillary tangles in the brain.

There are two types of Alzheimer's disease. Early-onset AD affects individuals under the age of 60 years, whereas late-onset AD is characteristically found in individuals over the age of 60 years. There is also a familial Alzheimer's disease, which has a pattern that tends to run in families. There is no singular diagnostic test for AD. The only positive diagnoses are the neuritic plaques and neurofibrillary tangles seen on autopsy. Clinical manifestations begin with a mild cognitive impairment. The Alzheimer's Association has developed a list of manifestations present in AD (Table 17.1).

Table 17.1 Early Warning Signs of Alzheimer's Disease

- Memory loss that affects job skills
- Difficulty performing familiar tasks
- Problems with language such as forgetting a word or speaking inappropriate words, making the person's language difficult to understand
- Disorientation to time and place
- Poor or decreased judgment, such as inappropriately dressing for the weather
- Problems with abstract thinking, such as difficulty recognizing numbers or performing basic calculations
- Misplacement of items followed by no memory of how they got there
- Significant changes in mood or behavior for no apparent reason
- Changes in personality, including becoming less tolerant or angry, suspicious, or fearful in an otherwise easygoing individual
- Loss of initiative or interest in many areas of life that the person was once engaged in

Treatment for Alzheimer's disease focuses on cholinesterase inhibitors such as donepezil (*Aricept*), rivastigmine (*Exelon*), and galantamine (*Razadyne*), which are responsible for the breakdown of acetylcholine in the synaptic cleft. Memantine (*Namenda*) is an N-methyl-D-aspartate (NMDA) receptor antagonist in which NMDA receptors are activated in the brain by glutamate, an excitatory amino acid. It is used in the treatment of moderate to severe Alzheimer's disease.

Other drugs have been useful in the treatment of Alzheimer's disease. Antidepressants such as sertraline (*Zoloft*), fluoxetine (*Prozac*), amitriptyline, and nortriptyline and antipsychotics such as loxapine (*Loxitane*), haloperidol, risperidone (*Risperdal*), olanzapine (*Zyprexa*), and quetiapine (*Seroquel*) may be used to alleviate manifestations. Zolpidem (*Ambien*) may also be prescribed for sleep disturbances.

Headaches

Headaches are the most common symptom of pain exhibited. The two most common types of headaches are tension-type and migraines. Tension-type headaches are characterized by a bilateral pressure feeling around the head that is generally worse with physical activity and may involve a sensitivity to light (photophobia) or sound (phonophobia). They may be treated with a nonnarcotic analgesic such as aspirin or acetaminophen alone or in combination with a sedative, muscle relaxant, tranquilizer, or codeine. Erenumab-aooe (*Aimovig*) is the first FDA approved therapy that prevents migraines by blocking the calcitonin gene-related peptide receptor (CGRP-R). Butalbital and aspirin (*Fiorinal*), butalbital and acetaminophen (*Fioricet*), and dichloralphenazone, acetaminophen, and isometheptene may be used for short-term treatment.

Migraine headaches are characterized by unilateral or bilateral throbbing pain that is recurrent. Generally there is an event that triggers the pain, or a strong family history of migraines, causing nausea, vomiting, irritability, sweating, photophobia, or phonophobia. They may be associated with a prodromal phase, which precedes the headache by hours to days. The prodrome may be followed by an aura, which is a sensation of light or warmth or a sense of a spreading depression. If analgesics or drug treatment for migraine headaches fails, a variety of other drugs may be used. Sumatriptan succinate (*Imitrex*) is an antimigraine drug administered subcutaneously at the first indication of an impending headache. It also comes in oral and nasal preparations. Topiramate (*Topamax*) is an anticonvulsant used in the prophylaxis of migraine headaches in adult patients. It is administered orally either by tablets or sprinkle capsules. Eletriptan hydrobromide (*Relpax*) is a serotonin receptor antagonist used in the treatment of migraine headaches with or without an aura.

Tumors

Any abnormal growth in the brain is dangerous, even though it may not be cancerous (malignant). The danger arises because the brain is encased in a hard covering, the skull. Any growth or swelling that presses on the healthy parts of the brain may cause damage or malfunctions. Surgery, antineoplastics, and radiation are three possible treatments for brain tumors. Diuretics and corticosteroids may be used to reduce edema.

Infections and Inflammations

Infections and inflammations have specific names, depending on which part of the nervous system they attack. Inflammation of the brain is called encephalitis. Inflammation of the linings of the brain and the spinal cord (meninges) is called meningitis. Nerve inflammations are called neuritis and are characterized by weakness, abnormal sensations, temporary paralysis, and loss of reflexes. Neuralgia is a painful condition of the nerves caused by inflammation or irritation. These conditions are treated with pain relievers (analgesics) and with antibiotics if the infection can be identified as not viral.

STROKE—CEREBROVASCULAR ACCIDENT (CVA) [LO 17-5]

A **cerebrovascular accident (CVA)**, commonly known as stroke, is the sudden onset of a neurologic deficit resulting from disease of the blood vessels that supply the brain. Strokes may happen with or without a warning. Patients who have had a **transient ischemic attack (TIA)** have a greater incidence of having a stroke. A TIA is a transient period of neurologic deficit. Strokes are currently the third leading cause of death in the United States and are a significant health problem, especially in the older adult population. Therefore, it is especially important for the healthcare provider to educate the older adult population on stroke prevention.

The cause of stroke can be a cerebral thrombus or embolus or a hemorrhage in part of the brain. Symptoms depend on the location of the interruption in the blood supply to the brain and can range from minor impairment to total incapacitation.

The treatment of a patient after a stroke depends on the type of stroke and the extent of injury. The goal is prevention of strokes, and measures have proved successful in decreasing the number of strokes. These measures include administration of aspirin or dipyridamole (*Persantine*), or tirofiban (*Aggrastat*), which prevents the formation of a thrombus or embolus.

Once a stroke has occurred, the goal is to preserve life and decrease and prevent further disability. Anticoagulants such as heparin sodium and enoxaparin sodium (*Lovenox*) may be used to prevent further clotting when a

Patient Education Stroke Prevention

- Have regular blood pressure checks.
- Take blood pressure medication as prescribed.
- Reduce dietary salt intake—both salt and food high in salt content.
- Stop smoking.
- Reduce and control weight within a normal range.

- Decrease intake of foods high in saturated fats and cholesterol, particularly fried foods.
- Avoid drinking alcohol.
- Be monitored by a provider if taking oral contraceptives.
- Increase daily activity.
- Increase fruits and vegetables in the diet.

Caution Signs of Stroke

- Memory loss
- Dizziness (vertigo)
- Headache
- Fainting

- Weakness
- Blurred vision
- Speech difficulty
- Partial paralysis

stroke is in progress. Long-term anticoagulation therapy is accomplished with warfarin sodium (*Coumadin*). The provider may prescribe acetylsalicylic acid (aspirin) to treat symptoms of a progressing stroke.

DRUGS THAT AFFECT THE CNS [LO 17-6]

Because they act on the body's control systems, nervous system drugs often affect the whole body. How they work is not well understood. They appear to influence the chemical changes that allow nerve impulses to be transmitted between nerve cells.

We will focus on drugs that affect mainly the CNS. These are divided into two major categories: CNS stimulants and CNS depressants. Stimulants speed up the cell processes and make it easier for nerve cells to transmit messages. Depressants slow cell activity and inhibit the passing of nerve impulses. Within these two broad categories are many specific types of drugs.

Some drugs affect the peripheral ANS and the automatic regulation of internal organs. These drugs (e.g., epinephrine and atropine) are described in other chapters (e.g., Chapters 10 and 11) because they are used to treat disorders affecting other body systems. You will see these drugs referred to in drug references as **sympathomimetic**, **sympatholytic (adrenergic blocking agent)**, **parasympathomimetic** or **cholinomimetic**, and parasympatholytic or **anticholinergic**. The names of the drug categories may be confusing; just keep in mind that they all affect the unconscious, automatic processes that keep the body functioning.

CNS Stimulants

Central nervous system stimulants have been commonly used for a variety of purposes. They were formerly used to treat obesity and to counteract overdoses of CNS depressant drugs. Today, however, they are essentially obsolete. Their use is limited in practice to attention-deficit disorder and episodes of excessive drowsiness and uncontrolled sleep attacks during the day (narcolepsy). Indiscriminate use of CNS stimulants may result in cardiac dysrhythmias, hypertension, convulsions, or violent behavior. Examples of CNS stimulants used for attention-deficit disorder and narcolepsy are methylphenidate hydrochloride (*Ritalin*), dextroamphetamine/amphetamine (*Adderall*), and methylphenidate (*Concerta*). Because of the high risk of toxicity, CNS stimulants are controlled substances (Schedule II). Although caffeine is not often thought of as a drug, it is a CNS stimulant, and healthcare providers should educate patients about the effects of caffeine.

Some CNS stimulants, such as doxapram (*Dopram*), are used in the treatment of respiratory depression induced by drug overdose. It is often administered intravenously, since immediate effect is needed in such emergencies.

 Pediatric Considerations CNS Stimulants

- If possible, avoid using CNS stimulants in children less than 3 years of age with attention-deficit hyperactivity disorder (ADHD). If used, carefully monitor to avoid excessive stimulation, anorexia, and insomnia.
- Monitor growth during administration of these drugs because a slowed growth rate may occur.

- Monitor children closely if they have psychosis or Tourette's syndrome because there can be an exacerbation of symptoms.
- Avoid overprescribing CNS stimulants. They might be overused.
- Suggest a drug holiday once a year to evaluate progress with therapy.

Older Adult Considerations | CNS Stimulants

- Because of slowed metabolism and excretion, use CNS stimulants cautiously. An increased risk of toxicity may occur.
- An increased incidence of anxiety, confusion, nervousness, insomnia, and cardiovascular effects may occur.
- Give the smallest possible dose to decrease side effects.

Patient Education | Caffeine

- Know which foods and beverages contain caffeine, such as chocolate, cocoa, coffee, tea, and soft drinks.
- Eliminate caffeinated beverages from your diet, and replace them with decaffeinated beverages such as decaffeinated coffee.
- Some medications, such as cold preparations, contain caffeine. Discuss their use with your provider.
- Avoid drinking caffeinated beverages, eating chocolate, or taking medications containing caffeine at bedtime (Figure 17.5).

- Avoid or limit caffeine consumption if you are pregnant because of the potential for birth defects.
- Avoid caffeine if you are breastfeeding because it is passed into the breast milk and causes the baby to be jittery.
- Drinking two or more cups of coffee may result in nervousness, irritability, or headache.

Figure 17.5

Caffeine is a CNS stimulant. The healthcare worker should educate patients about products that contain caffeine.

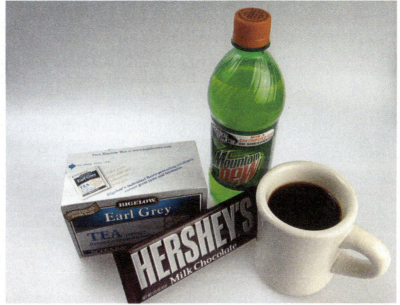

©McGraw-Hill Education/Jill Braaten, photographer

CNS Depressants

Drugs in this category can either depress the whole CNS (e.g., sedatives) or selectively depress only parts of the nervous system (e.g., analgesics, tranquilizers, anticonvulsants). CNS depressants are used in the treatment of both physical and psychological problems. Like CNS stimulants, the depressants have high potential for abuse. In addition, many of them can cause physical dependence. (Sedatives and tranquilizers will be discussed in Chapter 18.)

Analgesics. **Analgesics** are drugs that relieve pain either by affecting the brain itself or by interfering with the ability of pain receptors around the body to send pain messages to the brain. One large group of analgesics is the **narcotics**. Along with pain relief, these drugs bring euphoria and a sense of calm; therefore, they are often abused. Examples of narcotic analgesics are morphine, codeine, oxycodone (*OxyContin*), meperidine (*Demerol*), methadone, pentazocine (*Talwin*), hydrocodone with acetaminophen (*Vicodin*), and oxycodone with acetaminophen (*Percocet*). Morphine sulfate and naltrexone (*Embeda*) is an extended-release drug for pain. Tramadol (*Ultram*) is a centrally acting analgesic that is not chemically related to opiates. It is used in the treatment of moderate to moderately severe pain.

A common group of nonnarcotic analgesics has the ability to reduce fever (antipyretic) as well as relieve pain. This group includes the familiar drugs aspirin and acetaminophen (*Tylenol*). They reduce fever by eliminating heat through vasodilation and increased respiration. Aspirin also has anti-inflammatory effects, which are put to use in treating musculoskeletal disorders. Analgesic antipyretics are often combined with narcotic analgesics or sedatives in prescription pain relievers—for example, *Tylenol with Codeine,* and *Fiorinal* (butalbital with aspirin and codeine). Ibuprofen, a nonsteroidal anti-inflammatory drug (e.g., *Motrin IB, Advil*) is available by prescription and over the counter. Ibuprofen acts by inhibiting the synthesis of prostaglandin, a substance involved with mild to moderate pain. *Caldolor* is the first injectable form of ibuprofen to treat pain. such as arthritis. Aspirin, acetaminophen, and ibuprofen are the three major pain-relieving drugs available without prescription. Each has analgesic and antipyretic activity, and aspirin and ibuprofen also have anti-inflammatory activity.

Diclofenac potassium (*Zipsor*) is a nonsteroidal anti-inflammatory analgesic recently approved for treatment of mild to moderate pain such as osteoarthritis and arthritis. *Zipsor* comes in a liquid-filled capsule usually taken orally four times a day. The most common side effects are nausea, headache, and abdominal pain.

Anticonvulsants. Anticonvulsants are used to control or prevent seizures. Aside from cases of epilepsy, seizures may occur as reactions to high fever, drug overdose, or injury and for unexplained reasons.

Although the exact mechanism of action of anticonvulsants is unknown, it is thought to stabilize the cell membrane by altering the movement of sodium, potassium, and calcium across the membrane. Anticonvulsants often cause drowsiness and may be toxic to the liver. Because there is a small difference between enough drug to be effective and too much drug (causing serious side effects), anticonvulsant doses must be finely adjusted. This is done by monitoring drug concentrations in the blood. Phenytoin (*Dilantin*) is the major drug prescribed. Others include primidone (*Mysoline*), ethosuximide (*Zarontin*), valproic acid (*Depakene*), carbamazepine (*Tegretol*), clonazepam (*Klonopin*), and gabapentin (*Neurontin*).

Antiparkinsonian Agents. Several types of drugs are used to treat Parkinson's disease. Some of them control tremors by interrupting the nerve messages that cause them. Others are used for relaxing rigid muscles. Gentle stimulants help counteract slowness. A combination of levodopa and carbidopa, *Sinemet* is

Pediatric Considerations — Anticonvulsant Medications

- Oral anticonvulsant medications are slowly absorbed and inefficient in newborns, but IM phenobarbital is effective.
- Unlike newborns, oral drugs are rapidly absorbed and have short half-lives in infants and children. As a result of this, therapeutic serum drug levels occur earlier in children than in adults, which means that children need a higher dose per kilogram of body weight than do adults.

- The rapid rate of drug elimination persists until approximately 6 years of age, and then the rate slows to that of an adult by 10 to 14 years of age.
- The effects of most of the newer anticonvulsant drugs are unknown for use in children.
- All but *Keppra* and zonisamide are approved for use in children.

Older Adult Considerations — Anticonvulsant Medications

- Seizures that occur in older adults require drugs.
- Because of multiple conditions and multiple drugs, older adults usually have a decrease in liver and kidney function and are more sensitive to adverse drug reactions of anticonvulsants.
- A cardiac evaluation is indicated when a history of cardiac disease is present.

- A tremor may occur with *Depakote* that could be confused with Parkinson's disease. The usual recommendation is to reduce the dose or discontinue the drug.
- The most common adverse reactions of anticonvulsant medications are ataxia, confusion, dizziness, and drowsiness, but older adults are more likely to develop adverse reactions to specific individual drugs. For example, hyponatremia is more common with *Tegretol,* especially if diuretics that deplete the body of sodium are taken.

widely used because it can be given in smaller doses, with fewer side effects than levodopa alone. Other drugs for Parkinson's disease are benztropine (*Cogentin*), trihexyphenidyl, bromocriptine (*Parlodel*), selegiline (*Eldepryl*), and amantadine.

Dizziness, drowsiness, and blurred vision are common side effects of antiparkinsonian agents. Those that have an anticholinergic effect can cause dry mouth. This is relieved by giving the patient hard candy or gum or by rinsing the mouth with water.

Anesthetic Drugs. **Anesthetic drugs** interfere with the conduction of nerve impulses to produce a loss of sensation and muscle relaxation and may cause a partial or complete loss of consciousness. The two types are local and general anesthetics.

Pediatric Considerations — Antiparkinsonian Drugs

- Parkinson's disease is primarily an adult disease, so the drugs have not been sufficiently studied for use in children.

- Antiparkinsonian drugs are used for other reasons such as drug-induced extrapyramidal reactions.

Older Adult Considerations — Antiparkinsonian Drugs

- Caution must be used with amantadine because it is excreted through the kidneys, and renal function is generally reduced in older adults.
- The dose of levodopa/carbidopa (*Sinemet*) may need to be decreased because of an enzyme that is inhibited with this drug.

- Anticholinergic drugs may also be given but may cause blurred vision, dry mouth, tachycardia, and urinary retention.
- There is an increased risk of hallucinations with dopamine agonist drugs.

Local anesthetics produce a temporary loss of sensation or feeling to a specifically defined area. They are most frequently used to alleviate pain before and during minor surgeries, dental procedures, and delivery. Local anesthetics may also be found in over-the-counter products used to treat sunburns, insect bites, and hemorrhoids. Local anesthetics are administered either topically, by injection, or by infiltration. Topical anesthetics are available as creams, lotions, ointments, sprays, suppositories, eyedrops, and lozenges. Common examples include benzocaine (*Outgro*), dyclonine (*Sucrets Classic Sore Throat*), and lidocaine (*Xylocaine*).

EMLA (lidocaine/prilocaine) has been a huge development in dermal anesthetics. It is made up of lidocaine and prilocaine combined with a thickener and emulsifier, and it is applied as a thick layer to intact skin and covered with a clear wrap to promote penetration of the skin. EMLA allows higher concentrations of local anesthetics to be absorbed than is possible with other topical anesthetics. It may also be used to anesthetize the skin before biopsies, venipuncture, or intramuscular injections.

Injection of local anesthetics may be intradermal (under the skin) or spinal, epidural, or caudal (into the spaces around the spinal cord) or may be by infiltration (directly into tissue). Examples of injectable anesthetics are chloroprocaine (*Nesacaine*), and lidocaine (*Xylocaine*).

Infiltration anesthetics may be combined with epinephrine to double the duration of anesthesia. They may last for up to six hours. Examples of infiltration anesthetics include, mepivacaine (*Carbocaine*), dibucaine (*Nupercainal*), and bupivacaine (*Marcaine*).

Local anesthetics produce an anesthesia effect to a local area but occasionally may be absorbed into the bloodstream, affecting the blood vessels, heart, and brain. Generally, local anesthetics cause vasodilation, bradycardia, and central nervous system effects. A rash or itching may occur due to a release of histamine. A more serious adverse reaction that may develop is hypersensitivity. There are not many drug interactions with local anesthetics.

You should advise your patient that there will be a temporary loss of sensory perception or motor function. Instruct your patient to avoid exposing the skin or gums to extreme temperatures for an hour. Eating and drinking should also be avoided for an hour after topical anesthesia to the throat or after dental procedures.

General anesthetics suppress all sensations and are used primarily to prevent painful stimuli with surgery. They produce a deeper state of unconsciousness, resulting in the patient being unable to respond to stimuli. General anesthetics are administered by inhalation or intravenous injection. They provide rapid delivery of the drug into the bloodstream, facilitating general anesthesia. Although the majority of the effects of general anesthesia are on the central nervous system, they may also affect the cardiac system, salivary and bronchial secretions, skeletal muscles, gastrointestinal tract, and liver. A variety of other drugs may also be used with anesthetics to aid the induction of general anesthesia, counteract the side effects of anesthetics, or make the recovery process more comfortable. Most of the adverse effects that occur after a general anesthetic are related to the residual depression of the central nervous system.

 Caution Nonprescription Pain Relievers

New FDA Guidelines

- The FDA has issued organ-specific warnings for over-the-counter analgesic, antipyretic, and antirheumatic drug products.

Aspirin

- May cause gastrointestinal upset and bleeding.
- Possible allergies (shortness of breath, rash, swelling, hives, asthma, or shock).

Acetaminophen

- Risk of overdose greater than from either aspirin or ibuprofen.
- Individuals who have alcoholism, cirrhosis, or other serious liver diseases should consult their provider before taking acetaminophen.

Ibuprofen

- Should not be taken by individuals who have had a severe allergic reaction to aspirin.
- May cause renal failure.
- May cause gastrointestinal upset and bleeding.

GIVING MEDICATIONS FOR THE NERVOUS AND SENSORY SYSTEMS [LO 17-7]

To give medications that affect the nervous system, you will need to know how to administer drugs efficiently by all the usual routes. In addition, there are specific principles to follow in administering certain types of drugs.

Long-Term Medications

Patients on long-term drug therapy to control seizures and Parkinson's disease must be watched carefully for signs of toxicity (drug poisoning). Your observations may suggest that the patient needs blood and urine studies, and this may help avoid serious overmedication. Patients need to be educated as to the importance of taking their medicines regularly over a long period of time, even after symptoms disappear. Patients with Parkinson's disease may have tremors that make it difficult for them to care for themselves and even to take their medicines. You should stress the importance of continued drug treatment despite their difficulties.

Drugs for Pain

Unfortunately, the reality of actual clinical patient care is that there is often a long delay between the time when a patient feels pain severe enough to alert the nurse and the time when the pain medicine provides relief.

To be effective, analgesics must be given on time. The objective is to keep the patient as comfortable as possible. If you wait too long to give the next dose of analgesic, the last dose will have worn off, the patient will suffer needlessly, and the pain will be much harder to control. In an effort to reduce this time difference, **patient-controlled analgesia (PCA)** pumps may be used. As the name implies, PCA pumps are machines filled with analgesics—often IV morphine or meperidine (*Demerol*)—that patients themselves control.

When pain is felt, the patient simply pushes a button and a dose of analgesia is given. The immediate response puts patients at ease, and they may actually end up using fewer total daily doses of their narcotic. Pumps have a built-in safety mechanism to prevent overdosing.

Let patients know that the medication you are giving is for pain. The psychological effect of telling them their medication will decrease pain may help the drug work better (this is the placebo effect).

If the pain reliever is a narcotic, remember to discard the unused portion (chart this properly!) and the equipment used to administer it. There should be no chance of anyone else using the leftover medication.

Some analgesics have antipyretic (fever-reducing) effects. With these drugs, take the patient's temperature as ordered, give extra liquids, and chart these procedures so that the provider can review the patient's progress.

Pain medications ordered before surgery must be given on time so that they take effect before the procedure begins. Insist on undisturbed bed rest for the patient after giving a preoperative medication. This will help the medication take effect. Encourage the family to cooperate with your instructions. After surgery, check on the patient often and administer pain medications as needed. An anesthetic does not eliminate the pain of surgery. It only makes the patient drift in and out of consciousness. During conscious moments, the patient may feel pain.

Stimulants

Dryness in the mouth is a side effect of some stimulants and other CNS drugs. To counteract dryness, suggest using hard candy or sugarless gum or rinsing the mouth with water.

Emergency Drugs

Many medical emergencies are treated with drugs that affect the nervous system. Emergency drugs are powerful, and errors in dosage can be extremely hazardous. Be certain to check the dosage strength and the route before administering them. As a matter of routine, the supply of emergency drugs should be reviewed often to be sure all medications are in good condition and not discolored or expired.

Explain the possible effects of emergency nervous system drugs to the patient to avoid fear and worry when new symptoms appear. Support the patient's family in emergency situations.

Emergency patients often receive IV infusions. Be careful when moving these patients to avoid letting the fluids pass into surrounding body tissues. Check often to be sure the needle is in the vein.

 Healthcare for Today and Tomorrow Dosing of Analgesics

As a member of the healthcare team administering opioid analgesics to patients, you must assess your patient's response to the analgesic and determine if an alternative route of administration might control your patient's pain better. For example, the rectal route offers an excellent but often overlooked alternative method to administering an oral opioid to a patient who cannot take oral medications because of a difficulty in swallowing. Generally, the dosing of oral and rectal opioids is equal; however, some research supports decreasing the initial dose by approximately 25 percent.

The most common reason for failure in achieving analgesia with a rectal opioid is an insufficient dose. Therefore, your knowledge of the various methods of administering opioids will help match your patient's pain control needs with the most effective and least invasive route.

Somnolence, or falling asleep, has been proved to occur in patients taking pramipexole (*Mirapex*) or ropinirole (*Requip*), two antiparkinsonian drugs used in the treatment of Parkinson's disease. Patients have been reported to fall asleep while eating, talking, and even driving, with serious and often deadly consequences. When these patients discontinued the drug, the somnolence disappeared.

It is your responsibility to warn your patients who are to receive these dopamine agonists of this potential adverse reaction. Patients should be advised to avoid dangerous activities such as driving, drinking alcohol, and taking cimetidine (*Tagamet HB*) until their reaction to *Mirapex* or *Requip* is known.

Representative Drugs for the Nervous and Sensory Systems

Category, Name,[a] and Route	Uses and Diseases	Actions	Usual Dose[b] and Special Instructions	Side Effects and Adverse Reactions
Stimulants				
methylphenidate (*Ritalin*) Oral	Attention-deficit disorder in children, narcolepsy	Is a cerebral stimulant	20–30 mg/day in divided doses for adults; 10 mg/day for children; adjusted individually	Nervousness, insomnia, seizures, hypersensitivity, palpitations
Analgesics				
hydrocodone with acetaminophen (***Vicodin***) Oral	Moderate to moderately severe pain	Hydrocodone produces analgesic action on the CNS by the opiate receptors; acetaminophen analgesic action is produced by both peripheral and central mechanisms (narcotic analgesic)	1–2 tablets (5 mg/500 mg) every 4–6 hours; 1 tablet (7.5 mg/750 mg) every 6 hours (*Vicodin ES*)	Lightheadedness, dizziness, sedation, drowsiness, nausea, vomiting, respiratory depression related to dose
acetaminophen with codeine (***Tylenol with Codeine***) Oral	Mild to moderately severe pain	Inhibits CNS prostaglandin synthesis, producing analgesic effect (acetaminophen); attaches to specific receptors located in the central nervous system, resulting in various CNS effects, which decrease pain impulses (codeine) (narcotic analgesic)	1–2 tablets every 4–6 hours	Dizziness, headache, nausea, vomiting, constipation, rash
oxycodone and aspirin (*Percodan*) Oral	Moderate to severe pain	Relieves pain, sedates, reduces fever	1 tablet every 6 hours prn; give with food or with a full glass of water or milk	Dependence, respiratory depression (especially in elderly), dizziness, drowsiness, gastrointestinal upset, constipation

Representative Drugs for the Nervous and Sensory Systems (continued)

Category, Name,[a] and Route	Uses and Diseases	Actions	Usual Dose[b] and Special Instructions	Side Effects and Adverse Reactions
Analgesics (continued)				
pentazocine (*Talwin*) Oral, IM, subcutaneous, IV	Moderate to severe pain; preparation for surgery	Relieves pain, sedates	50–100 mg every 3–4 hours PO; 30 mg IM; caution patient to avoid alcohol and OTC drugs	Dependence, dizziness, drowsiness, euphoria, nausea, dyspnea, hypotension, dry mouth, urinary retention
meperidine (*Demerol*) IM, subcutaneous, IV, oral	Moderate to severe pain; preparation for surgery	Relieves pain, sedates	50–100 mg every 3–4 hours prn orally or parenterally; may cause drowsiness; caution patient to avoid alcohol	Dependence, dizziness, drowsiness, nausea, flushing, sweating, dry mouth, orthostatic hypotension, seizures
Anticonvulsants				
clonazepam (***Klonopin***) Oral	Absence, akinetic, myoclonic seizures	Controls seizures without impairing the normal functioning of the central nervous system; selectively depresses the hyperactive areas of the brain that cause seizures	0.5 mg tid, increase by 0.5–1 mg every 3 days until seizures under control	Rash; fever; headache; pain or swelling in the mouth, nose, urinary tract; sore throat; bruising; dark urine; loss of appetite; abdominal pain
gabapentin (***Neurontin***) Oral	Partial seizures	Controls seizures, anticonvulsant action unknown	900–1800 mg/day in 3 divided doses	Somnolence, ataxia, dizziness, fatigue, nystagmus, tremor, nervousness, dysarthria, amnesia, depression, abnormal thinking, twitching, headache
phenytoin sodium (*Dilantin*) Oral, IV	Grand mal epilepsy; psychomotor seizures; tonic-clonic seizures	Controls seizures	300 mg/day divided every 8 hours for liquid oral and IV administration	Back-and-forth eye movements (nystagmus); diplopia (double vision); swollen, tender gums; staggering walk (ataxia); slurred speech; constipation; dizziness; nausea and vomiting; rashes; anemia; sedation

Representative Drugs for the Nervous and Sensory Systems *(continued)*

Category, Name,[a] and Route	Uses and Diseases	Actions	Usual Dose[b] and Special Instructions	Side Effects and Adverse Reactions
Anticonvulsants (continued)				
carbamazepine (*Tegretol*) Oral	Tonic-clonic seizures; other seizure types	Is a prophylactic treatment of seizures	200 mg bid increased to 800–1200 mg/day; should not be used by pregnant women or nursing mothers	Dizziness, drowsiness, nausea, vomiting, ataxia, mouth sores
Antiparkinsonian Drugs				
carbidopa and levodopa (*Sinemet*) Oral	Parkinson's disease or Parkinson-like symptoms	Reduces rigidity of head and limbs; is a **dopaminergic** (involving activity of a neurotransmitter)	*Initial dose:* 1 tablet (10 mg carbidopa/100 mg levodopa or 25/100) tid *Maintenance dose:* 1–2 tablets (25/250) tid, individually adjusted; watch for symptoms of depression; give with food; may cause drowsiness	Mood changes; unusual, uncontrolled body movements; palpitations; difficult urination; dry mouth; nausea; vomiting; orthostatic hypotension
benztropine mesylate (*Cogentin*) Oral, IM	Parkinson's disease adjunct	Is an anticholinergic	0.5–6 mg/day	Dry mouth, blurred vision, constipation, palpitations
Alzheimer's Drugs				
donepezil (*Aricept*) Oral	Mild to moderate dementia of Alzheimer's disease	Enhances cholinergic function by increasing levels of acetylcholine	5 mg daily, may increase to 10 mg after 4–6 weeks	Nausea, vomiting, diarrhea, insomnia, dizziness, hypertension, headaches, muscle cramps, urinary incontinence, dyspnea
rivastigmine (*Exelon*) Oral	Mild to moderate dementia of Alzheimer's disease	Enhances cholinergic function by increasing levels of acetylcholine	1.5 mg bid	Nausea, vomiting, diarrhea, anorexia, weight loss, dizziness, headache, hypotension, rashes, arthritis, rhinitis, anemia
memantine (*Namenda*) Oral	Moderate to severe dementia of Alzheimer's disease	Affinity as an antagonist for N-methyl-D-aspartate receptors, preventing activation of glutamate (an excitatory amino acid)	5 mg daily; may increase in increment doses to 10 mg bid	Constipation, vomiting, melena, dizziness, headache, vertigo, hypertension, coughing, frequent micturition, cataracts, fatigue, pain

Representative Drugs for the Nervous and Sensory Systems (*continued*)

Category, Name,[a] and Route	Uses and Diseases	Actions	Usual Dose[b] and Special Instructions	Side Effects and Adverse Reactions
Antimigraine Drugs				
sumatriptan succinate (*Imitrex*) Subcutaneous, oral, inhalation	Migraine headaches	Agonist for vascular 5-HT₁ receptor subtype	6 mg subcutaneously but no more than 12 mg in 24 hours; 25 mg, 50 mg, or 100 mg orally at onset of migraine; may repeat in 2 hours but not more than 200 mg daily; 5 mg, 10 mg, or 20 mg as a nasal spray; may repeat in 2 hours up to 40 mg daily	Angina pectoris, flushing, hyper- or hypotension, bradycardia, tachycardia, palpitations

Note: Bolded trade names are among the 50 most commonly prescribed drugs.

[a]*Trade names given in parentheses are examples only. Check current drug references for a complete listing of available products.*

[b]*Average adult doses are given. However, dosages are determined by a provider and vary with the purpose of the therapy and the particular patient. The doses presented in this text are for general information only.*

Summary

Learning Outcome	Summary Points
17-1 List the main divisions and parts of the nervous system.	• *Central nervous system (CNS)* consists of the brain and spinal cord. • *Peripheral nervous system (PNS)* consists of cranial and spinal nerves and peripheral components of the autonomic nervous system (ANS).
17-2 Identify the basic function of the autonomic nervous system.	• Regulate the functions of the cardiac and smooth muscles.
17-3 Know the correct medical terms for symptoms of nervous system disorders.	• Tremor • Spasticity • Vertigo • Paralysis • Stupor • Insomnia • Bradykinesia and rigidity occur with Parkinson's disease • Convulsions occur with epilepsy

Learning Outcome	Summary Points
17-4 Recognize descriptions of the major nervous system disorders for which medications are given.	• *Parkinson's disease* is a syndrome characterized by bradycardia and rigidity, tremor, and impaired postural reflexes. • *Myasthenia gravis* is a disease of the neuromuscular junction characterized by a fluctuating weakness in certain skeletal muscle groups. • *Multiple sclerosis* is a chronic, progressive, degenerative disease that attacks the myelin sheath of the nerves. • *Epilepsy* is a set of disorders that cause periodic seizures. • *Cerebrovascular accident* is the sudden onset of a neurologic deficit resulting from disease of the blood vessels that supply the brain. • *Transient ischemic attack* is a period of neurologic deficit disease. • *Alzheimer's disease* is a chronic, progressive, degenerative disease of the brain. • *Migraine headache* is a unilateral or bilateral throbbing pain.
17-5 Articulate to patients how to prevent strokes.	• Have blood pressure checks. • Take blood pressure medications. • Reduce salt intake. • Stop smoking. • Reduce or control weight. • Decrease foods high in saturated fats and cholesterol. • Avoid drinking alcohol. • Inform the provider about oral contraceptives. • Increase daily activity. • Increase fruits and vegetables in the diet.
17-6 Describe the actions of the following drug groups: central nervous system stimulants, analgesics, anticonvulsants, antiparkinsonians, Alzheimer's drugs, and antimigraine drugs.	• *Central nervous system stimulants* are used primarily for attention-deficit disorders. An example is *Ritalin*. • *Analgesics* relieve pain either by affecting the brain itself or by interfering with the ability of pain around the body to send pain messages to the brain. *Demerol* is an example. • *Anticonvulsants'* exact action is unknown, but they are thought to stabilize the cell membrane by altering the movement of sodium, potassium, and calcium across the membrane. An example is *Dilantin*. • *Antiparkinsonian drugs* either interrupt the nerve messages that cause tremors or relax rigid muscles. An example is *Cogentin*. • *Alzheimer's drugs* (cholinesterase inhibitors) break down acetylcholine in the synaptic cleft. An example is *Aricept*. • Antimigraine drugs include alpha-adrenergic blocking agents.
17-7 Know the principles for administering pain medications, long-term medications, stimulants, and emergency drugs.	• Educate the patient on the administration of analgesics and what is being administered, and administer them on time. • Take the patient's temperature with some analgesics because of the antipyretic effects. • Take blood and urine samples to prevent serious overmedication with long-term medications. • Encourage patients to take medications until gone even after symptoms are gone. • Encourage patients to chew gum or suck on hard candy for dry mouth. • Ensure that emergency drugs are in good condition and are not discolored before use. • Explain the purpose of emergency drugs to the patient. • Move the patient carefully to avoid letting fluids pass into surrounding tissues.

Chapter 17 Review

Define each of the terms listed.

1. (LO 17-3) Tremor _____

2. (LO 17-3) Vertigo _____

3. (LO 17-3) Paralysis _____

4. (LO 17-3) Coma _____

5. (LO 17-3) Stupor _____

6. (LO 17-3) Insomnia _____

7. (LO 17-3) Bradykinesia _____

8. (LO 17-3) Seizure _____

Complete the statements by filling in the blanks.

9. (LO 17-1) The two main divisions of the nervous system are the _____ nervous system and the _____ nervous system.

10. (LO 17-1) The _____ carries messages from the peripheral nerves to the brain.

11. (LO 17-1) The organs of the chest and the abdomen are regulated automatically by a part of the peripheral nervous system called the _____ nervous system.

12. (LO 17-4) Foods high in saturated fat and cholesterol should be reduced in the prevention of _____.

Tell what these types of drugs do; for example, Cerebral stimulants speed up brain activity, which speeds up the whole body.

13. (LO 17-6) Analgesics _____

14. (LO 17-6) Antipyretics _____

15. (LO 17-6) Anticonvulsants _____

Match the drug categories to the drug names.

_____ 16. (LO 17-6) Caffeine, *Ritalin*

_____ 17. (LO 17-6) *Demerol, Percodan,* morphine

_____ 18. (LO 17-6) Aspirin, acetaminophen

_____ 19. (LO 17-6) *Dilantin,* valproic acid, phenobarbital

_____ 20. (LO 17-6) trihexyphenidyl, benztropine

_____ 21. (LO 17-6) *Xylocaine, Nupercainal, Marcaine*

_____ 22. (LOs 17-3, 17-4) Donepezil, *Exelon, Namenda*

_____ 23. (LOs 17-3, 17-4) *Imitrex, Topamax*

a. anesthetics

b. analgesic antipyretics

c. anticonvulsants

d. cerebral stimulants

e. Alzheimer's drugs

f. narcotic analgesics

g. antiparkinsonian drugs

h. antimigraine drugs

Complete the statements by filling in the blank.

24. (LO 17-7) Patients on long-term drug therapy should be encouraged to _____.

25. (LO 17-7) Patients should also be watched for any signs of drug _____.

26. (LO 17-7) To keep the patient as comfortable as possible, analgesics must be given _____.

27. (LO 17-7) Always _____ any leftover narcotic and the equipment used to administer it.

28. (LO 17-7) With analgesic antipyretics, take the patient's _____.

29. (LO 17-7) To soothe a dry mouth caused by stimulants or antiparkinsonian agents, give the patient _____ or rinse the mouth with water.

Drug Calculations—Fill in the blank with the answer.

30. (LO 17-6) The provider orders benztropine mesylate (*Cogentin*) 1.5 mg intramuscularly bid. Available is 1 mg/mL. Prepare to administer _____ mL to your patient.

31. (LO 17-6) The provider orders valproic acid (*Depakene*) syrup 0.75 g orally daily. Available is 250 mg/5 mL. Prepare to administer _____ mL to your patient.

32. (LO 17-6) The provider orders methylphenidate (*Ritalin*) 10 mg orally tid. Available are 20-mg tablets. You will give your patient _____ tablets.

33. (LO 17-6) The provider orders meperidine (*Demerol*) 75 mg intramuscularly stat. Available is 100 mg/mL. Prepare to administer _____ mL to your patient.

34. (LO 17-6) The provider orders phenytoin (*Dilantin*) 200 mg orally bid. Available are 100-mg capsules. You will give _____ capsules to your patient.

Multiple Choice—Circle the correct letter.

35. (LO 17-6) Which of the following are the major side effects of antiparkinsonian drugs?
    a. Diarrhea, abdominal cramping, hypertension
    b. Urinary frequency, bladder spasms, ataxia
    c. Dizziness, drowsiness, blurred vision
    d. Somnolence, tremor, amnesia

36. (LO 17-7) Which of the following drugs are often abused?
    a. Anticonvulsants
    b. Narcotic analgesics
    c. Anesthetic drugs
    d. Antiparkinsonian drugs

37. (LO 17-6) What is the patient education that you should provide about caffeine?
    a. Nervousness, irritability, or headache may result from drinking two cups of caffeine daily.
    b. Limit caffeine if breastfeeding.
    c. Drink only caffeine beverages before bedtime.
    d. Chocolate, cocoa, and soft drinks do not contain caffeine.

38. (LO 17-6) What controlled substance increases the risk of toxicity to the CNS?
    a. Schedule I
    b. Schedule II
    c. Schedule III
    d. Schedule IV

39. (LO 17-7) Which of the following nonprescription medications has a greater risk of overdose?
    a. *Motrin IB*
    b. *Advil*
    c. Aspirin
    d. *Tylenol*

Chapter 17 Case Studies

40. (LO 17-5) You have been instructed to watch for signs of a cerebrovascular accident as you work with a patient. What is the definition of a stroke? What are the signs to report? The nurse asks you to reinforce the prevention of stroke. What should you tell the patient? _____

_____

_____

_____

41. (LO 17-4) A patient's wife tells you she suspects her husband has Alzheimer's disease. What are the early warning signs of Alzheimer's disease? _____

_____

_____

_____

Critical Thinking

Select the disorder that best matches the patient description and write it in the blank.

epilepsy	stroke or CVA	meningitis
Parkinson's disease	multiple sclerosis (MS)	Alzheimer's disease

42. (LO 17-4) Mr. Brown has trouble getting dressed in the morning because his hands shake so badly. When he walks, he moves very slowly and has trouble keeping his balance.

_____

43. (LO 17-4) Dick Takei has blurred vision in his left eye, and his left leg is paralyzed. The provider says it is because the disease has destroyed some of the myelin sheath that covers the nerves.

_____

44. (LO 17-4) Mrs. Poston has a sudden hemorrhage in a part of the brain. This causes her to feel dizzy and have difficulty speaking.

_____

45. (LO 17-4) Sam Houston, an older adult, gets lost frequently and misplaces his personal belongings.

_____

46. (LO 17-4) Marta Weiss is taking *Dilantin* regularly. If she were to skip a dose, she knows she might have a seizure.

_____

47. (LO 17-4) George Thompson has a serious inflammation of the covering of the brain and the spinal cord.

_____

Applications

Obtain an electronic drug guide or a current copy of the *PDR®* from your school, health facility, or clinic. Use it to answer the following questions in a notebook or on file cards.

48. In Section 2 of the *PDR®*, Brand and Generic Name Index, find another product name for each of the drugs in the Representative Drugs for the Nervous and Sensory Systems table in this chapter.

49. In Section 3 of the *PDR®*, Product Category Index, find the subheading Serotonin Uptake Inhibitors. List all the drugs in this category.

chapter

18

PSYCHOTROPIC DRUGS

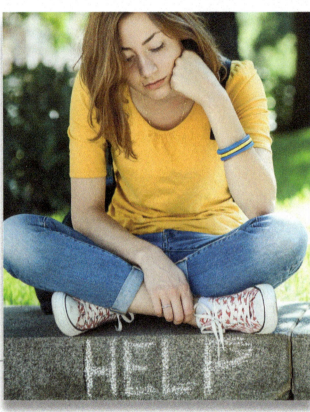

©Mixmike/Getty Images

In this chapter you will learn how the central nervous system and biochemical mechanisms relate to emotions. You will become familiar with the major mental disorders and the drugs used to treat them, how to properly administer them, and how to prevent unwanted side effects.

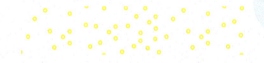

THE NERVOUS SYSTEM AND EMOTIONS [LO 18-1]

Knowledge of how the nervous system functions is essential to understanding the actions of psychotherapeutic drugs. You have already learned how the central nervous system controls bodily functions such as heart rate, blood pressure, respiration, temperature, and gastric secretions (Chapter 17). Now you will learn how the central nervous system is responsible for behavior, memory, learning, consciousness, imagination, and abstract thinking.

Biochemical Mechanisms

The functions of the central nervous system are dependent on the actions of neurohormonal agents in the brain. The neurohormones stimulate transmission of reactions. During activity, acetylcholine is released from nervous system tissue to the cerebrospinal fluid. Norepinephrine is also present in the central nervous system. Tyrosine and dopamine are normal constituents of the brain. Both norepinephrine and dopamine function as transmitters. They have both inhibitory and excitatory effects on functions such as sleep, arousal, and memory. Serotonin is another transmitter substance found in the central nervous system. Alterations in the level of serotonin are associated with changes in behavior. Other neurotransmitters include histamine, amino acids, and prostaglandin. There is strong evidence that dopamine, serotonin, and histamines play an important role in maintaining mental health. The role dopamine plays in psychotic disorders has received much attention over the years. Drugs such as the phenothiazines block the effect of dopamine.

MENTAL DISORDERS [LO 18-2, LO 18-3]

Depression

There are two types of **depression**. **Major depression** is a substantial psychological, social, and occupational disability in which the patient experiences considerable suffering and a significant change in usual functioning. Patients may have recurrent thoughts of suicide. Sixty percent of patients with a major depressive episode will have another episode.

The second type of depression is **dysthymia**. It is characterized by a minimal psychological, social, and occupational impairment. It occurs in early childhood to early adulthood. Patients with dysthymia are at risk for developing major depression.

Psychosis

Psychosis is an impaired ability to recognize reality, a demonstration of bizarre behaviors, and an inability to deal with life's demands. It is characterized by **hallucinations**, a disorder of perception involving one of the five senses, and **delusions**, false beliefs that are resistant to reasoning. **Schizophrenia** is a mental illness in which psychosis is the classic feature. In addition to hallucinations and delusions, patients may experience disorganized speech and grossly disorganized behavior or **catatonia**. Patients with schizophrenia may benefit from antipsychotic drugs.

Psychological Disorders

Disorders of the thought processes and emotions account for many uses of drugs that affect the nervous system. Psychological disorders range from mild depression or anxiety to severe changes in behavior. Drugs that energize, tranquilize, and control mood swings are among the types used for these conditions. They act by stimulating or depressing the CNS or specific parts of the brain. Mild tranquilizers, sedatives, and antidepressants are prescribed for people with temporary emotional problems or anxiety. For example, patients who are worried about upcoming surgery or about an illness might be given a mild sedative to help them sleep.

Much more powerful antipsychotic drugs are used to control symptoms in patients with severe behavior changes. These changes include psychotic depression, manic-depressive psychosis, and schizophrenia, which keep the patient from functioning in daily life.

Alcoholism

Alcoholism is a chronic, progressive disease that if left untreated can be fatal. It does not matter if a person is an occasional drinker or alcohol-dependent, the consequences are negative. Disulfiram (*Antabuse*) is used to prevent the ingestion of alcohol in chronic alcoholics and produces a severe hypersensitivity to alcohol. It inhibits liver enzymes that are part of a normal degradation of alcohol, which results in an accumulation of acetaldehyde in the blood. High levels of acetaldehyde produce a wide variety of symptoms referred to as a disulfiram-alcohol reaction. *Antabuse* is a tablet that may need to be given for months or years.

Vivitrol is a version of the drug naltrexone and is the first injectable drug to treat alcohol dependence. It is thought to decrease the urge to drink by blocking neurotransmitters in the brain associated with alcohol dependence. It does not affect alcohol withdrawal symptoms. It is administered intramuscularly monthly to patients who are also in counseling. The incidence of heavy drinking decreases more when the patient receives both *Vivitrol* and counseling than when the patient just receives counseling. Adverse reactions include **insomnia** (sleeplessness), nausea, vomiting, diarrhea, headache, dizziness, fatigue, and injection site discomfort. Depression and suicidal tendencies may occur in some patients and should be reported immediately.

Pediatric Concerns

Attention-deficit hyperactivity disorder (ADHD) and learning disability (LD) affect every aspect of a child's life but are most obvious in the classroom. Attention-deficit hyperactivity disorder refers to developmentally inappropriate degrees of inattention, impulsiveness, and hyperactivity. The symptoms are present before the age of 7 years. Learning disability refers to a group of disorders manifested by difficulties in listening, speaking, reading, writing, reasoning, mathematic abilities, or social skills. Frequently prescribed medications are dextroamphetamine (*Dexedrine*) and methylphenidate

(*Ritalin*). Not all children benefit from these medications. Side effects include nervousness, insomnia, decreased appetite, and weight loss. Long-term use of *Dexedrine* may cause suppressed growth.

Various salts of amphetamine and dextroamphetamine have been combined into a drug named *Adderall,* used in the treatment of ADHD. It is given in a morning dose, which eliminates a midday dose in the school setting. *Adderall* has been proved to be equivalent to *Ritalin. Adderall* does have a high potential for abuse. If prescribed for long periods of time, a drug dependency may occur. Therefore it should be prescribed sparingly.

SELECTION AND USE OF PSYCHOTROPIC DRUGS [LO 18-4, LO 18-5]

Drug therapy plays a major role in contemporary approaches to psychiatric care. The administration of drugs alleviates a patient's symptoms, such as disturbances in mood and behavior, and facilitates compliance with other forms of treatment, such as psychotherapy. Although the drugs exert changes in mood and behavior, the changes are only temporary. It is through psychotherapy that permanent changes in mood and behavior occur (**Figure 18.1**). The appropriate selection of psychotherapeutic drugs is made by a provider on the basis of the patient's diagnosis. The provider matches the patient's symptoms to a particular drug's therapeutic effects.

Antidepressants

These drugs intervene in the chemical processes in the brain. In so doing, they relieve severe depression. They work to normalize the chemical imbalance.

One group of antidepressants is called monoamine oxidase inhibitors (MAOIs). These drugs prevent an enzyme, monoamine oxidase, from metabolizing certain chemicals needed for nerve impulses to pass between neurons. By blocking the destruction of these chemicals, they aid the passage of nerve impulses, which appears to counteract depression. These drugs are used to treat depression with features that include hypersomnia, weight gain, mood swings, and sensitivity in interpersonal relationships. They have also been used with success for anxiety disorders, eating disorders, and migraine headaches. The major side effects of these drugs are orthostatic hypotension, dry mouth, blurred vision, urinary retention, constipation, and weight gain. These drugs

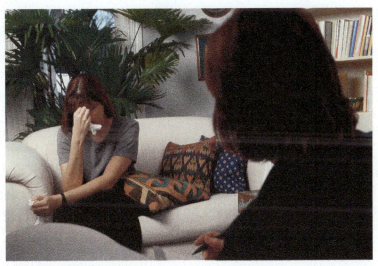

Figure 18.1

A combination of psychotherapy and drug therapy can benefit the patient and allow for permanent changes in mood and behavior.

©David Buffington/Getty Images

may have dangerous side effects, mainly hypertensive crisis, when mixed with certain other drugs (e.g., antiasthmatics, antihypertensives, allergy and cold medications) and certain foods (e.g., cheese, liver, alcohol). Examples of MAO inhibitors are tranylcypromine (*Parnate*), isocarboxazid (*Marplan*), and phenelzine (*Nardil*). Selegiline (*Emsam*) is a transdermal MAO inhibitor that may be prescribed for depression.

Another chemical group of antidepressants is the tricyclic antidepressants. These drugs increase the concentration of impulse-transmitting chemicals between neurons. Examples of tricyclic antidepressants are amitriptyline, doxepin, amoxapine, desipramine (*Norpramin*), nortriptyline (*Pamelor*), imipramine (*Tofranil*), and clomipramine (*Anafranil*). *Anafranil* is commonly used in the treatment of obsessive-compulsive disorder. Its effectiveness in the treatment of depression is still under investigation. Unfortunately, tricyclic antidepressants have frequent side effects, such as dry mouth, blurred vision, constipation, sedation, and orthostatic hypotension.

Other antidepressants classified as selective serotonin reuptake inhibitors (SSRIs) act to block the reuptake of serotonin. Serotonin is a potent vasoconstrictor that is important in sleep and sensory perception. Escitalopram oxalate (*Lexapro*) is an SSRI that has an antidepressant effect occurring as a result of the inhibition of the neuronal uptake of serotonin. Other examples include citalopram (*Celexa*), paroxetine (*Paxil*), fluoxetine (*Prozac*), and sertraline (*Zoloft*). Vilazodone hydrochloride (*Viibryd*) and duloxetine (*Cymbalta*) have been approved by the FDA to also treat osteoarthritic back pain. These serotonin inhibitors have fewer side effects and are better tolerated than tricyclic antidepressants. Their side effects include nausea, drowsiness, dizziness, headache, sweating, insomnia, and anorexia. Desvenlafaxine (*Pristiq*) is a serotonin-norepinephrine reuptake inhibitor (SNRI) indicated in the treatment of major depression.

Other miscellaneous antidepressants that may be prescribed for depression include trazodone, bupropion (*Wellbutrin XL*), and venlafaxine (*Effexor XR*). *Wellbutrin XL* has also received FDA approval to be used in the treatment of seasonal affective disorder.

Patients should be educated to avoid alcohol, OTC drugs, and restricted foods while on antidepressants. Close watch must be kept for serious side effects, especially changes in blood pressure, and dosages must be carefully individualized. The provider increases the patient's dose slowly while the body becomes accustomed to the drug.

 Pediatric Considerations | Antidepressants

- Depression increases after puberty.
- There is an increased risk of suicide with the use of antidepressants.
- Few antidepressants may be used in children.
- Drug therapy should be used only when nonpharmacological measures have failed.
- SSRIs are considered safer than tricyclic antidepressants and monoamine oxidase inhibitors and may be used for severe depression.

- Fluoxetine (*Prozac*) is used for major depression and obsessive-compulsive disorder.
- Sertraline (*Zoloft*) also is used for obsessive-compulsive disorder.
- Tricyclic antidepressants may be used for enuresis.
- Sexual dysfunction may occur with SSRIs.
- Lithium is not approved for children under the age of 12 years but may be used to treat bipolar disorder and aggressiveness.
- Risperidone (*Risperdal*) was recently approved for use in type I bipolar disorder.

Antianxiety, Sedative, and Hypnotic Drugs

Antianxiety drugs, also called anxiolytics, are **minor tranquilizers**. Generally, **anxiety** is a normal physiological and psychological mechanism that protects an individual from a threatening situation. This protective mechanism triggers the "fight or flight" reaction.

Sedatives and hypnotics are central nervous system depressants. The major difference between a sedative and a hypnotic is the degree of central nervous system depression. **Sedatives** produce a calming effect and decrease nervousness and excitability. **Hypnotics** are used to produce sleep. In the past, **barbiturates** were used as sedatives and hypnotics, but because of their many side effects, they have been replaced by benzodiazepines. **Benzodiazepines** do not cause a generalized central nervous system depressant effect. They have muscle relaxant, antianxiety, anticonvulsant, and hypnotic properties. The most frequent side effects are drowsiness and decreased coordination. Examples of benzodiazepines are alprazolam (*Xanax*), chlordiazepoxide, lorazepam (*Ativan*), diazepam (*Valium*), oxazepam, midazolam, flurazepam, temazepam (*Restoril*), and triazolam (*Halcion*). These drugs may cause drowsiness, so the patient must avoid tasks that require alertness. Flumazenil (*Romazicon*) is an antidote for benzodiazepine-induced sedation or benzodiazepine overdose.

There are many other drugs in the sedative/hypnotic category. Some of the better-known drugs are buspirone, hydroxyzine (*Vistaril*), eszopiclone (*Lunesta*), and zolpidem (*Ambien*).

- Because older adults have a slowed excretion of drugs, the dose will last longer.
- Dosages generally should be small.
- There is an increased risk of falls, and this should be carefully watched in older adults.
- Although SSRIs are antidepressants, they are considered to be the first-line drugs for anxiety because of their lower incidence of side effects.
- Short-acting benzodiazepines are recommended over long-acting ones. Examples include alprazolam (*Xanax*) and lorazepam (*Ativan*).

- Buspirone may be preferred over benzodiazepines because of a decreased risk of falls.
- Sedatives/hypnotics are not recommended for insomnia in older adults.
- If a sedative/hypnotic is used, short-acting benzodiazepines are recommended because there are fewer side effects.
- Avoid giving a sedative/hypnotic for more than a few days.

Ramelteon (*Rozerem*) is the first insomnia drug that acts by a mechanism other than central nervous system depression. It is a melatonin receptor antagonist and structurally similar to melatonin. It helps maintain the circadian rhythm underlying the normal wake-sleep cycle. Don't give drug with or immediately after a high-fat meal.

Antipsychotics

Antipsychotics are also known as neuroleptics, or **major tranquilizers**. They are used in patients with a psychotic disorder in which there is an inability to recognize reality and bizarre behaviors are exhibited. Schizophrenia is a psychotic disorder in which antipsychotics are beneficial. Antipsychotics are dopamine receptor blockers. Examples of antipsychotics are perphenazine, thiothixene, molindone, loxapine (*Loxitane*), haloperidol, clozapine (*Clozaril*), thioridazine, trifluoperazine, fluphenazine, chlorpromazine, and risperidone (*Risperdal*). Asenapine (*Saphris*), aripiprazole (*Abilify*), and lurasidone hydrochloride (*Latuda*) are atypical antipsychotics used in the treatment of schizophrenia and acute mania of a bipolar disorder.

The main side effects of antipsychotics are sedation, blurred vision, orthostatic hypotension, dry mouth, tachycardia, urinary retention, constipation, disorientation, and **extrapyramidal** symptoms. The major extrapyramidal symptoms include **dystonia** (muscle spasms of the face, tongue, neck, jaw, or back), **akathisia** (motor restlessness), **tardive dyskinesia** (abnormal involuntary muscle movements around the mouth, lips, and tongue), and Parkinson-like symptoms such as shuffling gait, drooling, tremors, and increased rigidity. Prevention of tardive dyskinesia is essential because this is a permanent side effect. Patients should be closely monitored for these side effects. The side effects are relatively predictable, and their likelihood increases with the size of the dose. The Parkinson-like symptoms may be prevented by simultaneously using either benztropine (*Cogentin*) or diphenhydramine (*Benadryl Allergy*). Patients who take tranquilizers must not drink alcoholic beverages because alcohol potentiates these drugs, and the results could be fatal.

Pediatric Considerations — Antipsychotics

- Antipsychotics are used for childhood schizophrenia, which is more chronic than schizophrenia in adults.
- Because children have less body fat than adults, more frequent administration may be necessary.
- A faster metabolism than that of adults may necessitate a higher dose for the child's size and weight.
- *Risperdal* is gaining popularity as the first atypical antipsychotic drug used for the treatment of schizophrenia.
- Quetiapine (*Seroquel*) carries a black-box warning of an increased risk of suicide.
- Prochlorperazine, trifluoperazine, and haloperidol may be used in children over the age of 2.
- Extrapyramidal symptoms occur more commonly in children than in adults.
- Hypotension is a common side effect.

Older Adult Considerations — Antipsychotics

- Use antipsychotics cautiously in older adults.
- Rule out psychiatric symptoms caused by organic disease.
- Medical conditions such as cardiovascular disease, liver damage, and Parkinson's disease contraindicate the use of these drugs.
- Antipsychotics should be used cautiously with diabetes mellitus, glaucoma, peptic ulcer disease, prostatic hypertrophy, and chronic respiratory disorders.
- Use the lowest possible dose.
- Antipsychotics may be used with dementia to relieve symptoms, but they do not improve memory loss.
- There is a black-box warning with atypical antipsychotics, or second-generation antipsychotics, because of increased risk of cardiovascular disorders or infections.
- Avoid excessive use in long-term care facilities to control agitation.
- Excessive use of antipsychotics increases the risk of side effects.

Antimanics

Antimanic drugs are used in the treatment of mood disorders or bipolar disorders such as **mania**. The most common bipolar disorder is manic depression. The drug of choice is lithium carbonate. Its exact mechanism of action is unknown. It is known that lithium is an element similar to the chemical properties of sodium. The body uses lithium like sodium; however, sodium is normally required for the conduction of nerve impulses and lithium interferes with nerve conduction. As a result of this, a decrease in the excitability of nerve tissue occurs. Lithium also increases the reuptake of norepinephrine and dopamine while decreasing the release of neurotransmitters.

Because lithium is a toxic drug, lithium blood levels are monitored one to two times a week during initiation of therapy and monthly thereafter. The lithium blood level is generally drawn 8 to 12 hours after taking a dose. It is important to understand that a patient's response to lithium may not be known for one to two weeks after treatment. The therapeutic blood level should be 0.4 to 1.0 mEq/L. Toxic blood levels begin to occur at 2.0 mEq/L. The most common side effects are fine hand tremors, polyuria, thirst, transient and mild nausea, and general discomfort. All of the side effects are dose related. Patient education is essential for compliance and effective lithium therapy.

Patient Education | **Lithium**

- Compliance, cooperation, and commitment are essential for stabilization of manic-depressive disorder.
- Signs of drug toxicity include diarrhea, vomiting, lack of coordination, drowsiness, tinnitus (ringing in the ears), and urinary frequency.
- Notify the provider immediately if any signs of toxicity appear.
- Lithium may produce sodium depletion, so you must follow a normal diet with a consistent sodium level.
- A daily fluid intake of 10 to 12 glasses of water is required.

- Avoid fluids such as coffee, tea, and cola because they aggravate the mania.
- Avoid strenuous exercise, saunas, and hot weather, which result in diaphoresis.
- Weigh yourself daily, and notify the provider of any weight gain. This may occur as a result of sodium retention.
- Report persistent diarrhea because you may need supplemental fluids or salt.
- Notify the provider when ill and experiencing vomiting, diarrhea, or sweating.
- Report for all appointments to check blood lithium levels.
- Carry a medical identification card.

 Pediatric Considerations | **Antimanics**

- Do not use lithium carbonate.
- Antimanics are approved for use in bipolar disorder and aggressiveness.
- Lithium is excreted quicker in children than in adults.
- Carefully monitor the lithium blood level.

- Administer the smallest possible dose.
- Risperidone (*Risperdal*) may be used in adolescents 10 to 17 years of age with type I bipolar disorder. It may be used by itself or with lithium.

 Older Adult Considerations | **Antimanics**

- Lithium is approved for use in the treatment of manic depression.
- Start with the smallest possible dose, and adjust or increase the dose as indicated by the blood serum level.

- Monitor the patient closely for adverse reactions.

GIVING MEDICATIONS [LO 18-6]

To give medications that affect the nervous system, you will need to know how to administer drugs efficiently by all the usual routes. In addition, there are specific principles to follow in administering certain types of drugs.

Sedatives/Hypnotics

When sedatives are being prescribed, the provider's concern is to order an amount that enables the patient to be quieted and comfortable but not so much that he or she is in a daze and unable to function normally. You can make sedatives more effective if you follow the guidelines given in **Table 18.1**.

Table 18.1 Guidelines That Make Sedatives More Effective

- Reduce the noise level in the patient's room.
- Avoid loud talking.
- Turn down the television.
- Offer the patient a warm bath or back rub.
- Encourage the patient to verbalize concerns or fears about taking sedatives.
- Ensure adequate exercise for the patient.
- Avoid overuse of hypnotics if possible.

When sedatives are ordered PRN, be sure to ask the patient for the reason when he or she requests a sedative. If the reason is pain, sedatives will not help. The patient will need an analgesic to relieve the pain that is interfering with sleep.

Do not be too concerned about the possibility of drug dependence with sedatives/hypnotics if a patient is hospitalized for an illness. This is a period of great concern and tension. The patient's worries may be greater because of the unfamiliar surroundings of the hospital. Do not withhold PRN medications unless you have carefully evaluated the situation. Withholding PRN medications when they are really needed is as bad as giving them too often.

On the other hand, avoid overuse of sedatives. Do not give sedatives just to avoid listening to the patient's complaints and worries. Sedatives are no substitute for good care. Also, do not leave sedatives at the bedside to take as needed. If the patient takes the drugs too often or all at one time, overdose is possible.

Be observant of patients who are taking CNS depressants. Check their vital signs (pulse, blood pressure, respirations, etc.) often, and report any notable changes. The dosage must be changed if a medication depresses the nervous system too much. Drugs such as the narcotics and barbiturates that depress the whole CNS tend to cause respiratory depression (very slow breathing) when an overdose is taken or given.

Look for idiosyncratic responses and drug interactions. Older adult patients often become confused while under sedation. Depressant drugs given during the day may unexpectedly potentiate a sedative given at night.

Allow the proper amount of time for drugs to show their effects. Long-acting sedatives/hypnotics, such as phenobarbital, may take 30 to 60 minutes to give the desired results.

If patients are confined to bed and are taking sedatives, help protect them from complications. Their medication will keep them from moving about. You will need to change their positions often to prevent bedsores and pneumonia. The medications may also dry mucous membranes. Lubricate the eyes, the mouth, and the nose to prevent sores caused by dryness. Sugarless chewing gum and rinsing the mouth with water also help relieve dryness.

Giving Drugs to Alcoholics

Be conscientious about giving medications to alcoholic patients. The medications are prescribed for their nutritional and psychological needs so that they can recover from their alcoholism. Be sure to explain what drugs you are giving and what they are supposed to do. This will calm the patients' fears and gain their support for treatment.

Psychiatric Patients

The care of psychiatric patients requires special training and knowledge. Medication handlers must fully understand the actions and the long-term side effects of antipsychotic drugs. Along with drug therapy, these patients often receive psychological therapy. As they begin to respond to drug therapy, there is sometimes a danger that they may attempt to commit suicide. You must be sure they do not manage to "pocket" their medications inside their cheeks and then spit them out when you are not looking. They may try to save pills in this way to take a fatal overdose later. Stay with patients until they swallow their oral medications, and watch carefully for signs of toxicity. Never forget to treat these patients kindly and with respect, despite any behaviors they may show.

DRUG ABUSE [LO 18-7]

Nervous system drugs are prone to abuse. This is true of aspirin as well as of narcotics, sedatives/hypnotics, and stimulants. Help educate patients about the dangers of drug overuse. Support their efforts to understand and cope with their disease so that they do not depend on drugs for their support. Be aware, too, of opportunities for the misuse of alcohol and amphetamines. These are the most commonly abused drugs:

- Hallucinogens (psychedelics): LSD, marijuana (aka "grass," "pot," "dope"), mescaline.
- Narcotics: heroin, methadone, morphine, opium, *Demerol*.
- Sedatives and tranquilizers: alcohol, barbiturates (aka "barbs," "phennies," "sleepees"), pentobarbital (*Nembutal*), secobarbital (*Seconal*).
- Stimulants: glue, cocaine ("crack"), methamphetamines ("ice").

 Healthcare for Today and Tomorrow | *Zyprexa Zydis* Administration

A vehicle for medication administration is a freeze-dried wafer that dissolves almost instantly on contact with saliva. Olanzapine (*Zyprexa Zydis*) is an antipsychotic drug administered by wafer to patients with schizophrenia or a bipolar mania. This is a safe and effective method of medication administration, especially to patients who may pocket their medications in the cheek and spit them out later to prevent taking them. It is important that you understand that the term *Zydis* always indicates the medication will be administered by wafer and nothing else. It does not designate an active ingredient.

 Legal and Ethical Issues | Providing Patient Medication Information

It has been reported that in some psychiatric facilities it is common practice to crush a patient's medications, mix them in food, and administer them without the patient's knowledge or consent. Healthcare members accept this as standard practice to ensure patient compliance with medication therapy and to prevent patients from refusing medications, which could lead to undesirable behavior such as acting out or confusion. You must recognize this as an unethical practice that violates the patient's right to know. It is important that you abide by medication policies that state your responsibilities to inform your patients about their medications, the risks, and the benefits. You must also be knowledgeable about policies dealing with the right to refuse medications and the appropriate steps to be taken with patients who refuse.

Representative Psychotropic Drugs

Category, Name,[a] and Route	Uses and Diseases	Actions	Usual Dose [b] and Special Instructions	Side Effects and Adverse Reactions
Miscellaneous Antidepressants				
venlafaxine (*Effexor XR*) Oral	Major depression	Inhibits uptake of serotonin, norepinephrine, and dopamine	75 mg bid or tid	Anxiety, nervousness, insomnia, hypertension, anorexia, nausea, vomiting, dry mouth, constipation, suicidal attempts
trazodone Oral	Depression without anxiety	May inhibit serotonin uptake by the brain cells, resulting in an increased serotonin concentration in the synapse; may also cause changes in binding of serotonin to receptors	150 mg bid initially, then increase by 50 mg daily to a total of 400 mg daily in divided doses	Hypertension or hypotension, syncope, diarrhea, nausea, vomiting, delayed urine flow, nightmares
bupropion (*Wellbutrin XL*) Oral	Major depression	Unknown, does not inhibit MAO, weakly blocks uptake of epinephrine, serotonin, and dopamine	*Immediate release:* 100 mg bid for 3 days, followed by 100 mg tid *Extended release:* 150 mg daily, followed by 300 mg daily	Headache, dizziness, insomnia, tachycardia, hypotension, excessive sweating, muscle spasms, dry mouth, nausea, vomiting
Tricyclic Antidepressants				
amitriptyline Oral, IM	Depression	Is a tricyclic antidepressant; inhibits serotonin reuptake	75 mg/day in divided doses; may increase to 150 mg daily; 20-30 mg qid IM, or 80-120 mg at bedtime	Dizziness, drowsiness, constipation, dry mouth, orthostatic hypotension, blurred vision
imipramine (*Tofranil*) Oral, IV	Depression	Is a tricyclic antidepressant; inhibits serotonin reuptake	75-100 mg/day in divided doses or in a single dose at bedtime; up to 300 mg given to hospitalized patients; caution patient to avoid alcohol, OTC drugs, prolonged exposure to sunlight, and hazardous activities that require alertness	Drowsiness, dry mouth, blurred vision, urine retention, constipation, weight gain, tachycardia, photosensitivity

Psychotropic Drugs   **483**

Category, Name,[a] and Route	Uses and Diseases	Actions	Usual Dose[b] and Special Instructions	Side Effects and Adverse Reactions
Selective Serotonin Reuptake Inhibitors (SSRIs)				
escitalopram (***Lexapro***) Oral	Major depression	Inhibits serotonin reuptake	10 mg daily	Insomnia, somnolence, dizziness, decreased appetite, nausea, vomiting, dry mouth, palpitation
Fluoxetine (***Prozac***) Oral	Depression	Inhibits serotonin reuptake	20–80 mg/day, given once or twice daily in divided doses	Anxiety, insomnia, weight loss, sexual dysfunction, nausea, headache, diarrhea, dry mouth
sertraline (***Zoloft***) Oral	Depression, obsessive-compulsive disorders	Inhibits serotonin reuptake	Begin with 50 mg PO and gradually increase every few weeks; range 50–200 mg	Headaches, nausea, diarrhea, insomnia, male sexual dysfunction
paroxetine (*Paxil*) Oral	Depression, obsessive-compulsive disorders	Inhibits serotonin reuptake	20–50 mg/day PO in divided doses	Headache, sedation, nausea, dry mouth
Monoamine Oxidase Inhibitors (MAOIs)				
tranylcypromine (*Parnate*) Oral	Depression	Increases concentration of epinephrine, norepinephrine, serotonin, and dopamine in the CNS by inhibition of MAO	10 mg bid; increase to 30 mg/day after 2 weeks; not to exceed 60 mg/day; avoid foods high in tyramine	Dizziness, drowsiness, constipation, weight gain, orthostatic hypotension, edema, urinary hesitancy
Antianxiety Agents and Sedatives/Hypnotics				
lorazepam (***Ativan***) Oral, IM, IV	Anxiety, tension, insomnia, agitation, premedication before operative procedure	Depresses the central nervous system	2–6 mg daily in divided doses; caution patient to avoid alcohol; may cause drowsiness; 2–4 mg IM	Drowsiness, lethargy, dependence
alprazolam (***Xanax***) Oral	Anxiety and tension	Is a benzodiazepine; depresses the central nervous system	0.25–0.5 mg tid	Drowsiness, lightheadedness, suicidal tendencies
diazepam (*Valium* - Oral only) Oral, IM	Anxiety, tension before surgical procedures, muscle spasms, adjunct in seizure disorders	Is a benzodiazepine; depresses the central nervous system	2–10 mg tid to qid PO, adjusted individually to the lowest effective maintenance dose; caution patient to avoid alcohol; give with food to avoid upset stomach	Drowsiness, slurred speech, blurred vision, pain at injection site, unusual fatigue, dependence

Representative Psychotropic Drugs (continued)

Category, Name,[a] and Route	Uses and Diseases	Actions	Usual Dose[b] and Special Instructions	Side Effects and Adverse Reactions
Antianxiety Agents and Sedatives/Hypnotics (continued)				
chlordiazepoxide Oral	Anxiety, tension before surgical procedures, alcohol withdrawal	Depresses the central nervous system	5-25 mg tid or qid PO; up to 100 mg IM or IV	Drowsiness, dizziness, confusion, lethargy, thrombophlebitis
flurazepam Oral	Insomnia	Acts on the central nervous system to produce hypnotic effects	15-30 mg at bedtime for hypnotic effect; may take 2-3 nights for medication to reach full effectiveness; caution patient to avoid alcohol and activities that require alertness	Dizziness, daytime sedation, headache, lack of coordination
triazolam (*Halcion*) Oral	Insomnia	Acts on the central nervous system to produce hypnotic effects	0.125-0.5 mg at bedtime	Headache, nausea, dizziness, lightheadedness
Sedatives and Hypnotics				
zolpidem (*Ambien*) Oral	Short-term treatment of insomnia	Nonbenzodiazepine central nervous system depressant	10 mg at bedtime	No clear evidence of withdrawal syndrome; may experience fatigue, nausea, flushing, lightheadedness, uncontrollable crying, abdominal cramps, nervousness
Antipsychotic Agents				
chlorpromazine Oral, IM, rectal	Psychotic disorders, schizophrenia, severe agitation, severe nausea and vomiting, intractable hiccups	Blocks dopamine receptors in the brain	30-75 mg tid or qid and increased as necessary	Extrapyramidal reactions, sedation, tardive dyskinesia, dry mouth, constipation, urine retention, orthostatic hypotension

Representative Psychotropic Drugs (continued)

Category, Name,ᵃ and Route	Uses and Diseases	Actions	Usual Dose ᵇ and Special Instructions	Side Effects and Adverse Reactions
Antipsychotic Agents *(continued)*				
fluphenazine Oral, IM	Psychotic disorders	Blocks dopamine receptors in the brain	0.5–10 mg PO daily in divided doses	Extrapyramidal reactions, tardive dyskinesia, dry mouth, constipation, urine retention, orthostatic hypotension
trifluoperazine Oral	Anxiety disorders, schizophrenia, other psychotic disorders	Blocks dopamine receptors in the brain	1–2 mg bid	Extrapyramidal reactions, tardive dyskinesia, dry mouth, constipation, urine retention, blurred vision
haloperidol Oral, IM	Psychotic disorders	Blocks dopamine receptors in the brain	0.5–5 mg bid or tid; may cause drowsiness	Severe extrapyramidal reactions, tardive dyskinesia, blurred vision, urine retention
Antimanics				
lithium carbonate Oral	Prevention or control of mania	Unknown; decreases excitability of nerve conduction; increases reuptake of norepinephrine and dopamine; decreases release of neurotransmitters	300–600 mg tid	Fine hand tremors, polyuria, thirst, mild and transient nausea, general discomfort

Note: Bolded trade names are among the 50 most prescribed drugs.

ᵃ*Trade names given in parentheses are examples only. Check current drug references for a complete listing of available products.*

ᵇ*Average adult doses are given. However, dosages are determined by a provider and vary with the purpose of the therapy and the particular patient. The doses presented in this text are for general information only.*

Summary

Learning Outcome	Summary Points
18-1 Describe the biochemical mechanisms of the central nervous system that affect emotions.	• The functions of the central nervous system are dependent on the actions of neurohormonal agents of the brain.

Learning Outcome	Summary Points
18-2 Define the symptoms of mental disorders.	• *Catatonia* is a state characterized by disorganized speech and behavior. • *Insomnia* is sleeplessness. • *Dystonia* is muscle spasms of the face, tongue, neck, jaw, or back. • *Akasthisia* is motor restlessness. • *Tardive dyskinesia* is abnormal involuntary muscle movements around the mouth, lips, and tongue.

18-3 Recognize descriptions of the major mental disorders.	• The two types of depression are major depression and dysthymia.
	  • *Major depression* is a substantial psychological, social, and occupational impairment.
	  • *Dysthymia* is a minimal impairment.
	• *Alcoholism* is a chronic, progressive disease that, if left untreated, can be fatal.
	• *Schizophrenia* is a mental illness in which psychosis is the classic feature.

18-4 Distinguish between when a sedative is recommended and when a hypnotic is recommended.	• *Sedatives* are prescribed to produce a calming effect and decrease nervousness and excitability. • *Hypnotics* are used to produce sleep.
18-5 Describe the actions of the following drug groups: antidepressants, sedatives/hypnotics, antipsychotics, antianxiety drugs, and antimanics.	• *Antidepressants* intervene in the chemical processes in the brain. They include monoamine oxidase inhibitors (*Parnate*), tricyclic antidepressants (amitriptyline), serotonin selective reuptake inhibitors (*Lexapro*), and miscellaneous antidepressants (*Wellbutrin XL*). • *Sedatives/hypnotics* are central nervous system depressants. *Benzodiazepines* have muscle relaxant, antianxiety, anticonvulsant, and hypnotic effects. An example is *Valium*. • *Antipsychotics* are used when patients aren't able to recognize reality. An example is *Risperdal*. • *Antianxiety drugs* act to decrease anxiety. Also called anxiolytics or minor tranquilizers. • *Antimanics* are used in the treatment of mood disorders. Lithium is the drug of choice.
18-6 Illustrate administering sedatives/hypnotics, antidepressants, antianxiety drugs, antipsychotics, and antimanics.	• When administering sedatives/hypnotics: Decrease the noise level in the patient's room. Avoid loud talking. Offer a warm bath or back rub. Encourage enough exercise. • Tell patients on antidepressants to avoid alcohol. • Monitor for side effects. • Tell patients on antipsychotics to avoid alcohol because these drugs potentiate the effects. • For antimanics, review the summary points for Learning Outcome 18-5.
18-7 Identify drugs that are often involved in drug abuse.	• Hallucinogens • Narcotics • Sedatives • Tranquilizers • Stimulants

Chapter 18 Review

Match the terms to their definitions.

_____ 1. (LO 18-2) False belief that is resistant to reasoning

_____ 2. (LO 18-2) Muscle spasms of the face, tongue, neck, or back

_____ 3. (LO 18-2) Disorder of perception involving one of the five senses

_____ 4. (LO 18-2) Motor restlessness

a. akathisia

b. hallucination

c. dystonia

d. delusion

Define each of the terms listed.

5. (LO 18-3) Anxiety _____

6. (LO 18-3) Depression _____

7. (LO 18-3) Mania _____

8. (LO 18-3) Schizophrenia _____

Complete the statements by filling in the blanks.

9. (LO 18-1) The two neurohormones present in the central nervous system that affect emotions are
   _____ and _____.

10. (LO 18-1) _____ stimulate transmission of reactions.

11. (LO 18-1) Both norepinephrine and dopamine have _____ and
    _____ effects on the functions of sleep, arousal, and memory.

Describe the purpose of each drug; for example, *Cerebral stimulants speed up brain activity, which speeds up the whole body.*

12. (LO 18-5) Antimanics _____

13. (LO 18-5) Antidepressants _____

14. (LO 18-5) Hypnotics _____

15. (LO 18-5) Antianxiety agents _____

16. (LO 18-5) Antipsychotics _____

17. (LO 18-5) Neuroleptics _____

Match the drug categories to the drug names.

_____ 18. (LO 18-5) *Ambien, Lunesta*

_____ 19. (LO 18-5) amitriptyline, imipramine

_____ 20. (LO 18-5) *Risperdal, Abilify, Latuda*

_____ 21. (LO 18-5) Alprazolam, oxazepam, halazepam

_____ 22. (LO 18-5) Lithium

_____ 23. (LO 18-5) *Ativan, Xanax, Valium*

a. antidepressants

b. sedatives/hypnotics

c. antianxiety agents

d. benzodiazepines

e. antimanics

f. antipsychotic agents (neuroleptics)

Complete the statements by filling in the blanks.

24. (LO 18-5) Patients on long-term antipsychotic therapy should be monitored for _____.

25. (LO 18-5) Patients taking tranquilizers should be cautioned not to drink _____.

26. (LO 18-5) To keep the serum lithium level stable, patients should have a consistent _____ _____ intake.

27. (LO 18-3) The drug used to prevent the ingestion of alcohol in chronic alcoholics and produce a severe sensitivity to alcohol is _____.

Answer the questions in the space provided.

28. (LO 18-4) What three things can you do to make sedatives/hypnotics more effective? _____

_____

_____

_____

29. (LO 18-7) What drugs are prone to abuse? _____

_____

_____

_____

_____

30. (LO 18-6) What two foods should a patient taking a monoamine oxidase inhibitor (MAOI) avoid?_____

_____

_____

31. (LO 18-3) What drug is given every month intramuscularly to treat alcohol dependence? _____

_____

Drug Calculations—Fill in the blank with the answer.

32. (LO 18-7) The provider orders lithium carbonate 300 mg orally tid. Available are 150-mg capsules. You will give your patient _____ capsules.

33. (LO 18-7) The provider orders haloperidol 2.5 mg intramuscularly stat. Available is 5 mg/mL. Prepare to administer _____ mL to your patient.

34. (LO 18-7) The provider orders bupropion (*Wellbutrin XL*) 0.2 g orally bid. Available are 100-mg tablets. You will give _____ tablets to your patient.

35. (LO 18-7) The provider orders quetiapine fumarate (*Seroquel*) 50 mg orally bid. Available are 100-mg tablets. You will give your patient _____ tablets.

36. (LO 18-7) The provider orders diazepam 3 mg intramuscularly stat. Available is 5 mg/mL. Prepare to give your patient _____ mL.

37. (LO 18-4) Which of the following is true?
    a. Sedatives produce sleep.
    b. Hypnotics produce a calming effect and decrease nervousness and excitability.
    c. Benzodiazepines do not cause a generalized central nervous system depressant effect.
    d. Antianxiety drugs are also known as major tranquilizers.

38. (LO 18-5) Which of the following medications is administered by a wafer to a patient with schizophrenia?
    a. Venlafaxine (*Effexor XR*)
    b. Zolpidem (*Ambien*)
    c. Tranylcypromine (*Parnate*)
    d. Olanzapine (*Zyprexa*)

39. (LO 18-5) Monitor a patient for which of the following side effects of amitriptyline?
    a. Dizziness, constipation, orthostatic hypotension
    b. Anxiety, nervousness, nightmares
    c. Syncope, hypertension, diarrhea
    d. Weight loss, tachycardia, photosensitivity

40. (LO 18-6) Which of the following instructions should you give to a patient taking lithium carbonate?
    a. Report constipation, nervousness, and urinary retention.
    b. Restrict fluids to 3 to 4 glasses a day.
    c. Avoid fluids such as coffee, tea, and cola.
    d. Exercise carefully in hot weather.

41. (LO 18-5) Which of the following are side effects of chlorpromazine?
    a. Extrapyramidal reactions, tardive dyskinesia, constipation
    b. Anxiousness, urinary frequency, GI upset
    c. Diarrhea, headache, hypertension
    d. Sexual dysfunction, blurred vision, slurred speech

Chapter 18 Case Studies

42. (LO 18-5) You are caring for a patient who is taking thioridazine and complains of muscle spasms of the face, tongue, and neck and motor restlessness. The patient also said he is having movements around the mouth, lips, and tongue that can't be controlled, a shuffling gait, and drooling and is scared. What are these side effects called? What should you do with this information? Are these side effects common? What are the most common side effects? _____

_____

_____

_____

43. (LO 18-6) A patient is taking phenelzine (*Nardil*). What does she need to know to safely take this drug? What kind of drug is this? _____

_____

_____

_____

Critical Thinking

Select the disorder that best matches the patient description and write it in the blank.

anxiety   psychosis   depression

44. (LO 18-3) Sandy Peters is feeling threatened at work and experiencing the "fight or flight" reaction.

_____

45. (LO 18-3) Karen Jones is out of touch with reality and experiencing hallucinations and delusions.

_____

46. (LO 18-3) Alma West has a psychological disorder that keeps her from fully living her life. Without medication, she sits with her head buried in her hands most of the day. But when she takes amitriptyline she is able to function almost normally.

_____

Applications

Obtain an electronic drug guide or a current copy of the *PDR*® from your school, health facility, or clinic. Use it to answer the following questions in a notebook or on file cards.

47. In Section 2 of the *PDR*®, Brand and Generic Name Index, find another product name for each of the drugs in the Representative Psychotropic Drugs table in this chapter.

48. In Section 3 of the *PDR*®, Product Category Index, find the subheading Serotonin Reuptake Inhibitors. List all the drugs in this category.

chapter

19

ANTINEOPLASTIC DRUGS

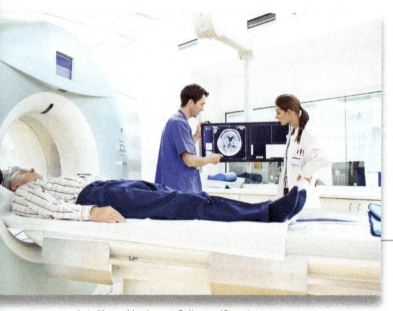

©Luis Alvarez/the Agency Collection/Getty Images

In this chapter you will learn basic facts about cells, tissues, organs, and systems. You will also learn about cancer, how it affects the body, and drugs that are used during treatment.

LEARNING OUTCOMES

19-1 Define cells, tissues, organs, and body systems.

19-2 Identify the characteristics of all cancers.

19-3 Describe how chemotherapy works.

19-4 List common antineoplastic drugs and their effects on the cell cycle.

19-5 List common side effects and associated care for patients receiving chemotherapy.

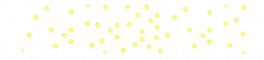

BODY SYSTEMS [LO 19-1]

Cells

Cells are the basic unit of structure of all living things. There are millions of them in every human body. Each cell carries out certain routine functions to keep itself alive—absorbing food; creating energy for heat, growth, or movement; excreting waste products; and reproducing itself when conditions are right. But each cell works with other cells, too, to carry out more complex activities that keep the whole body working smoothly.

For efficiency, cells are specialized to do certain jobs. Some are designed to form protective coatings and linings for body parts. Some specialize in producing chemicals that control body processes. Others are specialized for connecting body parts or creating body movement. Still others have the job of sending messages to and from the body's main control center, the brain. The four types of cells in the human body, each with its own special job, are epithelial cells, connective cells, muscle cells, and nerve cells (**Figure 19.1**).

Cells have the ability to divide into two when they reach a certain size. This is called cell reproduction. The two cells that result from division are

Figure 19.1

The four types of cells, with some of the body parts they make up.

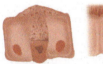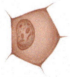

Epithelial cells
Linings of body tubes and cavities
Glands
Skin

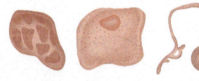

Connective cells
Bones, ligaments, cartilage
Scar tissue

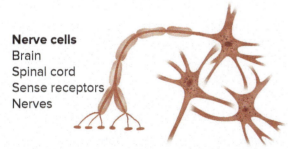

Nerve cells
Brain
Spinal cord
Sense receptors
Nerves

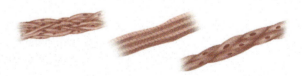

Muscle cells
Muscles that move bones
Smooth muscles in internal organs
Heart muscle

exactly alike. They will do the same job in the body as the original cell. Cell reproduction enables living things to grow. As cells divide and redivide, the body grows larger. At some point the growth process stops: The human body reaches its full adult size. From then on, cells reproduce themselves only to replace worn-out or damaged cells.

During disease and trauma, many cells may be damaged. But because cells can reproduce themselves, the body can often replace damaged cells. This is called healing.

As the body grows older, the process of cell division begins to slow. Cells are not able to replace themselves as easily as they did during youth. Consequently, the body takes longer to heal after an accident or illness. The routine processes of digesting, producing energy, and excreting waste all slow down, too. The slowing down of body processes is why older adults have special medical needs and why drug doses must be adjusted for age.

Tissues, Organs, and Systems

Cells are specialized to do certain jobs, but they do not do their jobs alone. They work together with other cells that have the same specialty. These groups of cells that together perform a certain function are called **tissues**.

Four basic types of tissues, corresponding to the four types of cells, make up all the body parts: epithelial tissue, connective tissue, muscle tissue, and nerve tissue. Each type of tissue has a different structure and function.

After cells and tissues, organs are the next most complex structures in the human body. **Organs** are made up of two or more types of tissue, organized to carry out a particular function. The heart, the liver, the stomach, the kidneys, and the skin are organs.

The important functions that keep the body alive—breathing, eating and digesting, eliminating, thinking, and regulating the body processes—are performed by well-organized groups of organs and tissues called body systems. Of the body's 10 major systems, each is responsible for one important body function.

Necessary Substances

The body is built of living cells, and it can manufacture many substances that it needs. However, there are some materials that the body must take in.

Water is the most important of these substances. In fact, about 66 percent of the body is composed of water. Water is the largest component of the fluid inside cells, or **cytoplasm**.

Water also surrounds the cells, bathing every tissue in fluid. This is important because water is the medium through which most of the body's chemical activities take place. Gases, liquids, and solids are dissolved in water before traveling through the body. The processes of absorption, distribution, biotransformation, and excretion all involve water. The water that surrounds the cells is known as **tissue fluid**.

Other substances that the body depends on for its life processes are minerals such as salt (tissue fluid is slightly salty) and calcium (for the hardness in bones and teeth), vitamins, fats, carbohydrates, and proteins. A well-balanced diet ensures that the body takes in a good supply of these necessary substances.

The Immune System

The immune system has two parts: external and internal.

External.   The external immune system gives protection from infection because of normal functioning defenses. The most important defense is the skin.

It provides a tough physical barrier to the entry of **pathogens**, or harmful microorganisms. When the skin barrier is damaged, as when cut or burned, many pathogens can enter the body and cause infection.

Internal.   The internal immune system is made up of microscopic substances whose specialized function is to fight infection.

Certain cells, called neutrophils, surround and digest the pathogens. **Leukocytes**, also called white blood cells, produce antibodies, which are proteins that help destroy pathogens as they enter the body.

Antibodies.   Antibodies are proteins that either destroy or stop the growth of certain types of pathogens. Antibodies are carried in the bloodstream and can readily move to the site of entry.

Specific antibodies act against specific pathogens. When an unfamiliar pathogen enters the body, proteins in the blood are stimulated to produce a special antibody to act against it. The next time the same pathogen enters the body, the antibody "remembers" it and proceeds to destroy it. Antibodies make the body immune to a great many infections.

Immunity can be either temporary or permanent, depending on the type of antibody. People who, for some reason, cannot form antibodies are at risk because they cannot defend themselves against the pathogens to which we are all constantly exposed.

CANCER AND CHEMOTHERAPY [LO 19-2, LO 19-3]

Cancer is not one disease but several hundred. The course of the disease and its treatment vary with the part of the body that is affected. The drugs used to treat cancer are best understood by looking at processes that take place at the cell level. All cancers have several characteristics in common, such as outlined in Table 19.1.

Rapid cell growth may give rise to **tumors**, which are lumps or masses of tissue. Not all tumors are cancerous, however. Noncancerous tumors are called **benign** tumors. They involve rapid cell growth, but the cells do not invade nearby tissues or spread to other parts of the body.

Cancerous tumors are called **malignant** tumors. As they grow, they put pressure on surrounding healthy tissues and organs and also invade them, causing destruction. Some cancers affect whole systems, such as the blood and lymph-forming organs, rather than causing a local tumor. In such cases, the cancer cells circulate throughout the body.

Early detection of cancer gives the best chance of curing the disease. The methods of treatment most often used first are surgery and radiation. Surgery is used to remove tumors and nearby lymph glands, where cancer cells that have spread from the tumor may be trapped. Radiation may be focused on a specific spot to kill cancer cells. It may also be implanted in nearby tissue or swallowed in a substance that is attracted to the site of the cancer.

Table 19.1 Characteristics of Cancer

- *Rapid cell growth and reproduction:* This is caused by changes in the genetic code governing normal cell reproduction and results in cancer cells reproducing at a much faster rate than normal cells.
- *Effects on adjacent cells:* Cancer cells can invade nearby tissues as they grow, causing destruction.
- *Seeding:* Cancer cells can seed or implant themselves in other parts of the body, starting new growths there (**metastasis**).

DRUGS FOR CHEMOTHERAPY [LO 19-4]

Drug treatment of cancer is called **chemotherapy**. Drugs can cure a few rare types of cancer, but they are more often used to control cancer symptoms in combination with surgery and/or radiation or after surgery and radiation have failed to bring about a cure. They are also used in systemwide invasions of cancer cells, such as leukemia and Hodgkin's disease.

The drugs used for chemotherapy are powerful and have strong effects on healthy cells as well as cancer cells. They are dangerous drugs whose use must be carefully planned and supervised by a provider. Some of the drugs are specifically attracted to cells that are multiplying rapidly. Thus they rush to the scene of a tumorous growth, killing cancer cells.

But, at the same time, they are attracted to the blood-forming centers of the body because there the cells are also multiplying rapidly. When the drugs kill blood cells, they weaken the body and destroy some of its defenses. Patients receiving chemotherapy often bruise easily because many platelets (parts of the blood that help stop bleeding) have been destroyed. They may be especially prone to infection because of the destruction of white blood cells. Their bones may break easily and heal slowly because the cancer drugs weaken the bone tissue where blood cells are produced.

Other areas of the body that have rapidly multiplying cells are the skin and the linings of the mouth, throat, stomach, and intestines because they are near blood vessels and the lymph canal, allowing easy penetration by the invading organism. These areas, too, are affected by chemotherapy. Side effects such as nausea, vomiting, and hair loss are common.

Doses must be carefully controlled because large doses can be toxic to healthy cells. Chemotherapeutic agents cannot differentiate between normal cells and cancer cells. Often some toxic effects are necessary to achieve the benefit of a drug's cancer-suppressing ability. Rather than giving a low dose continuously over a long period, cancer drugs are sometimes given in cycles—intensive treatment followed by a recovery period of 4 to 6 weeks, followed by another intensive treatment, and so on. This cyclical approach gives the body time to recover from the toxic effects and to build blood counts back up to normal levels.

No drug is able to kill all cancer cells at one time. But each successive dose kills a few more, so that the population is kept down to a level where the symptoms are under control. Without chemotherapy, after six generations a cancer cell would have produced 64 cancer cells. With two waves of chemotherapy, it would have produced only 6. During the same amount of time, a normal cell might have reproduced itself only one or two times.

Remission means the disappearance of symptoms (not just of cancer, but of any disease). The object of cancer chemotherapy is to bring about remission and to keep the symptoms from recurring. Chemotherapy is not guaranteed to cure cancer, but it can give a patient many years of quality of life.

Drugs used against cancer are called **antineoplastics**. The prefix *anti-* means "against," and **neoplasm** means "tumor." Antineoplastics slow down or kill growing cells by interfering with chemical processes or by substituting for nutrients in the cells so that the cells "starve" to death. Other terms used for anticancer drugs are **cytostatic**, which means that they stop all growth, and **cytotoxic**, which means that they are poisonous to cells.

Alkylating Agents (Nitrogen Mustards)

Alkylating agents are drugs that cross-link strands of cellular DNA and interfere with RNA, causing an imbalance of growth. This imbalance results in cell destruction. Nitrogen mustards are related to mustard gas, first used in World War I as a chemical weapon. In 1942, nitrogen mustard was first used to treat lymphosarcoma.

When nitrogen mustard is applied to the skin, the patient showers and thoroughly dries before each application and does not shower again until before the next treatment. You should wear plastic gloves and avoid contact with the eyes, nose, and mouth. When giving the drug IV, reconstitute it with sterile water or sodium chloride and administer within 15 minutes. Flush the vein with running IV solution for 2 to 5 minutes to clear the tubing of any remaining drug.

Alkylating agents function as cancer drugs by stopping the growth of many cancer cells. They also have toxic effects on the blood-building organs, the gastrointestinal system, and the sex glands. An immediate side effect is usually vomiting and nausea. But after a while, the patient's daily blood counts reveal that fewer lymph cells are being produced in the bone marrow, signaling remission. Examples of alkylating agents are temozolomide (*Temodar*), mechlorethamine hydrochloride (*Mustargen*), chlorambucil (*Leukeran*), cyclophosphamide, and carmustine (*BiCNU*).

An alkylator-like drug classified as a nitrosourea is cisplatin. Although the exact action of cisplatin is unknown, it appears to act similarly to the alkylating agents. It is used in the treatment of bladder, testicular, and ovarian cancer.

Antimetabolites

Antimetabolites are structurally similar to a building block necessary in the formation of DNA. The cell accepts this substance; however, since it is an imposter, it interferes with the normal production of DNA, resulting in cell death. Examples of antimetabolites are fluorouracil (*Adrucil*), mercaptopurine, cytarabine, and methotrexate. The major side effects include nausea, vomiting, and **alopecia** (hair loss). These drugs may cause a decrease in the white blood cell count and must be monitored carefully.

Antibiotic Antitumor Drugs

Antibiotic antitumor drugs are both antineoplastic and antibiotic drugs whose action as an antineoplastic drug is unknown but thought to bind DNA and inhibit RNA synthesis. Some antibiotics stop the growth of cancer cells and so are used in chemotherapy. Examples are dactinomycin (*Cosmegen*), bleomycin, doxorubicin, epirubicin (*Ellence*), mitomycin (*Mutamycin*), and daunorubicin. Because they interfere with the malignant cells' ability to grow and reproduce, they can be toxic.

Miotic Inhibitors

Miotic inhibitors are plant alkaloids that block cell division in the metaphase. Vinblastine and vincristine are examples. Patients receiving these drugs should be watched closely for neuromuscular side effects such as numbness, tingling, headache, muscle pain, loss of deep tendon reflexes, and double vision. These symptoms may indicate early signs of neurotoxicity.

Hormones

Hormones may be used in the treatment of neoplasms that are sensitive to the body's hormonal growth. Their exact mechanism of action is unknown. They are thought to interfere with growth-stimulating receptor proteins at the cellular membrane. Estrogens are used to treat postmenopausal cancer. Progestins are used with cancer of the kidney. Androgens are used to treat breast cancer in menopausal women. Tamoxifen is a synthetic antiestrogen drug used in metastatic breast cancer in women. It has proved beneficial in preventing the recurrence of breast cancer in postmenopausal women. Side effects include weakness, sleepiness, fluid retention, nausea, and vomiting.

Miscellaneous Antineoplastic Agents

Miscellaneous antineoplastic agents cannot be grouped by their action into any of the previously mentioned categories. Estramustine (*Emcyt*) is a combinaton of estradiol and nitrogen mustard. It is used in metastatic prostate cancer. Flutamide was the first oral anti-androgen available. It is also used to treat metastatic prostate cancer. It may cause leukopenia, thrombocytopenia, nausea, vomiting, diarrhea, and ataxia. Interferon alfa-2b (*Intron A*) has antiviral, antiproliferative, and immune properties. This medication appears to kill cancer cells and stimulate the immune system. This medication is used in certain types of leukemia and AIDS-related Kaposi's sarcoma. It is administered IM or subcutaneous. Side effects include GI effects such as anorexia, diarrhea, nausea, vomiting, and abdominal pain. Paclitaxel is used in the treatment of ovarian cancer unresponsive to other treatment. Imatinib (*Gleevec*) is used in the treatment of leukemia. Dasatinib (*Sprycel*) is used for patients with leukemia who don't respond to *Gleevec*. Gemcitabine (*Gemzar*) is a chemotherapeutic agent that may be prescribed in metastatic cancer of the pancreas. Cancer of the pancreas is hard to treat and has a poor prognosis. First line of treatment is cisplatin for inoperable cancer. *Gemzar* is the next line of treatment. Pembrolizumab (*Keytruda*) is an immunotherapy agent, not chemotherapy or radiation. It is indicated in treating various metastatic melanomas and Hodgkin lymphoma.

Immunomodulating Agents

Immunomodulating agents activate the immune defenses or modify a biological response to an unwanted stimulus such as a tumor. Interferon beta-1b is an example.

Lymphokines

Lymphokines are involved in the regulation of immune system functions. Some of these products are interleukin-1 and -2 and colony-stimulating factor (CSF). CSFs are proteins normally produced by the body that trigger production of more blood cells. G-CFS (*Neupogen*) or GM-CSF (*Leukine*) can be given to cancer patients with low blood counts caused by chemotherapy. These drugs, given by injection only, are extremely expensive.

Vomiting

Vomiting is a problem resulting from cancer chemotherapy. It can be such a serious problem that the doses of chemotherapy may have to be limited. Antiemetics are more effective in preventing vomiting than they are in treating it. They should be administered prophylactically before administering a chemotherapy drug. Frequently several antiemetic drugs with different actions are administered together to increase their effectiveness. Examples are metoclopramide (*Reglan*) and lorazepam (*Ativan*), dexamethasone, or prochlorperazine. *Reglan* has another action. It is used in delayed gastric

Pediatric Considerations — Antineoplastics

- There has been an increase in pediatric cancers in the last few years.
- Increased cure rates are resulting in more children being enrolled in clinical trials.
- Cytotoxic drug dosages should be based on body surface.
- Monitor closely for adverse reactions.

- The risk of adult cancers increases after treatment with chemotherapy as a child.
- The risk of breast, thyroid, or brain cancer increases after treatment with radiation.
- Newer cancer-fighting drugs are not used in children because little is known about their effects.

- The incidence of cancers in older adults increases with age, with a 10 times greater rate among those over the age of 65.
- Cytotoxic effects of drugs are greater in older adults because they generally have multiple chronic medical conditions.
- Physiological results of aging such as decreased renal and cardiac function make the management of cancers more difficult and increase the potential for toxicity.

- Older adults are more sensitive to adverse reactions of cancer treatment, particularly neurotoxic effects.
- Estrogen- and androgen-inhibiting drugs are commonly used to treat breast and prostate cancers because they are better tolerated.
- Newer biological drugs are used to treat colorectal and hematologic cancers.

emptying. Ondansetron (*Zofran*) is a serotonin antagonist approved for use in the prevention of nausea and vomiting associated with the use of antineoplastic drugs. It may cause a headache, which can be relieved by an analgesic. Granisetron is an injection for the prevention of nausea and vomiting associated with chemotherapy. It provides 24-hour antiemetic coverage. Its most common side effects are headache, sedation, diarrhea, or constipation. Dronabinol (*Marinol*) is an antiemetic used when other antiemetics have proved ineffective. A little known fact is it is a derivative of marijuana. It, too, has all the typical GI effects plus orthostatic hypertension, palpitations, and tachycardia.

Administration of Chemotherapy

It is important that you know there are specially designed guidelines for the administration of chemotherapeutic drugs and that these drugs may be hazardous for the healthcare professional. Because a person preparing or giving chemotherapy may absorb the drug through the inhalation of particles or nonintact skin, guidelines have been developed by the Occupational Safety and Health Administration (OSHA). Chemotherapy agents must be prepared in a specially ventilated room by only designated people using strict aseptic technique. Gowns, disposable gloves, and eye protection must be worn when handling chemotherapy drugs. Because there is some risk involved in the handling of the patient's vomit, urine, or feces, you should also wear the appropriate protective equipment.

SIDE EFFECTS OF CHEMOTHERAPY AND ASSOCIATED CARE [LO 19-5]

Patients undergoing chemotherapy need special care and emotional support from you. They are dealing not only with the cancer itself but also with the unpleasant, often dangerous side effects of chemotherapy. Although many of the drugs given for cancer therapy are administered parenterally by specially trained nurses or providers, you may be involved in giving some of the routine drugs for nausea or pain. You can provide emotional support by listening to your patient's fears and needs and by doing what you can to help make the patient comfortable. You should also observe your patient carefully for physical signs of the cancer itself and the following side effects of chemotherapy so that you may implement the appropriate care. Table 19.2 outlines the physical side effects of chemotherapy.

Fatigue is a common side effect of chemotherapy that you should let your patient know is anticipated and not a sign that the chemotherapy is not

Table 19.2 Physical Side Effects of Chemotherapy

1. Fatigue.
2. Nausea and vomiting.
3. **Stomatitis**—irritation of the mucous membranes of the mouth.
4. Anorexia.
5. **Leukopenia**—reduction in the number of leukocytes in the blood (4,000 L or less).
6. Alopecia—hair loss.

effective or that the cancer is spreading. Tell your patient that the fatigue may be less on certain days or certain times of day. Encourage your patient to rest before an activity and to pace himself or herself.

Anorexia, nausea, vomiting, and stomatitis are especially common and problematic side effects of chemotherapy in a patient who is losing weight or having trouble maintaining weight. Antineoplastics irritate the gastrointestinal tract from the mouth through the rectum, making eating both undesirable and uncomfortable. Vomiting may occur within 1 hour of administration of the chemotherapy and last for 24 hours or more. Encourage your patient to eat by providing a pleasant environment and helping him or her select desirable foods. Foods with strong odors such as onions and red meats should be avoided. A glass of wine with meals may help stimulate your patient's appetite. Help your patient with oral hygiene by rinsing the mouth often with water or mouthwash. A topical anesthetic such as viscous *Xylocaine* may be used with oral care. Instruct your patient to use a soft toothbrush to cleanse teeth and gums. Administer an antiemetic such as metoclopramide (*Reglan*) or ondansetron (*Zofran*) 30 minutes prior to meals to alleviate nausea. Aprepitant (*Emend*) is an antiemetic that is especially effective in treating delayed nausea and vomiting that may occur after the administration of some chemotherapies. Also, offer your patient small, frequent, high-protein meals that are high in calories and may be better tolerated. Avoid strong-smelling meats and difficult-to-digest foods.

Pain is a very disheartening side effect that may occur with chemotherapy. Your patient has to deal not only with the pain from the cancer but also with the discomfort associated with the chemotherapy because it may be irritating to the veins. Administer analgesics as prescribed and tolerated. Offer your patient diversional activities if helpful.

Leukopenia caused by depression of the bone marrow is a side effect that occurs secondarily to the chemotherapy. Monitor your patient's temperature and report if elevated. You may administer an antipyretic for fever. Instruct your patient to avoid large crowds, and explain the principles of good hand-washing techniques.

Alopecia occurs in response to the destruction of the hair follicles from chemotherapy, and it can produce considerable stress for your patient. Suggest the use of wigs, hairpieces, or scarves to help your patient cope. Explain the benefits of cutting hair before therapy is initiated. It is also helpful to tell your patient to avoid excessive shampooing, brushing, combing, and drying with hair dryers.

 Healthcare for Today and Tomorrow *Aredia* Warnings

A warning has been added to the breast cancer drug pamidronate. It is recommended that a single dose should not exceed 90 mg because of renal toxicity and potential kidney failure. As with other antineoplastic drugs, pamidronate should not be used by pregnant women because of the possibility of harm to the fetus.

Legal and Ethical Issues Indiscriminate Morphine Use

You observe a healthcare worker caring for a terminal patient with cancer who is in constant pain that is often excruciating. Morphine sulfate 10 mg IV is ordered every 4 hours. The patient's respirations have fallen to 8 breaths per minute, and the patient is requesting more morphine after only hours. You observe the healthcare worker administer an additional 10 mg of morphine 3 hours after the previous dose and with respirations of only 6 per minute. Realizing the patient is within days of death, you question whether you should let this incident go or report it. You should promptly report it, because it is not acceptable safe practice and it could be considered assisted suicide.

Representative Antineoplastic Drugs

Category, Name,[a] and Route	Uses and Diseases	Actions	Usual Dose[b] and Special Instructions	Side Effects and Adverse Reactions
Alkylating Drugs				
mechlorethamine (*Mustargen*) IV	Hodgkin's disease, lymphosarcoma	Inhibits rapidly growing cells	IV dosage according to body weight, adjusted to highest nontoxic dose; assist patient with oral hygiene; give adequate fluid; follow provider's orders carefully; note length of time for IV infusion; watch for pain at infusion site	Nausea, vomiting, anorexia, bleeding, bruising, metallic taste
carmustine (*BiCNU*) IV	Brain tumor, Hodgkin's disease, lymphomas, melanoma	Inhibits rapidly growing cells	IV dosage according to surface area; pain at injection site common	Blood and liver problems, nausea, vomiting, diarrhea
temozolomide (*Temodar*) Oral	Brain cancer	Inhibits rapidly growing cells	May be taken orally at home; adjust dose based on neutrophil and platelet counts	Thrombocytopenia, neutropenia, nausea, vomiting, constipation, headache, fatigue
Antimetabolites				
fluorouracil (*Adrucil*) IV, topical	Cancer of the breast, colon, rectum, stomach, pancreas, cervix, and bladder	Inhibits DNA synthesis	IV dosage according to body weight; avoid **extravasation** (discharge of blood or other substances into tissues)	Anorexia, nausea, vomiting, stomatitis, diarrhea, weakness, dermatitis
mercaptopurine Oral	Leukemias	Inhibits DNA synthesis	Oral dosage according to body weight, adjusted to highest nontoxic dose	Blood and liver problems, anorexia, nausea, vomiting

Representative Antineoplastic Drugs (continued)

Category, Name,[a] and Route	Uses and Diseases	Actions	Usual Dose[b] and Special Instructions	Side Effects and Adverse Reactions
Antibiotic Antitumor Drugs				
dactinomycin (*Cosmegen*) IV	Cancer of the testes and uterus, Wilms' tumor	Inhibits cell reproduction	IV dosage according to body weight, adjusted to highest nontoxic dose; drug is corrosive; avoid contact with skin; avoid extravasation	Nausea, vomiting, stomatitis, blood problems, bruising, loss of hair
epirubicin (*Ellence*) IV	Breast cancer as an adjunct therapy	Inhibits DNA synthesis	Administer IV slowly over 3–5 minutes	Leukopenia, neutropenia, anemia, nausea, vomiting, mucositis, alopecia, amenorrhea
Miscellaneous Antineoplastic Drugs				
tamoxifen Oral	Cancer of the breast	Acts as estrogen antagonist	10 mg PO bid to tid	Nausea, vomiting, anorexia, rash, vaginal discharge, depression, dizziness, hair thinning, or partial loss of hair

[a] *Trade names given in parentheses are examples only. Check current drug references for a complete listing of available products.*
[b] *Average adult doses are given. However, dosages are determined by a provider and vary with the purpose of the therapy and the particular patient. The doses presented here are for general information only.*

Summary

Learning Outcome	Summary Points
19-1 Define cells, tissues, organs, and body systems.	• *Cells* are the basic unit of structure for all living things. The four types of cells are epithelial, connective, nerve, and muscle. • Specialized cells are called *tissues*. • *Organs* are made up of two or more types of tissues organized to carry out a specialized function. • The 10 *body systems* are each responsible for one important function.
19-2 Identify the characteristics of all cancers.	• Rapid cell growth and reproduction • Effects on adjacent cells • Seeding

Learning Outcome	Summary Points
19-3 Describe how chemotherapy works.	• Chemotherapy cannot differentiate between cancer cells and normal cells—it has strong effects on both. • It kills blood cells. • The skin, lining of the mouth, throat, stomach, and intestines are also affected by chemotherapy. • No drug is able to kill all cancer cells at one time.
19-4 List common antineoplastic drugs and their effects on the cell cycle.	• *Alkylating agents* such as nitrogen mustards cause cell destruction (e.g., *Leukeran*). • *Antimetabolites* cause cell death (e.g., fluoruracil). • *Antibiotic antitumor drugs* stop the growth of cancer cells. • *Miotic inhibitors* block cell division in the metaphase (e.g., vinblastine). • *Hormones* have an unknown action.
19-5 List common side effects and appropriate care for patients receiving chemotherapy.	• *Fatigue:* encourage the patient to rest before activity to decrease fatigue. • *Nausea and vomiting:* encourage desirable foods to alleviate nausea and vomiting; avoid foods with strong odors. • *Stomatitis:* assist with oral hygiene. • *Leukopenia:* monitor temperature; administer an antipyretic; instruct the patient to avoid large crowds. • *Alopecia:* explain the benefits of cutting hair before therapy; tell patients to avoid excessive shampooing, brushing, combing, and drying hair with hair dryer; suggest the use of hairpieces and scarves. • *Pain:* offer diversional activities to alleviate pain.

Chapter 19 Review

Define each of the terms listed.

1. (LO 19-5) Leukopenia _____

2. (LO 19-1) Cell _____

3. (LO 19-4) Cytotoxic _____

4. (LO 19-2) Tumor _____

5. (LO 19-3) Chemotherapy _____

6. (LO 19-1) Metastasis _____

7. (LO 19-2) Malignant _____

8. (LO 19-5) Alopecia _____

9. (LO 19-2) Benign _____

10. (LO 19-2) Neoplasm _____

11. (LO 19-5) Stomatitis _____

Match the appropriate term to the characteristic or description.

_____ 12. (LO 19-1) Basic unit of structure of all living things   a. tissues

_____ 13. (LO 19-1) Groups of cells working together   b. water

_____ 14. (LO 19-1) Substance that makes up two-thirds of the body   c. cells

_____ 15. (LO 19-1) Groups of organs and tissues working together   d. systems

_____ 16. (LO 19-1) Fluid found inside cells   e. cytoplasm

_____ 17. (LO 19-1) Fluid surrounding cells   f. tissue fluid

Answer the questions in the space provided.

18. (LO 19-2) What are the characteristics of cancer cells? _____

_____

_____

_____

19. (LO 19-5) How long before meals should you administer an antiemetic to alleviate nausea?

_____

20. (LO 19-4) Antineoplastics harm healthy cells as well as cancer cells. Which parts of the body are especially affected by chemotherapy?_____

_____

_____

_____

Match the drug categories to the drug names.

_____ 21. (LO 19-4) *Mustargen, Leukeran,* cyclophosphamide   a. antimetabolites

_____ 22. (LO 19-4) fluorouracil, methotrexate   b. immunomodulating agents

_____ 23. (LO 19-4) doxorubicin, dactinomycin, epirubicin   c. alkylating agents

_____ 24. (LO 19-4) Interferon beta-1b   d. antibiotic antitumor drugs

_____ 25. (LO 19-4) Metoclopramide, *Zofran, Emend*   e. antiemetics

Drug Calculations—Fill in the blank with the answer.

26. (LO 19-4) The provider orders filgrastim (*Neupogen*) 210 μg subcutaneously daily. Available is 300 μg/1 mL. Prepare to administer _____ mL to your patient.

27. (LO 19-4) The provider orders methotrexate 15 mg intramuscularly for 5 days. Available is 50 mg/2 mL. Prepare to administer _____ mL to your patient.

28. (LO 19-4) The provider orders tamoxifen 15 mg orally bid. Available are 10-mg tablets. You will give your patient _____ tablets.

29. (LO 19-4) The provider orders temozolomide (*Temodar*) 150 mg orally daily for 5 days. Available are 100-mg tablets. You will give _____ tablets to your patient.

30. (LO 19-4) The provider orders mercaptopurine 100 mg orally daily. Available are 50-mg tablets. You will give your patient _____ tablets.

Multiple Choice—Circle the correct letter.

31. (LO 19-4) When administering a nitrogen mustard, what should you include in the care?
    a. Instruct the patient to avoid showering before each application when applied to the skin.
    b. Do not wear gloves when administering.
    c. Monitor for immediate side effects of nausea and vomiting.
    d. Reconstitute the IV drug with a dextrose solution.

32. (LO 19-4) A patient asks how an antibiotic works in chemotherapy. What is the best response?
    a. Helps fight infection
    b. Stops the growth of cancer cells
    c. Is a preventive therapy
    d. Calms the stomach when there is a GI upset

33. (LO 19-5) In the care of a patient undergoing chemotherapy, which of the following should be included to avoid irritating the gastrointestinal tract?
    a. Restrict calorie intake.
    b. Encourage strong foods.
    c. Offer red meats.
    d. Offer a glass of wine with meals.

34. (LO 19-4) Which drug will a healthcare worker administer to a patient with cancer of the breast?
    a. Tamoxifen
    b. Temozolomide (*Temodar*)
    c. Mercaptopurine
    d. Mechlorethamine (*Mustargen*)

35. (LO 19-4) A patient is taking temozolomide (*Temodar*). For which side effects should you monitor?
    a. Dermatitis, bruising, urinary frequency
    b. Diarrhea, allergic reaction, amenorrhea
    c. Vaginal discharge, depression, rash
    d. Fatigue, nausea, constipation

Chapter 19 Case Studies

36. (LO 19-5) You are caring for a patient with cancer of the breast who is receiving chemotherapy and is afraid of losing her hair. What is this side effect called? What causes it? What should you tell your patient to help with the hair loss? _____

_____

_____

_____

37. (LO 19-5) While receiving chemotherapy for cancer, a patient is experiencing nausea and vomiting and is losing weight. Why does this occur? What should you tell him that might help? _____

_____

_____

_____

Critical Thinking

Answer the questions in the space provided.

38. (LO 19-5) What signs should you look for when giving medications to cancer patients?

_____

_____

_____

39. (LO 19-5) Identify three interventions that you should implement when caring for a cancer patient.

_____

_____

_____

Applications

Obtain an electronic drug guide or a current copy of the *PDR*® from your school, health facility, or clinic. Use it to answer the following questions in a notebook or on index cards.

40. Use the *PDR*®, Section 2, Brand and Generic Name Index, to find another product name for each drug listed in the Representative Antineoplastic Drugs table in this chapter.

41. In Section 3, Product Category Index, of the *PDR*®, find the subheading Antimetabolites. List all the drugs named.

42. Section 3, Product Category Index, of the *PDR*® gives a page number for some drugs shown in Section 4, Product Identification Guide. Using the page numbers, identify the pictures of those drugs shown as antimetabolites.

43. Notice the different forms that Section 5, Product Information, displays for two products. If solid, state the form. If liquid, how is it administered?

44. For the same two drugs you identified in the previous question, name the manufacturer. In Section 1 of the *PDR*®, Manufacturers' Index, find the address of the manufacturer.

45. In Section 2 of the *PDR*®, Brand and Generic Name Index, identify the pages that give detailed information about these two drugs. Read about these two drugs in Section 5, Product Information.

46. In Section 5 of the *PDR*®, under Product Information, locate the information referring to children and older adults, and write it out.

47. In Section 6 of the *PDR*®, Diagnostic Product Information, find the name of the manufacturer that produced the two drugs you identified in question 43.

48. List the diagnostic drugs produced by one of the manufacturers you identified in the previous question.

If you have a problem answering any of these questions, look in the back of the *PDR*® under Discontinued Products to see if any of the drugs are listed there.

DRUGS FOR THE PEDIATRIC PATIENT

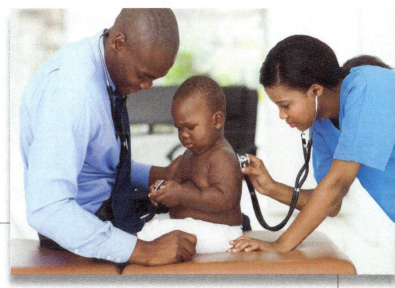

©michaeljung/Shutterstock

In this chapter you will learn how the physical changes that occur during the various stages of growth and development pose special problems for medication administration to the pediatric patient. Considering the alterations in growth and development, you will learn how to safely administer medications to infants and children.

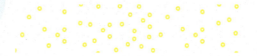

DRUGS AND THE PEDIATRIC PATIENT [LO 20-1]

Regardless of whether you work in a hospital or in a clinic, you are likely to find yourself working with a pediatric population. **Pediatrics** is the branch of medicine pertaining to the diseases and disorders of infants and children. A **pediatrician** is a provider trained in caring for infants and children. Pediatrics includes **infancy,** the period of life extending from birth to the end of the first year; **childhood,** the period of life extending from infancy to puberty; and **puberty,** the period of accelerated growth rate and sexual development generally occurring around age 12 in girls and age 14 in boys. You may not be directly administering medications to the pediatric patient in a provider's office or outpatient clinic, but you are responsible for educating the parents on how to administer medications to their child.

PHYSIOLOGICAL ALTERATIONS IN THE PEDIATRIC PATIENT [LO 20-2]

Infants and small children do not have fully developed bodies and are not able to metabolize and excrete drugs as an adult would. As a result, infants and children require smaller doses of medications. The processes of absorption, distribution, biotransformation, and excretion may significantly alter the effects of a drug. Infants have immature enzyme systems in the liver, lower plasma concentrations of protein for binding with drugs, and kidneys that function immaturely—all of which make them more vulnerable to the harmful effects of drugs. Children beyond infancy may metabolize drugs faster and will need larger doses of medications, but still not equivalent to those of an adult. An example of this would be pain control.

Other problems exist in the administration of drugs to small children. Infants and small children cannot tell you that they are experiencing symptoms that may be side effects of a drug. For example, a preverbal child cannot verbalize dizziness or ringing in the ears. With this population, perhaps more than any other, obtaining an accurate dose of a drug cannot be emphasized enough. Dehydration is another potential problem for children who are ill. In an ill child, water requirements and losses are both increased, with the fluid intake decreased. Because of an altered ability to excrete the drug, a toxic drug accumulation may occur.

SAFEGUARDS CRITICAL TO SAFE ADMINISTRATION OF PEDIATRIC MEDICATIONS [LO 20-3]

Checking the Dose and Drug

Checking the dose of a medication is a shared responsibility between the pediatrician ordering the drug and you administering the drug. As previously discussed, both healthy and ill infants and children are particularly sensitive to the effects of drugs. Because of this fact, you must know the safe range for drug administration.

To avoid an unpredictable response to the drug, double-checking the drug with another person is advised. You should check with the healthcare

> When a drug is ordered outside the safe range for administration of a drug to a child, you should contact the drug prescriber to verify the dose. Because you are legally responsible for the safe administration of the drug, you may need to refuse to administer the drug if you are still uncomfortable with a dose outside the safe range.

facility where you are employed for a list of drugs that should be double-checked. Generally, these include digoxin, heparin, insulin, opioids, sedatives, epinephrine, and chemotherapy drugs. The drug dose should be double-checked because the decimal point may make the difference between life and death. For example, there is a significant difference between administering a microgram and a milligram. A milligram is a thousand times larger than a microgram.

Identification

It is essential that you realize children are unreliable sources of information. As previously learned, the only reliable method of drug administration is to check the child's hospital identification band with the medication label. Parents may also be asked for the child's identity, but this is not considered the most reliable method of medication administration. A child should never be asked his or her identity. Infants are not able to state their identity. Toddlers and preschoolers may answer to any name, and school-age children may deny their identity to avoid administration of the medication.

Parents

Because almost all parents have administered a drug to a child, they may provide helpful information and offer techniques that may assist you in the successful administration of the drug. A parent may also inform you of the child's known allergies. Perhaps the most successful strategy would be for the parent to administer the oral and liquid drug forms. A child who has a medication administered by a parent may feel safer and be less likely to fuss.

METHODS OF ADMINISTRATION OF PEDIATRIC MEDICATIONS [LO 20-4]

Whenever possible, the oral route of medication administration is preferred in pediatric patients. Dissolved or suspended medications are preferred to solid (pills, tablets, capsules) medications because of a decreased risk of aspiration or choking. With solid medications, choking is an especially serious concern if the child is extremely fussy or crying. Many oral medications come in flavored suspensions to increase the child's acceptance. There are a variety of recommended strategies to enhance the acceptance of giving an oral medication to a child (Table 20.1).

Table 20.1 Strategies to Enhance Acceptance of Giving an Oral Drug to a Child

- Offer a Popsicle to numb the tongue before administering the medication.
- Offer a carbonated beverage such as 7-up before or after the drug to decrease nausea.
- Suggest pinching the nose and drinking through a straw to decrease the unpleasant taste and smell.
- Mix the medicine with approximately 1 teaspoon of a sweetened substance like jam or pudding (avoid mixing the drug with essential foods like cereals, formulas, or milk because this may result in the child refusing these foods).
- Offer water, juice, or a flavored drink immediately after the drug to decrease the unpleasant taste.

Because many oral drugs are ordered in teaspoons and teaspoons are inaccurate devices, the measurement should be converted to milliliters. The standard conversion is 1 teaspoon equals 5 mL. Drops and teaspoons may be the prescribed dose for some medications, leaving room for error. As long as the drug is administered by the dropper supplied with that drug, the dose is considered accurate. Avoid putting the liquid drug in a medicine cup because some of the drug would adhere to the sides of the cup and result in an inaccurate dose.

A very accurate means of administering a drug with a dose of less than 1 mL is a tuberculin syringe. Directly place the syringe in the child's mouth to ensure that the child receives the complete dose. An alternative technique to administering an oral medication in a liquid preparation is to ask the provider or pharmacist for another form of the drug, such as a chewable troche or lozenge. Remember, tablets and capsules are not generally given to a child because of the risk of aspiration. If a drug comes only in a tablet or capsule, certain precautions must be taken. The contents of a capsule should be emptied into a medicine cup after crushing the pill with a pill crusher, followed by mixing the medicine with 1 teaspoon of a sweetened substance. To avoid cross-contamination and administration of other medications, always wash and completely dry the crusher that comes with a pill crusher.

Never place a child on his or her back or side for oral medication administration because this results in aspiration. Blowing a small puff of air in the face of an infant up to 11 months of age or gently stroking the throat will stimulate the sucking reflex.

 Patient Education Parent Assistance with Medications

When administering oral medications, it is critical to have the parent hold the child in an upright position, with one of the child's arms firmly secured against the parent's side—the parent uses the hand without the medicine to hold the child's arm (**Figure 20.1**).

Intramuscular (IM) Administration

The small volume of prescribed medication administered in an intramuscular injection poses unique risks for the pediatric patient who has a small amount of tissue. Very small volumes, such as less than 1 mL, should be administered in a low-dose (0.5-mL) syringe to ensure accuracy. Such syringes, with specially designed needles, decrease the chance of administering inaccurate doses because of a **dead space,** space that allows fluid to remain in the syringe and needle after the plunger is completely pushed forward. Generally, a minimum of 0.2 mL is left in the standard needle hub, especially when two drugs are mixed in the same syringe. When mixing two drugs in the same syringe, such as insulin, it is recommended to always draw up the two drugs in the same order, use the same brand of syringe, and use the needle permanently attached to decrease the risk of dead space occurring. Furthermore, flushing the syringe is not recommended after medication administration because this practice may also result in dead space.

Medications such as iron and diphtheria and tetanus toxoid are specifically irritating and may result in irritation when tracked into the subcutaneous tissue; they should be administered by Z-track. Changing the needle after drawing up the medication and before giving it is a practice that also decreases tracking. Needle size and gauge are also specific considerations for infants and children (**Table 20.2**).

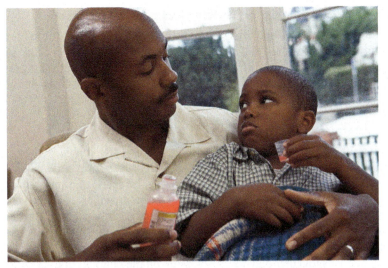
©BananaStock/Getty Images

Figure 20.1

A parent partially restrains the child for easy and comfortable administration of oral medication.

Because the response to an injection is unpredictable, it is recommended that someone assist you to hold the child.

Subcutaneous and Intradermal Administration

The most common sites for subcutaneous medication administration are the center third of the lateral aspect of the upper arm or abdomen or the center third of the anterior thigh. The volar surface of the forearm is the preferred site for administering an intradermal injection. The medial side of the arm should be avoided because the skin is more sensitive. These are the injection methods generally used to administer immunizations.

Intravenous Administration

The intravenous route is both a common and useful route of medication administration. It is the preferred route not only for children who have poor absorption, diarrhea, vomiting, dehydration, or peripheral vascular collapse but also for children who have resistant infections and need repeated parenteral medications and for children in need of emergency treatment or extended pain control. It cannot be stressed enough that because the effect of intravenous administration is immediate, it is critical that the dose be accurate to avoid life-threatening complications that can arise from administering too much of a drug. IV administration may be used for children who need fluid replacement and can tolerate the extra fluid. For very small children or children who need the drug administered intravenously but cannot tolerate the extra fluids, a special delivery system such as a syringe pump may be used.

Table 20.2 Location, Length of Needle, Gauge of Needle, and Fluid Amount for Administration of Drugs to Infants and Children

Child's Age	Location	Needle Length	Needle Gauge	Maximum Amount of Drug Given
Infant (less than 4 months)	Vastus lateralis Ventrogluteal	$\frac{5}{8}$ inch $\frac{5}{8}$ inch	25G for immunizations; 23G for thick drugs	1 mL 1 mL
Infant (older than 4 months)	Vastus lateralis Ventrogluteal	1 inch 1 inch	25G for immunizations; 23G for other injections	1 mL 1 mL
Toddler	Deltoid Vastus lateralis Ventrogluteal	$\frac{5}{8}$ inch 1 inch 1 inch	25G for immunizations; 23G for other injections	1 mL 1 mL
Preschooler and School Age	Deltoid Ventrogluteal	$\frac{5}{8}$ inch 1 inch	25G for immunizations; 23G for other injections	1 mL 1 mL
Adolescent	Deltoid Ventrogluteal	$\frac{5}{8}$ – 1 inch 1 inch	25G for immunizations; 23G for other injections	1 mL 1 mL

Nasogastric, Orogastric, or Gastrostomy Administration

Oral medications are given nasogastrically, orogastrically, or through a gastrostomy when the child has an indwelling feeding tube. As with all administration of medications through a feeding tube, a major disadvantage is the clogging of the tube by thick solutions. The most important intervention to prevent this complication is to flush the tube.

Rectal Administration

The rectal route of medication is a less preferred and less predictable method of administration. The dosage of a drug, usually in suppository form, ordered for a child is often less than the available form. The irregular shape of a suppository makes dividing or splitting the suppository to obtain an exact dose very difficult. If half a suppository is ordered, it is recommended to cut it lengthwise rather than in half. A child may not be able to follow the instructions to hold the suppository in place to avoid expelling. Holding the buttocks together or gently taping the buttocks together may relieve pressure on the buttocks until the urge to expel the suppository passes, generally in 5 to 10 minutes. A suppository may be administered in the home for a child who is vomiting or running a fever. Examples include acetaminophen, aspirin, or antiemetics.

Optic, Otic, and Nasal Administration

There aren't many differences in optic, otic, or nasal administration between a child and an adult. The biggest consideration is the child's ability to cooperate. The child's head must be immobilized or held to facilitate easier administration. As with all medication given to a child, an explanation should be given because a child should never be startled or surprised and an older child will be more likely to cooperate. Placing eyedrops in infants may be particularly challenging because they tend to squeeze their eyelids shut. It is recommended to administer an eye ointment before a nap because the child's vision will most likely be blurred.

When administering ear drops in children under the age of 3 years, the external auditory canal should be straightened by pulling the pinna downward and straight back. The pinna is pulled upward and back in children over the age of 3 years. Again, encouraging the child to lie still on the opposite side after instillation may be challenging. Nose drops in the child are administered much the same as with an adult. A small infant must be held much like a football to administer nose drops. An older child's head may be held over the end of the bed. A small pillow may be placed under the child's shoulders to aid in the flow of the medicine through the nasal passage. Again, cooperation is an issue because the child should be instructed to remain in the instillation position for 1 minute.

WHAT'S NEW IN PEDIATRIC MEDICATIONS [LO 20-5]

Acetaminophen (*Tylenol*)

Acetaminophen (*Tylenol*) has developed a meltaway *Tylenol* in a variety of flavors that will quickly melt in a child's mouth. There are two types: *Children's Tylenol Meltaways* for children 2 to 6 years of age and *Junior Tylenol Meltaways* for children 6 to 11 years of age.

Acetylsalicylic Acid (Aspirin)

Although this guideline is not necessarily new, it cannot be stressed enough that acetylsalicylic acid (aspirin) should never be used in children and teenagers because of Reye syndrome, which is a potentially life-threatening disorder.

Summary

Learning Outcome	Summary Points
20-1 Define terms pertinent to drugs for the pediatric patient.	• *Pediatrics* is the branch of medicine pertaining to the diseases and disorders of infants and children. • A *pediatrician* is a provider trained in caring for infants and children.
20-2 Describe the physiological alterations in the pediatric patient.	• Does not have a fully developed body to metabolize and excrete drugs as an adult does, thus requiring that smaller doses of medications be given. • Has immature enzyme systems in the liver. • Has lower plasma concentrations of protein for binding with drugs. • Has kidneys that function immaturely, making the child more vulnerable to the harmful effects of a drug. • Has an altered ability to excrete drugs, so a toxic accumulation may occur.
20-3 Identify the safeguards critical to safe administration of pediatric medications.	• Check the drug. • Check the dose, remembering that some medications must be double-checked. • Correctly identify the patient by checking the identification band and obtaining essential information from the parents.
20-4 Describe the methods of administration for oral, intramuscular, subcutaneous, intradermal, intravenous, optic, otic, nasal, rectal, nasogastric, or gastrostomy medication in the pediatric patient.	• *Oral:* Oral administration is the preferred route of medication administration. The parent holds the child in an upright position with one of the child's arms firmly secured against the parent's side while the parent uses the hand without the medicine to hold the child's arm. • *Intramuscular:* Caution must be used when administering an IM injection because of smaller amounts of tissue. • *Subcutaneous or intradermal:* Subcutaneous and intradermal injections are the methods of administration for immunizations. • *Intravenous:* The IV route is preferred for children who have poor absorption, diarrhea, vomiting, dehydration, or infections or who need pain control. • *Optic, otic, or nasal:* These drugs can be given only to a child who can cooperate. • *Rectal:* Less preferred and less predictable method of administration because a child may not be able to cooperate by holding a suppository for the directed length of time. • *Nasogastric or gastrostomy:* Oral drugs are given nasogastrically or through a gastrostomy when the child has an indwelling feeding tube. • Medication safety practices cannot be emphasized enough when administering medicine to a pediatric patient. • Checking the dose and drug, properly identifying the patient, and including the parents are all essential.
20-5 Know the newer pediatric medications.	• Discuss acetaminophen and acetylsalicylic acid.

Match the medical terms to their definitions.

_____ 1. (LO 20-1) Branch of medicine pertaining to disorders of children

_____ 2. (LO 20-1) Period of life extending from infancy to puberty

_____ 3. (LO 20-1) Provider trained in the care of infants and children

_____ 4. (LO 20-4) Area that allows fluid to remain in the syringe after the plunger is completely pushed forward

_____ 5. (LO 20-1) Period of accelerated growth rate and sexual development

_____ 6. (LO 20-1) Period extending from birth to the end of the first year

a. childhood

b. dead space

c. puberty

d. pediatrics

e. infancy

f. pediatrician

Place a T in the blank if the statement is true. Place an F in the blank if the statement is false.

_____ 7. (LO 20-2) Infants rapidly metabolize and excrete drugs.

_____ 8. (LO 20-3) When a drug is ordered outside the safe range of administration, you should contact the prescriber.

_____ 9. (LO 20-3) Always ask a child his or her name before giving a medication.

_____ 10. (LO 20-4) Never offer a carbonated beverage before or after administering a medication.

_____ 11. (LO 20-4) A 25G needle should be used to administer an immunization to an infant.

_____ 12. (LO 20-4) Clogging of a nasogastric tube is a major disadvantage to giving medications by this route.

_____ 13. (LO 20-4) When administering ear drops to a child under the age of 3 years, you should pull the pinna upward and backward.

_____ 14. (LO 20-2) Infants require smaller doses of medications than adults do.

_____ 15. (LO 20-2) Dehydration is a potential problem for children who are ill.

_____ 16. (LO 20-3) Asking a parent the name of his or her child before administering a medication is the most reliable procedure to follow in medication administration.

_____ 17. (LO 20-4) A medicine should be mixed with 1 teaspoon of cereal before it is administered to a child.

Complete the statements by filling in the blanks.

18. (LO 20-4) The preferred route of medication administration for children who have poor absorption, diarrhea, vomiting, dehydration, or peripheral vascular collapse is _____.

19. (LO 20-3) Checking the dose of a medication is a shared responsibility between the _____ and _____.

20. (LO 20-3) _____ is a serious concern when administering medications to a child who is extremely fussy or crying.

21. (LO 20-4) Because a teaspoon is an inaccurate medication administration device, the teaspoon should be converted to _____.

22. (LO 20-4) The preferred route of administration for iron is _____.

23. (LO 20-4) The gauge of the needle for injections other than immunizations to be used for toddlers is

_____.

24. (LO 20-4) The _____ side of the arm should be avoided when administering a subcutaneous or intradermal injection to a child because the skin is more sensitive.

25. (LO 20-2) A _____ child cannot verbalize side effects of medications such as dizziness or ringing in the ears.

26. (LO 20-4) To administer drops to a child, a(n) _____ should be used.

27. (LO 20-4) The route of medication administration that should never be used with a child who is at risk for aspiration is _____.

28. (LO 20-4) The route of medication administration for giving an immunization to a child is _____.

Drug Calculations—Fill in the blank with the answer.

29. (LO 20-4) The provider orders a drug 10 mg/kg orally daily for a child weighing 27 kg. Available is a 50-mg/mL suspension. Prepare to administer _____ mL to the child.

30. (LO 20-4) The provider orders a drug 3 μg/kg intramuscularly bid for a child weighing 21.36 kg. Available is 50 μg/mL. Prepare to administer _____ mL to the child.

31. (LO 20-4) The provider orders a drug 200 mg orally qid for a child weighing 55 lb. Available is 250 mg/5 mL. Prepare to administer _____ mL to the child.

32. (LO 20-4) Calculate the body surface area for a child who is 75 cm tall and weighs 10.2 kg.

33. (LO 20-4) Calculate the body surface area for a child who is 25 inches tall and weighs 10 lb.

Multiple Choice—Circle the correct letter.

34. (LO 20-2) Which of the following physiological alterations should you take into consideration when administering medications to a pediatric patient?
    a. Infants and children require larger doses of medications than do adults.
    b. The kidneys of pediatric patients dilute the drugs more, making effects weaker.
    c. Pediatric liver enzyme systems are immature, making children more vulnerable to harmful effects of the drug.
    d. Children have higher plasma concentrations of protein for binding of drugs.

35. (LO 20-3) What is the most important critical safeguard for safely administering pediatric medications and preventing an unpredictable response to the drug?
    a. Read the side effects of the drug.
    b. Double-check the drug with another person.
    c. Administer a smaller than prescribed dose.
    d. Ask the child's name.

36. (LO 20-4) What is the preferred route or form of medication for administering a drug to a pediatric patient?

 a. Dissolved or suspended oral medications

 b. Subcutaneous

 c. Intramuscular

 d. Intravenous

37. (LO 20-4) Which of the following strategies should you use to enhance acceptance of giving an oral drug to a child?

 a. Avoid carbonated beverages.

 b. Mix the medicine with cereal.

 c. Pinch the nose and drink through a straw.

 d. Avoid water immediately after giving the medicine.

38. (LO 20-4) In preparing to administer a medication to a child, which of the following principles should you consider?

 a. Medications that are irritating, such as iron, should be administered subcutaneously.

 b. Avoid administering an oral medication in a flavored suspension.

 c. A 1-mL syringe should be used to give a low-dose, small-volume drug.

 d. Use the intravenous route in a child experiencing diarrhea and dehydration.

Chapter 20 Case Studies

39. (LO 20-4) A mother asks you what she can do to help her son take his medicine. What will you tell her to do? _____

_____

_____

_____

40. (LO 20-4) An immunization has been ordered for a 2-month-old infant. At what location should you give this injection? What length and gauge of needle should you use? What is the maximum amount that may be given? _____

_____

_____

_____

Critical Thinking

41. (LO 20-4) What can you do to enhance acceptance of an oral medication by a child who is fussy and doesn't want the medication?

_____

_____

42. (LO 20-4) What should you tell a child to do when the child complains of an unpleasant taste and smell when taking a medication?

_____

_____

43. (LO 20-4) How should you prevent cross-contamination between medications after crushing a tablet in a pill crusher?

_____

_____

44. (LO 20-4) You have been assigned to administer digoxin and insulin to a child. What should you do before administering these drugs?

_____

_____

45. (LO 20-4) Before you administer a drug by any route, what is the most reliable method you should use to verify the identity of the child?

_____

_____

DRUGS FOR THE OLDER ADULT PATIENT

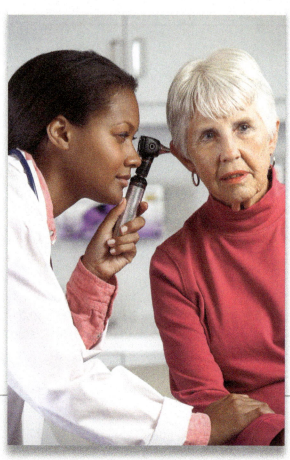

©Monkey Business Images/Shutterstock

In this chapter you will learn how the normal physical changes of aging affect pharmacokinetics and why this poses special problems for medication administration. You will learn about the social and psychological aspects of aging so that you can adjust your treatment to best meet older adult patients' needs.

DRUGS AND THE OLDER ADULT [LO 21-1, LO 21-2]

Regardless of whether you are employed in a long-term care facility or in another clinical setting, you are likely to find yourself working with an older adult patient population. The population aged 65 years and older is the fastest-growing segment of the population, increasing approximately 2 percent each year. Medication therapy is one of the most important ways in which geriatric medicine is different from medical care delivered to younger patients. Not only are there physiological alterations of advancing age, but multiple diseases, environmental factors, and genetic variations all affect a drug's effect, metabolism, and toxicity. Older adults make up the largest group of users of pharmaceuticals, accounting for over 30 percent of all written prescriptions and over 40 percent of all over-the-counter drugs and herbal remedies. In addition, older adults are two to three times more likely to experience adverse reactions to drugs than are younger patients. Medical assistance is required to help older adults maintain the best possible health. Drugs are part of the health maintenance program; they also play a large part in disease management.

The study of aging is called **gerontology,** and the study of diseases of older adults is called **geriatrics.** Because you will probably work with older adults in administering medications, it is important to understand their special problems and needs. It is especially important because older adults are often slighted in treatment. You want to be the best caregiver possible, and a thorough understanding of older adults and their drug-related needs is an important step toward that goal.

The Aging Process

As body cells are lost through aging, the organs that they compose slow down. Almost every organ loses some of its function, although this loss does not necessarily represent disease. Such changes are normal, anticipated changes in older adults. The body also loses some of its ability to cope with stress. Stress is longer-lasting and more extreme with aging. Disease and injury are forms of stress that put the body temporarily out of balance. The effect of aging is to make it harder for the older adult to "bounce back" after diseases—even minor diseases such as colds. Healing takes longer and complications are more likely to develop. That is why flu, pneumonia, and broken bones are much more serious for older adults than for younger adults.

Aging does not occur at exactly the same rate in everyone. Body systems age at different times and at different rates. There are also wide variations among individuals in the course of aging. For some people, the first sign of aging is loss of visual sharpness—requiring reading glasses, for example. For others, it is a slowdown of the digestive system and resulting constipation. These people find they must drink prune juice or eat more bran cereals to keep regular bowel habits. Fruits and vegetables are not only an excellent source of vitamins and minerals, but they also help maintain evacuation.

Many people react to aging by becoming less active. They take up less strenuous sports and reduce their workload. This is a normal adjustment to the changes of aging. But reducing the level of activity does not and should

Figure 21.1

Proper health maintenance can help older adults continue to lead active lives.

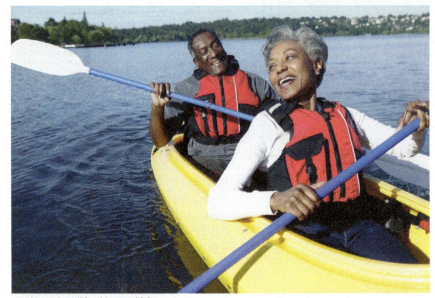

©Andersen Ross/Blend Images LLC

not mean giving up all activity. With proper health maintenance and proper attitudes in people around them, older adults can continue to lead active and rewarding lives (**Figure 21.1**). Walking even short distances is beneficial. Some health facilities have stretching exercises that are not strenuous.

The following is a discussion of specific changes that may be expected at some time in each body system. Now that you have studied these systems, you should be able to appreciate how the changes of aging affect their functioning.

Integumentary System. The skin becomes thinner, drier, and loses its suppleness. The fatty layer under the skin disappears, causing wrinkles and folds and giving less protection against cold and injury. Bruising is more common. Spots of color appear on the skin, and small vessels are likely to burst, causing "spiders." Sweating decreases, and there is less blood flow to the skin. Older adults who are bedridden are at high risk of developing decubitus ulcers (pressure sores). Lichen planus is more common in older patients. It is characterized by flat-topped, purple elevations that appear on the scalp, fingernails, toenails, or inside the mouth or genitalia.

Cardiovascular System. The heart becomes less efficient, pumping less forcefully and less blood with each beat, while the number of beats per minute increases. The heart has less ability to gear up for action when the body is under stress. Various parts of the heart and the blood vessels lose elasticity, and fatty substances may be deposited on the inner layers of arteries. These deposits give more resistance to the heart's pumping action, so hypertension may develop. There is less blood flow to all parts of the body.

Respiratory System. A protein called **collagen** settles in the lungs, lessening their ability to expand. Along with reduced blood flow to the lungs, reduced expansion makes respiration less efficient, and not as much oxygen is supplied to the body. To make up for this deficiency, an older adult may breathe faster than the normal 16 to 20 times per minute. Breathing is also shallower.

Nervous System. Brain cells die and brain weight decreases. Less blood flow to the brain affects memory and the ability to make decisions. Confused thinking and personality changes can also result from the decreased supply of oxygen to the brain.

Sensory System. The ability to perceive messages received through the senses decreases. The eyes have difficulty adjusting to changes in light.

The ears do not hear the higher sounds, and hearing aids may be needed. Taste and smell are dulled, so that eating becomes less pleasurable. The sense of touch is dulled. When the senses do not provide as much information as before, the older adult may become confused, especially in strange surroundings.

Gastrointestinal System. The secretions and muscular movements of the digestive tract slow down, and older adults produce less stomach acid than normal. These changes make food harder to digest and slower to move through the system. Indigestion and constipation are common problems. If teeth are lost or inflamed, eating may be difficult or uncomfortable. Absorption of nutrients from the intestines is less efficient, so nutrition may be affected.

Urinary System. There is less blood flow to the kidneys, and there are changes within the kidneys themselves. They do not filter the blood as efficiently, so wastes are excreted more slowly. The kidneys cannot adapt as quickly as before to changes in the fluid–electrolyte balance. Urgency and stress incontinence may occur in female patients from a decrease in perineal muscle tone. Urinary frequency may occur in males because of an enlarged prostate.

Endocrine System. All the glands secrete less of their hormones. As a result, body cell metabolism is not as well regulated and the body cannot react as quickly to stress.

Reproductive System. Usually between ages 45 and 52, females no longer menstruate and are no longer able to conceive. In both men and women, sex hormone production decreases, with resulting physical changes. However, because sexual enjoyment is determined by attitudes and emotions, not just hormones, older adults can still enjoy active sex lives.

Musculoskeletal System. Muscles lose strength and flexibility. There is also an increase in the percentage of body fat, replacing muscle. The bones are more prone to demineralization and become lighter and more porous. As a result, they are more apt to fracture easily and heal slowly. Ligaments and joints are subject to stiffening and thickening. Diseases of bones, joints, and ligaments are more common.

PHARMACOKINETICS IN THE OLDER ADULT [LO 21-3]

Let us look at what the changes of aging do to the actions of drugs in the body. Remember that drugs entering the body undergo four processes: absorption, distribution, biotransformation (metabolism), and excretion. Naturally, the aging of the body systems has an impact on how drugs are absorbed, distributed, metabolized, and excreted. In general, absorption, metabolism, and excretion become slower, and distribution becomes unpredictable. For a person administering medications to older adults, it is important to understand these pharmacokinetic effects of aging. This discussion will help you learn why you should be particularly watchful for side effects and unusual effects of drugs in older adults.

Slower Circulation, Slower Absorption

Absorption and distribution are affected mainly by two things: slower blood circulation and slower absorption of oral medications through the intestines. Slower circulation occurs because the heart pumps less efficiently and must work against blood vessels that have lost their elasticity. The stomach and intestines have fewer of the digestive enzymes needed to help drugs break down and be absorbed through the lining. Peristalsis is weaker, so drugs do not reach the intestine as quickly. As a result, drug absorption and distribution are slower and less predictable in older adults. Therefore, you cannot be sure that the proper dose is getting to where it is needed in the usual amount of time.

In addition, because of decreased circulation, the heart and brain compete with the rest of the body for the blood supply. They demand and get more blood, and other parts of the body get less. Distribution of drugs is affected, because more of the drugs end up in the heart and brain. This distribution can lead to abnormal drug reactions.

Biotransformation or metabolism of drugs is affected by the reduced capacity of the liver. Most drugs are biotransformed (metabolized) in the liver. In older adults, however, the liver produces fewer enzymes to break down drugs, so they are not biotransformed as quickly or as completely. The drugs stay in effect longer and can build up in the body with repeated doses. The result may be a cumulative effect and even drug toxicity.

Excretion is affected by changes in kidney function. Reduced blood circulation and changes in kidney cells combine to make blood filtration slower. Thus drugs are not excreted as quickly. Again, they can build up in the body and show cumulative or toxic effects. Some drugs, such as urinary antiseptics, do not become active until they are excreted by the kidneys. In older adults these drugs take longer than usual to show an effect.

Finally, because of the body's lessened ability to keep a balance among all the systems, drugs are more apt to throw the body into wide imbalances. Unusual and unexpected drug reactions may occur from time to time. Also, older adults are more sensitive to the effects of certain drugs.

Because of these changes in pharmacokinetics, one must be very careful in administering medications to older adults. As a general rule, medications for older adults are prescribed in lower doses and are to be given less frequently to help prevent cumulation and toxicity. To aid absorption, adjustments are made in the forms of medication given and their routes.

Diseases and Drug Interactions

Two other age-related factors have an impact on the effect of a drug: disease and other drugs. We have said that older adults are more prone to disease. By adding disease factors to the age changes already mentioned, the overall picture becomes complicated. For instance, a diseased kidney or liver, a heart condition, or hypertension can further slow the body's handling of drugs. Because older adults tend to have more diseases, there is a greater chance for adverse drug reactions, especially cumulation.

Consider also the possible drug interactions. Older adults have more ailments, both major and minor, than do younger adults. Thus they are likely to take more drugs together. For example, they may routinely take nonprescription laxatives, antacids, or mild stimulants. Any of these can interact with drugs that a provider may prescribe. It is extremely important for the medical staff to find out what other medications patients are taking on their own, especially OTC medications. For example, you may discover that a tetracycline has been prescribed for an infection for an older adult patient who is also taking bicarbonate of soda for an upset stomach. As you know, antacids decrease the absorption of tetracyclines.

As a situation that can be even more dangerous, consider the patient who is on corticosteroids for chronic rheumatoid arthritis, a condition common in the older adult population. Corticosteroids increase the excretion of potassium in the kidneys. Now suppose that the person develops a heart condition requiring digitalis, a cardiac stimulant. A normal dose of digitalis becomes dangerously strong (i.e., is potentiated) when there is little potassium in the body. Cardiac arrhythmias could result from the combined action of the corticosteroid and digitalis.

It is the provider's responsibility to avoid, wherever possible, prescribing drugs that could interact in a harmful way. But as an added safety precaution, you too should be aware of possible interactions. There are times when the provider must order drugs that are known to interact because the risk of drug interaction is less than the risk of not giving two drugs the patient needs. In these circumstances, all the people who are attending the patient must be especially careful to chart any unusual signs. Examples of important drug interactions that can occur with medications for older adults are listed in Table 21.1. Examples of drug and food interactions are listed in Table 21.2.

The complex pharmacokinetics in the older adult should suggest, then, that you be alert for possible adverse reactions and side effects. You must watch especially for signs of cumulation, toxicity, drug interactions, and unusual effects. All your skills of observation and communication are needed to ensure that older adult patients receive safe drug treatment. Talk with your patients, ask them questions, and carefully notice all their physical and psychological signs. Question your patients specifically about the use of a number of different drugs prescribed by different providers (**polypharmacy**).

Table 21.1 Common Drug Interactions with Older Adult Patients

Drugs That Interact	Results of Combination
Alcohol + sedatives	Both depress central nervous system and can result in toxicity
Antipsychotics + antiparkinsonian agents + antidepressants + antihistamines	All have anticholinergic effects; when combined, can cause dry mouth, blurred vision, urine retention, constipation, increased intraocular pressure
Nonsteroidal anti-inflammatory drugs (NSAIDs) + diuretics	Decrease effects of diuretics
Nonsteroidal anti-inflammatory drugs (NSAIDs) + anticoagulants + acetylsalicylic acid	Increased anticoagulant effect, increased bleeding
Bisacodyl (*Dulcolax*) + antacids	Enteric coating of bisacodyl dissolves in stomach, causing gastric irritation
Tetracycline + metals (milk, antacids, and other substances containing calcium, magnesium, aluminum, or iron)	Reduced absorption of tetracycline can lessen its effect
Cholestyramine (*Questran*) or colestipol (*Colestid*) (anticholesteremics) + acidic drugs	Poor absorption of acidic drugs may lessen their effects
Cathartics (laxatives)	Increased intestinal motility caused by cathartics can decrease absorption of any drug
Warfarin (*Coumadin*) + cimetidine (*Tagamet-HB*)	Warfarin is potentiated
Warfarin (*Coumadin*) + phenobarbital	Anticoagulant breaks down more quickly, so has less effect; increases risk of thrombus formation
Warfarin (*Coumadin*) + aspirin or nonsteroidal anti-inflammatory drugs (NSAIDs)	Increased action of warfarin
Vitamin D + anticonvulsants phenytoin (*Dilantin*) and phenobarbital	Vitamin D breaks down more quickly; patient may require vitamin D supplements

(continued)

Table 21.1 (continued)

Drugs That Interact	Results of Combination
Allopurinol (*Zyloprim*) + mercaptopurine or azathioprine (*Imuran*)	Allopurinol slows breakdown of the other drugs; can lead to toxicity
Salicylates (e.g., aspirin) + acidifiers	Prolongs and possibly increases effects of salicylates; can lead to toxicity
Penicillins + probenecid	Excretion of penicillin blocked
Monoamine oxidase inhibitors + sympathomimetics (e.g., beta agonists)	Releases large amounts of norepinephrine; can cause severe headache, hypertension, or arrhythmias
Digitalis + diuretics	Diuretics can cause potassium loss, making heart more sensitive to digitalis effects; can cause arrhythmias
Lithium carbonate + diuretics	Loss of sodium increases effects of lithium; toxicity (nausea, vomiting, weakness, sleepiness, seizures)
Digoxin + quinidine	Quinidine interferes with digoxin clearance; increases risk of digoxin toxicity (nausea, vomiting, weakness, heart rhythm changes)
Phenytoin (*Dilantin*) + enteral feedings	Reduced phenytoin absorption
Phenytoin (*Dilantin*) + cimetidine (*Tagamet-HB*)	Phenytoin is increased
ACE inhibitors + potassium-sparing diuretics (e.g., *Aldactone*)	Hyperkalemia (elevated potassium level)

Table 21.2 Common Drug–Food Interactions

Drug–Food Interaction	Results
Carbidopa/levodopa (*Sinemet*) + protein	Decreased absorption of *Sinemet*
Cyclosporine (*Sandimmune*) + grapefruit	Increased blood level of *Sandimmune*
Iron + tea, eggs, or bran	Decreased absorption of *Feosol*
Monoamine oxidase inhibitors such as phenelzine (*Nardil*) and tranylcypromine (*Parnate*) + foods high in amines such as wine, cheese, chicken, liver, avocados, pickled herring, figs	Hypertension
Quinolone antibiotics such as ciprofloxacin (*Cipro*) and ofloxacin + dairy products	Decreased absorption of quinolone antibiotics
Sedatives + alcohol	Increased sedation
Tetracycline + dairy products	Decreased absorption of tetracycline
Warfarin (*Coumadin*) + psyllium	Decreased absorption of *Coumadin*
Warfarin (*Coumadin*) + vitamin E	Increased effectiveness of *Coumadin*

OBTAINING A MEDICAL AND MEDICATION HISTORY [LO 21-4]

Obtaining a medical history is a standard and comprehensive way of collecting information about a patient to be used by various members of the healthcare team. Components of a medical history include demographic data, chief complaint, history of present illness, past health history, family health history, a list of all medications taken, and a review of systems. You may be asked to collect portions of the medical history of a patient upon admission to the hospital, at a long-term care facility, or in the provider's office. Before beginning a medical history, explain to your patient that it will provide information that will be used in the development of an individualized plan of care and also for health promotion.

The medical history includes both subjective and objective data. Subjective data are the information your patient tells you, such as demographic data, including age, address, marital status, occupation, and so on. The patient's chief complaint, history of present illness, past health history, family health history, and a review of medications are also examples of subjective data. The patient's chief complaint is what brought the patient to the healthcare facility. The history of the present illness includes what kinds of symptoms the patient is having and how long they have been a problem. Illnesses or surgeries the patient has had in the past are revealed under the patient's past health history. Taking a family health history reveals such illnesses as cancer or heart disease.

A review of medications is a particularly valuable piece of information for the older adult. It is recommended that the older adult patient bring a list of all medications or the bottles of all medications, including both prescription and over-the-counter medications, to the healthcare provider. Pay particular attention to the names of the prescribing providers. Often, an older adult patient may see different providers for the same condition and get similar medications to treat the same condition. This can be a very dangerous practice. Older adult patients may also be taking an over-the-counter medication to treat the same condition, resulting in overmedication. For example, a patient may see a provider for osteoarthritis and be taking celecoxib (*Celebrex*) while another provider prescribes naproxen (*Naprosyn*). The patient may also be self-medicating by taking over-the-counter ibuprofen (*Motrin IB*). The end result is the patient is taking three medications to treat the same condition. These medications may interact with each other, increasing the incidence of adverse reactions such as gastrointestinal bleeding.

It is essential that you question your patients about multiple providers and medications to treat the same conditions. It is only through an evaluation of all of your patient's medications that interactions between medications may be discovered. For example, a patient may be taking digoxin (*Lanoxin*) and furosemide (*Lasix*) for congestive heart failure. The combination of both drugs may put the patient at risk for potassium loss and arrhythmias. Being aware of all of your patient's medications allows you to monitor your patient's condition carefully or notify the appropriate resource of a change or concern so that you will be a safe practitioner.

Objective data obtained during a medical history consist of an assessment or a review of the patient's systems. Generally the review of systems is performed by the nurse or the healthcare provider. Skills such as inspection, palpation, percussion, and auscultation are necessary to perform the review of systems. However, you may be asked to assist or perform select procedures such as checking body temperature, pulse, respirations, and blood pressure.

ADMINISTERING MEDICATIONS TO OLDER ADULT PATIENTS [LO 21-5, LO 21-6]

Aging brings changes in the patterns of daily living. It also brings changes in your responsibilities as a giver of medications. Remember that you must individualize your treatment of each patient. The provider is responsible for adjusting dosages and routes, and you must adjust your care. You must be resourceful, caring, firm, patient, aware, and knowledgeable. The following suggestions may help you adjust your care to the older adult so as to achieve the best drug effect and maximize the patient's independence.

Identify the right patient. This is the first rule of the "seven rights." As previously discussed, never administer medication to a patient who does not have an identification bracelet. Remember, any patient may incorrectly respond to a name. If the patient does not have an identification bracelet, have another identification bracelet made. If for some reason a patient will not leave the bracelet on, secure it to the head of the bed.

Explain what you are doing. Explaining your actions to the patient is one of the most important general rules for administering medications. Everyone likes to be told what to expect, even if they may expect some discomfort. Older adults are sometimes fearful of medications. Explain cheerfully and positively why you are there, what medications you are giving, and how you will give them. Allowing older adult patients to take an active role in their own care helps them maintain their self-confidence and feeling of independence.

Be patient; do not rush. Encourage patients who are lying down to sit up before you administer medications. They will have an easier time swallowing the medication. Give one tablet at a time to swallow, and allow the patient time between tablets to rest. Take the time to treat each patient as an individual. A slow and easy approach on your part will encourage confidence and cooperation.

Explain what the drug is supposed to do. Explain in simple terms what the drugs are for. Encourage patients to ask questions about their medications. Questions and answers help enhance patient compliance and drug effectiveness.

Help a patient who has trouble swallowing pills. When a patient has difficulty swallowing tablets or capsules, ask the provider to substitute a liquid medication if at all possible. As a general principle, have the patient take a few sips of water before giving the medication to moisten the mouth and make swallowing easier. Do not cut or crush a tablet or place it in applesauce or fruit juice. This practice can reduce the dose and effectiveness of some drugs. It may also cause choking or aspiration of medication particles. Raise the head of the bed or have the patient sit up to facilitate swallowing. Encourage patients to drink 5 to 6 ounces of fluid after medication administration, unless a patient's condition, such as renal failure, contraindicates this. Encouraging fluids ensures that the medication leaves the esophagus and enters the stomach to speed its absorption. Always stay with the patient until you are sure the medication has been swallowed.

When a patient appears confused, assess the reason. Confusion about identity, location, last drug taken, and so on comes from many sources. There may be a lack of oxygen in the brain. Medication that affects the nervous system may cause confusion. Or the patient may have psychological problems. Do not automatically assume that a patient has dementia or has given up trying to communicate. Consider the drugs the patient is taking. Confusion and other mental status changes are frequent side effects of a number of medications. Help the patient focus on what you are saying. Encourage the patient to express his or her needs clearly and to stay in touch with reality.

Respect each patient's customs and beliefs. Be empathetic to patients' cultural and ethnic beliefs and traditions in regard to drug therapy. Be flexible, and try to adapt to the patient's requests as much as the provider's orders allow.

Adapt to hearing and vision problems. Older adults may have difficulty hearing or seeing, so you need to adapt your behavior to their special problems. Speak slowly and clearly when giving instructions, and wait for signs of understanding. Stand facing the patient when you speak, so that he or she can read your lips. Write things down, if necessary, and use large letters that are easy to read. Sometimes what seems like mental confusion is merely a sign that a patient cannot hear or see what you are saying or doing. Always keep this possibility in mind so that you adjust to the patient's situation.

Blood and urine tests are important. When ordered, make sure these tests are done and the results checked. Many drugs do not have a therapeutic effect until they reach a certain level in the body. Tests are necessary to find out when this point has been reached. A patient who is fearful of tests may accept them better if you explain their importance.

Help older adult patients with eye drops. Some patients prefer to administer their own eye drops; others do not. Support their wish for independence. If you administer the eye drops, take care not to contaminate the dropper by touching the eye or eyelashes. You may need to instruct the patient in self-administration. (See Practice Procedure 8.1, at end of chapter 8.)

Watch for dangers of OTC drugs. Seemingly harmless OTC drugs, which many older adult patients take, can be dangerous when they accumulate or interact with prescription drugs. Know the combined effects of OTC and prescription drugs so that you can be alert to adverse reactions.

Make sure that all ordered medications are given. A good charting system and proper organization will ensure that each patient receives all ordered medications.

Explain the need for medication to asymptomatic patients. A patient who has no obvious symptoms may refuse medications. Explain to patients why they must continue to take some medications (e.g., those for hypertension and infection) even after the symptoms are under control.

Help older adult patients remember their medications and instructions. Arrange for your older adult patients to take medications at certain times each day, such as before meals. Taking medications at regularly scheduled times makes it easier for the patient to remember. If special instructions go along with the medications, explain them clearly and simply and also write them out. If a patient has poor eyesight, label drug bottles with large letters. A daily pill box can also organize a patient's pills according to the day to help the patient remember to take all medications.

Never force a patient to take medication. Explain the purpose of the medication. If your positive, encouraging attitude and your explanations of the benefits of the drugs do not get the patient to accept a drug, do not push the issue. Instead, report the problem to the nurse in charge and wait for further instructions. In some cases, medications will have to be given parenterally until the patient's cooperation can be secured for oral medication.

Keep medications secure. Never leave the medicine room unlocked. Patients may wander by and take medications that can cause them harm. Never leave the medicine cart unattended. Because you may be spending more time with older adult patients in giving their medications, you will have less time to keep an eye on the cart. On the other hand, you do not want to rush each patient. A good solution is to get an attendant to watch the cart while you help patients. When possible, lock the cart while you work with patients.

Chart medications promptly. Do your charting as soon as you finish giving medications. You will have many medications to chart, and you may be tempted to leave charting until the end of the day. This is a dangerous practice that can lead to medication errors. It can and must be avoided by properly organizing your charting procedures. The only correct time to chart medications is right after you give them. When a cart is used, the charting form for medications is usually on it for immediate charting.

Use caution with prn medications. When a prn order has a range of doses, try giving the smallest dose first. This dose is often enough to bring about the desired effect. Because of slow absorption and metabolism, a higher dose may produce unpleasant side effects or adverse reactions. Guard against giving a higher dose of a prn medication just because a patient is confused. The prn medication may actually be causing the confusion through some effect on the oxygen supply to the brain. Make sure you chart prn medications immediately. If you put it off until later, someone else may give the patient another dose of the medication. The patient may not remember that you gave a previous dose. It is easy to overdose a patient accidentally by forgetting to chart prn medications. You should be aware that some patients may pretend to take their medications but actually put their pills and capsules in pockets, drawers, pillowcases, plants, or anywhere. Report this to the lead healthcare team member, and follow his or her instructions. Be aware that this can happen, and try to prevent it by staying with your patient until the medication is swallowed.

ENGAGING PATIENTS IN THEIR CARE [LO 21-7]

When you give medications to older adults, it is important to remember that they can and should take an active part in their medication therapy. They should be encouraged to take their own medications under your supervision. They can pour their own glass of water. They can apply their own ointments. They can help design a plan for remembering to take all their medications. The point is that their care includes concern for their mental health. Your treatment must leave room for independent effort. Let them do as much as they are capable of doing, even if you could do it more quickly and efficiently. Their mental health depends on your letting them care for themselves when they are willing and able to do so. Give medical care with the patient, not for the patient (**Figure 21.2**).

Figure 21.2

Take time to talk and listen to the patient. Encourage patients to take an active role in their medication therapy.

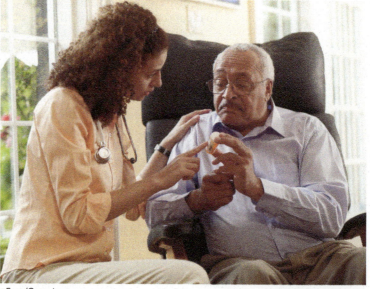

©Fuse/Getty Images

Finally, be prepared to meet many needs in individual older adult patients. Be supportive of their activities. Encourage them to get the most they can out of life. Show that you care about them, and help ease their physical and emotional burdens. You and your fellow workers have the power to influence your patients' lives, either positively or negatively. Do not abuse that power. The more you help them be independent and confident, the less older adults will feel like a burden, both to you and to themselves.

 Healthcare for Today and Tomorrow | **Anti-inflammatories and Alzheimer's**

Current research suggests that older adults who take aspirin and other anti-inflammatory drugs such as ibuprofen for at least two years have a significantly lower incidence of Alzheimer's disease than do older adults who do not take these drugs. The results show promise in preventing Alzheimer's if these drugs are taken during this critical period before the brain has been damaged enough to produce symptoms.

 Legal and Ethical Issues | **Older Adult Issues**

The United States has a severe shortage of **geriatricians,** geriatric-trained providers to treat older adults. Recent research indicates that there are not enough geriatricians to treat the rapidly growing older adult population. According to a recent study in the *Journal of the American Medical Association,* errors in prescribing drugs to geriatric patients are frequent. In addition, the average older adult patient takes seven or more drugs—often prescribed by different providers—and some may be deemed dangerous for older adults.

As a member of the healthcare team, it is your responsibility to report unexplained weight loss, decreased function, drowsiness, or frailty to your patient's provider. The provider will need to reevaluate the patient's prescriptions. You may be protecting your patient from medication errors or possible fatal drug combinations.

Summary

Learning Outcome	Summary Points
21-1 Describe the major changes that take place in the various body systems during aging.	• *Skin* becomes thinner and drier and loses suppleness. • The *heart* becomes less efficient, while the number of beats per minute increases. • Collagen accumulates in the *lungs,* lessening their ability to expand. Breathing becomes more rapid and shallow. • *Brain* cells die and brain weight decreases, affecting memory. • *Senses* decrease. • The *digestive tract* slows down, increasing constipation. • Less blood flows to the *kidneys,* so wastes are excreted more slowly. • All *endocrine glands* secrete less of their hormones, so the body cannot react as quickly to stress. • *Menstruation* stops, and *sex hormones* are decreased. • *Muscles* lose their flexibility. • *Bones* demineralize, and fractures are more common.

Learning Outcome	Summary Points
21-2 Describe the effects of aging on absorption, distribution, metabolism, and excretion of drugs.	• *Absorption* and *distribution* are affected by slower blood circulation and slower absorption of oral medications through the intestines. Thus drug absorption and distribution are slower and less predictable. As a result, the patient may not get the proper dose in the usual amount of time. Also, because the heart and brain compete with the rest of the body for blood, distribution can lead to abnormal drug reactions. • *Metabolism (biotransformation)* of drugs is affected by the decreased capacity of the liver. Drugs stay in effect longer and may build up in the body. • *Excretion* of drugs is slower because there is reduced circulation through the kidneys.
21-3 Explain why the presence of multiple diseases in older adults makes drug therapy more complicated, including adverse reactions.	• There is a greater chance of adverse reactions, especially cumulation. • Patients may take multiple drugs prescribed by multiple providers. Drug interactions are common.
21-4 Discuss an older patient's medical and medication history with him or her.	• Obtaining a medical history is a comprehensive way to gather information on a patient that will be used by members of the healthcare team. • The medical history is valuable because it provides both subjective and objective data.
21-5 Explain how older adults are affected by the attitudes and actions of healthcare workers.	• Older adult patients must feel comfortable and safe with the members of the healthcare team to honestly answer healthcare questions.
21-6 Describe safe medication administration practices and the principles that are specific for the older adult patient.	• Identify the right patient. • Adapt care to the patient's health status. • Consider vision and assist with eye drops. • Consider hearing problems. • Assist with methods that improve the swallowing of pills.
21-7 List ways that patients can take an active part in their own medication therapy.	• Allow older patients to be self-sufficient, such as pouring their own water and applying their own ointments. • Encourage patients to be independent and confident.

Chapter 21 Review

Define each of the terms listed.

1. (LO 21-2) Geriatrics _____

2. (LO 21-2) Gerontology _____

3. (LO 21-3) Polypharmacy _____

4. (LO 21-3) OTC medications _____

Briefly describe the major changes that occur in each body system as one ages.

5. (LO 21-1) Integumentary system _____

_____

_____

_____

6. (LO 21-1) Cardiovascular system _____

_____

_____

_____

7. (LO 21-1) Respiratory system _____

_____

_____

_____

8. (LO 21-1) Nervous system _____

_____

_____

_____

9. (LO 21-1) Sensory system _____

_____

_____

_____

10. (LO 21-1) Gastrointestinal system _____

_____

_____

_____

11. (LO 21-1) Urinary system _____

_____

_____

_____

_____

12. (LO 21-1) Endocrine system _____

_____

_____

_____

13. (LO 21-1) Reproductive system _____

_____

_____

_____

_____

14. (LO 21-1) Musculoskeletal system _____

_____

_____

_____

_____

True or False

Place a T in the blank if the statement is true. Place an F in the blank if the statement is false.

_____ 15. (LO 21-1) Older adults make up the largest group of users of pharmaceuticals.

_____ 16. (LO 21-1) Older adults are less likely to experience adverse reactions than are younger patients.

_____ 17. (LO 21-1) It is recommended that older adult patients bring a list of all prescription drugs, over-the-counter drugs, and herbal remedies they are taking to their healthcare provider.

_____ 18. (LO 21-3) Normally, an older adult patient has the same provider to treat all of his or her illnesses and conditions.

_____ 19. (LO 21-2) An older adult patient who takes cathartics will have increased absorption of any drug.

_____ 20. (LO 21-3) Older adult patients who drink alcohol and take sedatives will experience increased sedation.

Answer the question in the space provided.

21. (LO 21-3) How and why does a provider usually adjust the normal adult dose when ordering medications for an older adult patient? _____

_____

_____

_____

Drug Calculations—Fill in the blank with the answer.

22. (LO 21-3) The provider orders hydromorphone (*Dilaudid*) 3 mg intramuscularly prn. Available is 4 mg/mL. Prepare to administer ——————— mL to your patient.

23. (LO 21-3) The provider orders naproxen (*Naprosyn*) 250 mg orally bid. Available are 500-mg tablets. You will give your patient ——————— tablets.

24. (LO 21-3) The provider orders heparin 3000 units subcutaneously daily. Available is 5000 units/0.5 mL. Prepare to administer ——————— mL to your patient.

25. (LO 21-3) The provider orders verapamil (*Calan*) 80 mg orally tid. Available are 40-mg tablets. You will give your patient ——————— tablets.

26. (LO 21-3) The provider orders donepezil (*Aricept*) 10 mg orally daily. Available are 5-mg tablets. You will give your patient ——————— tablets.

Multiple Choice—Circle the correct letter.

27. (LO 21-1) Which of the following should you consider before administering medications to an older adult?
    a. Loss of visual sharpness is the last sign of aging.
    b. Most older adults are more active than they were when they were younger.
    c. The digestive tract speeds up with aging.
    d. The presence of disease makes it harder to regain health.

28. (LO 21-3) You should monitor an older adult for which of the following drug interactions?
    a. The absorption of tetracycline is reduced with antacids.
    b. *Tagamet-HB* decreases the effect of warfarin (*Coumadin*).
    c. Lithium decreases salt loss when given with diuretics.
    d. A potassium-sparing diuretic and an ACE inhibitor given together may result in hypokalemia.

29. (LO 21-4) Which of the following questions would be most beneficial to ask an older adult who takes a sedative and complains of increased sedation?
    a. "How much sleep do you get?"
    b. "Do you drink alcohol?"
    c. "Do you eat before bedtime?"
    d. "How many times do you get up during the night?"

30. (LO 21-6) Which of the following should you consider in the treatment plan when administering medications to an older adult?
    a. Ask the patient his or her name for identification.
    b. Administer all the medications at one time.
    c. Never administer a liquid medication when the patient has trouble swallowing.
    d. Administer medications at regularly scheduled times.

31. (LO 21-3) Why is it important to inform an older adult not to take bisacodyl (*Dulcolax*) tablets and an antacid together?
    a. The two drugs taken together cancel each other's effect.
    b. The action of the antacid is decreased.
    c. The enteric coating of the *Dulcolax* dissolves, resulting in gastric irritation.
    d. There is decreased action of *Dulcolax.*

Chapter 21 Case Studies

32. (LO 21-3) A patient who has multiple chronic health conditions and is taking a variety of medications complains of dry mouth, blurred vision, urine retention, and constipation. How should you determine what is causing these symptoms? What is the explanation for the cause of these symptoms? What should you do with this information? _____

_____

_____

_____

33. (LO 21-6) An older adult patient tells you he is starting to experience more constipation. He doesn't understand why this is suddenly a problem. What is the plausible cause? What advice can you give the patient that will help prevent constipation? _____

_____

_____

_____

Critical Thinking

The following are situations or scenes that might take place in a long-term care facility or in a hospital unit that has many older adult patients. Answer the questions briefly, using the information in this chapter.

34. (LO 21-2) Mr. Jones and Mr. Smith are both 80 years old. Mr. Jones is strong and physically active and enjoys taking walks. He wears glasses to correct his failing vision. He is forgetful sometimes and tends to tell the same jokes over and over again. Mr. Smith, on the other hand, is frail and walks with a cane, but his watchful eyes take in everything that goes on. His mind is sharp, and he entertains the nursing home staff with his views of current political and social events. Why are these men so different in their physical ability and mental alertness, even though they are the same age? What does this mean in terms of their medication therapy?

_____

_____

_____

35. (LO 21-1) Ms. Peach is taking life easier than she used to, because she finds that her energy runs out more quickly now that she is 72. Her breathing has become slightly faster and shallower than before, which the provider says is normal for a person her age. What changes has her respiratory system probably undergone as a result of aging?

_____

_____

_____

36. (LO 21-3) "Doc Webster" is a delightful older adult man who is full of stories about the days when he practiced surgery in a big city hospital. He is taking a number of medications for heart disease and a nervous condition. Today, when you go to his room, he does not answer to his name and has forgotten where he is. It's hard for you to give him his medication instructions, because he can't seem to concentrate on what you are saying. What possible reasons might explain why he appears confused?

_____

_____

_____

37. (LO 21-7) In giving Mrs. Nimitz, an older adult, her medications, you want to be sure to treat her as an independent, intelligent adult. How can you help her be responsible for taking her medications?

_____

_____

_____

38. (LO 21-3) Mr. Redbone is taking medication for an infection and several other minor disorders. Because of his advanced age, you know that his liver and kidneys are not working as well as they once did. What effect does a weakened kidney or liver have on how the body handles drugs? For what adverse reactions should you be on the lookout?

_____

_____

_____

39. (LO 21-3) Mrs. Mendoza is suffering from phlebitis and must take an anticoagulant to keep blood clots from forming. She keeps a bottle of aspirin in her purse for occasional arthritic pain. She also has an old bottle of tranquilizers her sister gave her. She hasn't mentioned the aspirin and tranquilizers to her provider, but she asks you if it would be all right to take them when necessary. What should you say?

_____

_____

_____

40. (LO 21-7) Your facility has recently admitted a number of new patients, so the staff's workload is heavier than usual. You are busy giving medications and carrying out your other duties. You would like to put off your charting until the end of the day, but you're not sure you should. How will your decision affect the welfare of your patients?

_____

_____

_____

41. (LO 21-6) A new older adult patient, Mr. Minassian, is getting his first dose of medicine. You are instructing him on the usual side effects of the drug. He is smiling and nodding, but he does not seem to understand what you are saying. What can you do to make sure he gets the information he needs?

_____

_____

_____

42. (LO 21-6) Ms. Brill sweetly declines any medications you offer her, saying that she doesn't need them. You are worried because you know that her blood pressure could become dangerously high if she fails to take the antihypertensive and she needs *Glucophage* to control a tendency toward high blood sugar. What should you do?

_____

_____

Abbreviations

Routes of Administration

Route	Abbreviations	Meaning
Buccal	buc	Inside the cheek
Intradermal	ID	Into the skin
Intramuscular	IM	Into the muscle
Intravenous	IV	Into the vein
Oral	PO, p.o.	By mouth
Rectal	R	By rectum
Subcutaneous	subcut	Under the skin (into the fatty layer)
Sublingual	subling, subl, SL	Under the tongue
Topical	No abbreviation	On the skin
Vaginal	vag	By vagina

Times of Administration

Abbreviations	Meaning
a.c.	Before meals
ad lib.	As desired
AM, a.m.	Morning
BID, bid	Twice a day
h., hr.	Hourly
n., noc.	Night
p.c.	After meals
PM, p.m.	After noon
PRN, prn	As necessary
q.h.	Every hour
q2h, q.2h.	Every two hours
q3h, q.3h.	Every three hours
q4h, q.4h.	Every four hours
QID, qid	Four times a day
stat	Immediately
TID, tid	Three times a day

Medical Terms

Abbreviations	Meaning
a	Before
c̄	With
°C	Degrees Celsius (centigrade)
c/o	complains of
DC, d/c	Discontinue
dil.	Dilute
°F	Degrees Fahrenheit
♀	Female
♂	Male
NKA	No known allergies
n.p.o.	Nothing by mouth
ophth, op	Ophthalmic
p̄	After
per	By means of
pH	Hydrogen concentration (acidity and alkalinity)
q	Every
®	Registered product name
Rx	Take
s̄	Without
sig.	Label

Abbreviations Prone to Error in Interpretation

Abbreviations	Current Recommendations
AD	Right ear
AS	Left ear
AU	Both ears
h.s.	Bedtime
MS4	Morphine sulfate
MgS	Magnesium sulfate
OD	Right eye
Os	By mouth, PO, orally
OS	Left eye
OU	Both eyes
q.d., QD	Daily
q.o.d., QOD	Every other day
SC, SQ, subq	Subcut, subcutaneously

Symbols Commonly Used in Medical Notations

Apothecaries' Weights and Measures

℥   minim
ʒ   dram
f ʒ   fluidram
f ℥   fluid ounce
lb   pound

Other Weights and Measures

lbs   pounds
°   degrees
′   foot; minute
″   inch; second
μm   micrometer
μ   micron (former term for micrometer)
mμ   millimicron; nanometer
μg   microgram
mEq   milliequivalent
mL   milliliter
dL   deciliter

Abbreviations

c̄   with
p̄   after
s̄   without
ss, s̄s̄   one-half (Latin *semis*)

Mathematical Functions and Terms

$+$ plus; positive; acid reaction
$-$ minus; negative; alkaline reaction
$\pm$ plus or minus; either positive or negative; indefinite
$\times$ multiply; magnification; crossed with, hybrid
$\div$ divided by
$=$ equal to
$\approx$ approximately equal to
$>$ greater than; from which is derived
$<$ less than; derived from
$\leq$ equal to or less than
$\geq$ equal to or greater than
$\sqrt{}$ square root
$\sqrt[3]{}$ cube root
$:$ ratio; "is to"
$\%$ percent

Chemical Notations

Δ change; heat
$\uparrow$ increase
$\downarrow$ decrease

Warnings

ⓒ   Schedule I controlled substance
ⓒ   Schedule II controlled substance
ⓒ   Schedule III controlled substance
ⓒ   Schedule IV controlled substance
ⓒ   Schedule V controlled substance
☠   poison
☢   radiation
☣   biohazard

Others

Rx   prescription
♂   male
♀   female
†   one
††   two
†††   three

Appendix B

Conversion Tables

The Household System

Weight (dry)	Volume (liquid)	Equivalents
ounce (oz)	drop (gt); drops (gtt)	16 ounces = 1 pound
pound (lb)	teaspoon (t, tsp)	3 teaspoons = 1 tablespoon = $\frac{1}{2}$ ounce
ton (t)	tablespoon (T, tbsp)	16 tablespoons = 1 cup = 8 fluid ounces
	teacup (6 oz)	2 cups = 1 pint
	cup (c) or glass (8 oz)	2 pints = 1 quart
	pint (pt)	4 quarts = 1 gallon
	quart (qt)	
	gallon (gal)	

Converting a Fahrenheit Temperature to the Celsius Scale

$$\frac{°F - 32}{1.8} = °C$$

Converting a Celsius Temperature to the Fahrenheit Scale

$$1.8 \times °C + 32 = °F$$

Common Measurement System Equivalents

	Apothecary	Metric	Household
Liquid Volume	minim (m) 1	0.06 mL (or cc)	1 drop (gt)
	minims 15	1 mL	15 drops (gtt)[a]
	fluidram (f℥) 1	4-5 mL	1 teaspoon (60 gtt)
	fluidrams 4	15 mL	1 tablespoon
	1 fluid ounce (f℥)	30 mL	2 tablespoons (1 oz)
		180 mL	1 teacup (6 oz)
		240 mL	1 cup or glass (8 oz)
		500 mL	1 pint (16 oz)
		750 mL	1.5 pints (24 oz)
		1000 mL (1 L)	1 quart (32 oz)
Dry Weight	gr $\frac{1}{60}$	1 mg	
	gr 1	60 mg	
	gr $7\frac{1}{2}$	500 mg (0.5 g)	
	gr 15	1000 mg (1 g)	
	gr (1 dram) 60	4 g	
	1 oz	30 g	1 oz
		500 g	1.1 lb
		1000 g (1 kg)	2.2 lb

Approximate Conversions between the Metric and Apothecary Systems

	Metric Amount	Apothecary Amount
	2 g (2000 mg)	gr 30
	1 g (1000 mg)	gr 15
	600 mg (0.6 g)	gr 10
	100 mg (0.1 g)	gr $1\frac{1}{2}$
	60 mg (0.06 g)	gr 1
	30 mg (0.03 g)	gr $\frac{1}{2}$
	1 mg (0.001 g)	gr $\frac{1}{60}$
	0.1 mg (0.0001 g)	gr $\frac{1}{600}$
Approximation Formulas	grains × 60 = milligrams	grams × 15 = grains
	milligrams ÷ 60 = grains	grains ÷ 15 = grams

ᵃThis figure varies; number of drops per milliliter depends on the substance being measured.

Glossary

A

abortifacients anything used to terminate pregnancy

abscess localization of pus in any part of the body

absorption passage of a substance into the bloodstream from the site of administration

acid substance with a low pH (below pH 7); opposite of base or alkali

acidifier drug that makes the body's pH more acidic

acidosis condition in which there is an excessive proportion of acid in the blood

acne inflammatory condition of sebaceous glands

acoustic pertaining to hearing or sound

acquired immune deficiency syndrome (AIDS) sexually transmitted disease caused by the human immunodeficiency virus (HIV)

acromion process an extension of the shoulder blade that can be felt at the point where the upper arm meets the shoulder; a landmark for locating the deltoid injection site

action a drug's chemical effects on body cells

active ingredient the ingredient in a drug that produces the therapeutic effect

acute short-term, usually less than six months

administration how a drug is given

adrenals paired glands covering the superior surface of the kidneys; made up of the adrenal cortex, which secretes steroids, and the adrenal medulla, which secretes epinephrine and norepinephrine

adrenergic drug that causes increased contractility of the heart and vasoconstriction of the blood vessels

adrenergic blocking agent (sympatholytic) drug that blocks the effects of impulses transmitted by the sympathetic nervous system

adverse reaction an unintended and undesirable effect of a drug

aerobic bacteria that can survive only in the presence of oxygen

air conduction function of the middle and external ear that conducts and amplifies sound waves from the environment

akathisia side effects characterized by motor restlessness, inability to sit or stand still, and the need to pace, rock, or tap the foot; usually occurs within 5 to 30 days (up to 90 days) of starting an antipsychotic drug

alcoholism chronic, progressive disease that if left untreated can be fatal

alkalizer drug that makes the body's pH more basic or alkaline

alkalosis condition in which there is an excessive proportion of alkali in the blood; opposite of acidosis

allergy reaction of the body cell to a foreign substance (antigen) to which it has previously developed antibodies

alopecia hair loss

alveoli tiny air sacs in the lungs that permit the exchange of oxygen and carbon dioxide through capillary walls (singular: *alveolus*)

Alzheimer's disease (AD) chronic, progressive, degenerative disease of the brain

amenorrhea failure to menstruate; missed menstrual period

ampule a small, sealed glass container holding medication for injection

anaerobic bacteria that can survive without oxygen

analgesic drug that relieves pain

anaphylaxis severe allergic reaction that may be fatal

anatomy the study of the structure of body parts

anemia any condition in which the oxygen-carrying capacity of the blood is reduced

anesthetic drugs drugs that interfere with the conduction of nerve impulses to produce a loss of sensation and muscle relaxation; may cause a partial or complete loss of consciousness

angina pectoris chest pain resulting from lack of oxygen in the heart tissue

angiotensin-converting enzyme (ACE) these inhibitors are the vasodilators of choice for congestive heart failure

anion negatively charged ion

antacid drug that neutralizes hydrochloric acid in the stomach

antagonism the interaction of two drugs to inhibit or cancel each other's effect

anthelmintic drug that eliminates intestinal parasites

antiarthritic drug that suppresses inflammation in degenerative diseases of the joints

antibiotic antimicrobial agent, either natural or synthetic, that kills or stops the growth of other organisms

antibody substance produced in the body that helps the body fight off foreign invaders like microorganisms and antigens

anticholinergic drug that acts on the autonomic nervous system to reduce intestinal motility and slow production of stomach acid

anticoagulant drug that inhibits or delays blood clotting

anticonvulsant drug that prevents, treats, and halts seizures

antidiabetic agents insulin and oral hypoglycemics

antidiarrheal drug that slows intestinal motility and helps produce formed stools instead of loose, watery stools

antiemetic drug that prevents or relieves nausea and vomiting

antiflatulent drug that relieves gassiness and bloating; also known as *carminative*

antifungal drug that kills or prevents the growth of fungi

antigen substance that stimulates production of antibodies and causes allergic reactions

antihistamine drug that counteracts the effects of histamine, relieving allergy symptoms

antihistaminic drug that works against the effects of histamine

antihypertensive drug that lowers high blood pressure

antihyperuricemic drug that reduces formation of uric acid

anti-inflammatory drug that suppresses inflammation

antilipemic drug that lowers the level of lipids in the blood

antimanic drug used to treat the mania episode of manic-depressive illness

antineoplastic drug that interferes with malignant cell replication or reproduction

antiplatelet drug that suppresses platelet aggregation and prevents thrombosis in arteries

antipruritic drug that relieves itching

antipsychotic drug used to treat serious mental illnesses, such as being out of touch with reality; it produces a state of tranquility and works on abnormally functioning nerves; also known as *neuroleptic* or *major tranquilizer*

antiseptic agent that inhibits the growth of microorganisms

antispasmodic drug that acts on the smooth muscle of the intestines to relieve cramping

antitussive drug that decreases coughing

anuria no measurable production of urine; less than 100 mL in 24 hours

anus distal (far-end) opening of the gastrointestinal tract through which feces are eliminated

anxiety state of feeling apprehensive, uneasy, uncertain, or in fear of an unknown or recognized threat

anxiolytic see **minor tranquilizer**

apical pulse heart rate measured with the bell or diaphragm of a stethoscope placed on the apex of the heart

apnea stoppage of breathing; may be temporary or fatal

apothecary system system of measurement in which the basic unit of volume is the minim and the basic unit of weight is the grain

aqueous thin and watery

Arabic numerals 0, 1, 2, 3, 4, 5, 6, 7, 8, 9

arteriosclerosis thickening of the walls of the arterioles with a loss of elasticity and ability to contract

artery blood vessel that carries blood away from the heart

arthritis name for several disorders of the joints, each having different causes and treatments (e.g., gouty arthritis, osteoarthritis, rheumatoid arthritis)

aseptic free of pathogens

aspirate to draw by suction; the process of pulling back on a syringe plunger to check for entry into a blood vessel during an injection

astringent drug that shrinks the blood vessels locally, dries up secretions from weepy lesions, and lessens skin sensitivity

atherosclerosis accumulation of cholesterol and lipids on the walls of the arteries

atrophy wasting away of body tissue (e.g., atrophy of a muscle from lack of use)

autoclave machine that sterilizes with steam under pressure, usually at 250°F, for a designated time

automated external defibrillator (AED) machine that shocks the heart back into a normal rhythm

automated medication dispensing system system used to provide access to medications that is configured to meet the needs of a specific facility, such as a patient care unit in a hospital, long-term care facility, surgery center, or provider's office, 24 hours a day; the most common is Pyxis

automatic sphygmomanometer device that has all the components for taking blood pressure in it instead of having to use both a stethoscope and blood pressure cuff

autonomic nervous system (ANS) part of the nervous system that regulates involuntary vital functions of cardiac and smooth muscles and glands

avitaminosis a condition that results from a deficiency or lack of absorption of vitamins in the diet; also known as *hypovitaminosis*

azotemia accumulation of nitrogenous waste in the blood

B

bactericide an agent that is destructive to bacteria

bacteriostatic an agent that inhibits the growth or multiplication of bacteria

barbiturates drugs that suppress the central nervous system; largely replaced by benzodiazepines

barrel hollow cylinder with graduated markings on it that makes up the body of a syringe

base substance with a high pH (above pH 7); opposite of acid; also known as *alkali*

benign referring to a well-defined tumor that is contained and will not spread to other parts of the body

benign prostatic hyperplasia or hypertrophy (BPH) increase in the epithelial and stromal tissue within the prostate

benzodiazepines drugs that do not exert a general central nervous system depressant effect; act as a muscle relaxant, antianxiety agent, anticonvulsant, and hypnotic

bile digestive juice produced by the liver and stored in the gallbladder; helps digest fats

biotransformation normal body process by which substances are chemically broken down into water-soluble form that the body can excrete; part of the cells' work of burning fuel for growth and energy; also known as *metabolism*

bladder muscular organ for storage of urine, and primary organ of secretion

blepharitis bacterial infection of the eyelid that causes crusting, redness, and irritation

blood pressure force of the blood against vessel walls

body surface area (BSA) a very reliable method of calculating doses of medication for infants and children up to 12 years of age using the child's height, weight, and a nomogram; generally used only in critical care and oncology environments

bone marrow depression disorder of the blood-forming tissue that produces erythrocytes (red blood cells), leukocytes (white blood cells), and platelets

bradycardia slow heartbeat (fewer than 60 beats per minute)

bradykinesia slowness of movement

brand name licensed name under which a drug prepared by a specific manufacturer is sold; also known as *proprietary* or *trade name*

broad-spectrum antibiotics antibiotics that are effective against a wide variety of pathogens

bronchi air passages leading from the trachea to the bronchioles in the lungs (singular: *bronchus*)

bronchiole branch of the bronchi leading to alveolar ducts

bronchodilator drug that increases the vital capacity of the lungs by dilating the bronchi and relaxing the smooth muscles

bronchopulmonary pertaining to the lungs and the air passages

bursa small, fluid-filled sac that cushions places where bones and muscles rub together (plural: *bursae*)

C

canthus angle at either end of the slit between the eyelids

capillaries tiny blood vessels with very thin walls that let certain substances pass through them

cardiac pertaining to the heart

cardiac arrest sudden cessation of breathing and of sufficient circulation of blood by the heart

cardiac catheterization test using a dye injected into the leg with the use of a wire to determine the extent of heart damage; also known as *cardiac angiogram*

cardiac glycoside drug that strengthens the force of the myocardial contraction, slows the heart, and improves the tone of the myocardium

cardiopulmonary resuscitation (CPR) chest compressions and breaths to reestablish circulation and breathing

cataract an opacity that appears in the crystalline lens

catatonia state of psychologically induced immobilization, at times interrupted by episodes of extreme agitation

catheter tube inserted through the urethra into the bladder to allow urine drainage, bladder irrigation, or instillation of medication

cation positively charged ion

cell the basic unit of structure of all living things

Celsius temperature scale in which there is a 100-degree difference between the freezing and boiling points of water

centimeter one-hundredth of a meter (0.01 m)

central hearing loss difficulty understanding the meaning of words heard; inability to understand the meaning of incoming sounds or words; caused by problems of the central nervous system from the auditory nucleus to the cortex

central nervous system (CNS) the part of the nervous system that consists of the brain and spinal cord

cerebral pertaining to the brain

cerebrovascular accident (CVA) hemorrhage or thromboembolism in the brain; also known as *stroke*

cerumen earwax

cervicitis inflammation of the cervix

cervix opening of the uterus

charting keeping records of all patient care on appropriate forms

chemical name name that describes the chemical structure of a compound

chemotherapy drug therapy for cancer symptoms

childhood the period of life extending from infancy to puberty

cholinomimetic drug that stimulates the release of acetylcholine (a neurotransmitter)

chronic long-term, usually more than six months

chyme food mixed with gastric secretions

cirrhosis chronic, progressive disease of the liver characterized by degeneration and destruction of the liver cells

Clostridium difficile Gram-positive, anaerobic, spore-forming bacteria that are the major cause of nosocomial infection

cochlea part of the inner ear; the primary organ of hearing

collagen protein making up fibers in connective tissue; builds up in the lungs during aging, thus decreasing lung elasticity

colon the main part of the large intestine

comedo blackhead

computerized order order transmitted via computer

concentration amount of drug in a certain amount of liquid

conductive hearing loss alteration in the perception of or sensitivity to sounds; occurs with problems in the external and middle ear

conjunctiva a thin mucous membrane lining the eye sockets and eyelids

conjunctivitis an inflammation of the mucous membrane that lines the back of the eyelids and the front of the eye except the cornea

contact dermatitis reaction to an irritating substance that has touched the skin

contraceptives drugs used to control fertility and prevent pregnancy

contracture abnormal, permanent shortening of a muscle caused by muscular atrophy

contraindications conditions in which the use of a certain drug is dangerous or ill-advised

controlled substances potentially dangerous or habit-forming drugs whose sale and use are strictly regulated by the Controlled Substances Act because of their potential for abuse

Controlled Substances Act of 1990 law that regulates manufacturing and distribution of controlled substances; also known as *Comprehensive Drug Abuse Prevention and Control Act*

convert to change from one unit of measurement to another

convulsion periodic, sudden attack of involuntary muscular contractions and relaxations

coronary pertaining to the heart vessels

corticosteroids drugs used on the skin because they suppress inflammation, tighten blood vessels, and relieve itching

cranial pertaining to the skull

cretinism hypothyroidism occurring in infancy and childhood

Crohn's disease chronic, nonspecific, inflammatory bowel disease generally affecting the terminal ileum, jejunum, and colon

culture and sensitivity test laboratory technique for finding out which, if any, microbes are present and which antibiotic will be effective against a specific pathogen

cumulative effect increased effect of a drug that is not completely metabolized or excreted before another dose is administered

cyanosis bluish color of the skin due to lack of oxygen

cystitis inflammation of the bladder caused by bacterial infection

cystoscopy direct visualization of the interior of the bladder through a flexible scope

cytoplasm the part of the cell that contains water, protein, lipids, carbohydrates, and inorganic solutes

cytostatic able to suppress cell growth and replication

cytotoxic poisonous to cells

D

dandruff scaling of the dead tissue of the scalp

dead space space that allows fluid to remain in a syringe and needle after the plunger is completely pushed forward

decongestant drug that reduces congestion or swelling, especially in nasal passages, by constricting blood vessels and restricting blood flow to the area

defecation passage of feces out of the body; bowel movement

dehydration excessive loss of water from tissues

delusions false beliefs that are resistant to reasoning

demulcent drug designed to coat and soothe tissues

denominator bottom number of a fraction

dependence a compulsion to continue taking a drug; can be physical and/or psychological

depression disorder characterized by a sense of worthlessness or hopelessness and often resulting in inability to carry out normal activities

dermatitis inflammation of the skin causing redness, irritation, and skin lesions; also known as *eczema*

dermis inner layer of skin that contains blood, lymph, nerves, glands, and hair follicles

detoxify eliminate substances that are toxic or poisonous to the body

diabetes mellitus most common pancreatic disorder, characterized by an inability to use carbohydrates; insulin production is ineffective or not available

diabetic coma unconsciousness caused by too little insulin accompanied by increased caloric intake, physical or emotional stress, or undiagnosed diabetes mellitus; also known as *diabetic ketoacidosis*

diagnostic drugs drugs used to diagnose disease

dialysis technique that moves substances from the blood through a semipermeable membrane and into a dialysis solution; used to correct fluid and electrolyte imbalances and remove waste products in case of kidney failure

diastolic pressure force of the blood when the heart is at rest between contractions; lowest point at which sounds are heard when taking blood pressure

digestant drug that aids digestion by replacing digestive enzymes that are missing due to diseases such as stomach cancer, pernicious anemia, or pancreatitis

diplopia double vision

disinfectant chemical capable of killing bacteria; used in the sterilization process

distribution transport of drugs to body cells and spaces between cells

diuretic drug that reduces fluid volume in the body by stimulating urine flow

dopaminergic involving the activity of a neurotransmitter (dopamine)

dosage range the different amounts of a drug that will produce therapeutic effects but not serious side effects or toxicity

drug chemical substance used in the diagnosis, treatment, cure, or prevention of a disease; also known as *medication*

drug abuse taking drugs for their mood-altering effects or taking too many drugs or too much of a drug

drug card index card on which you write drug information for your own reference

Drug Enforcement Administration (DEA) since 1973, the only legal U.S. drug enforcement agency

drug misuse overuse or careless use of any drug

duodenum first portion of the small intestine, just past the stomach

dysmenorrhea painful menstruation

dyspepsia indigestion

dyspnea difficult or labored breathing

dysrhythmia any deviation from the normal rhythm of the heartbeat; also known as *arrhythmia*

dysthymia depression characterized by a minimal psychological, social, and occupational disability

dystonia muscle spasms of the face, tongue, neck, or back; tongue may protrude, and facial grimaces usually occur after large doses of antipsychotic drugs

dysuria difficult or painful urination

E

eardrum round disk that vibrates and transmits sound from the outer ear to the middle ear; also known as *tympanic membrane*

ecchymosis discoloration of the skin or bruising caused by leakage of blood into the subcutaneous tissue

eczema dermatitis

edema swelling; abnormal accumulation of fluid in the interstitial tissues

effect a physical or psychological change in a patient brought about by a drug

electrocardiogram (ECG) graphic record showing the spread of electrical excitation to different parts of the heart

electrolyte a solution that carries an electrical charge

embolus small amount of fat or air or a blood clot that circulates in the blood until it lodges in a blood vessel

emesis vomiting; reversal of peristalsis

emetic drug that causes vomiting

emphysema condition in which the air sacs dilate and are unable to contract to their original size; the alveoli lose their elasticity, causing residual air to be trapped in them

endocardium innermost layer of the heart

endometriosis growth of endometrial tissue outside the uterus

endometrium lining of the uterus

endoscope a flexible, tubelike instrument used to view the inside of the body

engorgement filling up of a body part with blood or another fluid (e.g., penis engorgement prior to intercourse, breast engorgement with milk in nursing mothers)

enteric-coated coated with a substance that dissolves in the intestine but not in the stomach (enteric—pertaining to the small intestine)

enzyme a chemical that speeds up biotransformation

epidermis outer skin layer

epiglottis leaf-shaped structure on top of the larynx that seals off the air passages to the lungs during swallowing

eructation belching, burping

erythema reddening of the skin caused by dilation of superficial capillaries

esophagus portion of the gastrointestinal tract leading from the mouth and pharynx to the stomach

estrogen female hormone

excretion the removal of waste substances from the body

expectorant drug that breaks down mucus to enable the patient to cough it up more easily; also known as *mucolytic*

expiration date date after which a drug should not be used

external auditory meatus part of the external ear; the ear canal

external otitis an inflammation and infection of the epithelium of the auricle and ear canal

extrapyramidal referring to a group of clinical disorders characterized by abnormal involuntary movements of the muscles (e.g., Parkinson's disease)

extravasation discharge of blood or other substances into tissues

F

facsimile order order transmitted through a facsimile machine

Fahrenheit temperature scale in which 32 degrees is the freezing point of water and 212 degrees is the boiling point of water

fascia fibrous membrane that supports and covers muscles

fat-soluble vitamins vitamins that are soluble in fat; vitamins A, D, E, and K

feces solid waste products remaining after food is digested and nutrients are absorbed; also known as *stools*

fetus the developing child in utero from the third month after conception until birth

fibrillate to quiver or contract spontaneously, causing ineffective contractions of the heart

flange flared part of a syringe barrel; used to steady the syringe while pulling or pushing the plunger

flatulence gas in the stomach and intestines

floaters nontransparent specks that are small pieces of cells floating across the visual field

Food and Drug Administration (FDA) enforcement agency for the FDCA

Food, Drug, and Cosmetic Act (FDCA) of 1938 law that mandates that drug manufacturers test all drugs for potentially harmful effects and that drug labels must be complete

Fowler's position position in which the patient's upper body is raised 45 degrees to 60 degrees by means of pillows or by adjusting the head of the bed

fraction a way of expressing an amount that is part of a whole

frequency (urinary frequency) the need to urinate more often than normal

fungi plantlike parasitic microorganisms

G

gallbladder storage pouch for bile

gastric pertaining to the stomach

gastrointestinal (GI) tract body tube leading from the mouth to the anus, through which food passes, nutrients are absorbed, and solid wastes are eliminated; also known as the *alimentary canal* or *digestive tract*

gastrostomy tube tube inserted through a stoma into the stomach, used for tube feeding and administration of medications

gauge (G) diameter (width) of the lumen of a needle; the smaller the gauge number, the wider the lumen; selection of gauge depends on the viscosity of the solution to be injected

generic name official nonproprietary name assigned to a drug by the manufacturer, with the approval of the United States Adopted Names Council

genitalia internal and external reproductive organs

geriatrician physician trained in caring for people over 65 years of age, including their quality-of-life issues

geriatrics the branch of medicine pertaining to the diseases and disorders of people 65 years of age or older

gerontology the study of aging and problems of older adults

gland specialized epithelial tissue that secretes hormones

glaucoma condition characterized by increased pressure within the eye caused by failure of the aqueous humor to drain

glomeruli tiny structures in the kidney that filter acids, urea, uric acids, water, glucose, amino, creatine, and major electrolytes

glucagon hormone secreted by the pancreas that raises the level of blood sugar; counteracts effects of insulin

glucocorticoids adrenal corticosteroids that regulate the metabolism of carbohydrates and fats by body cells and have an inflammatory effect

gluteal arteries large arteries that supply the muscles of the buttock area

glycogen form of glucose stored in the liver or muscles for release as the body needs it

glycosuria glucose in the urine

gonadotropins pituitary hormones that stimulate the gonads (ovaries and testes) to secrete hormones

gonads sex glands in which reproductive cells are formed; ovaries and testicles

grain basic unit of weight in the apothecary system

gram basic unit of weight in the metric system

Gram stain laboratory test for identifying microbes

greater trochanter knob on the upper leg bone (femur) that can be felt where the leg joins the hip; one of the landmarks used for locating the dorsogluteal injection site

H

hair follicle a structure of the skin from which hair grows

hallucination impairment of the special senses (auditory, visual, tactile, olfactory) by which the individual perceives in response to his or her own inner stimulation; that is, beliefs, delusions, feelings, unfulfilled wishes, and needs

health maintenance process of developing a healthy lifestyle, keeping existing diseases under control, and getting regular checkups

hematinic drug that increases the hemoglobin content in the blood; also known as *antianemic*

hematoma a collection of blood in an organ or tissue caused by a break in a blood vessel

hematuria blood in the urine

hemoglobin iron-containing substance that carries oxygen from the lungs and to the tissues

hemoptysis the coughing up of blood

hemostatic drug used to help in the formation of blood clots

hepatitis inflammation of the liver

hepatitis B virus (HBV) an example of a blood-borne pathogen; a sexually transmitted viral disease that can be prevented by vaccination

herpes simplex (genital) sexually transmitted disease that results in painful genital lesions

histamine substance released from injured cells during an allergic reaction; responsible for allergic symptoms

histamine H$_2$-receptor antagonist drug that inhibits gastric acid secretion

hives lesions of the skin caused by exposure to an allergen or by various other factors, such as fatigue and emotions

homeostasis state of fluid balance within the body

hordeolum a hard cyst on the eyelid resulting from a blocked sebaceous duct; also known as a *sty*

hormone chemical substance secreted by glands that regulates many body functions; each hormone has specified functions

household system system of measurement in which the basic unit of fluid volume is the fluid ounce and the basic unit of weight is the ounce

hub broad part of an injection needle that attaches to the syringe

human immunodeficiency virus (HIV) causes the sexually transmitted disease acquired immune deficiency syndrome (AIDS)

hyperacidity too much acid (e.g., in the stomach, esophagus)

hypercalcemia high blood calcium level, greater than 11 mg/dL

hypercholesterolemia high blood cholesterol level

hyperkalemia high blood potassium level, greater than 5.5 mEq/L

hypernatremia high blood sodium level, greater than 145 mEq/L

hyperplasia actual increase in the number of cells

hyperpnea breathing too rapidly or deeply; also known as *hyperventilation*

hypersensitivity an exaggerated response to a drug or other foreign agent

hypertension high blood pressure; two or more systolic readings above 140 mm Hg

hyperthyroidism disorder caused by an increase and sustained release of thyroid hormones

hypervitaminosis a condition that results from taking large doses of vitamins over a period of time

hypnotic drug that produces sleep by depressing the central nervous system

hypocalcemia low blood calcium level, less than 9 mg/dL

hypoglycemia low blood sugar, can be the result of administering too much insulin

hypokalemia low blood potassium level, less than 3.5 mEq/L

hyponatremia low blood sodium level, less than 135 mEq/L

hypotension low blood pressure; the systolic reading falls to 90 mm Hg or below

hypothalamus portion of the pituitary gland linked to the brain; controls many body functions such as temperature, sleep, and appetite

hypothyroidism disorder caused by a decrease in circulating thyroid hormones

hypovitaminosis a condition that results from a diet lacking in vitamins; also known as *avitaminosis*

hypoxia absence of or decrease in oxygen

I

idiosyncrasy a peculiar, unusual, individual response to a drug

iliac crest highest point on the hip bone; one landmark used to locate the ventrogluteal injection site

immune able to resist damage from pathogens

immunization a way of stimulating production of antibodies by exposing the body to weakened or killed germs

improper fraction a fraction in which the value of the numerator is greater than or equal to the value of the denominator; the value of the improper fraction is greater than or equal to 1

impulse electrochemical message transmitted by nerve cells

incident report form used for giving information about a drug error, patient injury, or accident

incontinence inability to control urination

indications diseases and disorders for which a certain drug may be used

induration hardening of a tissue caused by inflammation or edema

indwelling catheter catheter designed to be held in place over a long period of time until the patient can urinate voluntarily; also known as *Foley catheter* or *retention catheter*

infancy the period extending from birth to the end of the first year

infection an invasion by pathogens that reproduce, multiply, and cause disease

infectious disease disease caused by direct or indirect spread of pathogens from one person to another

inflammation protective response of body tissues to irritation and injury; a process that results in swelling, reddening, heat, and pain

influenza flu

infusion placement of a tube into a vein for the purpose of slowly adding fluids to the body (e.g., dextrose, plasma); also known as *intravenous (IV) drip*

inhalation administration of drugs by way of droplets or mist that the patient breathes in

inhaler handheld and pocket-size device used to administer a breathing treatment

inoculation process of immunizing by administration of a vaccine

inorganic compounds that do not contain carbon, such as minerals and water

insertion placement of an object into a body cavity (e.g., putting a suppository into the rectum)

insomnia sleeplessness, or inability to fall asleep or stay asleep

instillation placement of drops of liquid into the eyes, ears, nose, or some other body cavity

insulin naturally occurring hormone secreted by the beta cells in the islets of Langerhans in the pancreas in response to increased blood glucose levels

insulin pump battery-operated insulin infusion system connected to a small computer worn on the belt or side that administers small amounts of insulin every hour based on an individual's daily need for diet and physical exercise

integumentary system skin and its appendages—hair, nails, and sweat and sebaceous glands

interstitial fluid fluid that fills most of the cells of the body and provides a large portion of the liquid environment of the body

intestinal motility movement or excitability of the smooth muscles lining the gastrointestinal tract; speed of peristalsis

intravenous therapy administration of fluids, electrolytes, medications, blood, or nutrients through a vein

iodine mineral needed by the thyroid to produce thyroxine

ion a particle that carries an electrical charge

irrigation process of rinsing a body cavity with water or other solutions

islets of Langerhans structures made up of beta cells that secrete insulin and alpha cells that secrete glucagon

isolation keeping a patient in an environment where pathogens cannot spread from patient to healthcare worker and/or vice versa

K

keratin hard protein contained in cells of the epidermis, nails, and hair that is waterproof and acts as a barrier to pathogens and chemicals

keratolytic drug that loosens and facilitates the shedding of the outer layer of skin

keratosis overgrowth and thickening of keratin in the skin

ketoacidosis acidosis caused by a surplus of fatty acids (ketones) in the bloodstream; a complication of diabetes mellitus

kilogram 2.2 pounds

L

labia two sets of tissue folds, the labia majora and labia minora, surrounding the opening of the vagina

lacrimal gland gland that produces tears

larynx voice box; joins the pharynx with the trachea

laxative drug that promotes defecation either to relieve constipation or to clear the bowel before surgery; also known as *cathartic* or *purgative*

legend drugs prescription drugs

lesion area of pathological tissue

leukemia general term referring to a group of malignant conditions affecting the blood-forming tissues of the bone marrow, lymph system, and spleen

leukocytes white blood cells that defend the body against bacteria and destroy germ cells

leukopenia reduction in the number of leukocytes in the blood (4000 μL or less)

libido sex drive

ligaments connective tissue fibers that attach one bone to another

liter basic unit of volume in the metric system

liver organ that filters blood, stores and releases nutrients into the blood, and is involved in biotransformation or excretion of some drugs and other substances

local having an effect in the immediate area of administration; for example, eye drops designed to affect only the eye

lumen hollow part of a needle through which medication flows

lymph clear, watery-appearing fluid found in lymphatic vessels, which carry fluid from the interstitial spaces to the blood

M

macerate soften a solid, such as the skin, by moistening, causing increased absorption through the skin

macrominerals minerals needed with a daily requirement of 100 mg or more

major depression depression characterized by a significant psychological, social, and occupational disability

major tranquilizer see **antipsychotic**

malignant cancerous; able to spread to other parts of the body or to invade locally

mania mood disorder characterized by grandiose behavior, flight of ideas, hyperactivity, poor judgment, and aggressiveness

medication administration record (MAR) form documenting drugs that are administered to a particular patient every day; each dose is checked off after it is given

medicine cart movable unit for dispensing medications

menopause naturally occurring end of menstruation, usually between the ages of 45 and 52

menorrhea normal menstruation; also known as *menses*

metabolism the rate at which cells produce energy such as heat and muscle strength; also known as *biotransformation*

metastasis spreading of malignant cells from one site to other parts of the body

meter basic unit of length in the metric system

metric system a decimal system of measurement in which the basic unit of length is the meter, the basic unit of volume is the liter, and the basic unit of weight is the gram

microminerals minerals needed with a daily requirement of less than 100 mg; also known as *trace elements*

microorganisms tiny, one-celled plants and animals; some are pathogenic/disease-producing and others are nonpathogenic; also known as *microbes*

milliliter one-thousandth of a liter (0.001 L); also known as a *cubic centimeter*

millimeter one-thousandth of a meter (0.001 m)

mineralocorticoid hormone secreted by the adrenal cortex that maintains normal blood volume and promotes sodium and water retention and urinary excretion of potassium

minerals inorganic elements essential to the body; classified as macrominerals or microminerals

minim basic unit of volume in the apothecary system

minor tranquilizer drug that is given to calm anxious or agitated individuals; also known as *antianxiety drug* or *anxiolytic*

miotics drugs that cause the pupil to constrict by decreasing the intraocular pressure, increasing the aqueous humor outflow, and contracting the ciliary muscle

miticides drugs that kill parasites on the skin

mixed number number written with both a whole number and a fraction

mucolytic drug that liquifies or breaks down tenacious mucus so that it can be coughed up more easily; also known as *expectorant*

muscle tone normal, slightly contracted state of skeletal muscles that keeps them prepared for action

myalgia muscle pain

mycoses infections caused by fungi

mydriatics drugs used to dilate the pupil

myelin sheath insulating covering of the nerve cells

myocardial infarction (MI) "heart attack" or death of a part of the heart muscle due to lack of oxygen

myocardium the heart muscle; the middle layer of the heart wall

myxedema severe and long-standing hypothyroidism; the term is often used synonymously with *hypothyroidism*

N

narcotics group of potent analgesic drugs whose use can lead to physical dependence

narrow-spectrum antibiotics antibiotics that are effective against specific pathogens

nasogastric tube tube inserted through the nose and down the esophagus into the stomach, used for tube feeding and administration of medications

necrosis death of tissue in a living body

needle cover protective cover on a disposable injection needle; never put it back on the needle after administration

neoplasm new or abnormal growth of tissue; tumor

nephritis kidney inflammation

nephrons functional units of the kidney responsible for homeostasis

neuroleptic see antipsychotic

neurons primary functional units of the nervous system

neurotransmitter a chemical substance released from nerve endings transmitting across synapses to other nerves, muscles, and gland impulses; can be inside or outside the nervous system

nicotine dependence a physical vulnerability of the body to the chemical nicotine; brought on by tobacco products

nomogram a graphic device showing the relationship between numerical values designed for healthcare providers in pediatrics to estimate the body surface area of a child according to height and weight

nonproprietary name generic name of a drug

nosocomial pertaining to an infection that occurs in a hospital or long-term care facility

numerator top number of a fraction

nurses' notes form for charting observations, stat and PRN medications, and special treatments given

O

occlusive dressing dressing that seals in drugs, body heat, and moisture

official name generally, the same as the generic name of a drug; name of a drug as it appears in the official reference, the *United States Pharmacopeia/National Formulary (USP/NF)*

oliguria decreased urinary output in a given time period (100–400 mL in 24 hours)

optic pertaining to the eyes or sight

oral hypoglycemics drugs that stimulate the beta cells of the pancreas to secrete insulin

organ two or more tissue types that perform a specific function

organic compounds that contain carbon, such as vitamins, carbohydrates, proteins, and fats

orthopnea abnormal condition in which the patient must sit or stand to breathe deeply and comfortably

orthostatic hypotension condition of low blood pressure that occurs when a person rises from a sitting or lying position

osteomyelitis infection inside a bone

osteoporosis condition in which there is a decrease in total bone mass; major cause of fractures in postmenopausal women

otalgia ear pain

otic pertaining to the ear

outpatient patient who is not hospitalized; a walk-in (ambulatory) patient

ova female reproductive cells (singular: *ovum*)

ovaries two almond-shaped glands located in the pelvis, one on each side of the uterus, that produce ova

over-the-counter (OTC) drugs drugs available without a prescription

overdose drug dose that is too large for a person's age, size, or physical condition

ovulation release of an ovum from an ovary

oxytocic drug that stimulates contractions of the uterus

P

package insert printed information about a pharmaceutical product

palliative drugs drugs used to improve quality of life but not to cure or treat a condition

palpitations: rapid and throbbing heartbeats that can be felt by the patient

pancreas organ that secretes strong digestive enzymes that empty into the duodenum; also secretes insulin that passes directly into the bloodstream

paralysis inability to move the muscles

parasite organism that lives on or in another organism (e.g., lice, mites, tapeworms) and obtains nourishment from it

parasympathetic nervous system part of the autonomic nervous system that functions mainly to conserve energy and restore the body; the system of rest and digestion

parasympatholytic drug that opposes the action of substances released by the parasympathetic nervous system; also known as *anticholinergic*

parasympathomimetic drug that simulates the action of substances released by the parasympathetic nervous system

parathyroid hormone (PTH) hormone secreted by the parathyroids; regulates the calcium content of the bloodstream

parathyroids four glands located behind the thyroid; secrete parathyroid hormone

pathogens disease-producing microorganisms

pathology study of the disease process, including changes in structure and function of the body

patient chart a permanent record of care received

patient-controlled analgesia (PCA) system by which patients control the administration of their own pain medication from machines filled with analgesics

patient history sheet form describing the development of a patient's symptoms and the course of the disease

peak flow meter a device that measures the air flowing out of the lung, called the peak expiratory flow rate (PEFR), when a patient with asthma forcefully blows into the device

pediatrician physician trained in caring for infants and children

pediatrics the branch of medicine pertaining to the diseases and disorders of infants and children

pediculicide drug that kills lice

pediculosis infection caused by lice

penicillinase enzyme produced by microbes that makes them resistant to penicillin

penis part of male external genitalia that introduces sperm into the vagina

peptic pertaining to digestion in the stomach

percussion physical therapy for respiratory patients; tapping of various body organs and structures

pericardium sac that encases the heart

perineum skin-covered muscular area between the vulva and anus in the female and between the scrotum and anus in the male

peripheral nervous system (PNS) the thoracolumbar (sympathetic) and craniosacral (parasympathetic) divisions of the autonomic nervous system, as well as the sensory and motor nervous systems and all the nerves of the body that come and go to the brain and spinal cord

peristalsis rhythmic contractions of the smooth muscles lining the gastrointestinal tract that move food and waste materials through the system

petechiae tiny, purplish-red spots on the skin resulting from small hemorrhages

pH measure of the acidity or alkalinity of a solution

pharmacodynamics study of the body's response to a drug

pharmacokinetics the absorption, distribution, metabolism, and excretion of drugs

pharmacology study of drugs (uses, preparation, routes, laws, etc.)

pharmacy requisition form form on which to order supplies and medications from the pharmacy

pharynx tubelike structure that extends from the base of the skull to the esophagus; serves both respiratory and digestive tracts

phlebitis inflammation of a vein

photodermatitis irritation caused by skin sensitivity to light

photophobia abnormal intolerance to light

photosensitivity sensitivity to light, often a side effect of certain drugs; can cause a rash

Physicians' Desk Reference (PDR®) a widely used drug reference book that gives information about the drug products of major pharmaceutical companies

physiology the science that deals with the functions of cells, tissues, and organs of living organisms

pituitary gland at the base of the brain that regulates many body activities and stimulates other glands to secrete their own hormones; known as the master gland

placebo an inactive substance that has no pharmacological effect (a placebo can be a pill containing sugar or an injection of normal saline/sterile water)

plasma the liquid part of blood and lymph

platelets cells that aid in blood clotting

pleura membranes lining the lungs and lung cavities

plunger solid rod of a syringe that fits inside the barrel and pushes medication out under pressure

pneumococcal disease serious disease leading to infections of the lungs, the blood, and the meninges

point of maximum impulse (PMI) heartbeat felt at the fifth intercostal space, about 2 inches left of midline

polydipsia excessive thirst

polyphagia excessive hunger

polypharmacy the use of a number of different drugs by a patient who may have several different health problems

polyuria excessive urination

postpartum period after giving birth

postural drainage physical therapy for respiratory patients; use of positioning along with vibration and percussion to drain secretions from specific areas of the lungs, bronchi, and trachea

potentiation two drugs administered at the same time wherein one drug increases the effect of the other

pound 0.454 kilogram

precautions warnings to use care when giving drugs under certain conditions

precipitate solid particles that separate out from a solution as a result of a chemical reaction

preparation form in which a drug is available; determines route of administration

presbycusis decreased ability to hear high-pitched sounds

presbyopia farsightedness brought about by decreased accommodation of the eye as a result of the aging process

prescription drugs drugs that can be dispensed only with a provider's order or the order of another designated healthcare provider such as a nurse practitioner or physician's assistant

pressure ulcer bedsore, pressure sore, decubitus ulcer

PRN order drug order to administer a drug as needed

problem-intervention-evaluation (PIE) method of organizing information for charting patient progress

problem-oriented medical record (POMR) method of documenting in which the chart is organized according to a numbered list of problems or diagnoses

productive cough cough that brings up large amounts of mucus

progesterone female hormone

proper fraction a fraction in which the value of the numerator is less than the value of the denominator; the value of a proper fraction is less than 1

proprietary name brand name of a drug

prostate gland gland surrounding the male urethra and ejaculatory duct; secretes a thin alkaline substance that makes up the largest part of the seminal fluid

prostatitis inflammation of the prostate gland

protective soothing, cooling preparation that forms a film on the skin

provider's order sheet form for writing medication orders, located in the patient chart

pruritus itching

psoriasis chronic skin disease of unknown cause; characterized by itching, red macules, papules, or plaques covered with silvery scales

psychology study of the normal and abnormal processes of the mind

psychosis mental disorder in which the patient loses touch with reality

puberty age at which the reproductive organs become functional and secondary sex characteristics appear

pulmonary referring to the lungs

pulse oximeter a device that monitors oxygen saturation by placing a probe on the finger, toe, ear, forehead, or bridge of the nose

pulse rate the number of heartbeats that can be felt by touching the radial, carotid, femoral, or pedal arteries

pyelonephritis kidney infection

pyuria pus in the urine

R

rebound effect reappearance of symptoms in even stronger form after a drug dose has worn off

recommended daily allowance (RDA) daily level of intake for essential nutrients considered to be adequate to meet the nutritional needs of healthy individuals

reconstituting the process of adding the recommended amount of fluid to dissolve; usually with a powdered drug

rectum distal (far-end) portion of the large intestine

remission period during which disease symptoms disappear

reservoir a tissue in which drugs tend to collect; different drugs tend to collect in different tissues

residual urine urine remaining in the bladder after voiding (volumes of 100 mL or more)

resistance the ability of a particular microorganism to resist the effects of a specific antibiotic

respiration breathing

retention inability to urinate even though urine is present in the bladder

rigidity stiffness

Roman numerals I, II, III, IV, V, or i, ii, iii, iv, v, and so forth

routine order drug order by which the ordered drug is administered until a discontinuation order is written or until a specified termination date is reached

S

saliva digestive juice secreted by salivary glands in the mouth; breaks down certain sugars, moistens and coats food for easy swallowing

scabicide drug that kills mites

scabies infestation caused by mites

scaling an excess of keratin in the epidermis

schizophrenia mental illness in which psychosis is the classic feature; characterized by hallucinations, delusions, disorganized speech, and disorganized behavior

sciatic nerve largest nerve in the body; pierces the buttocks and runs down the back of the thighs

sclera fibers meshed together to form the opaque structure referred to as the "white" of the eye

scored the surface of a tablet is bisected by a groove to make for breakage into halves

scrotum skin-covered pouch containing the testes; part of the male external genitalia

sebaceous glands glands in the skin that produce sebum or oil

seborrheic dermatitis inflammatory irritation of the scalp, face, or groin, producing greasy scales

sebum oil that lubricates the skin, produced by the sebaceous glands

sedative drug that calms and decreases nervousness and excitability

seizure temporary loss of consciousness during which there is overactivity of part of the brain, often resulting in uncontrolled body movements

semi-Fowler's position position in which the patient's upper body is elevated to 30 degrees

sense receptor structure that picks up sensations of hot, cold, touch, pain, or pressure in the skin

sensorineural hearing loss alteration in the perception of or sensitivity to high-pitched sounds; occurs with problems in the inner ear

sexually transmitted disease (STD)/sexually transmitted infection (STI) infectious disease spread by intimate sexual contact; among the STDs are syphilis, gonorrhea, genital herpes, chlamydia, and AIDS

shaft the long portion of a needle that extends from the point to the hub and through which the medication passes

side effects desirable or undesirable drug effects apart from the primary purpose of giving the drug

site rotation the practice of injecting into different locations to avoid damaging tissue by repeated injections

skeletal muscles muscles responsible for body movement

sloughing shedding of dead tissue from a wound or sore

small intestine organ in which most absorption takes place after food intake; composed of the duodenum, jejunum, and ileum

soluble capable of being dissolved

solution liquid containing a dissolved drug

somatotropin growth hormone secreted by the pituitary gland

spasticity abnormal increase in muscle tone

spermatozoa male reproductive cells; also known as *sperm*

sphygmomanometer device for measuring blood pressure

spinal cord part of the central nervous system; carries messages between the brain and the peripheral nerves

spleen organ of the lymphatic system that works in the body's defenses, produces red blood cells, stores platelets, and serves as a reservoir for blood

sputum abnormally thick fluid formed in the lower respiratory tract that may contain blood, pus, or bacteria

Standard Precautions primary strategies for prevention of infection transmitted through blood, body fluid, nonintact skin, and mucous membranes

standards rules ensuring uniform quality, strength, and purity

standing order drug order that is to be continued until further notice

stat order a single drug order that is administered immediately

sterile free of microorganisms

stethoscope instrument for listening to the heartbeat and breathing sounds

stoma surgically produced opening in the stomach or the abdomen

stomatitis irritation of the mucous membranes of the mouth

stroke a loss in the supply of blood to any part of the brain; also known as *cerebrovascular accident (CVA)*

stupor state of mental dullness, confusion, or being in a daze

subcutaneous tissue loose connective tissue that attaches skin to underlying muscle and bone

subjective-objective-assessment-plan (SOAP) method of organizing information for charting patient progress

sudden cardiac death (SCD) unexpected death from cardiac causes in which there is a disruption in cardiac function that produces an abrupt loss of cerebral function

sudoriferous glands glands that produce sweat

superinfection secondary infection that occurs while an antibiotic is destroying the first infection

suspension liquid containing undissolved particles of a drug

sympathetic nervous system part of the autonomic nervous system that involves expenditure of energy and increases the blood sugar, heart activity, and blood pressure; the "fight or flight" system

sympatholytic drug that blocks the effects of impulses transmitted by the sympathetic nervous system; also known as *adrenergic blocking drug*

sympathomimetic drug that simulates the action of substances released by the sympathetic nervous system

symphysis pubis junction of the pubic bones in front on the midline

synapse gap between neurons

synergism drug interaction in which the effect of two drugs in combination is greater than the effect of each drug given separately

synovial capsule enclosed space between a bone and a joint

synthetic drugs drugs created in the laboratory from various chemicals

syringe device used to inject or withdraw fluids from the body; consists of a plunger, barrel, and hub

systemic having an effect throughout the body

systolic pressure force of blood pushing against the artery walls when the ventricles contract; the first taplike sound heard when measuring blood pressure

T

tachycardia rapid heartbeat (more than 100 beats per minute)

tachypnea rapid breathing

tardive dyskinesia potentially irreversible neurologic side effects of antipsychotic drugs in which there are involuntary repetitious movements of the face, limbs, and trunk

telephone order type of verbal order that is communicated via telephone

tendons connective tissue fibers that form a cord and connect muscles to bones

testes male reproductive glands (singular: *testis*)

testosterone male hormone that influences development of masculine characteristics; androgen that occurs naturally in the testes

tetany muscle spasms caused by a lack of calcium in the bloodstream

therapeutic effect desired or predicted physiological response caused by a drug

thrombolytic drug that is capable of dissolving blood clots

thrombophlebitis inflammation of a vein blocked by a thrombus

thrombosis condition in which a blood clot, or thrombus, is formed within a blood vessel

thrombus blood clot formed in a blood vessel

thyroid gland below the larynx that produces, stores, and releases thyroid hormone

thyroxine hormone secreted by the thyroid gland; regulates the speed of metabolism in body cells

tinnitus ringing in the ears

tissue group of cells of the same type, working together to perform some function

tissue fluid fluid found in spaces between cells; also known as *intercellular fluid*

tolerance need for increased dose of a drug to produce the same physical and/or psychological effect

toxicity poisonous effect of prolonged exposure to high doses or too-frequent administration of a drug

trachea windpipe; connects the larynx to the bronchi

tracking backing up of medication in the channel through which a needle enters tissue

tragus small cartilage projection in front of the entrance (exterior meatus) to the ear

transdermal passing, entering, or penetrating the skin

transdermal patch patch containing medication that is absorbed continually through the skin and acts systemically

transient ischemic attacks (TIAs) transient periods of neurologic deficit

tremor trembling, shaking

tumor abnormal lump or mass of tissue

type 1, insulin-dependent diabetes mellitus (IDDM) disorder wherein there is an inability to metabolize carbohydrates as a result of insulin deficiency; insulin must be given for treatment

type 2, non-insulin-dependent diabetes mellitus (NIDDM) disorder that usually affects individuals who are obese and over the age of 35; insulin may be part of treatment

U

ulcer open sore or break in the lining of the stomach (peptic ulcer) or duodenum (duodenal ulcer); can break through the gastrointestinal lining into the abdominal cavity (perforated ulcer)

ulceration open sore

ulcerative colitis disease of the colon and rectum characterized by inflammation and ulceration

United States Adopted Names (USAN) Council organization that adopts the generic name of a drug

United States Pharmacopeia Dispensing Information (USPDI) official reference for pharmacists or persons administering medications

United States Pharmacopeia/National Formulary (USP/NF) official book listing standardized drugs

Universal Precautions safety measures that consider all patients potentially infectious with blood-borne pathogens

unproductive cough cough that brings up nothing from the lungs; a dry cough

urea a waste product contained in urine

ureteritis inflammation of the urethra

ureters two tubes that carry urine from the kidneys to the bladder

urethra tube leading from the bladder to the outside of the body

urethritis inflammation of the urethra

urge incontinence (overactive bladder) condition caused by uncontrolled contraction or overactivity of the detrusor muscle

urgency feeling the need to urinate immediately

uricosuric drug that prevents reabsorption and increases excretion of uric acid through the kidneys

urinary catheter a device used to empty the bladder of urine or insert medication into the bladder

urination release of urine through voluntary control of the bladder; also known as *voiding* or *micturition*

urine fluid formed in the kidney that flows through the ureters to the bladder, where it is stored and then expelled voluntarily from the body; consists of 95 percent water and 5 percent solutes

uterus organ that contains and nourishes the embryo from time of fertilization until birth of the fetus; located between the bladder and rectum

V

vaccination introduction of an infectious agent for the purpose of establishing resistance to an infectious disease

vagina part of the female internal genitalia connecting the uterus to the outside of the body; passage into which sperm are introduced; canal through which a baby is born

vaginitis inflammation of the vagina

vasoconstrictive/venous insufficiency treatment drugs drugs that tighten blood vessels in an area of inflammation and reduce swelling

vasodilator drug that expands blood vessels; used to treat angina pectoris and hypertension

vein vessel that carries blood toward the heart

ventilator machine that assists breathing

ventricular fibrillation no organized heart rhythm; results in the heart quivering and imminent death if not treated

verbal order order that is expressed orally and not written down

vertigo dizziness; a whirling feeling in the head

vial small, glass, single-dose or multiple-dose, vacuum-sealed container with a rubber seal that must be punctured with a needle to fill a syringe for injection

vibration physical therapy for respiratory patients; a fine, shaking pressure applied to the chest wall during exhalation

villi small, fingerlike projections of the intestinal lining that provide a large surface area for absorption of nutrients into the bloodstream

viscosity thickness

viscous thick and sticky

vitamins organic substances essential for normal metabolism; classified as fat soluble or water soluble

voiding act of urination

W

water-soluble vitamins vitamins that are soluble in water; vitamin B complex and vitamin C

withdrawal symptoms set of physical reactions that occur when a person stops taking a drug on which he or she is physically dependent

Z

Z-track method of injection that minimizes tissue irritation by sealing the drug within muscle tissues

Note: Generic names are in roman type; product names are in *italic* type. Page numbers followed by f indicate figures; those followed by t indicate tables.